Biomedical Sc
Foundations

Cynthia A. Standley
Editor

Biomedical Science and Clinical Foundations

A Case-Based Approach

Springer

Editor
Cynthia A. Standley
Department of Bioethics and Medical Humanism
University of Arizona College of Medicine-Phoenix
Phoenix, AZ, USA

ISBN 978-3-031-98352-8 ISBN 978-3-031-98353-5 (eBook)
https://doi.org/10.1007/978-3-031-98353-5

This Springer imprint is published by the registered company Springer Nature Switzerland AG
The registered company address is: Gewerbestrasse 11, 6330 Cham, Switzerland

To the contributors of this edition, who took the time to take a case-based elective during their 4th year of medical school and share their knowledge and insight with all those who walk in their footsteps.

Preface

Medicine is an intricate interplay of foundational scientific principles and their real-world clinical applications. At the heart of every medical breakthrough, diagnostic insight, and therapeutic intervention lies the seamless integration of basic science with clinical reasoning. This book is designed to bridge that gap, bringing the mechanisms of disease and treatment to life through carefully selected case studies. This book is intended to provide students with the most useful way to study and learn basic science concepts—by integrating them with clinical science in a case-based approach.

By structuring each case around core scientific principles, we aim to demonstrate how physiological mechanisms and pathological changes translate into clinical presentations and medical decision-making. This approach fosters a deeper understanding of disease processes, moving beyond memorization to cultivate a problem-solving mindset essential for students, trainees, and practitioners alike.

Each case study is crafted to highlight the fundamental concepts that underpin clinical practice—whether it be the biochemistry behind metabolic disorders, the immunology of infectious diseases, or the pharmacodynamics guiding drug selection. Through this integration, we hope to reinforce the importance of scientific literacy in patient care while making complex concepts more tangible and applicable. This edition represents an outstanding effort by a talented group of authors. Our goal is not just to educate but to inspire curiosity and critical thinking. We invite you to engage with these cases, reflect on their implications, and appreciate the profound impact of basic science on everyday medical practice.

Phoenix, AZ, USA — Cynthia A. Standley

Introduction

The inspiration for this case book came from my Small Group Teaching Elective for fourth year medical students at the University of Arizona College of Medicine-Phoenix. One of the requirements for the elective is for students to author their own case, typically in an area of medicine that they have a particular interest. After 10 years of running this elective, there were more than 70 cases to choose from. From this, 35 were chosen to become the chapters of this book. Case-based learning is one of the fundamental pedagogies at The University of Arizona College of Medicine-Phoenix. Students learn by working through cases where they can integrate and apply their growing basic science knowledge with the clinical sciences.

First and second year medical students must first work their way through the preclerkship curriculum, much of which is basic science facts and figures they think has little relevance to the clinic. Yet, this basic science knowledge is foundational to the practice of clinical medicine. Since students are anxious to see how the basic science applies to the clinic, integrating it into weekly clinical cases is a practical way to do this. These cases have been written in such a way as to anchor basic science principles in the practice of clinical science. The basic sciences encompass a number of the disciplines including physiology, pharmacology, pathology, anatomy, and microbiology. The cases are arranged based on an organ system approach. Each case includes

- Basic science learning objectives
- Clinical science topics
- Integration of theme material, such as ethics, social determinants of health, and behavioral science
- Thought-provoking prompt questions
- Complete answers to all learning objectives
- United States Medical Licensing Examination® (USMLE)-based test questions

To encourage broad thinking, open-ended prompts are added throughout the cases. The explanations to the case learning objectives dive into the mechanisms to continue to help students build a foundation of knowledge that can continually be added to. In addition, USMLE-style board questions are included at the end of each case so students can test their knowledge.

By working through these cases, students will not only strengthen their understanding of basic and clinical sciences but also develop the critical thinking skills necessary for patient care. The integration of foundational science with real-world clinical scenarios fosters a deeper appreciation for the interconnectedness of medical knowledge. It is our hope that this book serves as a valuable resource for medical students and educators alike, inspiring curiosity, reinforcing key concepts, and ultimately enhancing patient-centered learning.

Acknowledgments

This has been a collaborative project. We greatly appreciate the helpful comments and feedback from faculty who have supported the authors during their training.

Thanks to the publisher, Springer for the valuable assistance.

While every effort has been made to ensure information is up to date, medical science is continually evolving.

Contents

Part IV Respiratory

Part V Renal/Acid Base

Contributors

Andrew Albert Department of Emergency Medicine, New York University Langone Health, Brooklyn, NY, USA

Evan Austin, MD Department of Obstetrics and Gynecology, University of Arizona College of Medicine, Phoenix, AZ, USA

Abbey Bayless University of Arizona, Anesthesiology Residency, Tucson, AZ, USA

Abigail Cantwell Department of Anesthesiology and Perioperative Medicine, Oregon Health and Science University, Portland, OR, USA

Philip Yue-Cheng Cheung Department of Radiology, Lewis Katz School of Medicine at Temple University/St. Luke's University Health Network, Bethlehem, PA, USA

Abel De Castro Internal Medicine – Pediatrics, UT Southwestern, Dallas, TX, USA

Sandeep Dhadvai Department of General Pediatrics & Adolescent Medicine, University of North Carolina School of Medicine, Chapel Hill, NC, USA

Joshua I. Gordon Department of Internal Medicine, Division of Pulmonary, Critical Care and Sleep Medicine, Wexner Medicine Center, The Ohio State University, Columbus, OH, USA

Center for the Advancement of Team Science, Analytics, and Systems Thinking in Health Services and Implementation Science Research (CATALYST), The Ohio State University, Columbus, OH, USA

Soham Gupta Oregon Health and Science University, Resident Physician, Multnomah Pavilion, Portland, OR, USA

Steven Osmond Han Department of Radiology, Lewis Katz School of Medicine at Temple University/St. Luke's University Health Network, Bethlehem, PA, USA

Chirag V. Kapadia Department of Hematology / Oncology, Andrew Weil Center for Integrative Medicine, University of Arizona College of Medicine, Tucson, AZ, USA

Sean P. Kelly Department of Orthopaedic Surgery, Tripler Army Medical Center, Honolulu, HI, USA

Jennifer Kirkpatrick Department of Emergency Medicine, The Permanente Medical Group, Sacramento, CA, USA

Jessie L. Koljonen Institute for Plastic Surgery, Southern Illinois University School of Medicine, Springfield, IL, USA

Alyssa Korenstein, MD Family Physician, One Medical, New York, NY, USA

Amaris Lestinsky Phoenix Children's Pediatric Residency Program Alliance, Phoenix Children's Hospital, Phoenix, AZ, USA

Ashley Lukefahr Department of Pathology, The University of Arizona College of Medicine – Phoenix, Phoenix, AZ, USA

Jacob K. Lythgoe Department of Radiology, University of Vermont Medical Center, Burlington, VT, USA

Patrick C. Mayolo Department of Orthopaedic Surgery, Tripler Army Medical Center, Honolulu, HI, USA

Sarah Monks Emergency Department, Hu Hu Kam Memorial Hospital, Sacaton, AZ, USA

Joseph Neely Internal Medicine, UC Davis Medical Center, Sacramento, CA, USA

George Nguyen Department of Internal Medicine, University of Arizona College of Medicine Phoenix – Banner University Medical Center, Phoenix, AZ, USA

Karen Pho Department of Emergency Medicine, HCA Houston Kingwood/University of Houston, Houston, TX, USA

Jasper Puracan Department of Psychiatry, Banner University Medical Center, Phoenix, AZ, USA

Leeann Qubain Banner University Medical Center-Phoenix, Phoenix, AZ, USA

Patrick Sarette The University of Arizona College of Medicine-Phoenix, Phoenix, AZ, USA

Kelby Schaeffler Emergency Physician, University of Arizona College of Medicine Phoenix, Phoenix, AZ, USA

Melanie Schroeder University of Arizona College of Medicine, Phoenix, AZ, USA

George Washington University Emergency Medicine, Washington, DC, USA

Cynthia A. Standley Department of Bioethics and Medical Humanism, University of Arizona College of Medicine-Phoenix, Phoenix, AZ, USA

Paul R. Standley Department of Basic Medical Sciences, University of Arizona College of Medicine-Phoenix, Phoenix, AZ, USA

Jeffrey Kyaw Wang Kaiser Permanente, San Leandro, CA, USA

Robert Yang Department of Psychiatry, University of Arizona College of Medicine Phoenix, Phoenix, AZ, USA

Part I

Neuroscience

1 Progressive Arm Weakness

Cynthia A. Standley

Learning Objectives

1. Differentiate upper motor neuron signs from lower motor neuron signs. Localize the problem in this patient to either the upper motor neuron, lower motor neuron, or both.
2. Explain the difference between a single muscle action potential and a compound muscle action potential (CMAP). Describe how this relates to the "all or none" principle of action potential generation.
3. Describe the steps in normal neuromuscular transmission and explain how these steps are affected in a patient with ALS.
4. Explain how to differentiate axonal from demyelinating disorders.
5. Develop a comprehensive management plan including multidisciplinary team involvement for a patient with ALS.
6. Recognize ethical considerations in ALS care and reflect on the impact of the disease on patients and their families.

Chief Complaint

"My left arm has gotten weaker, and I don't know why."

C. A. Standley (✉)
Department of Bioethics and Medical Humanism, University of Arizona College of Medicine-Phoenix, Phoenix, AZ, USA
e-mail: cstand@arizona.edu

Prompt: Construct a broad differential for this chief complaint.

A differential diagnosis for a weak left arm could include:

- Nerve compression issues like cervical radiculopathy (pinched nerve in the neck)
- Rotator cuff injury
- Muscle strain or injury
- Arthritis in the shoulder
- Thoracic outlet syndrome
- Peripheral neuropathy (nerve damage from diabetes)
- Demyelinating disorder (multiple sclerosis)
- Motor neuron disease (amytrophic lateral sclerosis)
- Spinal cord lesion
- Trauma to the arm or shoulder
- Stroke
- CNS tumor
- Lambert Eaton syndrome
- Lyme disease
- Myasthenia gravis

Prompt: What are some key factors to consider to help focus the differential?

- Onset: Was the weakness sudden or gradual?
- Location of weakness: Is it isolated to the shoulder, elbow, wrist, or hand?

C. A. Standley (ed.), *Biomedical Science and Clinical Foundations*,
https://doi.org/10.1007/978-3-031-98353-5_1

- Associated symptoms: Are there any accompanying sensations like numbness, tingling, pain, or muscle cramps?
- Medical history: Do they have any pre-existing conditions like diabetes, arthritis, or neurological disorders?

History of Present Illness

A 74-year-old right-handed male is referred to a neurologist for a 2-month history of arm weakness that has been progressively worsening. He has noted that he is not able to lift with his left arm. He has been having a hard time carrying groceries or bags of dog food, and his wife must help him. He denies similar symptoms in the past. He exercises when he "feels like it" and has noted that he has been unable to lift his typical 150-pound dumbbell weight with his left arm. He likes to golf, but he can't hold the golf club. He also notes that his muscles "jump" in his left arm.

He denies any numbness, tingling, or pins/needle sensation. He denies any radicular symptoms. He denies any bowel/bladder changes. He denies any muscle loss. He has been feeling "clicking" in his left shoulder and is worried that he might have to have shoulder surgery. He has lost 10 pounds in the last 3–4 months, but he attributes it to loss of taste. He denies any change in his sense of smell. He denies any vision changes, speech changes, trouble swallowing, or difficulty breathing. Regarding his lower extremities, he feels weak in the right leg, but that has been chronic due to a torn ACL. At times, he feels wobbly if he stands up too quickly, but he denies any recent falls.

Past Medical History
- Epiretinal membrane
- Essential hypertension
- Macular hole
- Posterior vitreous detachment
- Retinal hemorrhage

Past Surgical History
- Cataract extraction with intraocular lens implant, right/left, age 68
- Pars plana vitrectomy with repair of macular hole, age 65

Medications
- Fluticasone (Flonase) nasal spray
- Triamcinolone (Kenalog) ointment

Allergies
No known allergies

Family History
- Father prostate cancer
- Brother throat cancer
- Mother hypertension, hypothyroid
- No history of heart attack or stroke; no history of neurological disease

Social History
- Married
- 4 children
- Highest Level of Education: Detroit College of Applied Science Tool and Die Certificate
- Worked as a model maker at General Motors
- Former Smoker: 30 pack years
- Alcohol use: 2 cases (24 beers) per week
- Drug use: no

Review of Systems (ROS)
Gen: 10-pound weight loss, no fever, chills
Skin: Dry spots on knees and elbows, no other skin lesions
Head: No headache, no head trauma
Eyes: Presbyopia, corrected with reading glasses
Ears: Reduced hearing in right ear, no hearing aids
Nose: Occasional runny nose, no epistaxis or obstruction
Throat: No pharyngitis or dysphagia
Chest: Clear to auscultation
GI: No nausea, vomiting, diarrhea, constipation, or changes in bowel movements

GU: No dysuria, polyuria, or frequency
MSK: + lower back pain, non-radiating; left arm weakness, right leg weakness; no muscle or joint tenderness; no history of injury
Neuro: + lightheadedness, no syncope, paresthesia, or coordination issues
Endo: No hair changes, no facial or hand swelling, no changes in appetite
Psych: No mood changes, sleep issues

Physical Examination
Vitals:

- BP 156/91 mmHg
- Pulse 99 bpm
- Height 1.753 m (5′ 9″)
- Weight 82.9 kg (182 lb. 11.02 oz)
- BMI 26.98 kg/m^2

General The patient is in no apparent distress. Pleasant and cooperative.

Neurological Examination
Higher Cortical Function—Mental Status

- The patient is alert and oriented to person, place, and time. Attention and concentration are good. Speech is fluent with no dysarthria and no aphasia. Recent and remote memory function is intact. Fund of knowledge is within the average range.

Cranial Nerves II Through XII

- II—Pupils are mitotic but equal and reactive without afferent pupillary defect. Visual fields are intact to confrontation. Funduscopic examination is poorly visualized
- II, IV, and VI—No ptosis; extraocular movements are full with normal pursuit and saccades; no nystagmus
- V—Light touch is intact in all three divisions; motor V is intact
- VII—No facial asymmetry or weakness
- VII—Acuity intact to finger rubbing
- IX—Tongue rises symmetrically in the midline
- XI—Shoulder shrug is normal
- XII—Tongue protrudes in midline

Motor Examination

Muscle	Right	Left
Deltoid	5	4
Biceps Brachii	5	4-
Triceps	5	4-
Wrist extension	5	4+
Wrist flexion	5	4
Interossei	5	4-
Abductor Pollicis brevis	5	4
Hip flexion	5	5
Hip extension	5	5
Hip abductors	5	5
Hip adductors	5	5
Quadriceps	5	5
Hamstrings	5	4
Toe extensors	3	3
Ankle dorsiflexion	5	5
Ankle plantar flexion	5	5
Ankle inversion	5	5
Ankle eversion	5	5
Extensor Hallicus	5	5

Increased tone is noted throughout, worse on the left upper extremity and lower extremity. Fasciculations are noted throughout, most pronounced in the entire left arm but also seen in the right arm and bilateral lower extremities. No tongue fasciculations were appreciated on exam. Contracture of the 4th and 5th digits is seen. No pronator drift. Postural tremor is noted in hands.

Prompt: How is motor strength assessed?

Motor strength can be assessed by testing muscle strength in the upper and lower extremities. The Medical Research Council Manual Muscle Testing scale is a common method for evaluating muscle strength [1]. Muscle strength is graded on a scale from 0 to 5, with 0 indicating no movement and 5 indicating normal power.

Sensory Examination
Sensation is equal and symmetric to light touch in all four extremities.

Reflexes

Deep Tendon Reflexes (DTRs)

Upper Extremities	Right	Left
Brachioradialis	2+	3
Biceps	2+	3
Triceps	2+	3
Lower extremities		
Patellar	3	3
Achilles	3	4

Plantar response is extensor on left and flexor on right. Left ankle clonus and left Hoffman's reflex are present.

Prompt

How are reflexes graded?

Reflexes are graded on a scale of 0–4 as follows: [2]

0	Absent
1+	Reduced
2+	Normal
3+	Increased
4+	Increased with clonus

In an otherwise healthy person, when a muscle tendon is tapped, there is a reflex reaction and the muscle immediately contracts. This indicates normally functioning and is graded as a 2+. Hyporeflexia is evident when the contraction is less than normal, and hyperreflexia is evident when the contraction is greater than normal. This patient has ankle clonus on the left, a neurological sign where the ankle repeatedly flexes and extends in a rhythmic, involuntary manner when the foot is briskly dorsiflexed, indicating damage to the upper motor neurons. The presence of Hoffman's reflex, where flicking the nail of a person's middle finger causes involuntary flexing of the thumb and index finger, is another indication of damage to upper motor neurons.

Coordination

Difficulty with rapid alternating movements is seen.

Gait and Station

Gait is wide-based. Spastic gait is noted. Romberg is negative. Difficulty with tandem gait.

Prompt: What are the different descriptions for gait assessment?

When describing gait assessment, the following terms are used: [3]

- antalgic gait -limping to avoid pain
- ataxic gait -unsteady, wide-based walk
- Parkinsonian gait -small steps, stooped posture
- steppage gait -high foot lift due to foot drop
- Trendelenburg gait -trunk listing to one side due to weak gluteus medius
- Spastic (hemiplegic) gait -circumduction of affected leg
- waddling gait -exaggerated hip movement
- scissor gait -legs crossing inward
- equinus gait -walking on toes due to ankle stiffness

Spastic hemiparesis is characterized by a dominance of the tonus in the upper limb flexor muscles.

Laboratory

Routine Chemistry	Patient	Reference
Sodium	131 mmol/L	135–145 mmol/L
Potassium	4.1 mmol/L	3.5–5.0 mmol/L
Chloride	95 mEq/L	98–107 mmol/L
Carbon Dioxide	29 mmol/L	23–29 mmol/L
Anion Gap	7 mEq/L	4–12 mEq/L
Blood Urea Nitrogen	12	6–12 mg/dL
Creatinine	0.92	0.7–1.3 mg/dL
Calcium	9.7 mg/dL	8.5–10.5 mg/dL
C-reactive protein	0.2 mg/dL	<0.3 mg/dL
Glucose	106 mg/dL	<140 mg/dL
Liver panel		
ALT	27 U/L	7–56 U/L
AST	24 U/L	5–40 U/L
Albumin	4.6 g/dL	3.5–5.5 g/dL
Total protein	8.1 g/dL	6.0–8.3 g/dL
Total bilirubin	0.8 mg/dL	0.3–1.9 mg/dL
Alkaline phosphatase	37 IU/L	30–120 IU/L
Globulin	3.5 g/dL	2–3.5 g/dL
A/G ratio	1.3	1.1–2.5
TSH	2.48 mico U/L	0.5–5 mico U/L

Routine Chemistry	Patient	Reference
Iron/anemia studies		
Folate	11.6 ng/mL	2.5–20 ng/mL
Vitamin B-12	528 pg/mL	200–900 pg/mL
CBC		
WBC count	7.9	5000–10,000 cells/mm^3
RBC count	5.05	4.35–5.65 million cells/mm^3
Hemoglobin	16.9	13.0–16.0 grams/dL
Hematocrit	48.4	40–55%
MCV	95.9	80–100 fl
MCH	33.5	27–34 pg/cell
MCHC	35.0	32–36 g/dL
RDW	12.3	11.8–14.5%
Platelet count	217	150,000–400,000/mm^3
Sed rate	23	< 20 mm/h

Prompt: Interpret the laboratory data

Hyponatremia, low chloride, hemoglobin slightly elevated could suggest a state of dehydration or fluid imbalance. All other lab values are normal.

Prompt: What is on your differential now? What are next steps?

The patient's symptoms are concerning (prominent left upper extremity weakness, whole body fasciculations, increased tone L > R, with brisk reflexes, Hoffman's and clonus). It is important to order further testing. On the differential are motor neuron disease, multifocal motor neuropathy. He has both upper motor neuron and lower motor neuron findings, thus, more concern for a motor neuron disorder. EMG/NCS to rule out motor neuron disorder. MRI of the brain and cervical spinal cord.

The Case Continues

The patient is referred for an MRI of the brain and cervical spinal cord, as well as an EMG and nerve conduction testing.

Imaging Studies: MRI

Multiplanar, multisequence MRI of the brain and cervical spinal cord was obtained without the administration of intravenous gadolinium.

Brain

- Diffusion-weighted images demonstrate no evidence of an acute ischemic lesion in the brain.
- T2 and FLAIR images demonstrate a mild to moderate burden of periventricular and subcortical white matter hyperintensities as well as a few foci within the brainstem.
- Midline sagittal images demonstrate the craniocervical junction to be normal.
- There is no evidence of an acute intracranial hemorrhage, infarct, mass, mass effect, or an extra-axial fluid collection.
- There is cerebral and cerebellar volume loss, compatible with advanced age. There is prominence of the lateral ventricles, concordant with adjacent parenchymal volume loss.
- There is mucoperiosteal thickening within the paranasal sinuses. The mastoid air cells are clear.

Cervical Spine

- There is a grade 1 retrolisthesis of C3 on C4, C4 on C5, and C5 on C6.
- There is a grade 1 anterolisthesis of C7 on T1 and T1 on T2.
- Vertebral body heights are maintained.
- There are multilevel spondylotic changes, most pronounced at C6-C7.
- There is hemangioma within the C7 vertebral body. Marrow signal is otherwise within normal limits.
- The cervical cord demonstrates a normal course and caliber without abnormal signal intensity.

Impression

1. No acute intracranial abnormality.
2. Degenerative changes of the cervical spine are most pronounced at C4-C5, where there is mild central canal stenosis and moderate right

and mild to moderate left neural foraminal stenosis.

Prompt: How do these results help refine your hypothesis?

There is evidence of chronic small vessel ischemic damage in deep white matter, likely age-related, and likely not causing the patient's current complaint. There is no evidence of stroke or cancer. There is age-related brain tissue loss with ventricular enlargement in compensation. The patient shows sinus issues, but not related to current complaint. There is degenerative disease in the cervical spine related to arthritic changes. Grade 1 retrolisthesis (a mild spinal disorder that occurs when one vertebra slips up to 25% backward on another vertebra) is likely contributing to the patient's back pain.

EMG and Nerve Conduction Studies

The left sural-to-radial sensory amplitude ratio is 0.43 (normal >0.4). The left medial sensory nerve action potential amplitude is reduced. There is a 19% drop on the right and a 24% drop on the left between the ulnar compound muscle action potential amplitude (CMAP) at the wrist and below the elbow. The left ulnar CMAP amplitudes are reduced. There is mild, right ulnar motor conduction velocity slowing at the right elbow. The left tibial F-wave latency is slightly prolonged.

Needle electrode examination of selected muscles demonstrates increased insertional activity, positive sharp waves, fibrillations, and fasciculations in most of the muscles sampled and thoracic paraspinals. Reduced recruitment with an increased proportion of polyphasic motor unit action potentials (MUAPs) is present in the muscles in the left upper extremity. Reduced recruitment and an increased proportion of high-amplitude, long-duration polyphasic MUAPs are present in L2 myotomes.

Interpretation

This is an abnormal electrodiagnostic study. There is evidence of a diffuse. Neurogenic process. In the correct clinical context, this study meets the electrodiagnostic El Escorial criteria for motor neuron disease with involvement in three areas.

Prompt: Discuss the EMG and nerve conduction study results.

In the absence of a reliable marker for idiopathic amyotrophic lateral sclerosis (ALS), EMG forms the cornerstone of diagnosis. A low CMAP amplitude usually indicates damage to the nerve axons, leading to fewer motor neurons firing and a weaker muscle contraction [4]. When comparing the CMAP amplitude at different points along a nerve, a significant drop in amplitude between two recording sites suggests a nerve conduction block, which can occur due to compression or damage at a specific location. A drop in CMAP amplitude between 10–30% is often considered indicative of mild to moderate neuropathy. A slightly prolonged left tibial F-wave latency could indicate nerve damage, such as demyelination or polyneuropathy. F-wave latency is a measurement of how long it takes for a nerve impulse to travel.

A needle electrode examination showing "increased insertional activity, positive sharp waves, fibrillations, and fasciculations" on EMG indicates significant muscle denervation, meaning the muscle fibers are not receiving proper signals from the nerve due to damage or disease.

- Increased insertional activity: When the needle is inserted into the muscle, a brief burst of electrical activity is normal, but increased activity suggests muscle membrane instability, often an early sign of denervation.
- Positive sharp waves: These are small, positive-going electrical potentials seen at rest, representing spontaneous firing of individual muscle fibers due to denervation.
- Fibrillations: These are rapid, repetitive, small electrical discharges from single muscle fibers, also indicating denervation.
- Fasciculations; Larger, irregular spontaneous muscle contractions visible on the skin, which can be seen with both nerve damage and sometimes in normal individuals; their pres-

ence in an EMG with other denervation signs is significant.

When a muscle is asked to contract harder, normally more motor units are activated (recruitment). A reduced recruitment means fewer motor units are available to fire, indicating nerve damage. A normal motor unit action potential (MUAP) has a clean, predictable waveform, while a polyphasic MUAP has extra "phases" or peaks, signifying irregular firing of muscle fibers within a motor unit, often due to reinnervation after nerve damage. These EMG results are often seen in conditions like nerve root compression, peripheral neuropathy, or motor neuron disease (i.e. ALS).

Prompt: What are the El Escorial criteria?

The El Escorial criteria are a set of guidelines used to diagnose amyotrophic lateral sclerosis (ALS) [5]. The criteria include clinical and electrophysiological findings and are used to establish a diagnosis of ALS. The criteria include:

- Evidence of lower motor neuron degeneration in at least two muscles
- Evidence of upper motor neuron degeneration
- Progressive spread of symptoms
- Absence of other disease processes that could explain the observed signs

Prompt: What is this patient's diagnosis?

Amyotrophic lateral sclerosis

Prompt: What are the next steps?

The patient must choose what is right for him. Provide him and his family with information on group clinics. People with ALS who attend specialized group clinics, generally experience better outcomes, including extended survival and improved quality of life compared to those who do not access this type of care. This is because these clinics provide coordinated care from a team of specialists addressing the complex needs of ALS patients across various aspects of the disease [6].

Medication: 2 approved by FDA:

- Radicava (edaravone)—may reduce the speed of decline in daily functioning
- Riluzole (Rilutek, Tiglutik, and Exservan): may increase life expectancy by about 25%

ALSUntangled® https://www.alsuntangled.com/– good source of information

Clinicaltrials.govis a place to learn about clinical trials that the patient may be eligible for.

Modifications of house—ramps, handlebars, walk-in shower

Gait training and balance—for safety and to walk independently longer.

Physical therapy

A conversation about ventilators and feeding tubes with an ALS patient should begin early in the disease progression, ideally before any significant breathing or swallowing difficulties arise, allowing the patient to make informed decisions about their care as their condition progresses; this is crucial to ensure they have time to understand the implications and discuss their wishes with their healthcare team and loved ones.

Management

The patient is counseled on symptom management through a multidisciplinary approach. He is given prescriptions for Riluzole, physical therapy, and occupational therapy and a referral for respiratory care.

Pulmonary Function Testing

8 months later, the patient is seen by a pulmonologist to assess lung function.

	FEV1	FVC	FEV1/FVC ratio	Quality
Forced test 1	1.84	2.09	88%	Slow start
Forced test 2	1.55	1.59	97%	Good blow
Forced test 3	–	–	–	–

Insufficient number of good forced tests, 3 or more are required.

Selected Indices of the Best Blow

Index	Patient	% Predicted
FEV1	1.55 L	53%
FVC	1.59 L	39%
FEV1/FVC ratio	97%	–
PEF	162 L	36%

Prompt: What is the prognosis? What should be done next?

The most common cause of death for people with ALS is respiratory failure. This happens when the disease attacks the muscles used for breathing. ALS is considered a restrictive lung disease as it primarily affects the muscles involved in breathing, limiting the lungs' ability to fully expand, causing difficulty inhaling air, rather than obstructing airflow within the airways; this is due to its impact on the neuromuscular system. The patient's pulmonary function is significantly affected signifying disease progression and impacting life expectancy. Next steps include discussions regarding initiating noninvasive positive pressure ventilation (NIV) therapy, as well as exploring other supportive measures like airway clearance techniques, pulmonary hygiene practices, and advanced care planning discussions.

End of Case

Learning Objective Answers

1. **Differentiate upper motor neuron signs from lower motor neuron signs. Localize the problem in this patient to either the upper motor neuron, lower motor neuron, or both.**

Table 1.1 shows the characteristics of lower motor disorders compared to upper motor neuron disorders [7]. In a patient with ALS, both upper motor neuron and lower motor neuron signs are evident:

- Upper motor neuron signs: hyperreflexia, Babinski sign, increased muscle tone, slowed movement, poor balance, and coordination.
- Lower motor neuron signs: muscle weakness, muscle atrophy, fasciculations.

2. **Explain the difference between a single muscle action potential and a compound muscle action potential (CMAP). Describe how this relates to the "all or none" principle of action potential generation.**

CMAP stands for compound muscle action potential. The CMAP measures the sum of the electrical activity of all activated muscle fibers and is an evaluation of neuromuscular transmission [4]. It is recorded during an electromyographic (EMG) study that measures the voltage over a period of time of the muscle contraction when stimulated by a certain frequency. On the EMG, the amplitude of the CMAP evoked by a single nerve stimulus from a muscle at rest will

Table 1.1 Features of Lower Motor Neuron and Upper Motor Neuron Disorders

	Lower motor neuron	Upper motor neuron
Site	Anywhere from anterior horn cell to muscle	Brain Spinal cord
Distribution	Segmental (number)	Diffuse or patchy
Reflexes	Absent or reduced Babinski absent	Exaggerated Babinski present
Strength	Decreased	Decreased
Tone	Decreased	Increased, clonus
Atrophy	Severe	Mild, not prominent
Fasciculations	Present	Not present
Paralysis		
Type Location	Flaccid Paresis limited to specific muscles	Spastic and rigid Contralateral hemiparesis
Pattern of weakness	Depends on site of lesion	Extensors in arms Flexors in legs

be normal (~8 mV in amplitude), but this is variable and dependent on stimulation voltage and the muscle being activated. The CAMP is biphasic (upward deflection as the depolarization moves toward an electrode and downward as the depolarization moves away from it) and can be narrow (reflective of homogenous diameter of muscle fibers) or wide (heterogenous diameter). The shape of the CMAP (or, more importantly, the amplitude) is reflective of the number of individual muscle fibers that are activated. Individual muscle fibers express the "all or none" principle (they will either be brought to the threshold and generate an action potential or not be brought to the threshold and thus, no action potential will occur). CMAPs are not all or none. The larger the CMAP, the more muscle fibers have been activated.

3. **Describe the steps in normal neuromuscular transmission and explain how these are affected in a patient with ALS.**

Sequence of Events in Skeletal Muscle Neuromuscular Transmission

1. Action potential depolarizes presynaptic motor axon terminals
2. Increase in Ca^{2+} permeability and influx of Ca^{2+} into axon terminal
3. Exocytosis of acetylcholine from vesicles into the synaptic cleft
4. Diffusion of acetylcholine to postjunctional membrane
5. Binding of acetylcholine with nicotinic receptors
6. Increase in permeability of postjunctional membrane to Na^+ and K^+
7. Depolarization of postjunctional membrane: production of end plate potential in the muscle
8. Depolarization of muscle membrane adjacent to endplate and initiation of propagated sarcolemmal action potential.
9. Termination of transmission: Hydrolysis of acetylcholine by acetylcholinesterase and diffusion away from synapse.

In ALS, the steps of neuromuscular transmission are affected primarily by the degeneration of the neuromuscular junction, leading to a disruption in the release of acetylcholine from the motor neuron, impaired acetylcholine receptor binding on the muscle fiber, and ultimately muscle weakness and paralysis due to faulty signal transmission at the synapse; this is considered an early feature of the disease, often occurring before noticeable symptoms appear [8].

The primary pathology in ALS is the progressive loss of motor neurons, which directly affects the presynaptic terminal at the neuromuscular junction, causing decreased acetylcholine release. Motor neurons in ALS may also have fewer synaptic vesicles, further limiting the amount of acetylcholine available for release. As motor neurons degenerate, muscle fibers become denervated, leading to a loss of functional neuromuscular junctions and reduced muscle contraction. The impaired transmission of nerve impulses to muscle fibers results in decreased muscle strength and progressive weakness. Affected muscles tend to fatigue quickly due to the compromised neuromuscular transmission.

4. **Explain how to differentiate axonal from demyelinating disorders.**

To diagnose ALS, lower motor neuron abnormalities must be documented in at least 3 of 4 anatomic regions [5]. To reduce patient discomfort and anxiety, the number of muscles examined should be minimized but sufficient to reach the correct diagnosis. Start with the most severely affected limb, looking for abnormalities in at least 2 muscles with different innervations. Then move to another anatomic region, preferably in a limb with strength abnormalities. When changes have been identified in three anatomic regions, the EMG study can be concluded.

In demyelinating disorders, there is early loss of deep tendon reflexes, loss of large fiber sensation such as vibration and proprioception, and preservation of muscle bulk in the face of severe weakness. In axonal disorders, there is relative preservation of deep tendon reflexes until there is severe weakness and atrophy of the muscle, and large fiber sensation is not preferentially involved. Clinical differentiation can be difficult, and the distinction is made based on conduction slowing seen on nerve conduction studies in demyelinating disorders.

ALS is primarily considered an axonal disorder rather than a demyelinating one, as the primary pathology involves the degeneration and loss of axons rather than the myelin sheath that insulates them; however, some cases of ALS may show features of demyelination in peripheral nerves, though this is not the defining characteristic of the disease.

Multiple sclerosis (MS) is a classic demyelinating disease, while ALS is primarily an axonal disorder.

5. **Develop a comprehensive management plan including multidisciplinary team involvement for a patient with ALS.**

Patient-centered, interdisciplinary, and comprehensive rehabilitation is vital for individuals with ALS and has been shown to significantly improve their care and quality of life [9]. People who may be involved in the care of individuals with ALS include the patient's family and friends, family physician, neurologist, physiotherapists, occupational therapists, registered dieticians, speech-language therapists, social workers, and palliative care specialists. Table 1.2 lists the various symptoms of ALS and the management strategies that can be utilized. The goal is to improve both survival and quality of life for ALS patients [10]. When respiratory decline significantly affects quality of life, a referral to hospice can be discussed.

Table 1.2 Symptom management

Symptom	Management strategies
Muscle weakness	PT/OT, bracing, assistive devices, home modifications
Spasticity	Baclofen, tizanidine, stretching, PT
Respiratory decline	NIV, secretion management (cough assist, suction), tracheostomy if needed
Dysphagia	SLP-guided strategies, dietary modifications, PEG tube if needed
Speech difficulties	AAC devices (text-to-speech, eye-tracking systems)
Pain and fatigue	PT, massage, analgesics, energy conservation strategies
Depression/anxiety	Counseling, SSRIs, support groups
Drooling	Anticholinergics, botulinum toxin injections
Constipation	High-fiber diet, laxatives, increased fluids

PT Physical therapy, *OT* Occupational therapy, *NIV* Non-invasive positive pressure ventilation, *SLP* Speech-language pathologists, *PEG* Percutaneous endoscopic gastrostomy, *AAC* Augmentative and alternative communication, *SSRIs* Selective serotonin reuptake inhibitor

6. **Recognize ethical considerations in ALS care and reflect on the impact of the disease on patients and their families.**

Ethical considerations in ALS care focus on patient autonomy, informed decision-making, quality of life, and end-of-life care [11]. Helping the patient navigate complex decisions regarding advanced care planning, including artificial ventilation and feeding tube placement, is very important. The principle of respect for autonomy requires that patients retain control over decisions, even as their disease progresses. Advance directives and early discussions about care preferences help ensure patient wishes are honored. Ethical dilemmas arise when families and healthcare teams disagree about life-prolonging interventions. The ethical principle of beneficence supports early palliative care integration to maximize comfort. Ethical dilemmas may occur when patients' wishes evolve or if family members resist palliative care recommendations. Additional ethical dilemmas include family members' differing views on aggressive treatments versus comfort care.

The physical and emotional impact of ALS on patients is tremendous. ALS leads to a progressive loss of independence, paralysis, inability to speak, and respiratory failure. Family members also experience the emotional and psychological impact of a terminal diagnosis. Families often provide 24/7 care, leading to stress, exhaustion, and burnout. There is potentially a financial strain on the family, as the costs of home care, adaptive equipment, and lost income can be overwhelming. Access to multidisciplinary ALS clinics improves care but may be limited. Finally, not all patients have equal access to assistive devices, home modifications, or palliative care services.

This case is dedicated to my father who passed away from ALS at the age of 75.

Exam Questions

1. A 63-year-old male presents with complaints of twitching in his left arm that has been chronic over the last few months. Physical examination shows marked atrophy of the muscles in his left arm, hyperactive reflexes, Babinski sign, and unsteadiness on his feet. MRI shows normal age-related changes. An EMG and nerve conduction study are ordered. To diagnose ALS in this patient, which of the following would be seen in these tests?
   A. Abnormal sensory nerve responses
   B. Fibrillations and positive sharp waves
   C. A high CMAP amplitude
   D. Reduced F-wave latency
   E. Decreased insertional activity

Answer: B

Learning Objective: Explain the difference between a single muscle action potential and a compound muscle action potential (CMAP). Describe how this relates to the "all or none" principle of action potential generation.

Explanation: This patient shows both upper and lower motor neuron findings; thus, the diagnosis of ALS is very likely. As there is no reliable marker for ALS, EMG forms the cornerstone of diagnosis. EMG and NCS exams show evidence of active denervation on needle EMG, evident by fibrillations and positive sharp waves. A is incorrect, as sensory nerve conductions are usually preserved throughout the disease. C is incorrect, as CMAP amplitudes would be reduced due to loss of viable axons supplying the muscles. D is incorrect, as in ALS, F-wave latency would be prolonged, indicating nerve damage. E is incorrect, as there is increased activity in the ALS patient when the needle is introduced, suggesting muscle membrane instability.

2. A 68-year-old male presents with moderate dysarthria, fasciculations, muscle weakness, and gait imbalance. Definite ALS was diagnosed based on neurological abnormalities and electromyography results. Which of the following is consistent with the pathophysiology of the disease process in this patient?
   A. Degeneration of upper and lower motor nerves
   B. Degeneration of peripheral sensory nerves
   C. Demyelination of the myelin sheath of peripheral sensory nerves
   D. Antibody attack on acetylcholine receptors
   E. Antibody attack on presynaptic calcium receptors

Answer: A

Learning Objective: Differentiate upper motor neuron signs from lower motor neuron signs. Localize the problem in this patient to either the upper motor neuron, lower motor neuron, or both.

Explanation: While the cause of ALS is unknown, the pathophysiology involves degeneration of both upper and lower motor neurons. B is incorrect, as sensory nerves are usually preserved. C is incorrect, as in demyelinating disorders, there is early loss of deep tendon reflexes, loss of large fiber sensation such as vibration and proprioception, and preservation of muscle bulk, which is not consistent with ALS but more likely in a patient with multiple sclerosis. D is incorrect, as this describes the pathophysiology of a patient with myasthenia gravis. E is incorrect, as this describes the pathophysiology of a patient with Lambert-Eaton Syndrome.

3. A 68-year-old woman was hospitalized due to dizziness, gait disorders, decreased grip strength, and fasciculations. Upon physical examination, the patient was observed to

have speech difficulties, dysarthria, and drooling. A specialized neurological examination was requested, and the patient was placed under observation for amyotrophic lateral sclerosis. Which of her symptoms could best be managed with an anticholinergic medication?

A. Muscle weakness
B. Spasticity
C. Dysphagia
D. Drooling
E. Speech difficulties

Answer: D

Learning Objective: Develop a comprehensive management plan including multidisciplinary team involvement for a patient with ALS

Explanation: Anticholinergics can be helpful for a patient with ALS who is experiencing drooling by blocking muscarinic receptors. A is not correct, as anticholinergics are primarily used to manage excessive saliva (drooling) caused by muscle weakness, not directly to treat muscle weakness itself. B is not correct, as the medication of choice to treat spasticity would be baclofen or tizanidine. C is not correct, as treatment for dysphagia is not medication-based but rather through dietary modifications and referral to a speech-language pathologist. E is not correct, as treatment for speech difficulties is not medication-based but rather through the use of augmentative and alternative communication devices.

References

1. Naqvi U, Sherman AL. Muscle strength grading. [Updated 2023 Aug 28]. In: StatPearls [Internet]. Treasure Island (FL): StatPearls Publishing; 2025. Available from: https://www.ncbi.nlm.nih.gov/books/NBK436008/.
2. Walker HK. Chapter 72: Deep tendon reflexes. In: Walker HK, Hall WD, Hurst JW, editors. Clinical methods: the history, physical, and laboratory examinations. 3rd ed. Boston: Butterworths; 1990. Available from: https://www.ncbi.nlm.nih.gov/books/NBK396/.
3. Pirker W, Katzenschlager R. Gait disorders in adults and the elderly : a clinical guide. Wien Klin Wochenschr. 2017;129(3–4):81–95.
4. Barkhaus PE, Nandedkar SD, de Carvalho M, Swash M, Stålberg EV. Revisiting the compound muscle action potential (CMAP). Clin Neurophysiol Pract. 2024;9:176–200.
5. Joyce NC, Carter GT. Electrodiagnosis in persons with amyotrophic lateral sclerosis. PM R. 2013;5(5 Suppl):S89–95.
6. Miller RG, Jackson CE, Kasarskis EJ, et al. Practice parameter update: the care of the patient with amyotrophic lateral sclerosis: multidisciplinary care, symptom management, and cognitive/behavioral impairment (an evidence-based review): report of the Quality Standards Subcommittee of the American Academy of Neurology. Neurology. 2009;73(15):1227–33.
7. Zayia LC, Tadi P. Neuroanatomy, motor neuron. [Updated 2023 Jul 24]. In: StatPearls [Internet]. Treasure Island (FL): StatPearls Publishing; 2025. Available from: https://www.ncbi.nlm.nih.gov/books/NBK554616/.
8. Verma S, Khurana S, Vats A, et al. Neuromuscular junction dysfunction in amyotrophic lateral sclerosis. Mol Neurobiol. 2022;59:1502–27.
9. Paganoni S, Karam C, Joyce N, Bedlack R, Carter GT. Comprehensive rehabilitative care across the spectrum of amyotrophic lateral sclerosis. NeuroRehabilitation. 2015;37(1):53–68.
10. Miller RG, Jackson CE, Kasarskis EJ, et al. Practice parameter update: the care of the patient with amyotrophic lateral sclerosis: multidisciplinary care, symptom management, and cognitive/behavioral impairment (an evidence-based review). Neurology. 2009;73(15):1227–33.
11. Oliver DJ, Borasio GD, Caraceni A. A consensus review on the development of palliative care for patients with chronic and progressive neurological disease. Eur J Neurol. 2016;23(1):30–8.

Difficulty Urinating

2

Karen Pho

Learning Objectives

1. Review basic spinal vertebrae anatomy, and explain the pathophysiology associated with spinal cord compression.
2. Describe the gold standard for diagnostic evaluation in a spinal cord compression patient and explain the grading criteria.
3. Compare and contrast UMN vs. LMN pathology presentations. Identify when it is a neurological emergency associated with UMN and LMN processes.
4. Identify the clinical features associated with spinal cord compressions, and what maneuvers are utilized to assess neurological function, and explain its relevance.
5. Identify the gold standard treatment for spinal cord compression. Explain the mechanism of action and support why this treatment is the treatment of choice. Predict possible negative consequences of this treatment. Outline other treatment modalities and support its use.
6. Describe the epidemiology and risk factors associated with spinal cord compressions secondary to metastases.
7. Identify potential long-term physical and mental sequelae of spinal cord compression. Describe what social support a patient may need with spinal cord compression.

Chief Complaint Mrs. Juanita Garcia is a 56-year-old female presenting to the emergency department complaining that "I can't pee."

You were swiftly asked to evaluate this patient by the resident when she came into the ED. Thus, you did not have a chance to chart review this patient.

Prompt: What is your differential diagnosis?

Using the vindicaters mnemonic, the following differentials are suggested:

V—Vascular—stroke
I—Infectious/inflammatory—UTI, CMV cystitis, Guillain-Barre
N—Neoplastic—metastasis
D—Drug reaction/dermatologic/degenerative—anticholinergic toxicity, antipsychotics/TCAs, Herpes
I—Idiopathic/iatrogenic/intoxication—Fowler syndrome
C—Cardiac/congenital—horseshoe kidney
A—Abdominal/allergic/autoimmune/anatomical—pelvic organ prolapse, uterine fibroid
T—Traumatic—MVA, s/p recent abdominal surgery
E—Endocrine—diabetes mellitus
R—Renal/respiratory—bladder/ureteral stone, bladder cancer
S—Something else, pSychological—antipsychotics/TCAs, postoperative/postpartum, malingering

K. Pho (✉)
Department of Emergency Medicine, HCA Houston Kingwood/University of Houston, Houston, TX, USA

C. A. Standley (ed.), *Biomedical Science and Clinical Foundations*,
https://doi.org/10.1007/978-3-031-98353-5_2

History of Presenting Illness

Mrs. Juanita Garcia is a Spanish-speaking-only female who presented to the ED today for acute urinary retention for the past 3 days. The patient reports abdominal pain and distension secondary to not being able to pee for the past 3 days. She also reports that she has not been able to walk for the past 4 days. She states that she felt weak about 4 days ago but was able to move around with assistance. Additionally, the patient reports that she is not able to feel her legs, and that her appetite has decreased, along with worsening shortness of breath from her baseline. She denies any recent fever, chills, chest pain, lower extremity swelling, nausea, vomiting, diarrhea, or constipation. However, her last normal bowel movement was 3–4 days ago. She reports no new medications or recent travel.

Prompt: How does this expanded HPI help with your differential diagnosis?

Students should be able to narrow the differential down significantly with the classic symptoms this patient is presenting. However, it is still imperative to stress the importance of keeping a broad differential in the beginning, especially since the patient's history of stage IV lung cancer was not provided in the HPI. This may occur with patients who have language barriers. Without knowledge of a prior neoplastic disorder, the bolded differentials should still be highly considered.

V—Vascular—**stroke**
I—Infectious/inflammatory—**spinal epidural abscess**, UTI, CMV cystitis, **Guillain—-Barre**
N—Neoplastic—metastasis
D—Drug reaction/dermatologic/degenerative—anticholinergic toxicity, antipsychotics/TCAs, Herpes
I—Idiopathic/iatrogenic/intoxication—Fowler syndrome
C—Cardiac/congenital—horseshoe kidney
A—Abdominal/allergic/autoimmune/anatomical—pelvic organ prolapse, uterine fibroid
T—Traumatic—MVA, s/p recent abdominal surgery
E—Endocrine—**diabetes mellitus**
R—Renal/respiratory—bladder/ureteral stone, bladder cancer
S—Something else, pSychological—antipsychotics/TCAs, postoperative/postpartum

Past Medical History

Upon further questioning in the exam room, nursing staff informs you that the patient was recently diagnosed with stage IV pulmonary adenocarcinoma.

G2P2002 *(Gravida = total pregnancy; Para—TPAL = termed, preterm, abortion/miscarriages, living). So, 2002 breaks down to 2 termed pregnancies, and no preterm or abortions/miscarriages, with 2 living children out of a total of 2 pregnancies)*

LMP: July 2013

Medications:
None—patient reports that she was supposed to see her oncologist to start chemotherapy tomorrow

Allergies:
No known drug allergies

Surgeries:
None

Prior Hospitalization:
None, besides giving birth

Family History:
Father with diabetes mellitus II
Mother with HTN
Children are both healthy
Siblings' health is unknown

Social History:
Lives with husband and 2 children at home
Does not work
Never smoked

Negative EtOH screen
No RX or hx of recreational drug use
One sexual partner, no history of STI

Review of Systems:
General: +Decrease in appetite. No fever, chills, diaphoresis, or night sweats
Hematopoietic: No enlarged or tender lymph nodes, abnormal or excessive bleeding or bruising
Head: No headache and head trauma
Eyes: No vision changes, diplopia, or blurry vision
Ears: No hearing changes
Nose: No nasal discharge
Pharynx: No pharyngitis
Lungs: +Dyspnea. No cough or wheezing
Heart: No chest pain, lightheadedness, or palpitations
GI: +Abdominal discomfort and distension, constipation? No nausea, vomiting, melena, or hematochezia
Urinary: +Retention. No dysuria, frequency, urgency prior to retention symptoms. No gross hematuria
Endocrine: No hx of thyroid issues or DM. No changes to sensitivity to heat or cold
Musculoskeletal: No pain, tenderness, or stiffness of joints
Neurological: +Bilateral lower extremity weakness, paresthesia, difficulty ambulating, and saddle anesthesia
Psych: No prior hx or tx for psychiatric illness

Prompt: What critical information from the patient's past medical history, social history, family history, and ROS helps you change the likelihood of your differential diagnosis?

Patient's medical history of a stage 4 pulmonary adenocarcinoma raises the concern for metastatic disease to the spinal cord leading to urinary retention, paresthesia, sensory changes, and weakness.

No new foods or recent diarrheal illness decreases the likelihood of an infectious process leading to Guillain-Barre. Additionally, besides urinary retention, she did not have any urinary symptoms prior or any prior history of UTIs, consequently, the likelihood of a urinary tract infection is low. The same idea can be applied to nephrolithiasis, and even if she were to have nephrolithiasis, she should be making urine in her other kidney that would be able to pass into her bladder.

Her lack of medications decreases the likelihood of anticholinergic toxicity leading to urinary retention. Additionally, if anticholinergic toxicity is the cause of her urinary retention, she would likely present with more than just 1 symptom associated with anticholinergic toxicity. This includes increase in body temperature, rapid pulse, dry mouth, flushed skin, cycloplegia, and constipation:

- Hot as a bare
- Dry as a bone
- Red as a beet
- Blind as a bat
- Mad as a hatter
- Full as a flask

Lastly, her lack of surgical history decreases the likelihood of adhesions causing obstruction and her lack of personal history of diabetes mellitus makes it unlikely to be the cause. Although diabetes mellitus is often associated with polyuria, long-term effects include impaired detrusor activity, which is less likely in this case.

Physical Examination
Vitals:
T = 36.2 °C (97.8 °F)
P = 117 bpm
BP = 140/84 mmHg
RR = 24 breaths/min
Resting O_2 sat = 93%
General: Mrs. Juanita is lying in bed in mild distress likely 2/2 to abdominal discomfort. She is alert and conversant.
Skin: Warm and moist
Head: NC/AT
Eyes: PERRLA 3 mm
Ears: TM with normal light reflex
Nose: Moist mucous membrane. Septum is midline.
Throat: Uvula is midline. No erythema, edema, or exudates.

Neck: Unremarkable, no lymphadenopathy appreciated

Chest/Lungs: Tachypneic. Diminished breath sounds in all lung fields with mild rales, worse on the right. No wheezing or rhonchi appreciated.

Cardiovascular: Tachycardic rate, regular rhythm, normal S1 and S2, no murmurs appreciated

Abdomen: Mild distension. TTP to generalized abdomen, worse in suprapubic region. Bowel sounds difficult to appreciate, soft, no hepatosplenomegaly

Extremities: No edema, DP/PT pulses 2+ bilaterally

Neurological: Strength is 5/5 in BUE, sensation is intact from C5 to T2. Biceps and triceps reflexes are 2+ bilaterally. Strength is 2/5 to the RLE and 0/5 to LLE. Diminished sensation to BLE. Patellar reflex is 3+ bilaterally. Babinski sign bilaterally. CN II–XII intact.

Psych: Answers questions appropriately.

Prompt: What is remarkable from the patient's exam and how does this change your differential diagnosis?

Patient is tachycardic and tachypneic, with borderline O_2 saturation and diminished breath sounds bilaterally. Mild distention in the abdomen, tender to percussion. Reduced strength in both lower extremities, with positive reflexes and presence of Babinski.

Revisit the vindicaters mnemonic above—neoplastic rises in priority.

V—Vascular—stroke

I—Infectious/inflammatory—spinal epidural abscess, UTI, CMV cystitis, Guillain-Barre

N—**Neoplastic—metastasis**

D—Drug reaction/dermatologic/degenerative—anticholinergic toxicity, antipsychotics/TCAs, Herpes

I—Idiopathic/iatrogenic/intoxication—Fowler syndrome

C—Cardiac/congenital—horseshoe kidney

A—Abdominal/allergic/autoimmune/anatomical—pelvic organ prolapse, uterine fibroid

T—Traumatic—MVA, s/p recent abdominal surgery

E—Endocrine—diabetes mellitus

R—Renal/respiratory—bladder/ureteral stone, bladder cancer

S—Something else, pSychological—antipsychotics/TCAs, postoperative/postpartum

Patient's ROS and PE are highly suggestive of a neurological cause of urinary retention. Plus learning her history of a recent diagnosis of a high-grade adenocarcinoma is highly concerning for metastatic spinal cord compression.

Prompt: What are your concerns at this point?

Concerns for metastasis OR expanding pulmonary neoplasm into spinal processes and theca space, compressing on the spinal cord.

Concerns for how to preserve remaining neurological function, if patient will regain any function, prognosis, etc.

Prompt: What can you do at bedside right now to further evaluate this patient?

1. Bladder scan—can definitively determine if the patient is truly having urinary retention
   (a) How is retention defined in a female patient?
      (i) Bladder with ~150 cc of urine after urination
      (ii) Urinary retention is defined when bladder shows more than 300 cc of urine in men or women
2. Place a Foley catheter
   (a) Foley was placed and 300 cc of urine was drained

Prompt: What do you want to order next?

Order CXR (Fig. 2.1), MRI full spine w/ and w/o contrast, complete blood count (CBC) w/ differential (Table 2.1), complete metabolic panel (CMP) (Table 2.2), urinalysis (UA) (Table 2.3).

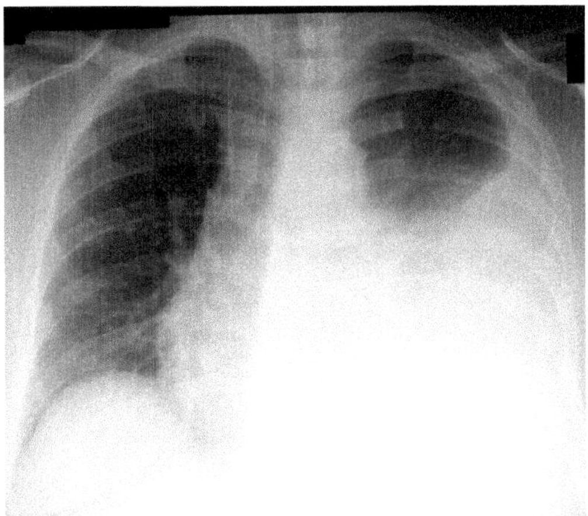

Fig. 2.1 Chest X-ray (https://commons.wikimedia.org/wiki/File:Left-sided_Pleural_Effusion.jpg)

Table 2.1 CBC

Component	Patient	Reference
Hemoglobin	13 g/dL	12–15 g/dL (13.6–17.7 g/dL for males)
Hematocrit	35%	33–43% (39–49% for males)
White blood count	7.0×10^9/L	$3.2–9.8 \times 10^9$/L
Platelet count	180×10^9/L	$130–400 \times 10^9$/L
MCV	96	80–100
MCH	33	27–31
MCHC	35	33–37
Platelet count	180×10^9/L	$130–400 \times 10^9$/L
Segmented neutrophil %	55	50–70
Lymphocyte %	23	20–40
Monocytes %	9	0–15
Eosinophils %	2	0–6
Basophils %	0.6	0–2

Table 2.2 CMP

Component (units)	Patient	Reference
Sodium (mEq/L)	139	136–144
Potassium (mEq/L)	4	3.6–5.1
Chloride (mEq/L)	103	101–111
HCO_3 (mEq/L)	26	22–32
Glucose (mg/dL)	90	74–106
Creatinine (mg/dL)	1.1	0.6–1.3
Calcium (mg/dL)	9.8	8.9–10.3
Total protein (g/dL)	7	6.5–8.1
Albumin (g/dL)	4	3.5–5
Total bilirubin (mg/dL)	1	0.3–1.2

Table 2.3 Urinalysis

Component (units)	Patient	Reference
pH	6	5–9
Specific gravity	1.105	1.000–1.060
Glucose (mg/dL)	0	<20
Protein (mg/dL)	0	<20
Bilirubin (mg/dL)	0	<1.80
Urobilinogen (mg/dL)	0	<1.60
Red blood cells (cell/hpf)	0	<3
Ketone (mg/dL)	0	<3
Nitrite (mg/dL)	Negative	0–1
Leukocytes	0	15–40
Color	Yellow	Yellow/amber/red/colorless/straw
Clarity	Clear	Clear/cloudy/turbid

Laboratory Results (Tables 2.1, 2.2 and 2.3)

Prompt: Interpret the CXR. What is your method of reading CXRs?

Interpretation of CXR:

- A—airway: overall appears patent
- B—bones: clavicles are symmetrical, visualized humeral heads appear within normal limits. Eight ribs visualized, perhaps not the best inspiratory effort, but decent
- C—cardiac silhouette: right border appears appropriate without signs of pericardial effusion. Unable to evaluate left border of heart
- D—right costovertebral angle is well visualized. Unable to visualize the left secondary to pleural effusion
- E—everything else: right lung parenchymal appears within normal limit. Left lung parenchymal obliterated secondary to pleural effusion

MRI Spine

MRI shows cord metastasis and rapidly progressive lower-limb weakness. Sagittal T2-weighted MR image shows the presence of a small, ovoid mass at T11/12 measuring 14 mm in craniocaudal length. The mass is mildly heterogeneous, with both isointense and hyperintense areas to cord. There is associated extensive abnormal increased T2 signal within the cord above and below the lesion, with cord expansion. There is abnormal increased T2 signal within the T11 vertebral body, with central compression in height. Contrast-enhanced T1-weighted MR image in the same patient shows intense enhancement of the mass with central hypointensity, in keeping with necrosis or cystic change. The margins are well defined. There is abnormal enhancement within the T11 vertebral body, in keeping with a metastasis.

Sagittal T1-weighted MR image shows abnormal hypointensity related to invasion by a paraspinal mass. The cortical margins of the pedicles are attenuated in keeping with erosive changes of the mass invading through the neural foramina into the lateral epidural space.

Prompt: What are your immediate next steps?

1. Give glucocorticoids—*specifically which one? What dose?*
   (a) Dexamethasone 16 mg. Other resources indicate a minimum of 10 mg IV.
2. Neurosurgery consult—*what is a one-liner you can provide to the neurosurgeon to support your reasoning for consulting neurosurgery?*
   (a) Patient is a 56-year-old female with stage 4 pulmonary adenocarcinoma who presented with 3 days of acute urinary retention, reported saddle anesthesia, sensory changes up to T10, and motor exam findings concerning for cord compression.

The Case Continues

Neurosurgery was consulted and will evaluate the patient in the ED for admission to the neurosurgery team for emergency surgery if the patient is stable enough.

Neurosurgery examined the patient and determined that she is currently not a surgical candidate as her pleural effusion would make it dangerous for her to undergo anesthesia and to place her in a prone position for surgery. The patient was consulted with general surgery, who placed a chest tube for fluid drainage and will be re-evaluated in the morning to assess her candidacy for surgical debulking for her spinal cord compression. The patient was kept in the hospital for 2 days, with constant re-accumulation of pleural fluid making her not a good surgical candidate. The patient was ultimately transferred to another facility for radiation therapy.

End of Case

Learning objective 1: Review basic spinal vertebrae anatomy, and explain the pathophysiology associated with spinal cord compression.

Key Points

1. Spinal cord is protected within the protective ring of bones comprising the vertebrae body anteriorly, pedicles laterally, and lamina/spinal processes posteriorly [4] (Fig. 2.2a).
2. Within the ring lies the thecal sac, which is the outermost layer of the dura. Between bone and dura is the EPIDURAL space (Fig. 2.2b).
3. Each spinal level, the nerve roots exit posteriorly to the vertebral body and laterally of the spinal cord (Fig. 2.2a).
4. Epidural spinal cord compression is usually the result of metastatic disease or direct cord compression from extension of the tumor.

Epidural spinal cord compression (ESCC) occurs when tumors or some external factor invades the epidural space and subsequently compresses on the thecal sac. The degree of compression will result in clinical features varying from asymptomatic to paraplegia. A high percentage of ESCC cases are due to metastatic disease to the vertebral bones. However, the mechanism of spread can vary. There are various methods that metastasis can occur, which include [7]:

1. Arterial seeding accounts for majority of cases.
2. Pelvic tumors, particularly prostate cancer, which has the Batson venous plexus, suspected to play an important role. This is because when abdominal pressure is increased for any reason, for example, a Valsalva maneu-

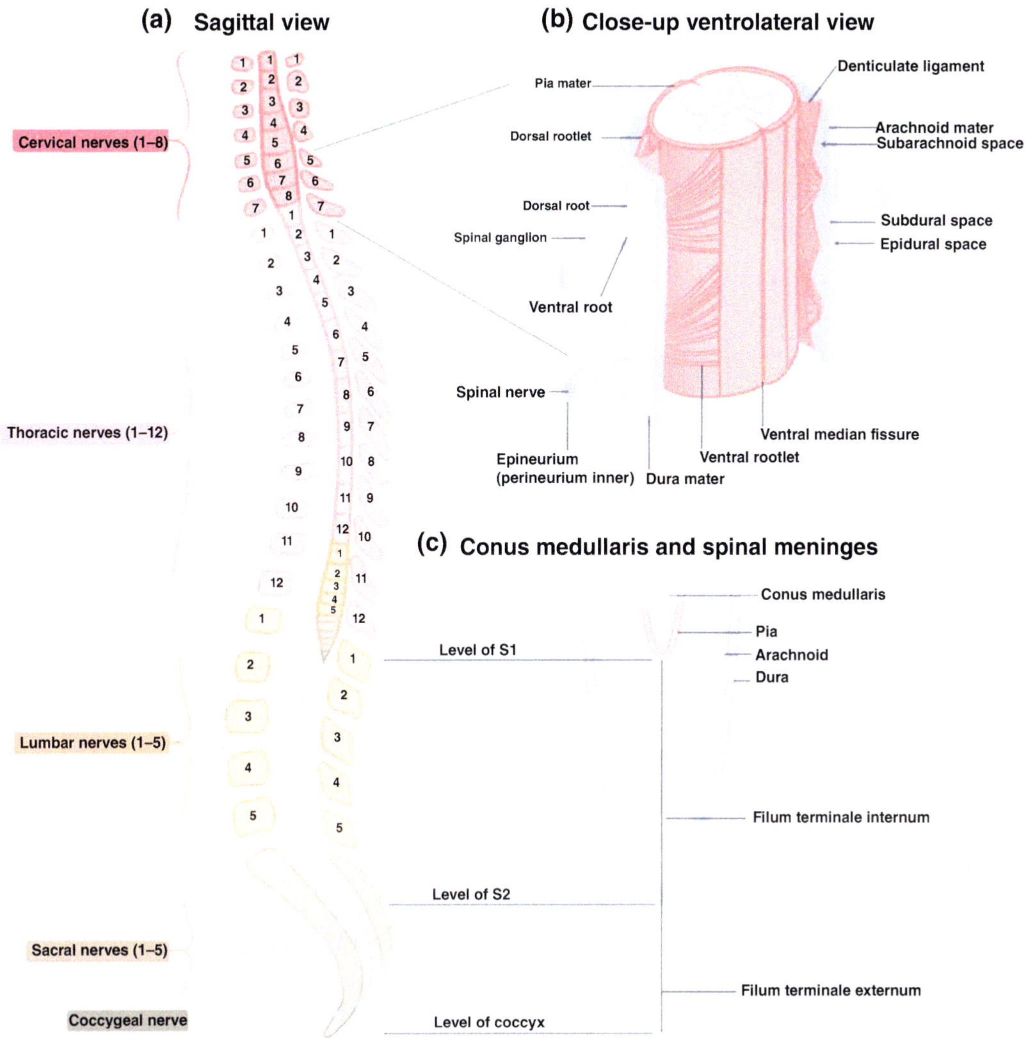

Fig. 2.2 Spinal Cord. (**a**) Spinal cord segments, (**b**) vertebral view, and (**c**) conus medullaris. Sheryl Tan, Faull L, Curtis A, CC BY 4.0 https://creativecommons.org/licenses/by/4.0, via Wikimedia Commons (https://commons.wikimedia.org/wiki/File:Spinal_cord_details.jpg)

ver will redirect venous drainage from the abdomen/pelvis to the epidural venous plexus. This in turn can increase vertebral metastases.
3. Approximately 10% of cases, paraspinal masses are able to gain access to the epidural space via the neural foramen. This is especially common with lymphoma.
4. Lastly, a rare component of ESCC tumors is that it can spread from the epidural space without a bony or paraspinal component.

As the tumor grows in any area of the body, it will take the path with the least resistance. As a result, oftentimes, the tumor will surround the thecal sac. Consequently, as the epidural venous plexus blood supply is compromised, vasogenic edema may occur in the white matter and eventually the gray matter of the spinal cord. If this is left untreated, spinal cord infarction can eventually develop and fully compromise all neurological function beyond the lesion.

Learning objective 2: Describe the gold standard for diagnostic evaluation in a spinal cord compression patient and explain the grading criteria.

Key Points

1. MRI full spine with and without contrast is the gold standard.
2. If MRI is contraindicated—such as those who have an electromagnetic cardiac device, or metallic foreign bodies—then CT myelography of the entire spine is second line.
3. Grading scale helps us communicate the extent of the disease process and gives clinicians an idea of the extension of the tumor. This further helps delineate treatment plans and estimate prognosis.

MRI of the entire spine is an urgent matter; it is recommended to complete this series of images within 24 h of suspecting ESCC. As such, if the facility the patient is currently at does not have these capabilities, it may require transferring the patient to another facility for a higher level of care.

Specifically, MRI sagittal T1 and/or short tau inversion recovery (STIR) sequences are utilized to look for metastases of the spinal cord. Additionally, a series of sagittal T2-weighted sequences may also be used to evaluate the degree of cord compression and to look for lesions within the cord itself (Fig. 2.3). If there are abnormalities seen on the T2 sagittal view, then dedicated axial images will be obtained to further evaluate. When it comes to tumor invasion of the bony processes, it is often well defined on noncontrast MRI sequences, but IV contrast is often given to further define the extent of the metastases of the epidural, foraminal, and paraspinal regions for tumor and to evaluate the presence of intramedullary or leptomeningeal disease.

Whole spine MRI with and without contrast will give the best depiction of the extent of the disease involving the vertebra, spinal canal, neural foramina, and paravertebral soft tissues. When lesions are found, axial T2-weighted images at the level are obtained to assign an ESCC score, which is widely used to describe the degree of disease process and extent of the epidural tumor. The grading is as follows:

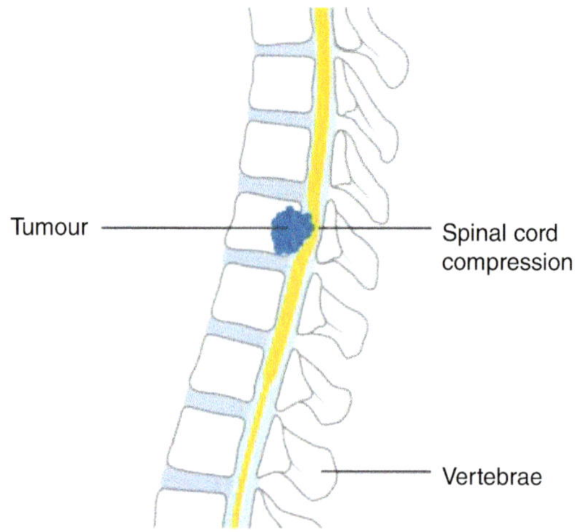

Fig. 2.3 Diagram showing a tumor causing spinal cord compression. Cancer Research UK, CC BY-SA 4.0 https://creativecommons.org/licenses/by-sa/4.0, via Wikimedia Commons (https://commons.wikimedia.org/wiki/File:Diagram_showing_a_tumour_causing_spinal_cord_compression_CRUK_081.svg)

- Grade 0—Tumor confined to the bone—not considered ESCC
- Grade 1—Tumor WITH epidural extension but WITHOUT contact to the spinal cord OR spinal cord abutment but no displacement of the cord.
  - Grade 1a: Epidural tumor *without* thecal sac compression
  - Grade 1b: Epidural tumor *with* thecal sac compression but NO cord contact
  - Grade 1c: Epidural tumor *with* thecal sac compression AND cord contact but no cord compression
- Grade 2—Tumor that displaces or compresses the spinal cord.
  - But NO circumferential tumor extension OR obliteration of the CSF space
- Grade 3—Tumor WITH circumferential extension and/or that causes spinal cord compression WITH obliteration of the CSF space

In hindsight, grades 2 and 3 represent high-grade spinal cord compression, whereas grade 1 is considered low grade

Learning objective 3: Compare and contrast UMN vs. LMN pathology presentations. Identify when it is a neurological emergency associated with UMN and LMN processes.

Key Points

1. UMN and LMN tend to have opposite findings. As such, physical exams that support a UMN or LMN process will help clinicians narrow down where the lesion and/or disease process is located at

UMN disease presentation:

- Deep tendon reflexes—HYPERACTIVE, tend to be 3+ or more
- Babinski sign—POSITIVE, where the toes fan upward toward the patient when the plantar surface is stroked from lateral side upwards to the balls of the feet going medially
- Weakness in the FLEXORS of the lower extremities
- Weakness in EXTENSORS of the upper extremities
- Supination of upper extremities will be weaker than pronation—pronator drift.
  - Someone with pronator drift has a relatively sensitive exam finding to support a subtle UMN process
- Muscle tone—UMN presents with spasticity

LMN disease presentation:

- Deep tendon reflexes—HYPOACTIVE, tend to be 1+ or lower
- Babinski sign—ABSENT = downgoing toes
- Weakness—depending on where the disease process is, you can see weaknesses either distally or more proximally.
  - Distal muscle weakness usually indicates a peripheral nerve disease
  - Proximal muscle weakness usually indicates a muscle disorder or NMJ disorder
- Fasciculations will be positive = muscle twitching
- Tone will be DECREASED
- Flaccid paralysis will be observed

UMN vs. LMN tends to describe the "location" of a lesion. LMN disease is usually in the periphery, which describes diseases including Guillain-Barre, Myasthenia, Lambert-Eaton, etc. On the contrary, UMN disease is thought of to be a "central" lesion anywhere from the cerebral cortex to the anterior horn cell; these tend to be thought of as an emergency.

Learning objective 4: Identify the clinical features associated with spinal cord compressions, and what maneuvers are utilized to assess neurological function, and explain its relevance.

Key Points

1. Pain is usually the first symptom patients will experience.
2. Bladder or bowel dysfunction is usually a late finding.
3. ESCC occurs 60–70% within the thoracic spine, 20–30% in the lumbosacral spine, and 10% in the cervical spine. However, if metastasis is noted in the thoracic spine, then the entire spinal column needs to be evaluated because there is a small chance that metastasis will be missed at the cervical or lumbosacral region.

Clinical features:

- Pain—usually the first symptom patients will experience. Tends to be worse at night, can be due to various reasons, including compression of the lesion on the back and decreased endogenous corticosteroid levels. Abrupt worsening of pain can be indicative of pathological vertebral fractures.
- Pain only with movement can indicate mechanical instability
- Unstable cervical metastases—can cause neck or scapular pain with extension/flexion/rotation of the neck
- Unstable thoracic metastases—usually causes pain when lying down
- Unstable lumbar metastases—usually causes radiculopathy, that can worsen with axial loading while ambulating or standing
- Spine instability neoplastic score (SINS)—developed to help aid in the detection of

potential spinal instability that may require urgent surgical evaluation
- Motor findings—any motor findings usually represent an advanced stage of ESCC and the severity of weakness tends to be greatest in those with compressive thoracic metastases. However, in order to do a full motor examination, if the patient still has neurological function intact, walking and standing must be a part of the exam in order to be complete.
  - Motor examinations:
    - Gait
      - Evaluate for normal gait, tandem gait, heel and toe walks
    - Coordination—cerebellar and cortical evaluation
      - Finger-to-nose test
    - Rapid alternating movement—cerebellar evaluation
      - Pronate and supinate the hands rapidly against their own thigh
    - Heel to shin test—cerebellar evaluation
      - Have patient lie supine, run the heel of one foot along the surface of the other shin proximally to distally
    - Involuntary movements
      - Tremors
      - Myoclonus
      - Chorea
      - Dystonia
      - Tics
    - Pronator drift—UMN lesion evaluation
      - Have patients extend both arms out while supinated, and evaluate if one arm starts to pronate and drift downwards
    - Strength test—UMN and LMN lesion evaluation
      - Test shoulder abduction, elbow flexion/extension, wrist extension/flexion, grip strength, finger abduction
      - Test hip flexion, knee extension/flexion, plantarflexion and dorsiflexion, great toe flexion/extension, hip adduction/abduction
  - Progression of motor weakness usually presents as increasing weakness →loss of gait → paralysis
- Sensory findings
  - Usually an ascending numbness and paresthesia. Spinal sensory deficits may present 1–5 levels below the level of lesion
  - Saddle anesthesia often present when cauda equina is present
  - Thoracic ESCC—usually presents with bilateral lower extremity weakness and back pain
  - Lumbar ESCC—usually presents with radicular pain and sensory complaints
- Bladder and bowel dysfunction
  - Usually a late finding, and is rarely the only finding in ESCC

Learning objective 5: Identify the gold standard treatment for spinal cord compression. Explain the mechanism of action and support why this treatment is the treatment of choice. Predict possible negative consequences of this treatment. Outline other treatment modalities and support its use.

Key Points

1. Gold standard—first treatment offered is glucocorticoids, specifically, dexamethasone
2. Dexamethasone is a long-acting corticosteroid with minimal sodium-retaining potential. Decreases inflammation by suppression of neutrophil migration and decreases inflammatory mediators, and reverses the increased capillary permeability
3. Goals for epidural spinal cord compression (ESCC) patients are pain control, avoidance of complications, and neurological preservation. As such, this in turn will help guide clinicians and patients to establish the goal for the patient and tailor treatment appropriately
4. Pain control often will require opioid analgesics

If epidural spinal cord compression (ESCC) is suspected, it is imperative that the patient is given glucocorticoids [1]. Prior studies suggested a minimum of dexamethasone 16 mg IV push. However, a recent systematic review in 2017 indicated that dexamethasone 10 mg IV push, followed by 16 mg daily PO had fewer complications than higher boluses [2]. This treatment is used to bridge to definitive treatment and for palliation of pain. Additionally, glucocorticoids may help with the vasogenic edema and help with compressive features. It is imperative to ensure that the patient's clinical signs are from metastases cord compression and not spinal epidural abscess, as corticosteroids may worsen immune function.

Dexamethasone is a synthetic adrenocortical steroid with potent anti-inflammatory effects in many organs within the body. It has a low mineralocorticoid activity but lacks the sodium-retaining property of hydrocortisone [3]. Corticosteroids inhibit multiple inflammatory cytokines resulting in decreased edema, fibrin deposition, capillary leakage, and migration of inflammatory cells. Therefore, all the total effects contribute to suppressing the inflammation and immune response.

Corticosteroids have been given in high doses to ESCC patients, but multiple studies did not show that it offered any better outcome compared to lower doses. Instead, at higher doses, there were more adverse outcomes for the patient. These adverse effects include:

- Psychosis
- Perforated gastric ulcer
- Death from infections
- Hypertension
- Cushing's syndrome
- Pulmonary TB
- Hyperglycemia
- Osteoporosis

In addition to glucocorticoid steroids, pain management is imperative for ESCC patients. The most common family for pain management is using pure mu agonists, which include morphine, oxycodone, hydrocodone, hydromorphone, and fentanyl. When using mu agonists, it is important to remember common side effects that we must watch out for as clinicians, including respiratory depression and constipation.

Other therapies for ESCC patients include:

- Surgical debulking or stabilization, depending on the patient's current prognosis
- Radiation therapy

Learning objective 6: Describe the epidemiology and risk factors associated with spinal cord compressions secondary to metastases.

Key Points

1. Metastases to the spinal column occur in 3–5% of patients with cancer.
2. Patients with breast, lung, and prostate cancer account for 50% of spinal cord metastases cord compression.

Major risk factors associated with spinal column compression are a well-known complication associated with certain oncologic disease. When epidural spinal cord compression occurs secondary to neoplasm, it is often an oncological emergency. The overall risk associated with metastatic spinal cord compression is approximately 3–5% of all patients with cancer [5, 6]. Those specifically with breast, lung, and prostate are at higher risk for metastatic epidural spinal cord compressions. The incidence may be as high as 19% for these cancer patients. However, of all metastatic cord compressions, 50% of the cases arise from patients with breast, lung, or prostate cancer. Additionally, the risk of metastatic spinal cord compression is associated with the duration of disease. As such, if cancer survival time increases, this may also contribute to increased incidence of metastatic spinal cord compression.

Keeping in mind the pathophysiology of epidural spinal cord compression, neurological deficits occur when either metastases occurred or direct compression via tumor growth. Consequently, understanding the three top neoplastic diseases that contribute to metastatic spinal cord compression will be critical to outlining a patient's care. It further helps increase the clinician's vigilance in evaluating for any neurological changes, with hopes to preserve as much function as possible if/when metastatic spinal cord compression occurs.

Learning objective 7: Identify potential long-term physical and mental sequelae of spinal cord compression. Describe what social support a patient may need with spinal cord compression.

Key Points

1. Once paraplegia sets in, it is usually irreversible which in turn affects the quality of life for the patient and their family.
2. Sudden changes to daily life have drastic consequences that can lead to depression.
3. Pain management and day-to-day life management will be critical after acute treatment of epidural spinal cord compression.
4. Bladder and bowel maintenance. If patients preserve any bladder function, it is important to continue timed voiding and intermittent catheterization; otherwise, long-term indwelling Foley catheters. Bowel regimens needed to maintain soft stools for normal evacuation.

When paraplegia is the presenting symptom for a patient with metastatic spinal cord compression, the likelihood to obtain neurological function again is low, despite surgical intervention. Each patient is unique; consequently, a true estimate of regaining neurological function varies. However, the range has not exceeded 5–10%, whether that is with surgical treatment or radiation treatment. Paraplegic patients will require 24-h nursing care either in hospital or in the community setting, or even at home caretakers.

Oftentimes, once metastatic spinal cord compression occurs, many of the treatments will be tailored for comfort/palliative care. As such, long-term pain management will be required for these patients, and the adverse effects of opioid use will need to be mitigated among clinicians. Other options include neuropathic pain medications, which will also require monitoring for adverse effects. Additionally, if patients present with bladder or bowel dysfunction, the likelihood of recovering these autonomic functions is slim. Consequently, long-term Foley catheter and/or colostomy placement and maintenance may be required. Patients with metastatic spinal cord compression present with UMN disease, which often leads to constipation secondary to inadequate emptying. Compounding the fact that opioids further decrease gut motility, consequently, a rigid bowel program needs to be a part of the treatment plan to prevent constipation/pain with defecation.

- These medications include:
  - Stool softener
  - Stimulant laxatives
  - Suppositories
  - Digital stimulation—must be used with caution secondary to mucosal fragility

Additionally, as patients lose their mobility *and* have a neoplastic disease, both of which increase their likelihood of developing blood clots, prophylactic measures will likely be instituted based on each specific patient. If a patient is not mobile, then consistently turning the patient on a regular basis will be imperative to maintain skin integrity, as pressure ulcers are preventable.

From a physical standpoint, there are many factors to consider and maintain. Therefore, all the changes may contribute to a decrease in mental health and depression. However, if patients present with depression-like symptoms, it is still important to rule out organic causes such as vitamin B12 deficiency, anemia, hypercalcemia, or radiation/chemotherapy side effects. SSRI may be something to consider; however, it will not be appropriate for every patient. As such, it is important to establish realistic expectations with the patient, determine what their goals are, and discuss the likely gains and/or toxicities associated with treatment interventions. Also, determining what the patient's overall goals will help guide what rehabilitation facilities will be best, and establishing a case manager can help facilitate advanced directive discussions.

Exam Questions

1. A 77-year-old man with a history of prostate cancer treated with radiation therapy is brought into your emergency department complaining of worsening back pain that started 3 weeks ago. He complains that the pain has acutely worsened over the past 12–18 h. He endorses difficulty ambulating and noted difficulty urinating this morning. Vitals are within normal limits except tachycardia with a rate of 110 bpm. On examination, patient appears uncomfortable with point tenderness over T9-T11. Upper extremity strength and reflex are normal. Strength in lower extremities is 2/5 bilaterally, with 3+ patellar reflexes. Babinski sign is present. Foley catheter drained 700 cc of urine. What is the next best step in management of this patient?
   A. MRI total spine
   B. Radiation to the spine
   C. Intravenous glucocorticoids
   D. Skeletal survey
   E. Fentanyl for pain control

Answer: C

Learning Objective: 5 and 1.

Explanation: IV glucocorticoid will be the gold standard as the immediate intervention given to patients who are suspected to have metastatic spinal cord compression. This patient has the risk factors with a history of prostatic cancer, along with new acute low back pain and neurological dysfunction. A is incorrect as although this will be part of the treatment plan, it is not the best initial step in a patient with concerns for metastatic spinal cord compression. Patient is presenting with new concerns of neurological deficits, the first immediate step with this concern is to treat the patient with IV glucocorticoids to decrease the inflammatory response and vasogenic edema; B is incorrect as while this may be an appropriate treatment option for a patient who is not a surgical candidate, this is not the best immediate step as the patient has not received the appropriate glucocorticoid treatment or MRI spine to evaluate the extent of the metastases; D is incorrect: Skeletal survey is not an appropriate answer as this is often ordered to evaluate for concerns of bony disease or concerns with child abuse. This is an elderly patient and the immediate concern is to preserve as much neurological function as possible; E is incorrect: Although pain management is one of the forefronts of managing patients with metastatic spinal cord compression, this is not the best immediate intervention. As mentioned previously, the first step is to give IV glucocorticoids to preserve the remaining neurological function.

2. A 55-year-old male with a history of stage 4 lung cancer was admitted to the hospital for acute low back pain and neurological deficits. Patient has a Foley catheter placed for urinary retention and has been receiving treatment and pain medications Q6 hrs and PRN doses. Overnight, the nurse pages you with concerns of acute behavioral changes that she noted in the patient, where he appears hyperactive and hypervigilant. What is the most likely etiology contributing to the patient's condition?
   A. Sundowning
   B. Opioid toxicity
   C. Delirium
   D. SSRI withdrawal
   E. Glucocorticoid adverse effects

Answer: E

Learning Objective: 5.

Explanation: The patient in the stem presents with signs and symptoms concerning metastatic spinal cord compression. The first step is to give IV glucocorticoids. Some patients may experience adverse effects of psychosis with low dose or high dose, especially concerning high-dose steroids. A is incorrect: Although this can be a plausible option for an elderly patient, especially someone with a history of dementia. This patient is relatively young in his 50 s with a red flag history of lung cancer. His history and clinical findings are most consistent and concerning for metastatic spinal cord compression, making this answer not the best explanation of the patient's acute behavioral changes. B is incorrect: Pain management is a critical component to a patient with metastatic spinal cord compression. However, these patients often require opioid medications to manage their pain. As such, the side effects for these medications are more likely associated with respiratory depression and CNS depression. These patients are more likely to have altered mental status or coma rather than acute psychosis. C is incorrect: Delirium is a common concern for patients who are elderly and in the hospital for an extended period of time. Also especially concerning if there is polypharmacy involved. This patient was admitted recently, with concerns of neurological changes consistent of upper motor neuron disease. This option is less likely when the main treatment options for these patients are glucocorticoids and opioid for pain management. D is incorrect: While SSRI withdrawal can produce acute symptoms consistent with anxiety, irritability, insomnia, etc., this patient does not have a history of psychiatric disorder, or any history of SSRI treatment. Consequently, this answer choice is very unlikely to be the explanation of the patient's acute psychosis.

3. A 49-year-old female with a history of breast cancer treated with radiation therapy is brought into your emergency department complaining of progressively worsening bilateral lower extremity weakness. Patient denies any new medications or any recent illnesses. On examination, upper extremity strength and reflex are normal. Strength in lower extremities is 2/5 bilaterally, with 3+ patellar reflexes. Babinski sign is present. Clonus is elicited with spasticity noted. What is the most likely pathology explaining this patient's presentation?
   A. Guillain-Barre
   B. Myasthenia gravis
   C. Lambert-Eaton
   D. Upper motor neuron disease
   E. Anticholinergic toxicity

Answer: D

Learning Objective: 3 and 1.

Explanation: Patient's history of breast cancer who is now presenting with bilateral lower extremity weakness is concerning for metastatic spinal cord compression disease. This is further supported with her upper motor neuron findings consisting of hyperreflexia, Babinski, clonus, and spasticity. A is incorrect: The patient's presentation is concerning for upper motor neuron disease with the hyperreflexia, Babinski sign, and clonus. Additionally, the patient has a history of breast cancer with radiation therapy, which can indicate she may have recurrence of disease along with metastasis. Regardless, Guillain-Barre is a lower motor neuron disease, usually presenting with an ascending pattern. The patient's history also notes no recent illness, decreasing the likelihood of GB. B is incorrect: Myasthenia gravis is a neuromuscular junction disease where antibodies block acetylcholine transmission. Instead of presenting with strictly lower extremity weakness and hyperreflexia, MG presents with muscle fatigue with continued usage. Additionally, ptosis, diplopia, and generalized weakness may be appreciated. To evaluate for myasthenia gravis, an edrophonium test or ice pack test may be used to confirm suspicion. C is incorrect: Similar to myasthenia gravis, Lambert-Eaton is a neuromuscular junction disease where antibodies attack the presynaptic Ca^{2+} channel, preventing depolarization. Patients present with proximal muscle weakness, and muscle weakness tend to improve with continued use. Patient's presentation is concerning for upper motor neuron disease and not Lambert-Eaton; E is incorrect - Anticholinergic toxicity presents with mydriasis, increase in body temperature, dry skin, tachycardia, constipation, etc. Additionally, the patient's history denied any new medications or current medications, which decreases the likelihood of having exposure to anticholinergic properties.

References

1. Loblaw DA, Mitera G, Ford M, Laperriere NJ. A 2011 updated systematic review and clinical practice guideline for the management of malignant extradural spinal cord compression. Int J Radiat Oncol Biol Phys. 2012;84(2):312–7. https://doi.org/10.1016/j.ijrobp.2012.01.014. Epub 2012 Mar 13

2. Kumar A, Weber MH, Gokaslan Z, Wolinsky JP, Schmidt M, Rhines L, Fehlings MG, Laufer I, Sciubba DM, Clarke MJ, Sundaresan N, Verlaan JJ, Sahgal A, Chou D, Fisher CG. Metastatic spinal cord compression and steroid treatment: a systematic review. Clin Spine Surg. 2017;30(4):156–63. https://doi.org/10.1097/BSD.0000000000000528. PMID: 28437329.
3. Dexamethasone (Systemic): Drug Information. UpToDate LexiDrug, Wolters Kluwer, www.uptodate.com/contents/dexamethasone-systemic-drug-information?search=dexamethasone&source=panel_search_result&selectedTitle=1%7E145&usage_type=panel&showDrugLabel=true&display_rank=1#F8015721. Accessed 6 June 2024.
4. Moore D. Spinal cord anatomy. Orthobullets, 1 May 2024, www.orthobullets.com/spine/2004/spinal-cord-anatomy. Accessed 6 June 2024.
5. Mak KS, Lee LK, Mak RH, Wang S, Pile-Spellman J, Abrahm JL, Prigerson HG, Balboni TA. Incidence and treatment patterns in hospitalizations for malignant spinal cord compression in the United States, 1998-2006. Int J Radiat Oncol Biol Phys. 2011;80(3):824–31. https://doi.org/10.1016/j.ijrobp.2010.03.022. Epub 2010 Jul 12. PMID: 20630663.
6. Loblaw DA, Laperriere NJ, Mackillop WJ. A population-based study of malignant spinal cord compression in Ontario. Clin Oncol (R Coll Radiol). 2003;15(4):211–7. https://doi.org/10.1016/s0936-6555(02)00400-4. PMID: 12846501.
7. Laufer I, et al. UpToDate. In: Clinical features and diagnosis of neoplastic epidural spinal cord compression. Wolters Kluwer; 2022. www.uptodate.com/contents/clinical-features-and-diagnosis-of-neoplastic-epidural-spinal-cord-compression?search=spinal%20cord%20compression&source=search_result&selectedTitle=2%7E150&usage_type=default&display_rank=2#H2. Accessed 6 June 2024.

Seeing Double

3

Amaris Lestinsky

Learning Objectives

1. Explain the immune mechanisms and pathogenesis of Miller Fisher syndrome, a GBS clinical variant. Where is the lesion? How is this different from other variants of GBS?
2. Create a flow chart or a table that outlines the differences between Miller Fisher syndrome, brainstem stroke, Wernicke encephalopathy, and myasthenia gravis. Include which part of the CNS is involved, clinical features, and diagnostic testing.
3. Identify the extraocular muscles and nerves involved in eye movement. Discuss common medical conditions that can cause binocular diplopia.
4. Discuss the diagnostic evaluation of Miller Fisher syndrome (CSF analysis, EMG testing, nerve conduction studies, antiganglioside antibody testing, and imaging).
5. Discuss the treatments that are available for Miller Fisher syndrome. Describe the mechanism of action, effectiveness, and side effects for each treatment.
6. Discuss the prognosis of Miller Fisher syndrome and reflect on the ways an interprofessional team is involved in the acute recovery and long-term care of patients.
7. Identify the risk factors and triggers for Miller Fisher syndrome (and more broadly, Guillain-Barré syndrome). Discuss the incidence and prevalence in the US population.

Chief Complaint

Imagine you are a neurology resident at New Haven Hospital. You have been called to do a consult on Mr. Glial, a patient transferred from an outside hospital.

Patient complaint: "I have double vision, my coordination is off, and the right side of my face is drooping".

Prompt: What else do you want to know? What are possible differential diagnoses?

Additional questions to ask: Onset and duration of symptoms (acute vs. chronic), progression of symptoms (are symptoms getting worse?), associated symptoms (dysarthria, sensory changes, headache, fever, seizures, changes in bowel/bladder control, etc.)

Differential diagnoses for diplopia, ataxia, muscle weakness: [1]

Inflammatory/Immune:

- Guillain-Barré syndrome (GBS): Acute inflammatory demyelinating polyradiculoneuropathy form or a different GBS clinical variant such as Miller Fisher syndrome

A. Lestinsky (✉)
Phoenix Children's Pediatric Residency Program Alliance, Phoenix Children's Hospital, Phoenix, AZ, USA

C. A. Standley (ed.), *Biomedical Science and Clinical Foundations*, https://doi.org/10.1007/978-3-031-98353-5_3

- Myasthenia gravis
- Lambert-Eaton syndrome
- Amyotrophic lateral sclerosis
- Transverse myelitis
- Neuromyelitis optica
- Poliomyelitis

Metabolic
- Diabetes
- Porphyria
- Electrolyte disorder

Nutritional
- Thiamine deficiency; Wernicke-Korsakoff syndrome, dry beriberi peripheral neuropathy

CV
- Acute stroke, brainstem stroke

Toxic
- Botulism
- NMJ blocking agents
- Organophosphates

The Case Continues

You are given his medical packet from the outside hospital. You review his records while the nurses set up IVs and make Mr. Glial comfortable.

History from Outside Hospital

Mr. Glial is a 40-year-old man with a PMH of alcohol use disorder who presents with diplopia and ataxia for 2 days. He developed diplopia and ataxia a few hours after he had three beers with a friend. He did not feel intoxicated. He reports that while he was driving home, he had a "hard time moving both eyes." He also felt like his coordination was "off." When the symptoms did not resolve after staying at home, he went to an outside hospital to be evaluated.

Prompt: What else do you want to know? How does this information modify your diagnostic possibilities?

His history of alcohol use disorder makes a diagnosis of Wernicke's encephalopathy more likely, and this is an emergency medical condition. Other important diagnoses include stroke, multiple sclerosis, myasthenia gravis, transverse myelitis, neoplasm, aneurysm, and Guillain-Barré syndrome.

History from Outside Hospital Continued

At the outside hospital, he was treated for presumed Wernicke's encephalopathy. He was given IV thiamine for 7 days and then converted to oral thiamine. His diplopia and ataxia did not improve despite receiving thiamine. Three days after he finished IV thiamine treatment, he was noted to have new right-sided facial weakness. He was transferred to New Haven Hospital for further evaluation.

Prompt: Why was his presentation presumed to be Wernicke's encephalopathy? Why is this urgent to treat?

His history of alcohol use disorder and acute onset ataxia and ophthalmoplegia makes a diagnosis of Wernicke's encephalopathy more likely. Wernicke's encephalopathy is an emergency medical condition caused by thiamine (vitamin B1) deficiency, which leads to dysfunction of energy metabolic pathways [2]. The nervous system is especially sensitive to thiamine deficiency because of the high metabolic demand of neuronal cells. It is an urgent condition to treat since it can result in neuronal death in the mammillary bodies and the dorsal medial nucleus of thalamus.

What do you want to ask the patient about now?

Prompt: How does this information modify your diagnostic possibilities?

Questions to ask: Is the facial weakness affecting the upper and lower parts of the face? Does he have muscle weakness in his limbs?

Is his speech slurred or nonsensical?

Are his symptoms improving, how long did they last?

Is there any change in his mental status?

Any changes in bowel or bladder control?

Any difficulty with respiration?

Important diagnoses include stroke, multiple sclerosis, myasthenia gravis, neoplasm, aneurysm, Guillain-Barré syndrome, electrolyte imbalance, poorly controlled diabetes, botulism, among others.

History at New Haven Hospital

He reports acute R-sided facial weakness x 1 day. It involves the upper and lower parts of the face. He denies other muscle weakness in his limbs.

No dysarthria or nonsensical speech.

No changes in alertness or orientation.

He reports some difficulty with swallowing.

He denies history of nausea and vomiting.

Prompt: What do you make of this history?

Bell's palsy is a **lower** motor neuron lesion that involves damage to the facial nerve in the brainstem, or after it exits the brainstem. It results in **ipsilateral** facial weakness involving **BOTH the upper and lower face**. Patients will be unable to raise their eyebrows, tightly close their eyes, or smile on the affected side. In comparison, a patient with a stroke has an **upper** motor neuron lesion that will typically present with contralateral lower facial weakness and **sparing** of the upper facial muscle function. This is because the **upper** face has **bilateral** upper motor neuron (UMN) cortical innervation which allows it to receive signals from the hemisphere of the brain that was not damaged by a stroke [3].

Prompt: How does this information influence your diagnostic thinking?

Some diagnoses that may be more likely now:

- Guillain-Barré syndrome because it involves acute onset progressive motor or sensory dysfunction.
- Myasthenia gravis because it can present with diplopia and bulbar symptoms.

Metabolic

- Diabetes: poorly controlled diabetes can damage the eye and peripheral nerves.

Nutritional

- Thiamine deficiency; Wernicke-Korsakoff syndrome is a possible diagnosis because of his history of alcohol use disorder, and symptoms of ophthalmoplegia and ataxia. However, he does not appear to have altered mental status.

CV

- Acute stroke and brainstem stroke symptoms are acute onset, and they can present with facial weakness, ataxia, and changes in vision.

History at New Haven Hospital (Continued)

PMH: Alcohol use disorder, presumed Wernicke's encephalopathy

Medications: None

Allergies to medication: None

Surgical history: None

Family history: Unknown

Social History

Mr. Glial lives alone. He calls his friends often, who are his emotional support. Mr. Glial is a senior manager at a local restaurant.

He does not smoke. He used to drink quite a lot (20–25 beers during the weekends) in the past, but he has recently cut down over the last 2 years to 3–6 beers over the weekend. He denies illicit drug use.

He reports his diet mainly consists of fast food.

Prompt: Let's review what we have gathered so far. What are additional questions we can ask?

We can ask questions to evaluate for infectious causes such as fever, chills, neck pain, or questions to evaluate for central nervous system malignancy such as weight loss, headaches, loss of bowel, or bladder control. Given the broad differential, it is also important to assess for additional symptoms such as limb muscle weakness, sensory changes, or psychological symptoms such as depression or anxiety.

Review of Systems at New Haven Hospital

General: No fever, chills, or weight loss; generally feels well

HEENT: Binocular vertical diplopia. R-sided upper and lower facial weakness, mild difficulty swallowing

Cardio/pulmonary: no chest pain, palpitations, shortness of breath
Gastrointestinal: no abdominal pain, hematochezia, diarrhea, constipation
Genital/urinary: no dysuria or hematuria
Musculoskeletal: no limb muscle weakness
Endocrine: denies heat/cold intolerance
Psych: no symptoms of depression or anxiety
Neuro: no headache, head trauma, neck pain, loss of bowel or bladder control, neuropathic pain, or numbness in extremities. Right-handed

Prompt: What is binocular vertical diplopia?

Binocular diplopia is present with both eyes open and absent when either eye is closed.

Often, patients will close the eye with the dysfunctional muscle unless that is the eye with better vision. Patients with vertical diplopia see two displaced images, one higher than the other.

Physical Exam at New Haven Hospital

Vitals **T:** 36.6 °C (Oral) **HR:** 90 **RR:** 18 **BP:** 122/80 **SpO$_2$:** 98% **Oxygen Method:** Room air **WT:** 92 kg, **HT:** 69 in **BMI**: 30 kg
General: Nontoxic, no acute distress
HEENT: Normocephalic, atraumatic, no scleral icterus or conjunctival injection
Lungs: CTA bilaterally. Nonlabored breathing, normal chest expansion
EXT: No cyanosis, clubbing or distal pitting edema, well perfused
Skin: Warm and dry, no ulcerations

Neurological Exam

Mental status: Alert. Oriented to person, place, time
Speech: Clear and fluent with good comprehension
Cognition: Comprehends 2-step commands
Memory: Registers new information and is able to articulate details well
No left/right confusion, no apraxia, no visual or sensory neglect

Cranial Nerves

II, III: Visual fields full to confrontation (VFFTC), pupils are equal, round, and reactive to light
VI: Ophthalmoplegia of both eyes, some ability to look up and down
V: Sensation intact to light touch bilaterally
VII: R-sided upper and lower facial weakness
VIII: Hearing grossly intact
IX, X: Voice normal, elevates palate symmetrically
XI: Trapezius 5/5 bilaterally
XII: Tongue protrudes midline without atrophy or fasciculations

Motor: No involuntary movements, tremor, hypokinesia, muscle fasciculations. Normal Bulk and tone. No pronator drift.

Upper Extremity Motor:
Deltoid: 5/5 right, 5/5 left
Biceps: 5/5 right, 5/5 left
Triceps: 5/5 right, 5/5 left
Grip, interossei: 5/5 right, 5/5 left

Lower Extremity Motor

Hip flexion: 5/5 right, 5/5 left
Knee extension: 5/5 right, 5/5 left
Plantar flexion: 5/5 right, 5/5 left
Dorsiflexion: 5/5 right, 5/5 left

Sensation

Intact light touch in all extremities

Reflexes:
Biceps: 1+ right, 1+ left
Brachioradialis: 1+ right, 1+ left
Patellar: 0 right, 0 left
Coordination and gait:
Finger-nose-finger: Ataxia on the left
Heel-to-shin: Ataxia on the right.

What are the key subjective and objective findings?

Prompt: What tests do you want to order and what are the priorities?

Key historical elements and exam findings:

- PMH of alcohol use disorder and presumed Wernicke's encephalopathy
- Binocular vertical diplopia and ataxia not responsive to thiamine treatment

- Ophthalmoplegia of both eyes, slight ability to look up and down
- One day of R-sided upper and lower facial weakness
- Hyporeflexia and areflexia for all DTRs tested
- No altered mental status

Tests to order: Complete blood count with differential (CBC with diff), complete metabolic panel (CMP), cerebrospinal fluid (CSF) studies, electromyography (EMG) and nerve conduction studies, Magnetic resonance imaging (MRI), antibody testing for antiganglioside antibodies seen in Guillain-Barré and acetylcholine receptor antibodies seen in Myasthenia gravis.

MRI brain with and without contrast is within normal limits. No hemorrhage, masses, hydrocephalus, or cerebral edema.

With a normal brain MRI, it is safe to do a lumbar puncture next to perform CSF analyses. CSF shows elevated protein of 100, elevated glucose of 100, and nucleated cell count of 0.

CBC and CMP were unremarkable.

Serologic antibody testing:

Acetylcholine antibodies: not detected
Ganglioside GQ1b antibodies: detected

Electromyography testing: normal
Nerve conduction studies: normal

Prompt: What is the most likely diagnosis? How would Mr. Glial be treated?

In meningitis you would expect CSF to show: Low glucose and high white blood cell count (WBC).

In Guillain-Barré syndrome, CSF studies may be normal early in disease course, or may show evidence of albuminocytologic dissociation (normal WBC and raised protein level)

Anti-GQ1b antibodies are sensitive testing for Miller Fisher syndrome.

Anti-Ach receptor antibodies are helpful to evaluate for myasthenia gravis.

The Case Continues

Mr. Glial was diagnosed with Miller Fisher syndrome (a clinical variant of Guillain-Barré syndrome that presents with acute onset of ophthalmoplegia, ataxia, and areflexia).

Treatment:

- Five-day course of IVIG
- Physical and occupational therapies

Prompt: What is Mr. Glial's prognosis? What are the discharge plans? What would comprise your discussion with Mr. Glial?

There is a favorable prognosis [4]. Involvement of interprofessional teams is an essential aspect of care and discharge planning. Physical therapy, speech therapy, and occupational therapy evaluations are recommended to help assist in the patient's recovery and adjustment into day-to-day life and work activities.

Discharge Plans and Follow-Up

Mr. Glial was discharged after completion of his 5-day course of IVIG and inpatient physical therapy. He was scheduled for outpatient physical therapy appointments to continue improving his muscle strength and coordination.

Over the next 8 weeks, his oculomotor dysfunction, ataxia, and facial paralysis slowly improved to full recovery.

End of Case

Answers to Learning Objectives

1. Explain the immune mechanisms and pathogenesis of Miller Fisher syndrome, a GBS clinical variant. Where is the lesion? How is this different from other variants of GBS?

Guillain-Barré syndrome (GBS) is broad category of acute immune-mediated polyneuropathies (dysfunction of many nerves) with many variant forms. Miller Fisher syndrome is GBS variant that classically presents with ophthalmoplegia, ataxia, and areflexia.

The pathophysiology of Miller Fisher syndrome GBS variant is thought to involve molecular mimicry. Molecular mimicry occurs when the immune system mounts a response against a bacterial or viral infection that cross-reacts with similar antigens on peripheral nerves [1]. Demyelination is thought to begin at the level of the nerve roots, where plasma proteins can leak into cerebrospinal fluid through deficiencies in the blood-nerve barrier. An inflammatory response involving complement and immunoglobulin develops against Schwann cells (glial cells that produce myelin) or peripheral myelin. Activated T cells infiltrate the area, followed by macrophages; the result is immune-mediated demyelination of peripheral nerves.

A respiratory tract or gastrointestinal illness often precedes the development of GBS. *Campylobacter jejuni* gastroenteritis is the most common preceding infection [5]. An immune response to *C. jejuni* can lead to the production of antibodies against gangliosides which are components of neuronal cell membranes; specifically, GQ1b gangliosides are a component of oculomotor nerve myelin [1].

Anti-GQ1b syndromes include Miller Fisher syndrome (ophthalmoplegia, ataxia, areflexia), Bickerstaff brainstem encephalitis (ophthalmoplegia, ataxia, and encephalopathy), and pharyngeal-cervical-brachial variant (swallow dysfunction, weakness of oropharyngeal, neck, and shoulder muscles).

2. Create a flow chart or a table that outlines the differences between Miller Fisher syndrome, brainstem stroke, Wernicke encephalopathy, and myasthenia gravis. Include which part of the CNS is involved, clinical features, and diagnostic testing for each diagnosis.

Miller Fisher syndrome, brainstem stroke, Wernicke encephalopathy, and myasthenia gravis are examples of conditions that can present with symptoms that mimic each other, making accurate diagnosis challenging. Table 3.1 lists features that help to distinguish among them.

3. Identify the extraocular muscles and nerves involved in eye movement. Discuss common medical conditions that can cause binocular diplopia.

There are six extraocular muscles controlling eye movement that are innervated by three cranial nerves: CN III (oculomotor), CN IV (trochlear), and CN VI (abducens) (Table 3.2). Binocular diplopia (double vision) can arise from problems with these muscles, nerves, or the brain's control of eye movement.

Table 3.1 Diseases that mimic each other

Disease	CNS area involved	Clinical features	Clinical testing that supports diagnosis
Miller fisher syndrome [6]	Dysfunction of neuromuscular junction between the 3rd, 4th, 6th cranial nerves and ocular muscles	Triad: Ophthalmoplegia, areflexia, and ataxia Often associated with a preceding infection Gradual onset Symptom progress for 4 weeks or less Other associated symptoms: diplopia, facial paresis, distal hyporeflexia without signs of UMN dysfunction. Some may develop fixed, dilated pupils	Serum antibodies against GQ1b ganglioside (a component of oculomotor nerve myelin) are found in 85–90% of cases Lumbar puncture with CSF studies shows an albuminocytologic dissociation (normal WBC and elevated protein level)

(continued)

Table 3.1 (continued)

Disease	CNS area involved	Clinical features	Clinical testing that supports diagnosis
Brainstem stroke [7]	Lateral medullary (Wallenberg syndrome): infarction of the posterior inferior cerebellar artery (PICA) or the vertebral artery Usually caused by atherosclerotic disease, hypertension, dissection, or embolism Areas affected: inferior cerebellar peduncle, dorsolateral medulla, spinothalamic tract, trigeminal nerve, vagus and glossopharyngeal nerves, sympathetic fibers, vestibular nuclei Lateral pontine syndrome: Infarction of the anterior inferior cerebellar artery (AICA) Areas affected: inferior and middle cerebellar peduncle, lateral pons, facial nucleus, spinothalamic tract, trigeminal nerve, vagus and glossopharyngeal nerves, sympathetic fibers, vestibular nuclei	Ophthalmoplegia with ataxia Acute onset of: Dysphagia Hoarseness Decreased gag reflex Vertigo Decreased pain and temperature sensation of ipsilateral face and contralateral body Horner's syndrome Ataxia	CT scan noncontrast to exclude intracerebral hemorrhage in patients with presentation concerning for stroke CT angiography is used to assess for a thrombus MRI/MRA can assess infarct volume
Wernicke encephalopathy [8]	Neurologic condition that affects the central and peripheral nervous system. Secondary to thiamine (vitamin B1) deficiency, which is a cofactor for enzymes involved in metabolism such as alpha-keto-glutamic acid oxidation and pyruvate decarboxylation Neuronal death occurs in areas such as the mammillary bodies and thalamus	Encephalopathy (confusion), ophthalmoplegia, nystagmus, ataxia More common in patients with alcohol use disorder and malnutrition	Clinical diagnosis that does not require imaging MRI imaging may show hyperintense signaling in the periventricular thalamus, mammillary bodies, periaqueductal gray matter
Myasthenia gravis [9]	Autoantibodies against neuromuscular junction receptors. Most commonly, Ab will target acetylcholine receptors (anti-AChR), and, less commonly, muscle-specific kinase (anti-MuSKAb)	Fluctuating muscle weakness, worsens throughout the day Ocular symptoms such as ptosis or diplopia Bulbar symptoms such as dysphagia or dysarthria Associated with thymoma	Placing an ice pack on the patient's eyelids will show improved ptosis due to decreased activity of acetylcholinesterase Edrophonium chloride (acetylcholinesterase inhibitor) test in patients with ptosis will show improvement in muscle strength CT chest to evaluate for a thymoma Serologic testing for anti-AChR and anti-MuSK Repetitive nerve studies may show a decremental decrease in CMAP (compound muscle action potential)

Table 3.2 Extraocular muscles and nerves involved in eye movement [10]

Muscle	Cranial nerve innervation	Action
Lateral rectus	VI (abducens)	Abduction
Superior oblique	IV (trochlear)	Incyclotorsion (inward rotation of eye), depression, and abduction
Medial rectus	III (oculomotor)	Adduction
Superior rectus	III (oculomotor)	Elevates eye, intorsion, adduction
Inferior rectus	III (oculomotor)	Depresses eye, extortion, adduction
Inferior oblique	III (oculomotor)	Excyclotorsion (outward rotation of eye), elevates eye, and abduction

Diplopia is the perception of two images of a single object (double vision). If diplopia persists after one eye is covered, then it is called monocular diplopia. Monocular diplopia is usually caused by eye pathology such as astigmatism and cataract [11].

If the diplopia resolves with one eye closed, then it is called binocular diplopia. Patients with vertical diplopia see two displaced images, one higher than the other.

Miller Fisher syndrome presents with binocular vertical diplopia.

Causes of binocular vertical diplopia: [11]

(A) Nerve dysfunction:
- 3rd cranial nerve palsy, possibly from tumor, vascular event, inflammation, or infection
- 4th cranial nerve palsy
- 6th cranial nerve palsy, possibly from uncontrolled diabetes or elevated ICP
- Guillain-Barré syndrome
- Multiple sclerosis
- Wernicke's syndrome

(B) NMJ disease:
- Myasthenia gravis: ptosis and diplopia worsen as the day goes on and improve with rest. Other symptoms include dysphagia, dysarthria, and dyspnea
- Botulism

(C) Eye muscle disease:
- Thyroid ophthalmopathy: inferior rectus is usually affected. Vertical diplopia is worse in the morning.
- Congenital causes
- Trauma
- Postsurgical complication of cataract, glaucoma, retinal detachment surgery

Third nerve (oculomotor) palsy: presents with ptosis, down and lateral gaze, +/− presence of a fixed dilated pupil (may indicate PCA aneurysm causing compression of nerve) [11].

Fourth (trochlear) nerve palsy: usually caused by microvascular disease or trauma [11].

Sixth (abducens) nerve palsy: most common nerve palsy, often due to microvascular disease [11].

4. Discuss the diagnostic evaluation of Miller Fisher syndrome (CSF analysis, EMG testing, nerve conduction studies, antiganglioside antibody testing, and imaging).

Clinical Features

The initial diagnosis of GBS is based on clinical features using the National Institute of Neurological Disorders and Stroke criteria (NINDS). NINDS criteria include **required** features of:

- Progressive weakness of limbs, trunk, bulbar facial, or ocular muscles
- Decreased or absent reflexes in affected limbs
- Symptom progression of equal to or less than 4 weeks [1]

Patients who do not meet the NINDS-required criteria may have a GBS variant, such as Miller Fisher syndrome. Patients with MFS may present with progressive ophthalmoplegia and hyporeflexia but not limb muscle weakness.

CSF Studies

Lumbar puncture for cerebrospinal fluid (CSF) analysis should be used to confirm the diagnosis and exclude other possibilities [1]. CSF analysis includes cell count with differential, protein, glucose, Gram stain, and culture. CSF studies show an albuminocytologic dissociation (normal white blood cell count and elevated protein level) in about 90% of cases at peak disease. Ten percent of patients will have normal CSF studies, especially early in the disease, so it cannot exclude the diagnosis.

If CSF studies are not diagnostic or if atypical symptoms are present, then electrodiagnostic studies and imaging are used to help evaluate for alternative diagnoses [1].

Electrodiagnostic Studies

These include nerve conduction studies (NCS) and electromyography (EMG). These tests give information about the nature and severity of nerve dysfunction. Results may be normal during the early stages of the disease. Electrodiagnostic studies may show decreased or absent sensory responses, but may not have slowing of sensory conduction velocities.

Serum Antibody Testing Is Useful in Diagnosing MFS

Presence of antibodies against **GQ1b ganglioside in serum** (85–90% sensitivity) in MFS [1].

Labs: CBC with diff, CMP, ESR, serum glucose, and hemoglobin A1c are obtained to evaluate for differential diagnoses of acute muscle weakness.
Imaging is obtained for patients with atypical symptoms, or nonconfirmatory electrodiagnostic studies.

MRI of the brain and cervical spine is obtained for patients with bulbar weakness and MRI of thoracic spine and lumbar spine is obtained for lower extremity weakness.

MRI of the spine may show thickening and enhancement of intrathecal spinal nerve roots and cauda equina.

5. Discuss the treatments that are available for Miller Fisher syndrome. Describe the mechanism of action, efficacy, and side effects for each treatment.

Disease-modifying treatments for GBS include treatment with IV immunoglobulin (IVIG) or plasma exchange (PLEX) immunotherapy; however, these treatments are less firmly established in MFS [4]. MFS symptom severity and duration are used to help guide the decision of whether to begin immunotherapy.

Immunotherapy is not suggested for patients with MFS who are stable and have symptoms limited to ophthalmoplegia, areflexia, and ataxia. This is due to a lack of evidence that immunotherapy will modify outcomes in these patients. One systematic review found that in patients with typical MFS, there were 60–100% rates of complete clinical recovery after 6 months without receiving treatment [12].

However, MFS symptoms can progress over time. Immunotherapy **is** suggested for patients with MFS who develop **severe** symptoms such as respiratory issues, or bulbar or limb weakness [4].

Immunotherapy with IVIG or PLEX should begin as early as possible, within the first 2 or 4 weeks of onset of symptoms, respectively.

IVIG: 0.4 g/kg/day for 5 days
Adverse effects: hypotension, nausea, headache with or without aseptic meningitis, rash, acute kidney injury (AKI), hypersensitivity reactions, anaphylaxis, and, rarely, stroke or myocardial infarction.

Plasma Exchange (PLEX): given in 4–6 treatments over 8–10 days.
Adverse effects: hypotension, sepsis, transfusion reactions.
Mechanism of action: Plasma exchange involves removing plasma from the patient's blood to remove antibodies and inflammatory mediators. Then, fluid replacement is given using donor plasma, colloid, or crystalloids [13].

Efficacy

One systematic review of the efficacy of treatment with PLEX showed treatment was associated with significantly shorter time to recovery of walking with assistance.

Further research is needed to compare treatment of IVIG vs. placebo to evaluate IVIG treatment effectiveness. A Cochrane review found that plasma exchange hastens the onset of recovery compared to supportive care alone [14].

In clinical settings where both treatments are available, IVIG is preferred because it is easier to administer and less likely to be discontinued due to side effects [4].

6. Discuss the prognosis of Miller Fisher syndrome and reflect on the ways an interprofessional team is involved in the acute recovery and long-term care of patients.

Patients with GBS typically show recovery of function in the first several weeks. Long term, there is a favorable prognosis for patients who received appropriate treatment for GBS. In fact, a literature review found that more than 80% of patients were able to walk without assistance within 6 months [15]. Rehabilitation for acute and long-term care of GBS and MFS variants depends on a patient's severity of symptoms and level of function. A case report of a patient with MFS saw symptom improvement with the use of exercise programs that enhance strength, range of motion, postural control, coordination, and equilibrium [16]. In addition to a physical therapist, interprofessional teams may also involve meetings with a nutritionist, speech therapist, and occupational therapist. Additionally, patients with bulbar weakness may need assistive communication devices [4].

7. Identify different antecedent events that are associated with increased risk of developing Miller Fisher syndrome (more broadly, Guillain-Barré syndrome). Discuss the incidence and prevalence in the US population.

Preceding Infections: *Campylobacter jejuni* gastroenteritis is the most common preceding infection [1]. About 76% of patients reported a triggering event (such as an upper respiratory infection or gastroenteritis) that occurred in the 4-week time frame prior to GBS symptoms according to results of the International Guillain-Barré Syndrome Outcome Study (IGOS).

Other antecedent infections associated with GBS include:

Cytomegalovirus
Influenza A and B
HIV
COVID-19 virus
Zika virus
Epstein-Barr virus
Varicella-zoster virus
HSV
H. influenzae
E. coli
M. pneumoniae

Vaccinations
Influenza, respiratory syncytial virus, meningococcal, recombinant zoster, and COVID-19 vaccines have been associated with a risk of GBS cases.

- Influenza vaccine: Several epidemiologic studies have shown that the risk of GBS after influenza vaccination is low or negligible. A case-centered analysis in the Vaccine Safety Datalink found no evidence for elevated GBS risk following 2009–10 MIV/2010–11 TIV influenza vaccines [17].
- Adenovirus vector COVID-19 vaccines: A statistically significant safety concern was identified for GBS following receipt of the Ad26.COV2.S vaccine [18]. Now the adenovirus vector COVID-19 vaccine is no longer available [1].

Other Surgery, trauma, and immunosuppressive medications have also been linked as triggering events for GBS cases.

Epidemiology
According to a systematic literature review of the epidemiology of GBS, the annual incidence of GBS in Europe and North America ranges between 0.84 and 1.91 cases per 100,000 per-

sons per year, and incidence of GBS increases with age after 50 years [19]. There is a higher incidence of GBS cases in males compared to females [1].

Exam Questions

1. A 42-year-old white male with no PMH presents with acute onset of diplopia and ataxia that has worsened over 3 days. He denies headache or neck pain. On examination, he is afebrile, alert, and oriented. DTR testing of biceps, brachioradialis, and patellar reflexes all show areflexia. Over the next several days, he developed bulbar weakness and UE muscle weakness bilaterally. Which of the following is the appropriate treatment for this patient?
   A. IVIG
   B. Systemic glucocorticoids
   C. Broad spectrum antibiotics
   D. No treatment

Answer: A

Learning Objective: #5 Discuss the treatments that are available for Miller Fisher syndrome. Describe the mechanism of action, efficacy, and side effects for each treatment.

Explanation: Immunotherapy is suggested for patients with MFS who develop severe symptoms such as respiratory issues, or bulbar or limb weakness. Immunotherapy with IVIG should begin as early as possible, within the first 2–4 weeks of onset of symptoms. Plasma exchange could also be considered. B is incorrect as there is no benefit to glucocorticoid treatment in GBS or MFS; they are not effective and may even slow down recovery. C is incorrect as antibiotics will not be effective against severe symptoms in this case. D is incorrect as the patient in this case has severe symptoms and should be treated with IVIG or plasma exchange. While there is no cure, and MFS can be treated with supportive care, when there are severe symptoms, treatment can help improve symptoms faster.

2. A 42-year-old white male with no PMH presents with acute onset of diplopia and ataxia that has worsened over 3 days. He denies headache or neck pain. On examination, he is afebrile, alert, and oriented. DTR testing of biceps, brachioradialis, and patellar reflexes all show areflexia. He undergoes a lumbar puncture as part of his evaluation. His CSF studies show abnormal findings. Which of the following are likely to be seen on his CSF studies?
   A. Normal WBC, elevated protein level
   B. Elevated WBC (neutrophils), elevated protein, low glucose
   C. Elevated WBC (lymphocytes), elevated protein, normal glucose
   D. Elevated WBC (lymphocytes), elevated protein, low glucose

Answer: A

Learning Objective: #4 Discuss the diagnostic evaluation of Miller Fisher syndrome (CSF analysis, EMG testing, nerve conduction studies, antiganglioside antibody testing, and imaging).

Explanation: This patient presentation is most likely Miller Fisher syndrome (acute and progressive ophthalmoplegia, ataxia, and areflexia). In Guillain-Barré syndrome and GBS variants such as Miller Fisher syndrome, CSF studies may show evidence of albuminocytologic dissociation (normal WBC and raised protein level) in 90% of cases at peak disease. B is incorrect as these would be typical CSF findings in bacterial meningitis. C is incorrect as these would be typical CSF findings in viral meningitis. D is incorrect as these would be typical CSF findings in tuberculosis meningitis. The patient has no headache, neck pain, or fever.

3. A 64-year-old Caucasian male with PMH of COVID-19 6 months ago, a flu-like illness 2 months ago, and a gastroenteritis 3 weeks ago presents with acute onset of diplopia, poor coordination, and difficulty swallowing. On examination, he has normal motor

strength in upper and lower extremities bilaterally, but all DTRs are absent. He is diagnosed with a Guillain-Barré syndrome (GBS) variant called Miller Fisher syndrome. Which of the following is the most common infection that preceded his current neurological syndrome?

A. *Campylobacter jejuni* gastroenteritis
B. COVID-19
C. Influenza A and B
D. *E. coli* gastroenteritis
E. Cytomegalovirus

Answer: A

Learning Objective: #7. Identify different antecedent events that are associated with increased risk of developing Miller Fisher syndrome (more broadly, Guillain-Barré syndrome). Discuss the incidence and prevalence in the US population.

Explanation: *Campylobacter jejuni* gastroenteritis is the most common preceding infection in patients with GBS variant of Miller Fisher syndrome. B is incorrect as while COVID-19 is a possible antecedent event to Guillain-Barré syndrome, it is less common than *C. jejuni* gastroenteritis. C is incorrect as Influenza A and B is a possible antecedent event to Guillain-Barré syndrome but it is less common than *C. jejuni* gastroenteritis. D is incorrect as *E. coli* gastroenteritis is a possible antecedent event to Guillain-Barré syndrome but it is less common than *C. jejuni* gastroenteritis. E is incorrect as Cytomegalovirus is a possible antecedent event to Guillain-Barré syndrome but it is less common than *C. jejuni* gastroenteritis.

References

1. Chandrashekhar S, Dimachkie MM. Guillain-Barré syndrome in adults: pathogenesis, clinical features, and diagnosis. UpToDate. 2025. Retrieved from www.uptodate.com/contents/guillain-barre-syndrome-in-adults-pathogenesis-clinical-features-and-diagnosis?search=miller%20fisher%20syndrome&source=search_result&selectedTitle=1~34&usage_type=default&display_rank=1. Accessed 15 Feb 2025.
2. So YT. Wernicke encephalopathy. UptoDate. 2025. https://www.uptodate.com/contents/wernicke-encephalopathy?search=miller%20fisher%20syndrome&topicRef=5137&source=see_link#H4. Accessed 15 Feb 2025.
3. Ronthal M, Greenstein P. Bell's palsy: pathogenesis, clinical features, and diagnosis in adults. UptoDate. 2025. https://www.uptodate.com/contents/bells-palsy-pathogenesis-clinical-features-and-diagnosis-in-adults?sectionName=CLINICAL%20FEATURES&topicRef=144452&anchor=H4&source=bqp#H4. Accessed 15 Feb 2025.
4. Muley SA. Guillain-Barré syndrome in adults: treatment and prognosis. UpToDate. 2025. https://www.uptodate.com/contents/guillain-barre-syndrome-in-adults-treatment-and-prognosis?search=miller%20fisher%20syndrome&topicRef=5137&source=see_link#H1. Accessed 15 Feb 2025.
5. Hahn AF. Guillain-Barré syndrome. Lancet. 1998;352(9128):635–41.
6. Rocha Cabrero F, Morrison EH. Miller fisher syndrome [2023]. In: StatPearls [Internet]. Treasure Island (FL): StatPearls Publishing; 2025. https://www.ncbi.nlm.nih.gov/books/NBK507717/. Accessed 16 Feb 2025.
7. Saleem F, Das JM. Lateral medullary syndrome. [Updated 2023 Aug 7]. In: StatPearls [Internet]. Treasure Island (FL): StatPearls Publishing; 2025. https://www.ncbi.nlm.nih.gov/books/NBK551670/. Accessed 16 Feb 2025.
8. Vasan S, Kumar A. Wernicke Encephalopathy. [Updated 2023 Aug 14]. In: StatPearls [Internet]. Treasure Island (FL): StatPearls Publishing; 2025. https://www.ncbi.nlm.nih.gov/books/NBK470344/. Accessed 16 Feb. 2025.
9. Nair AG, Patil-Chhablani P, Venkatramani DV, Gandhi RA. Ocular myasthenia gravis: a review. Indian J Ophthalmol. 2014;62(10):985–91.
10. Brazis PW. Overview of diplopia. UpToDate. 2024. www.uptodate.com/contents/overview-of-diplopia?search=diplopia&source=search_result&selectedTitle=1~150&usage_type=default&display_rank=1. Accessed 17 Feb 2025.
11. Iliescu DA, Timaru CM, Alexe N, et al. Management of diplopia. Rom J Ophthalmol. 2017;61(3):166–70. https://doi.org/10.22336/rjo.2017.31.
12. Overell JR, Hsieh ST, Odaka M, Yuki N, Willison HJ. Treatment for fisher syndrome, Bickerstaff's brainstem encephalitis and related disorders. Cochrane Database Syst Rev. 2007;2007(1):CD004761.
13. Chevret S, Hughes RA, Annane D. Plasma exchange for Guillain-Barré syndrome. Cochrane Database Syst Rev. 2(2):CD001798. 2017;2017:CD001798.
14. Hughes RA, Swan AV, van Doorn PA. Intravenous immunoglobulin for Guillain-Barré syndrome. Cochrane Database Syst Rev. 2014;2014(9):CD002063.
15. Rajabally YA, Uncini A. Outcome and its predictors in Guillain-Barre syndrome. J Neurol Neurosurg Psychiatry. 2012;83(7):711–8.
16. Boob MA, Dadgal R, Salphale VG. Emphasis on the optimal functional recovery through a struc-

tured inpatient rehabilitation program along with a home exercise regime in an individual with miller-fisher syndrome: a case report. Cureus. 2022;14(10):e29919.
17. Greene SK, Rett MD, Vellozzi C, et al. Guillain-Barré syndrome, influenza vaccination, and antecedent respiratory and gastrointestinal infections: a case-centered analysis in the vaccine safety datalink, 2009–2011. PLoS One. 2013;8(6):e67185.
18. Woo EJ, Mba-Jonas A, Dimova RB, Alimchandani M, Zinderman CE, Nair N. Association of Receipt of the Ad26.COV2.S COVID-19 vaccine with presumptive Guillain-Barré syndrome. JAMA. 2021;326(16):1606–13.
19. McGrogan A, Madle GC, Seaman HE, de Vries CS. The epidemiology of Guillain-Barré syndrome worldwide. A systematic literature review. Neuroepidemiology. 2009;32(2):150–63.

4 Trouble Swallowing

Abigail Cantwell

Learning Objectives

1. Describe the pathophysiology of nausea and vomiting and the role of neurotransmitters in this process. Explain the neurological mechanism of nausea and vomiting involving the chemoreceptive trigger zone.
2. Describe the general functions and signaling transduction pathways of the following autonomic receptors: alpha 1, alpha 2, beta 1, and beta 2.
3. Review the generic over-the-counter and prescription anti-nausea medications and their mechanisms of action. Identify which ones are used in the operating room setting.
4. Outline the presentation of a patient with anticholinergic toxicity and discuss its current treatment and management options.
5. Describe the physiological mechanism behind the ocular findings in our patient.
6. Explain what demographic of people and which surgeries put people at risk for postoperative nausea and vomiting.

Chief Complaint

"I can't swallow, and I feel dizzy".

A. Cantwell (✉)
Department of Anesthesiology and Perioperative Medicine, Oregon Health and Science University, Portland, OR, USA
e-mail: amcantwell@arizona.edu

JM is a 47-year-old white male who is brought to the ED by his wife with the chief complaint presented above.

Prompt What would you like to ask him?

Prompt the students to ask open ended questions starting with the "OPQRSTU" acronym they learned in doctoring. Here are examples of questions they should generate:

O—Onset—"When did you first notice these symptoms?"
P—Provocation—"Does anything make your symptoms better or worse?"
Q—Quality—"Describe your dizziness to me. Which direction do you feel the room is spinning?"
R—Radiation—"Do these sensations occur anywhere else in your body?"
S—Severity—"How severe is your dizziness on a scale of 1 to 10?"
T—Timing—"Does the dizziness come and go? Is it constant?"
U—Unassociated symptoms—"Do you have any other symptoms you feel are associated with this?"

Prompt: What other questions would you like to ask?

1. What is your past medical history?
2. What is your past surgical history?

C. A. Standley (ed.), *Biomedical Science and Clinical Foundations*,
https://doi.org/10.1007/978-3-031-98353-5_4

3. Any falls recently?
4. Do you have any allergies?
5. What do you do for a living?
6. Have you ever experienced any symptoms like this before?

History of Presenting Illness

JM is a 47-year-old male with a past medical history significant for hypertension, type II diabetes, obesity, and seasonal allergies who presents to the ED with complaints of inability to swallow and dizziness. He first noticed the symptoms this morning around 8 AM, and they are getting progressively worse, which prompted him to come into the ED this afternoon at about 3 PM. He feels his mouth is extremely dry. He also noted dry eyes and decreased urination despite adequate hydration. When he stood up from a chair quickly this afternoon, he found himself to be extremely dizzy. He has never had symptoms like this before. He did report being released from the hospital yesterday following a knee replacement surgery. He stated the surgery went well, and he was discharged on the same day.

Prompt: What are your differential diagnoses at this point?

At this point, guide the students through the VINDICATE acronym to try to identify the most likely differential diagnoses. Students should pick out symptoms that are related to the autonomic nervous system. Encourage the use of symptoms from the acronym for anticholinergic toxicity "red as a beet, dry as a bone, blind as a bat, mad as a hatter, hot as a hare, full as a flask." If a student recognizes these symptoms, please congratulate them. Here are some options for things the students might toss out for the VINDICATE pneumonic.

Vascular: stroke, fluid loss after surgery, orthostatic hypotension, polycythemia vera.
Infectious: meningitis
Neoplastic: brain metastasis, brain tumor
Degenerative: n/a
Iatrogenic: medication side effects
Intoxication: pain meds, alcoholism
Congenital: AV malformations
Autoimmune: SLE
Traumatic: a fall leading to intracranial bleed
Endocrine: hypoglycemia, hypothyroidism

Prompt: What other information do you want from JM?

The other information they should want from JM would be his past medical history, past surgical history, allergies, family history, and review of systems questions.

Past Medical History

Knee replacement surgery yesterday morning, hypertension for the past 8 years, and type 2 diabetes for the past 5 years.

Past Surgical History

Appendectomy 30 years ago.

Social History

One pack per day smoker for the past 20 years.

He reports "having a few beers on the weekends" and no drug use. He reports being a construction worker who is insured.

Prompt: Why is it important to ask for a social history?

The students should identify at this point that it is important to ask for a social history for a variety of reasons. First of all, the patient could have substance use issues and it is important to factor that into the differential diagnosis. Especially after a surgery when he would have most likely been given narcotics. The other thing I would like for them to identify is the cost of a neurological workup if he were not insured. At this point it would be a good time to have them look up online the cost of a CT non-contrast of the head and neck as well as the cost of an MRI of the head.

Medications

Lisinopril, metformin

Allergies

Peanuts, sulfa

Family History
Dad had a stroke at 65
Mother has diabetes

Prompt: What stands out about his family history?

The students should mention at this point that he has a familial history of cardiovascular disease which makes us more concerned for a stroke.

Review of Systems
General: No fevers, chills, night sweats, or weight loss
HEENT: +trouble swallowing, + dry mouth; no ear pain, changes in vision, congestion, or sore throat
Cardiopulmonary: Negative for pain or pressure with exertion
GI: +constipation
Urinary: +oliguria, no pain with urination
Endocrine: Negative for heat/cold intolerance, changes in hair/skin/nails, and night sweats
Skin: +flushed cheeks
Neurological: +dizzy.
Psych: no history of depression or anxiety

Prompt: Are there any signs or symptoms related to dysfunction in the autonomic nervous system?

This is another good spot to try to prompt the student to connect the symptoms of anticholinergic toxicity or try to pick out those related to autonomic nervous system function. Similarly to previously, it is okay if they do not full understand these concepts. They are fairly advanced but it will be a great review of the autonomic nervous system for them.

Prompt: What will you look for in the physical exam?

The students should all agree that the most important part of this physical exam is the neurological examination. This is a good spot to remind them the important details of a neuro exam including orientation to person, place and time. Talk to them about how you check each cranial nerve. Lastly, motor movement in the extremities as well as reflexes.

Physical Examination
Vital signs:

T: 98.3 °F
RR: 18 (normal = 12–18/min)
P: 110 (normal = 60–100/min)
BP: 130/80 (normal = below 110–130/60–80)
Wt: 220 lbs. Ht: 5′10″

General: Pleasant, interactive, flushed appearance
HEENT: +right pupil significantly larger than the left pupil, no oral ulcers or ocular inflammation,
Heart: regular rate and rhythm, no murmurs
Lungs: clear to auscultation
Gastrointestinal: nontender/nondistended, no organomegaly or masses
Genitourinary: normal anal sphincter tone
Skin: flushed appearance
Extremities: feet warm, well perfused with good cap refill; no edema, pulses 2+/2+ (B) LE
Neuro: A & O X 4, CN 2–12 grossly intact, normal motor movement for UE and LE bilaterally, normal sensation bilaterally

Prompt: Why is the neuro exam normal yet the pupils are asymmetric?

It is okay if the students are a bit confused on why the patient has a normal neurological status (although pupils are asymmetric). Try to guide them to think of reasons for the presentation without it being a stroke. This is a very important part of this case. Many times, patients that get scopolamine patches will accidentally touch the patch and then touch their eyes resulting in this ocular finding. They often have code strokes called on them and get very expensive neurological workups.

Prompt: What tests do you want to order?

This is a good time to engage the students in a conversation about cost of ordering various lab work. They will most likely immediately mention CBC and CMP. The next conversation would most likely be about neuroimaging.

Laboratory Data

Results from the patient's comprehensive metabolic panel and complete blood count are shown in Tables 4.1 and 4.2, respectively.

Prompt: After reviewing this lab work, what is your next step?

Since the lab work is all within the normal range, the next step would be to get some imaging studies.

Table 4.1 Comprehensive metabolic panel

Test	Patient	Reference
Glucose (mg/dL)	75	65–99
BUN (mg/dL)	18	6–24
Creatinine (mg/dL)	1.1	0.76–1.27
BUN/creatinine ratio	16	9–20
Sodium (mmol/L)	140	134–144
Potassium (mmol/L)	4.1	3.5–5.2
Chloride (mmol/L)	100	96–106
Carbon dioxide, Total (mmol/L)	23	20–29
Calcium (mg/dL)	9.0	8.7–10.2
Protein, Total (g/dL)	6.5	6.0–8.5
Albumin (g/dL)	4.0	3.5–5.5
Globulin, Total (g/dL)	2.5	1.5–4.5
A/G ratio	2.5	1.5–4.5
Bilirubin, Total (mg/dL)	0.9	0.0–1.2
Alkaline phosphatase (IU/L)	44	39–117
AST (IU/L)	40	0–40
ALT (IU/L)	39	0–44

BUN Blood urea nitrogen, A/G albumin/globulin, AST aspartate aminotransferase, ALT alanine aminotransferase.

Table 4.2 Complete blood count

Test	Patient	Reference
Hb (g/L)	40	135–175
RBC (L)	5.0	4.5–6.5 x10^{12}
Hct	0.48	0.40–0.52
MCV (fl)	83	80–95
MCH(pg)	28	26–34
MCHC (g/dL)	31	30–35
Reticulocytes (%)	1.0	0.5–20
WBC, Total (L)	6.8	4.0–11.0 × 10^9
Platelets (L)	300	150–400 × 10^9

Hb Hemoglobin, *RBC* Red Blood Cell count, *Hct* Hematocrit, *MCV* Mean Corpuscular Volume, *MCH* Mean Corpuscular Hemoglobin, *MCHC* Mean Corpuscular Hemoglobin Concentration, *WBC* White Blood Cell count

Prompt: What are the pros and cons of ordering neuro imaging?

Engage the students in a conversation about pros and cons of neuro imaging. The cost of a non-contrast CT of the head and neck can range all the way from $800–$5000. This often results in further follow-up with an MRI and an MRI of the head costs roughly $1600–$9000. Reflect on how expensive this is for the patient. Other points to discuss are radiation exposure and time of both healthcare providers as well as the time of the patient. See if students can come up with other options besides neuroimaging.

Next Steps

To save JM from a big hospital bill, you decide to order his medical records from his surgery, and they fax them over immediately.

Anesthesia Operative Note from Yesterday's Knee Surgery

HPI: JM is a pleasant 47-year-old male with past medical history significant for hypertension and diabetes who presents for knee replacement surgery. He denies any history of stroke, MI, angina, GERD, neuropathy, asthma, or COPD. He is a chronic tobacco user. He reports having surgery in the past and not having any issue with anesthesia, but he does report severe postoperative nausea and vomiting after his prior surgery.

Plan

- Pre-op: 2 midazolam, 2 fentanyl, and scopolamine patch for nausea
- Intraop: inhaled anesthetic gas, dexamethasone, and ondansetron
- Postop: PO and IV Dilaudid PRN for pain control

Prompt: Is there any medication from his surgery that could be causative of his current condition?

Guide the students through each medication given in the list and try to see if they figure out that the scopolamine is the most likely reason for the anti-cholinergic toxicity symptoms.

Prompt: JM's wife is angry because she truly wants to rule out a stroke. How do you explain to her that imaging is not necessary?

This is a great place to do a role play with the students to practice managing an angry patient or an unreasonable patient.

Assessment

After reviewing the anesthesia operative notes, you realize your patient is having reactions to their scopolamine patch! You decide to not order any imaging studies and instead, check behind his ear, and lo and behold, you find a patch!

Prompt: How will you manage the patient now?

Immediately remove the scopolamine patch to stop further absorption. Treatment for scopolamine patch-induced anticholinergic toxicity focuses on supportive care, Focus on maintaining airway, breathing, and circulation (ABCs). Closely monitor heart rate, blood pressure, temperature, and mental status. Be vigilant for signs of hyperthermia, rhabdomyolysis, and seizures. Intravenous benzodiazepines (e.g., lorazepam, diazepam) can be used for agitation. In severe cases, where agitation and delirium are refractory to benzodiazepines, physostigmine may be considered.

End of Case

Learning Objectives Explained

1. **Describe the pathophysiology of nausea and vomiting and the role of neurotransmitters in this process. Explain the neurological mechanism of nausea and vomiting involving the chemoreceptive trigger zone.**

Nausea and vomiting are protective reflexes that prevent the ingestion or absorption of harmful substances. These processes are coordinated at the level of the medulla oblongata in the brainstem, where there are chemoreceptors sensitive to emetic agents [1]. There are complex interactions between the central nervous system, autonomic nervous system, and gastrointestinal system. The primary neurological structures involved include the **vomiting center** (VC) in the medulla oblongata and the **chemoreceptor trigger zone (CTZ)** in the area postrema of the brainstem.

Several neurotransmitters play key roles in nausea and vomiting by modulating signals within the brainstem structures: [1]

1. **Dopamine (D2 receptors)**—Predominantly found in the CTZ, dopamine is a major mediator of nausea and vomiting, particularly in response to drugs such as opioids and chemotherapy agents.
2. **Serotonin (5-HT3 receptors)—**Released from enterochromaffin cells in the gastrointestinal tract in response to toxins or irritants, serotonin activates vagal afferents, which stimulate the VC. It is a primary target for antiemetic drugs like ondansetron.
3. **Histamine (H1 receptors)**—Involved in motion sickness and vestibular-induced nausea; antihistamines such as diphenhydramine block this pathway.
4. **Acetylcholine (M1 receptors)**—Plays a role in motion sickness and vestibular-mediated vomiting, acting via the vestibular nuclei and the VC.
5. **Substance P (NK1 receptors)**—A neuropeptide that binds to neurokinin-1 (NK1) receptors in the VC and is implicated in chemotherapy-induced nausea and vomiting.
6. **Gamma-aminobutyric acid (GABA) and cannabinoids (CB1 receptors)**—Act as modulatory neurotransmitters that can suppress nausea and vomiting, explaining the antiemetic effects of benzodiazepines and cannabinoids.

The **CTZ, located in the area postrema of the medulla**, is highly vascularized and lacks a well-developed blood-brain barrier, allowing it to detect circulating toxins, drugs, and metabolic disturbances. It transmits signals to the **VC**, which coordinates the motor and autonomic responses required for emesis.

The vomiting reflex consists of

1. **Afferent signals** from the CTZ, vestibular system, gastrointestinal tract, and higher brain centers (e.g., cortex, limbic system).

2. **Integration** of these signals within the medullary VC.
3. **Efferent signals** to the pharynx, esophagus, diaphragm, and abdominal muscles, leading to vomiting.

The vomiting reflex, controlled by the brainstem, specifically the area postrema and the nucleus tractus solitarius, is a crucial protective mechanism that expels harmful substances from the body, preventing potential damage from ingested toxins or irritants.

2. **Describe the general functions and signaling transduction pathways of the following autonomic receptors: alpha 1, alpha 2, beta 1, and beta 2.**

The autonomic receptors alpha 1, alpha 2, beta 1, and beta 2 are known as adrenergic receptors [2]. These are G-protein-coupled receptors (GPCRs) that mediate the effects of catecholamines, primarily **epinephrine (E) and norepinephrine (NE),** within the autonomic nervous system (ANS). These receptors are broadly classified into **α (alpha) and β (beta) receptors**, each with distinct functions and intracellular signaling mechanisms.

Adrenergic receptors play a crucial role in the **sympathetic division** of the ANS. Their activation modulates physiological responses such as

- **Cardiovascular regulation**—Heart rate, contractility, and vasoconstriction/dilation
- **Respiratory control**—Bronchodilation
- **Metabolic processes**—Glycogenolysis, lipolysis, insulin secretion
- **Smooth muscle tone**—Contraction or relaxation of vascular, gastrointestinal, and urinary smooth muscle

α-Adrenergic Receptors [3]

Alpha 1: Stimulation of this receptor causes arterial vasoconstriction, resulting in increased mean arterial pressure. It is attached to the Gq receptor, which in turn activates IP3-DAG cascade to increase intracellular calcium and activate protein kinase C. It also causes venoconstriction and pupillary dilation. Lastly, it can cause constriction at the venous level. It can also cause constriction of the urinary tract, creating a full bladder. It causes urethral sphincter and prostate muscle contraction.

Alpha 2: The primary mechanism of action of this receptor is to inhibit the release of neurotransmitters. It also acts at a central level to decrease sympathetic tone. Furthermore, stimulation of this receptor leads to decreased aqueous humor production and decreased lipolysis. Stimulation of this receptor can also inhibit insulin. It is connected to the Gi receptor, which inhibits adenylate cyclase, leading to a decrease in cAMP and reduced protein kinase A activation.

β-Adrenergic Receptors [4]

Beta 1: This receptor is heavily present on cardiac myocytes, and when this receptor is stimulated, it leads to increased contractility of the heart. It also causes increased chronicity of the heart and an elevated heart rate. Together, these actions increase cardiac output. This receptor also leads to increased renin release from the juxtaglomerular cells. It is attached to the Gs receptor, which activates adenylate cycles, leading to increased cAMP release and activation of protein kinase A.

Beta 2: The primary mechanism of action of this receptor is to relax smooth muscle, leading to bronchodilation. It also increases lipolysis and increases aqueous humor production. It causes an increase in the release of insulin. It can cause hypokalemia through intravascular shifting of potassium and results in increase in gluconeogenesis. This receptor is attached to the Gs receptor, which activates adenylate cycles, leading to increased cAMP release and activation of protein kinase A.

3. **Review the generic over-the-counter and prescription anti-nausea medications and their mechanisms of action. Identify which ones are used in the operating room setting.**

Table 4.3 Over-the-counter anti-nausea medications

Generic name	Drug class	Mechanism of action	Common uses
Dimenhydrinate	Antihistamine	Blocks H1 receptors in the CZT and vestibular system	Motion sickness, vertigo
Meclizine	Antihistamine	Blocks H1 receptors in the brainstem	Motion sickness, vertigo
Diphenhydramine	Antihistamine	Blocks H1 receptors and has anticholinergic properties	Motion sickness, mild nausea
Bismuth subsalicylate	Antidiarrheal	May coat the stomach lining and reduce gastric irritation	Nausea related to indigestion, mild gastritis
Ginger	Herbal remedy	Modulation of serotonin receptors in the GI tract	Motion sickness, mild nausea

Table 4.4 Prescription Anti-Nausea Mediations

Generic name	Drug class	Mechanism of action	Common uses
Ondansetron	Serotonin receptor antagonist	Blocks 5-HT3 receptors in the CZT	PONV, CINV
Metoclopramide	Dopamine receptor antagonist	Blocks D2 receptors in the CZT	PONV, nausea from migraine
Aprepitant	Neurokinin receptor antagonist	Blocks NK1 receptors in the brainstem	PONV, CINV
Scopolamine	Anticholinergic	Blocks muscarinic receptors in the vomiting center and vestibular system	PONV, motion sickness
Dexamethasone	Corticosteroid	Reduces inflammation and modulates neurotransmission in the vomiting center	PONV, CINV
Dronabinol	Cannabinoid	Activates CB1 receptors to inhibit nausea and vomiting signals	CINV, appetite stimulation

POVN Postoperative nausea and vomiting, *CINV* chemotherapy-induced nausea and vomiting

Nausea and vomiting are treated with various medications based on the underlying cause. These drugs act on different neurotransmitter receptors in the **chemoreceptor trigger zone (CTZ), VC, and gastrointestinal tract** [5]. Over-the-counter medications to treat nausea are shown in Table 4.3, while prescription medications are shown in Table 4.4 [5, 6].

The medications listed in Table 4.4 for PONV are often combined for multimodal prophylaxis in high-risk surgical patients. Of note, almost every surgical patient gets both dexamethasone and ondansetron before wakeup for preventative nausea and vomiting treatment.

4. **Outline the presentation of a patient with anticholinergic toxicity and discuss its current treatment and management options.**

Anticholinergic toxicity occurs due to excessive inhibition of **muscarinic acetylcholine receptors (M1–M5)** in the central and peripheral nervous systems. It is commonly caused by overdoses of medications with anticholinergic properties, such as **antihistamines, tricyclic antidepressants (TCAs), atropine, and scopolamine.**

Scopolamine functions by competing with acetylcholine and other muscarinic agonists for a common binding site on the muscarinic receptor. It has been suggested that scopolamine acts in the central nervous system (CNS) by blocking cholinergic transmission from the vestibular nuclei to higher centers in the CNS and from the reticular formation to the VC. The symptoms of anticholinergic toxicity are shown in Table 4.5, according to a classic mnemonic that is used for remembering them [7].

The CNS signs and symptoms (i.e., central anticholinergic toxicity) are the most worrisome, and, if present, the patient can be considered to have "severe" anticholinergic toxicity [8].

Table 4.5 Classic symptoms of anticholinergic toxicity

Mnemonic	System	Symptoms	Mechanism
Red as a beet	PNS	Flushing	Cutaneous vasodilation
Dry as a bone	Skin, glands, PNS	Dry skin	Sweat gland inhibition
Hot as a hare	Skin, glands, PNS	Hyperthermia	Interference with normal heat dissipation mechanisms
Blind as a bat	Ocular	Pupillary dilation, blurred vision	Pupillary sphincter inhibition
Mad as a hatter	CNS	Agitation, delirium, hallucinations, seizures, coma	Blocked central muscarinic receptors, reduced acetylcholine
Full as a flask	Urinary	Urinary retention	Detrusor muscle inhibition

Treatment and management of an anticholinergic crisis involves immediate supportive care, securing airway, breathing, and circulation, which includes monitoring temperature and providing cooling measures (IV fluids, external cooling) for hyperthermia. Benzodiazepines can be administered for agitation, IV fluids to maintain perfusion, and bladder catheterization to relieve urinary retention.

5. **Describe the physiological mechanism behind the ocular findings in our patient.**

The ocular findings in our patient occur very frequently in post-surgical patients. This happens specifically when patients touch their medicated patch and then touch their eyes. As patients are coming out of anesthesia, they tend to be very drowsy and unaware of their actions. Thus, they often do this, and that results in the ocular findings as seen in this patient. The ANS controls pupil size through the iris muscles, with the sympathetic system causing dilation (mydriasis) via adrenergic receptors and the parasympathetic system causing constriction (miosis) via muscarinic receptors [9]. When scopolamine is on a patient's hands, it gets absorbed through the eyes, and scopolamine will inhibit the muscarinic receptors. This prevents the iris from moving and will result in pupillary dilation.

6. **Explain what demographic of people and which surgeries put people most at risk for postoperative nausea and vomiting.**

Individuals who are female, have a history of motion sickness or previous nausea and vomiting episodes, are non-smokers, and those who received opioids postoperatively are at a higher risk for postoperative nausea and vomiting (PONV) [10]. While not as strong as these other factors, younger patients (especially children) may be at a slightly higher risk. Additionally, high levels of preoperative anxiety can also increase the risk.

Certain types of surgeries, such as gynecological, maxillofacial, and thyroid operations, have higher incidence of PONV [11]. Importantly, ear, nose, and throat (ENT) surgery is associated with a very high incidence of PONV compared to the general surgical population, potentially reaching up to 70% in some cases [12]. Longer surgeries are also associated with higher risk. While not always a major factor, some types of anesthesia, such as nitrous oxide or volatiles, may increase the risk.

The challenging part is confounding variables between gynecological surgery and young women being most at risk for postoperative nausea in the first place.

Exam Questions

1. A 40-year-old female is experiencing severe postoperative vomiting after her hysterectomy. Which area of the brain controls this?
   A. Nucleus tractus solitarius
   B. Frontal cortex
   C. Edinger-Westphal nucleus
   D. The spinothalamic tract

Answer: A

Learning Objective: #1Describe the pathophysiology of nausea and vomiting and the role of neurotransmitters in this process. Explain the neurological mechanism of nausea and vomiting involving the chemoreceptive trigger zone.

Explanation: The neuroanatomical site controlling nausea and vomiting is in a region called the "VC" within the medulla of the brainstem, specifically the area postrema and the nucleus tractus solitarius. B is incorrect: while the sensation of nausea often precedes vomiting and involves the cerebral cortex, the act of vomiting is primarily controlled in the brainstem. C is incorrect: while the Edinger-Westphal nucleus is known to control pupillary reflexes and pupils dilate when the ANS is activated, there is not a direct link between this nucleus and the VC. D is incorrect, as this tract conveys nociception, temperature, and crude touch but does not involve the vomiting reflex.

2. A 57-year-old male is prepped for surgery for a tympanic membrane repair. He has past medical history significant for hypertension, vertigo, and diabetes. What is his biggest risk factor for postoperative nausea and vomiting?
   A. Gender
   B. Age
   C. Type of surgery
   D. Past medical history

Answer: C

Learning Objective: #7 Explain what demographic of people and which surgeries put people at risk for postoperative nausea and vomiting.

Explanation: In reviewing this patient's specific information, the type of surgery in his case (i.e., ENT surgery) poses the highest risk for him to experience PONV. A is incorrect, as females have a higher risk than males. B is incorrect, as younger patients have a higher risk than older patients. D is incorrect, as while he has some health issues, these are not known to increase the risk of PONV.

3. A 35-year-old female with a medical history of asthma presents for an ovarian cyst removal. She is waiting in the pre-op area and being connected to the monitors. The EKG leads are reading heart rate of 180 bpm. What is the most likely explanation for this?
   A. She has an underlying heart condition
   B. She recently used her beta-2 agonist inhaler
   C. She is experiencing anxiety about her surgery
   D. She thought she was late for her appointment and ran to the clinic

Answer: B

Learning Objective: #2 Describe the general functions and signaling transduction pathways of the following autonomic receptors: alpha 1, alpha 2, beta 1, and beta 2.

Explanation: Inhaled beta-2 agonists, while effective for bronchodilation in an asthma attack, can cause tachycardia (i.e., heart rate of 180 bpm) as a side effect. A is incorrect: while tachycardia can be a symptom of an underlying heart condition, the most likely explanation in this patient with a medical history of asthma is use of a rescue inhaler, not the discovery of an underlying heart condition. C is incorrect: when someone is anxious about surgery, their heart rate typically increases, sometimes reaching 100 bpm or higher, but the most likely explanation for a heart rate of 180 bpm in this patient with a history of asthma is use of a rescue inhaler. D is incorrect: while running to an appointment would cause the heart rate to increase, it would likely be returning toward normal as she has moved from the waiting reception area to pre-op.

References

1. Zhong W, Shahbaz O, Teskey G, Beever A, Kachour N, Venketaraman V, Darmani NA. Mechanisms of nausea and vomiting: current knowledge and recent advances in intracellular emetic signaling systems. Int J Mol Sci. 2021;22(11):5797.
2. McCorry LK. Physiology of the autonomic nervous system. Am J Pharm Educ. 2007;71(4):78.

3. Taylor BN, Cassagnol M. Alpha-adrenergic receptors. [Updated 2023 Jul 10]. In: StatPearls [Internet]. Treasure Island (FL): StatPearls Publishing; 2025. Available from: https://www.ncbi.nlm.nih.gov/books/NBK539830/.
4. Wallukat G. The beta-adrenergic receptors. Herz. 2002;27(7):683–90.
5. Heckroth M, Luckett RT, Moser C, Parajuli D, Abell TL. Nausea and vomiting in 2021: a comprehensive update. J Clin Gastroenterol. 2021;55(4):279–99.
6. Cao X, White PF, Ma H. An update on the management of postoperative nausea and vomiting. J Anesth. 2017;31(4):617–26.
7. Broderick ED, Metheny H, Crosby B. Anticholinergic toxicity. [Updated 2023 Apr 30]. In: StatPearls [Internet]. Treasure Island (FL): StatPearls Publishing; 2025.
8. Lo A, Ho R. Anticholinergic toxicity: recognition and management. Emerg Med Clin North Am. 2021;39(2):227–44.
9. Levine MC, Gill RS. Pharmacologic mydriasis: mechanisms and clinical implications. Surv Ophthalmol. 2018;63(3):347–54.
10. Admass BA, Tawye HY, Endalew NS, Mersha AT, Melesse DY, Workie MM, Gashaw M, Ferede YA. Assessment of post-operative nausea and vomiting prophylaxis usage for cesarean section, 2021: a cross sectional study. Ann Med Surg (Lond). 2022;75:103399.
11. Koivuranta M, Läärä E, Snåre L, Alahuhta S. A survey of postoperative nausea and vomiting. Anaesthesia. 1997;52(5):443–9.
12. Yosief PK, Beraki GG, Mayer D, Mengistu MB, Tesfamariam EH. Incidence and risk factors of postoperative nausea and vomiting after ENT surgery. Int J Anesthetic Anesthesiol. 2022;9:132.

Part II

Muscle/Bone

5 Intermittent Leg Pain

Patrick C. Mayolo and Sean P. Kelly

Learning Objectives

1. Describe the common clinical presentation, physical examination, imaging, and lab findings consistent with osteosarcoma.
2. Discuss a differential of primary bone tumors of adolescence, highlighting key similarities and differences between osteosarcoma, Ewing sarcoma, giant cell tumor, and other benign tumors.
3. Discuss treatment options for osteosarcoma.
4. To understand the epidemiology of osteosarcoma to include a discussion of age, sex, and geographic location on incidence.
5. Understand the histologic hallmarks of osteosarcoma and the various subtypes.
6. Describe the genetic predisposition to the development of osteosarcoma.
7. Explain how risk factors such as radiation therapy, chemotherapy, and Paget disease of the bone can influence the development of osteosarcoma.

Histology imaging provided courtesy of Dr. Karen Thompson, University of Hawaii

P. C. Mayolo (✉) · S. P. Kelly
Department of Orthopaedic Surgery, Tripler Army Medical Center, Honolulu, HI, USA
e-mail: Patrick.c.mayolo.mil@health.mil; Sean.p.kelly10.mil@health.mil

Case Presentation

Today you are working in a community family medicine clinic. The first patient you are asked to see is a 14-year-old female, Emma Davis, accompanied by her mother, who is presenting with the following chief complaint:

Chief Complaint

My right leg has been hurting lately.

Facilitator Prompt

A thorough clinician will always establish a broad differential of potential diagnoses when a patient presents with a complaint. A helpful mnemonic to create this differential is VINDICATES (Vascular, Infectious/Inflammatory, Neoplastic, Degenerative/Deficiency/Drugs, Iatrogenic/Idiopathic/Intoxication, Congenital, Autoimmune/Allergic/Anatomic, Traumatic, Endocrine/Environmental). Using this mnemonic, prompt the students to create a list of potential causes of our patient's leg pain. As the case progresses, remind students to re-visit their differential diagnosis list frequently and modify the list as needed. An example differential diagnosis for this chief complaint is provided in Table 5.1.

C. A. Standley (ed.), *Biomedical Science and Clinical Foundations*,
https://doi.org/10.1007/978-3-031-98353-5_5

Table 5.1 Example differential diagnosis list using the VINDICATE mnemonic for an adolescent female with knee pain

System	Differential diagnosis
Vascular	Deep venous thrombosis
Infectious/Inflammatory	Cellulitis, abscess, septic arthritis
Neoplastic	Primary soft tissue tumor, primary bone tumor, metastatic disease
Degenerative/Deficiency/Drugs	Myopathy
Iatrogenic/Idiopathic/Intoxication	n/a
Congenital	Bipartite patella, lateral patellar instability
Autoimmune/Allergic/Anatomic	Juvenile idiopathic arthritis, reactive arthritis, patellofemoral pain syndrome, chondromalacia, quadriceps tendinitis, referred hip pain, slipped capital femoral epiphysis
Traumatic	Stress fracture, acute trauma, ligamentous sprain, muscle contusion/strain
Endocrine/Environmental	n/a

History of Presenting Illness

Emma Davis is a 14-year-old female with no known past medical history who developed intermittent right leg pain beginning 3 months ago. She states that she first noticed the pain after dance practice one afternoon, but now the pain seems to occur spontaneously without strenuous activity. The pain is mostly localized to her distal thigh and knee, but she is unable to discern if the pain starts in her knee and travels up her thigh or vice versa. Her mother, who is accompanying her, is convinced that she is experiencing growing pains since she grew 4 inches over the last year. When asked to describe the quality of the pain, she states, "It is dull and periodically throbs."

The patient denies any trauma to her right lower extremity. She denies any buckling, abnormal popping, or sensation of her knee "giving out." She also denies redness and warmth but does think her knee and thigh have been a little swollen.

Facilitator Prompt

Musculoskeletal pain is a common complaint in active adolescents. Symptoms are often vague and do not point to a clear etiology. It is important to keep a broad differential. Consider prompting the students what additional information they would ask the patient for given her history of the presenting illness before proceeding with the case.

Past Medical History

No known medical history
No past surgical history
Menarche at age 14; menses occur monthly.

Facilitator Prompt

Consider asking the students why menarche status is important to know. How does menarche relate to peak height velocity in females?

Menarche status is important to clinicians as it provides insight as to where the patient may be on their growth rate curve. Peak height velocity (PHV) typically occurs around age 12 years in females. Classically, after the onset of adolescent growth spurt females will begin developing breast tissue and pubic hair. Menarche occurs rather late in the growth spurt, roughly one year after PHV is reached [1].

Medications

No daily medications

Patient states that she has taken ibuprofen as needed for her leg pain with minimal relief.

Allergies

No known drug allergies

Social History

Lives at home with mother, father, and younger brother
Enrolled in the 9th grade, performs well in school.
Denies tobacco, alcohol, or recreational drug use.

High Risk Behaviors/Habits

Patient enjoys ballet and competes competitively at the national level. Practices 3 h a day, 5–6 days per week.

Family History

Father: HTN
Mother: Breast Cancer (diagnosed at age 38)

Facilitator Prompt
Ask the students to discuss the significance of a mother with a history of breast cancer. Direct students to the mother's age at time of diagnosis; what is the significance of early onset breast cancer versus late onset?

The development of early onset breast cancer raises concern for germline mutations that predispose to the disorder. BRCA1, BRCA2 and Li Fraumeni syndrome are a few known conditions that carry increased risk of breast cancer in women. These germline mutations may carry risks of developing other cancers. At some point the patient and her family should consider genetic counseling [2].

Review of Systems

General: no fever, chills, sweating, loss of appetite, malaise, sedation, weight gain/loss, or insomnia.
Eyes: no double vision, but no vision loss, eye pain, or light sensitivity.
ENT: No earache, ringing in ears, hearing loss, nasal congestion, neck pain or stiffness, no difficulty swallowing.
Cardiovascular: No chest pains, palpitations, fainting spells, or ankle swelling.
Respiratory: No cough or wheezing, no dyspnea.
Skin: No rash, itching, suspicious lesions, or alopecia.
GI: No nausea, vomiting, diarrhea, constipation, change in bowel habits, abdominal pain, blood, or black stool.
GU: No pain on urination, blood in urine, frequent urination, frequent urination at night, unusually large quantity of urine, or loss of bladder control.
Musculoskeletal: Pain and swelling in right lower extremity per HPI, but no joint pain, swelling of joints, muscle cramps, stiffness, or arthritis.
Neurological: No headaches, seizures, dizziness, or tremors; no sensory or motor deficits
Psychiatric: No depression, anxiety, hallucinations, paranoia, or panic attacks.
Endocrine: Denies heat/cold intolerance, increased thirst, or increased appetite.
Heme/Lymphatic: No abnormal bruising, bleeding, or enlarged lymph nodes.
Allergy/Immunology: No persistent infections or HIV exposures.

Facilitator Prompt
Challenge a student to summarize the important subjective information we have received into a concise statement. How does this information affect your differential? What would you be looking for on physical exam?

Physical Examination

Vitals: Blood pressure: 104/78, heart rate: 64, respiratory rate: 14, temperature: 98.6, BMI: 19
General: Alert and conversant in no acute distress
Skin: Warm and dry; no lesions
HEENT: Normocephalic, atraumatic, conjunctiva clear, pupils equal and reactive to light and accommodation, extraocular muscles intact, fundoscopic exam benign, hearing intact bilaterally, nasal passages clear.

Neck: no thyromegaly, lymphadenopathy, or carotid bruit bilaterally.
Chest: Clear to auscultation and percussion bilaterally
Cardio: Regular rate and rhythm, normal S1 S2 without murmurs or rub
Abdomen: Non-tender, non-distended, positive bowel sounds in all four quadrants, no hepatosplenomegaly
Genital/rectal: Deferred

Musculoskeletal
Right Hip
Inspection: No lesions, abrasions, erythema, ecchymosis, or edema.
Palpation: Non-tender over greater trochanter or anterior superior iliac spine. Negative compression test.
Range of motion: full range of motion in flexion, extension, internal rotation, external rotation, abduction, and adduction.
Motor: 5/5 hip flexion, extension, abduction, and adduction.
Special tests: Negative flexion, abduction, and external rotation test (FABER). Negative flexion, adduction, and internal rotation test (FADIR). No Trendelenburg sign.

Right Knee
Inspection: No lesions, abrasions, erythema, ecchymosis, or edema. Distal thigh mildly swollen compared to contralateral side.
Palpation: diffusely tender to palpation around distal thigh. Non-tender over the tibial tubercle, infrapatellar tendon, patella, quadriceps tendon, and joint line.
Sensation: Intact distally to light touch over deep and superficial peroneal, sural, saphenous, and tibial distributions.
Range of motion: full range of motion in flexion and extension.
Motor: 5/5 knee extension and flexion
Vascular: Warm and well perfused
Special tests: negative patellar apprehension test, patellar compression test, and patellar crepitus. Negative McMurray's test. No laxity to valgus or varus stress at 0 or 30 degrees. Stable to anterior drawer, no pivot shift, 1A Lachman. Stable to posterior drawer, negative quad activation test, no posterior sag. Dial test is symmetric at 30 and 90 degrees compared to contralateral side.
Neuro: no sensory or motor deficits, reflexes 2+ symmetrical diffusely
Gait: negative Romberg; normal gait

Facilitator Prompt
Discuss the components of a thorough musculoskeletal exam with the students.

A thorough musculoskeletal exam is typically comprised of visual inspection, palpation, range of motion, neuro examination (including sensation and motor strength testing), and any special tests pertinent to the area of interest. In this patient with a complaint pertaining to the distal thigh, it is necessary to examine the hip and knee. Special tests are used to examine for a specific pathology or injury and are essential to the physical examination. Some of the special tests used on this patient include FABER, FADIR, Trendelenburg exam, patellar apprehension test, McMurray's test, Lachman, and Dial test among others. Encourage the students to review the examination maneuvers performed on this patient and verify that they understand how to perform these tests and what pathology each positive test would indicate.

Imaging

Your team decides to order some plain radiographs of the patient's femur (Fig. 5.1).

Facilitator Prompt
Ask the students to read this X-ray as they would before an orthopedic surgeon on rounds. The standard approach to reading an X-ray is the following:

(a) Describe the views (i.e. AP and lateral views)
(b) Describe the joint or extremity (i.e. right femur)
(c) Assess the skeletal maturity of the patient (i.e. skeletally immature vs mature, assessed by looking at the physis)
(d) Describe pertinent positive and negative findings in a concise, objective manner.

An example description of the above radiographs would be

> These are AP and lateral views of a right femur in a skeletally immature patient. Examination of the right distal femur demonstrates a multilobulated osteolucent lesion with diffuse sclerosis, irregularity, and cortical thinning. There is associated periosteal reaction on the medial diaphysis and metaphysis with elevated periosteum. There is associated soft tissue edema surrounding the lesion.

After attempting to describe the radiographs, provide the students with the description above.

Facilitator Prompt

This is the first sign that the patient has an underlying disease that may require intervention. Encourage the students to revisit their differential diagnosis and refine it based on these radiograph findings. What further tests might you order now?

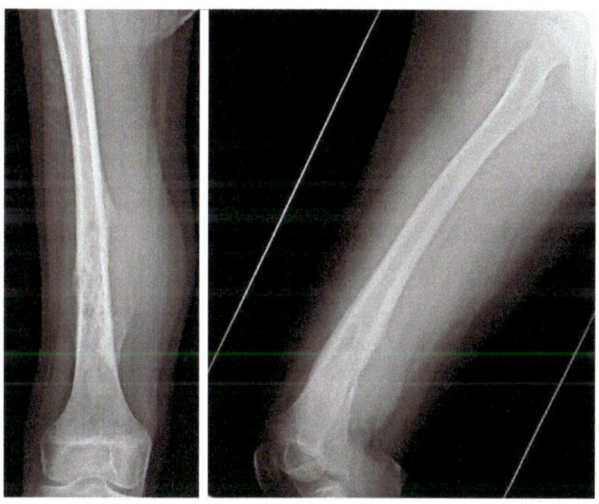

Fig. 5.1 Plain anteroposterior and lateral radiographs of the patient's right femur demonstrating an osseous lesion at the distal metaphysis of the femur

Laboratory/Pathology Data

Your team decides to order some baseline labs, including a complete blood count, lactate dehydrogenase, and alkaline phosphatase, which are shown below.

WBC: 6,500 (normal 4,500–11,000 per microliter)
Lactate dehydrogenase (LDH): 494 (normal 105–333 IU/L)
Alkaline phosphatase (ALP): 272 (normal 44–147 IU/L)

Given the mass discovered on the radiograph, the patient is referred to an orthopedic oncologist who decides to perform a biopsy of the lesion. The pathology report reads:

> Significant atypia, lacey osteoid, stroma cells with high nuclear-to-cytoplasmic ratio, and abnormal mitotic figures. Findings most consistent with osteosarcoma.

Histology images from the patient's biopsy are provided below (Fig. 5.2)

Facilitator Prompt

Leukocytosis could be indicative of either osteomyelitis or a tumor that causes abnormal white blood cell proliferation. LDH and ALP are often elevated in osteosarcoma and have been correlated with more aggressive disease. Ask the students to identify the irregularities displayed in the histology slides. Important things to highlight are the osseous matrix (pink stain), high nuclear to cytoplasmic ratio, and abnormal mitotic figures.

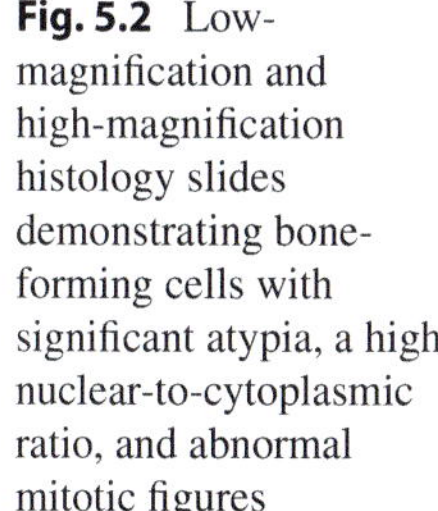

Fig. 5.2 Low-magnification and high-magnification histology slides demonstrating bone-forming cells with significant atypia, a high nuclear-to-cytoplasmic ratio, and abnormal mitotic figures

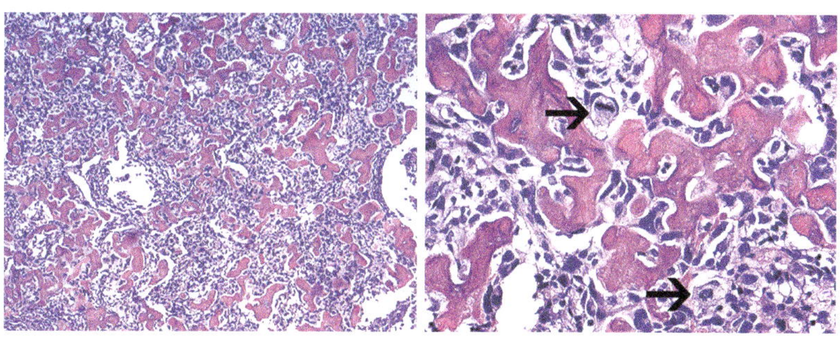

Additional Imaging

Facilitator Prompt
Ask the students if they would like to order any additional imaging.

The orthopaedic oncologist ordered an MRI of the right lower extremity (Fig. 5.3) and a total body radionucleotide bone scan (Fig. 5.4).

MRI of the right lower extremity obtained; no other lesions in right femur (T1 shown)

Total body radionuclide bone scanning with technetium showing prominent focal radiotracer uptake at the site of the primary tumor. No distant areas of abnormal increased radiotracer uptake. A chest CT was negative for pulmonary metastases.

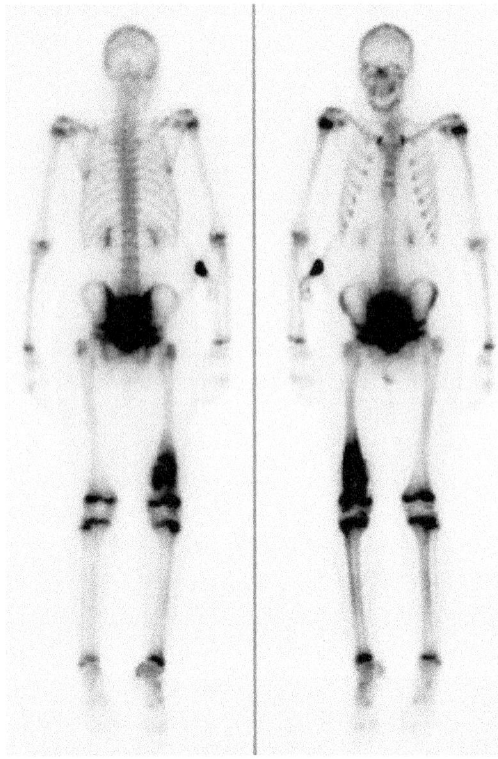

Fig. 5.4 Radionucleotide skeletal survey with increased uptake at the right distal femur indicating increased metabolic activity

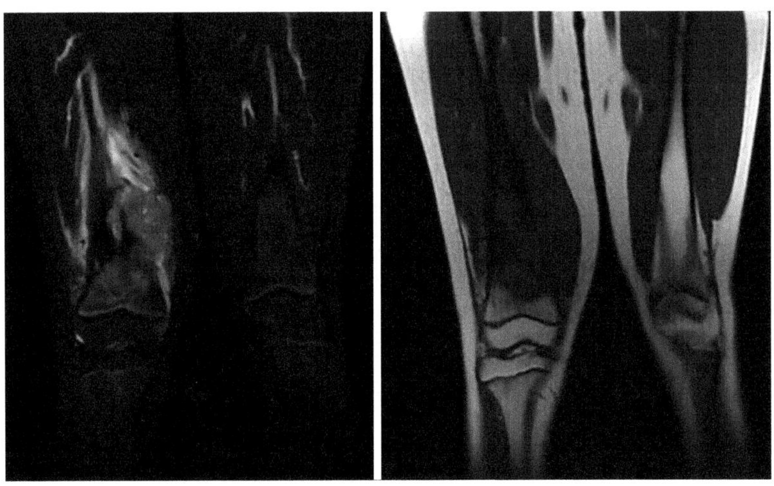

Fig. 5.3 T2 and T1 coronal MRIs of the bilateral lower extremities redemonstrating the osseous lesion at the medial distal femoral metaphysis with associated soft tissue edema

Treatment

The patient was appropriately counseled on the nature of her disease and the standard treatment regimen. She and her family decided to proceed with neoadjuvant chemotherapy, limb salvage resection, followed by adjuvant chemotherapy.

End of Case

Learning Objective Review

1. **Describe the common clinical presentation, physical examination, imaging, and lab findings consistent with osteosarcoma.**

Clinical Presentation
Most patients with osteosarcoma will present with nonspecific symptoms. Commonly, individuals will endorse focal tenderness and pain at the site of the primary tumor that may be exacerbated by strain [3]. Duration of pain will vary by patient, often lasting for several weeks to months before seeking medical attention [3]. Patients with osteosarcoma may have disruption of sleep secondary to the pain and may endorse swelling, a palpable mass, and localized warmth or erythema at site of the tumor [4]. Approximately 5–10% of undiagnosed patients will present with pain secondary to a pathologic fracture [5]. Osteosarcomas most commonly occur at sites of rapid bone turnover, such as the metaphysis of long bones. The most common sites of involvement, in descending order, are distal femur (32%), proximal tibia (19%), proximal humerus (10%), middle and proximal femur (10%), and other bones such as the mandible (8%) and pelvis (8%) [6].

Physical Exam
Oftentimes the only positive physical exam finding is a soft tissue mass, which is frequently large and tender to palpation. The mass may be erythematous and warm on examination, with increased vascularity of the skin. Range of motion may be affected if the mass is near a joint and can affect ambulation if the site of the tumor is in the lower extremities. Other positive exam findings may include regional lymphadenopathy. Systemic symptoms are generally absent in patients with osteosarcoma.

Imaging/Labs
The first diagnostic test in a patient with a suspected bone tumor is plain radiographs [7]. At a minimum, two orthogonal radiographs are required for any suspected bone lesion [4]. Classic radiograph findings include destruction of the normal trabecular bone pattern, irregular margins, and absent endosteal bone response. There is a mixture of radiodense and radiolucent areas, destruction of the cortex, and periosteal new bone formation, with the formation of Codman triangle (an incomplete response of host periosteal bone) (Fig. 5.5) [8].

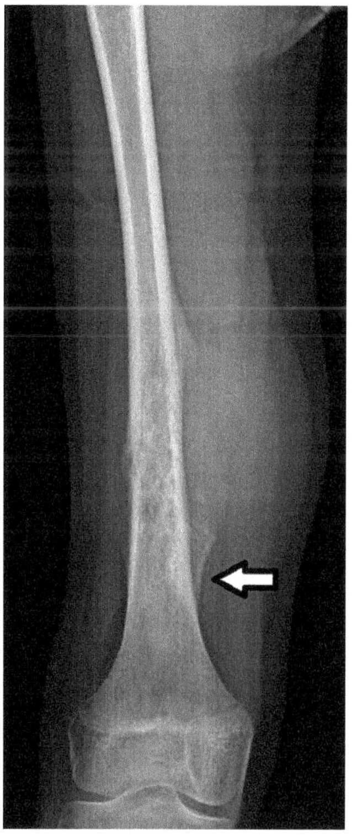

Fig. 5.5 AP radiograph of an osteosarcoma with an arrow identifying a periosteal reaction in which new bone is rapidly trying to form and contain the expansile neoplasia. This new bone formation is known as Codman's triangle

Once a lesion is identified, an MRI of the affected limb is warranted. MRI is the primary mode of evaluation and can demonstrate the extent of bone marrow replacement, tumor invasion of the surrounding soft tissues and neurovascular structures, and presence of discontinuous metastasis [4, 9, 10]. While the correct diagnosis can be deduced in up to two-thirds of patients based on clinical presentation and imaging, a biopsy and pathologic evaluation of the tumor are essential for definitive diagnosis [11]. Once diagnosis has been confirmed, a whole-body bone scan or PET-CT may be obtained to assess for metastases. CT chest is typically obtained to evaluate for pulmonary metastases.

Laboratory tests are not needed to diagnose osteosarcoma but can be helpful once the diagnosis has been established. Baseline laboratory values should be obtained to assess organ function before initiating chemotherapy; these typically include complete blood count with differential, basic metabolic panel, renal and liver function tests, and urinalysis [3]. Alkaline phosphatase and lactate dehydrogenase can show increased osteoblastic and osteoclastic activity, respectively [3]. Elevated lactate dehydrogenase and alkaline phosphatase are associated with a worse prognosis [12, 13].

2. **Discuss a differential of primary bone tumors of adolescence, highlighting key similarities and differences between osteosarcoma, Ewing sarcoma, giant cell tumor, and other benign tumors.**

Ewing Sarcoma

Ewing sarcoma is a peripheral primitive neuroectoderm tumor. This tumor most often arises in the long bones of the extremities and bones of the pelvis. It is the second most common bone tumor occurring in children and adolescents, accounting for approximately 10% of all primary malignant bone tumors [14, 15]. Presentation is not dissimilar from osteosarcoma, usually consisting of localized pain or swelling of a few weeks or months' duration [16]. Unlike osteosarcoma, which typically occurs in long bones, Ewing sarcoma occurs at nearly equal rates in both flat and long bones [17].

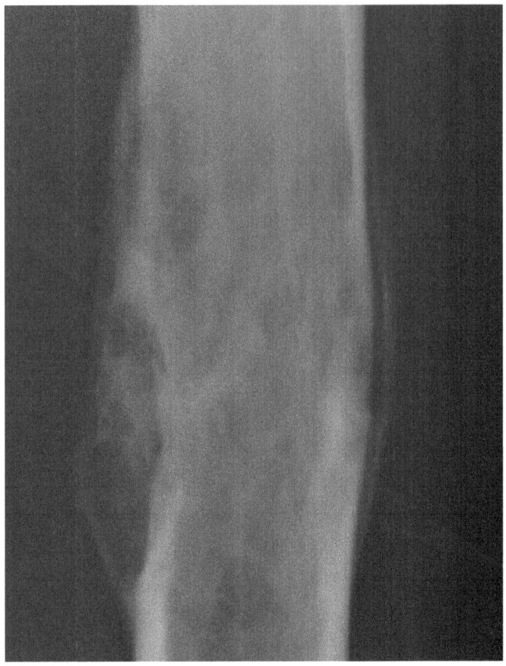

Fig. 5.6 AP radiograph of an Ewing sarcoma tumor in the distal with the classic multilayered reaction that resembles "onion skin"

Ewing sarcomas in long bones tend to occur in the diaphysis or metadiaphysis compared to osteosarcomas, which more frequently arise in the metaphysis [18]. Radiographic appearance of the lesion is classically described as permeative, mottled, "moth-eaten," with a multilayered reaction that resembles "onion skin" appearance (Fig. 5.6) [19]. It is important to realize that these radiographic findings are not pathognomonic for the disease and may be seen in other disease processes.

Tumor biopsy is necessary for histologic staining and diagnosis. As with osteosarcoma, a surgeon should be consulted before obtaining the biopsy. Grossly, the tumor is a gray-white tumor with variable amounts of necrosis and hemorrhage; morphologically, it is composed of sheets of small round blue cells with a high nuclear-to-cytoplasmic ratio [19].

Chondroblastoma

A chondroblastoma is a non-malignant cartilage-forming tumor that typically presents during adolescence. These lesions usually arise in the epiphyses or apophyses of long bones, with 30% occurring around the knee [20, 21]. On plain radiographs these tumors appear as small, well-defined epiphyseal lesions with a sclerotic border that may cross the physis with or without chondroid matrix calcification [22]. Treatment is curettage and bone grafting.

Osteoblastoma

Osteoblastomas are uncommon benign tumors that typically present during the second decade of life. These most commonly occur in the posterior column of the spine [23]. Patients will often complain of chronic pain that is less responsive to NSAIDs [24]. Radiographic findings are variable, but it may have the appearance of an aggressive lesion [25]. Treatment is generally curettage and bone grafting.

Giant Cell Tumor of Bone

Giant cell tumor of bone is a rare, benign tumor that is most commonly found in young adults that can cause local destruction to bone and soft tissue structures. Like many bone tumors, patients will often present complaining of pain, swelling, and possible limitations in range of motion near the primary tumor site. These tumors most frequently arise at the meta-epiphysis of the long bones, commonly at the knee. Radiographs of these tumors show expansile, lytic lesions without evidence of reactive periosteum that is commonly seen in aggressive neoplasms such as osteosarcoma [26].

Osteomyelitis

Osteomyelitis is an infection located in the bone. While the etiology of osteomyelitis is unrelated to neoplasia, it is important to always consider infection in your differential when you encounter lesions of the bone or soft tissue, given the high incidence. Microorganisms may enter the bone hematogenously or by inoculation. Patients will often present with pain, warmth, and erythema over the infected region. Some patients, particularly adolescents, may present with a subacute or chronic osteomyelitis that has been walled off by sclerotic bone to form a Brodie abscess. These infections tend to have a more insidious onset of mild symptoms [27]. Radiographic findings may include deep soft tissue swelling, periosteal reaction, periosteal elevation, and lytic sclerosis. Example imaging of a Brodie abscess in the proximal tibia is presented in Fig. 5.7.

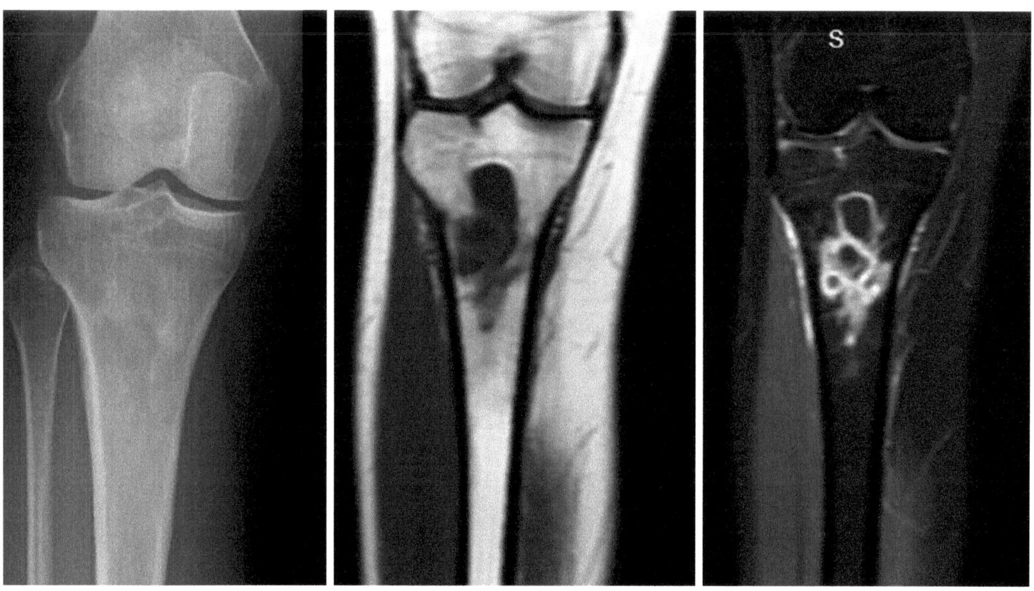

Fig. 5.7 AP radiograph and T1 and T2 MRI of a proximal tibia with a Brodie abscess

Aneurysmal Bone Cysts

Aneurysmal bone cysts are benign expansile vascular lesions that most commonly occur in the first two decades of life [28]. Like many of the benign and malignant tumors discussed in this chapter, they tend to occur around the knee. Patients with an aneurysmal bone cyst may report pain and soft tissue swelling at the site of the lesion [28]. The lesions consist of blood-filled channels that may grow rapidly and destroy bone. Imaging of the lesions classically depicts a radiolucent cystic lesion that is locally destructive with expansion into the surrounding cortical bone with or without elevation of surrounding periosteum [28].

3. **Discuss treatment options for osteosarcoma.**

Treatment for osteosarcoma requires a multidisciplinary approach, including surgical and oncologic specialists. In metastatic disease, survival rates significantly improve, surpassing 70% when a multidisciplinary approach is utilized [29–32]. Treatment for osteosarcoma consists of preoperative (neoadjuvant) chemotherapy, wide surgical resection, and postoperative chemotherapy (adjuvant). Patients without clinically detectable metastasis are presumed to have micrometastatic disease, which is why chemotherapy is an essential component of the treatment regimen [29]. Preoperative chemotherapy may also decrease the size of the primary tumor, making limb salvage surgery more feasible by promoting demarcation from surrounding tissues [33–35]. The chemotherapeutic agents that are most effective against osteosarcoma are doxorubicin, cisplatin, methotrexate, and ifosfamide; combining multiple drugs serves to decrease chemoresistance and increase tumor necrosis [29, 31, 32, 36, 37].

Surgical resection is performed 3–4 weeks following the last dose of preoperative chemotherapy. Postoperative chemotherapy is initiated around 2 weeks after surgery if the surgical wound is healed and follows the same multi-drug regimen as the preoperative course [4]. Radiation therapy for osteosarcoma is reserved for palliation, as the neoplasm is highly resistant to radiation [4].

The mainstay of treatment is complete surgical resection of all detectable tumor, including metastasis. Long-term survivability has a five-fold increase with complete resection of both primary and metastatic lesions compared with primary site excision alone [38]. Surgical options include limb salvage or amputation. Prior to the development of limb salvage surgery in the 1970s, amputation of the affected limb was considered the definitive surgical management; today, amputation remains the preferred surgical intervention when resection of disease-free margins leaves a non-functional limb. Many reconstruction techniques can be used for limb salvage surgery and include allograft, arthrodesis, or prosthetic implantation [4]. No significant differences exist between the survival rates of amputation versus limb salvage surgery in patients with osteosarcoma [33, 37, 39]. Current literature has shown that patients adapt equally well psychologically to either intervention [40].

In the skeletally immature patient, limb reconstruction can be particularly challenging. Surgeons must create a functional limb while avoiding limb-length discrepancy. Many osteosarcomas violate the physis of a long bone, requiring resection. Limb-length discrepancy can be counteracted with the use of an extendable endoprosthesis that allows for interval lengthening of the limb [41]. Rotationplasty, in which the ankle of the affected leg is rotated 180° and attached to the distal femur at the site of the above-knee amputation to serve as a functional knee joint for prosthesis attachment and ambulation, is another viable option in the skeletally immature patient. Gait analysis studies have shown improved kinematics in patients treated with rotationplasty compared with above-knee amputations [42].

4. **To understand the epidemiology of osteosarcoma to include a discussion of age, sex, and geographic location on incidence.**

Osteosarcoma is an uncommon neoplasm. Approximately 500 children and adolescents in the United States are diagnosed with this disease each year [43]. Osteosarcoma incidence peaks in the second decade of life during periods of rapid bone growth and is the most common primary malignancy of bone in children and adolescents aged 15–19 [44, 45]

The incidence of osteosarcoma has a bimodal age distribution. The first peak incidence occurs in children between 13 and 16 years of age, which coincides with peak growth velocity [6]. Adult peak incidence occurs over the age of 65 [46].

Males are slightly more predisposed to osteosarcoma than females, with an incidence ratio of 1.4–1 [46, 47]. In children, the disease affects Black individuals and other ethnicities more frequently than Caucasian children; in adults, however, osteosarcoma occurs more frequently in Caucasian individuals than Black individuals or other ethnicities [46–48].

Osteosarcoma incidence in children varies by geographic region. Regions of Africa, South Asia, and Central and South America are estimated to have nearly twice the number of new cases each year compared to regions of Europe and North America [49].

5. **Understand the histologic hallmarks of osteosarcoma and the various subtypes.**

The diagnosis of osteosarcoma is a histopathologic diagnosis based on morphology and the presence of malignant cells that form osteoid [50]. There are no specific immunostains or molecular tests to identify an osteosarcoma. The neoplasm is subcategorized based on clinical, radiographic, and histologic features. There are intramedullary subtypes, which include conventional, telangiectatic, low-grade intramedullary, and small cell osteosarcomas, and surface subtypes, which include parosteal, periosteal, and high-grade surface osteosarcomas [4].

Intramedullary Osteosarcomas

Conventional

Conventional osteosarcomas are the most common variant and account for approximately 80% of all osteosarcoma cases [29]. These primarily affect individuals in the first or second decade of life. These tumors arise from the intramedullary cavity of the bone, are typically high-grade, and most commonly occur in the metaphysis or diaphysis of long bones [30]. On histologic examination there will be malignant mesenchymal cells that are spindle- to polyhedral-shaped with pleomorphic nuclei and occasional mitotic figures [50, 51]. Conventional osteosarcomas can be further subdivided based on the predominant cellular component into osteoblastic, chondroblastic, or fibroblastic [7].

Telangiectactic

Telangiectatic osteosarcoma accounts for less than 4% of all osteosarcoma cases and is more common in children or adolescents than adults [51]. Approximately 25% of patients with this subvariant will present with a pathologic fracture [52]. The lesion is composed of multiple blood-filled sinusoids, which can be detected as high signal intensity on a T2-weighted MRI scan and may resemble an aneurysmal bone cyst [53]. Histologic examination will demonstrate multiple hemorrhagic cavitations with small amounts of osteoid and high-grade osteosarcoma cells within the septa [50, 51]. Foci of giant cells may occasionally be found, and the lesion may have the appearance of an aneurysmal bone cyst with the exception of clearly demonstrated high-grade sarcoma cells [50].

Low-Grade

Low-grade osteosarcomas only account for 1-2% of all osteosarcomas and typically occur in the 3rd or 4th decade of life [51, 54]. On imaging, these tumors are relatively non-aggressive in appearance, with mixed lytic and blastic patterns, and may even resemble a fibrous dysplasia [54]. On histologic examination there will be well-differentiated cells within woven microtrabeculae of bone and fibrous stroma; small amounts of osteoid, atypia, and mitotic figures can also be seen [50, 51].

Small Cell

This variant of osteosarcoma is rare, accounting for approximately 1.5% of all osteosarcomas [55]. Histologic examination will reveal small, round, malignant cells within an osteoid matrix [50, 51]. This lesion can have the appearance of an Ewing sarcoma and even stains positive for CD99 like Ewing sarcoma, but the production of osteoid and the occasional spindling of tumor cells distinguish the neoplasm as a small cell osteosarcoma [50, 51].

Surface Osteosarcomas

Parosteal Osteosarcoma

Surface osteosarcomas arise on the surface of long bones and spare the medullary canal. Parosteal osteosarcomas' peak incidence occurs in the third decade of life and affects more females than males [50, 56]. These lesions are composed of low-grade, well-differentiated fibrous stroma with osseous components [50, 51]. They commonly have bony trabeculae with a parallel orientation, and approximately 25–30% of these tumors will have a cartilaginous cap [50, 51].

Periosteal Osteosarcoma

This variant of surface osteosarcomas constitutes 1–2% of all cases [51, 57]. These neoplasms are more aggressive than the parosteal variant, and histologic examination reveals an intermediate-grade tumor that is composed of a cartilaginous matrix with areas of calcification and small amounts of osteoid [51].

High-Grade Surface Osteosarcoma

High-grade surface osteosarcomas constitute less than 1% of all osteosarcomas. These surface lesions resemble conventional osteosarcomas with high-grade spindle cells and atypia with varying amounts of osteoid deposition [50, 58].

6. **Describe the genetic predisposition to the development of osteosarcoma.**

Most cases of osteosarcoma occur sporadically with no known genetic predisposition to the disease. With that in mind, it is approximated that 70% of osteosarcoma tumor specimens have some chromosomal abnormality [44]. Mutations in tumor-suppressor genes or DNA helicases can predispose individuals to osteosarcoma.

Li-Fraumeni Syndrome is a heritable cancer syndrome that is the result of germline pathogenic variants of the TP53 tumor-suppressor gene, which is integral to proper cell cycle regulation. Patients with this syndrome are predisposed to a spectrum of cancers, to include breast, soft tissue, leukemias, brain tumors, and osteosarcoma [59].

Retinoblastoma is a germline pathogenic mutation in the RB1 gene, which can cause hereditary retinoblastoma. Patients with this condition are also predisposed to the development of soft tissue sarcomas and osteosarcomas. It is an important distinction that individuals with a history of non-hereditary retinoblastoma are not at an increased risk for sarcoma development [44, 60].

Bloom syndrome and Rothmund-Thomson syndrome, which occur from mutations in DNA helicase genes BLM and RECCQL4, respectively, are also associated with the development of osteosarcoma [59]. While identifiable genetic conditions that predispose a patient to the development of an osteosarcoma are rare, it is imperative that a thorough history and family history be taken when interviewing patients with a soft tissue or bone lesion.

7. **Explain how risk factors such as radiation therapy, chemotherapy, and Paget disease of the bone can influence the development of osteosarcoma.**

Any osteosarcoma that occurs in the setting of prior radiation or chemotherapy is considered secondary osteosarcoma. Radiation therapy can increase the risk of osteosarcoma development, albeit the risk is generally considered to be low. Current literature estimates that 3–6% of all sarcomas are secondary to prior radiation therapy

[61–63]. Osteosarcoma is the most common secondary malignant neoplasm to occur during the first 20 years following radiation therapy for a solid cancer in childhood [63]. Secondary soft tissue sarcomas and osteosarcomas are more common in patients with prior exposure to alkylating chemotherapy [63, 64].

Paget disease of the bone is a skeletal disorder characterized by increased turnover of bone that increases the risk of developing osteosarcoma [65]. While the incidence of bone tumors is significantly increased in patients with a history of Paget disease, osteosarcoma only occurs in 0.7–1% of these patients [66]. There is no consensus on how Paget disease predisposes to osteosarcoma development, but it is thought that genetic factors play a role [67, 68].

Exam Questions

1. A 9-month-old male is brought into the pediatrician's office for a wellness visit. During physical examination, the physician notices an abnormal red light reflex in the patient's left eye. The patient has no known medical history. Family history is significant for an uncle who was diagnosed with colon cancer at age 58. Further testing discloses that the patient has a germline mutation in his RB1 gene. Which of the following conditions is this patient at higher risk for developing compared to the general population?
   A. McCune-Albright syndrome
   B. Ewing Sarcoma
   C. Osteosarcoma
   D. Paget Disease of the Bone
   E. Langerhans Cell Histiocytosis
   F. Adenocarcinoma of the Colon

Answer: C

Learning Objective: Describe the genetic predisposition to the development of osteosarcoma

Explanation: This patient is exhibiting classic physical exam findings for a retinoblastoma. The question stem further explains that genetic testing is significant for a germline mutation in RB1, indicating that this is a hereditary retinoblastoma. Patients with mutations in RB1 have an increased risk of developing subsequent primary tumors, of which 60% are soft tissue and osteosarcomas (Answer C).

McCune-Albright syndrome (Answer A) is a rare mosaic disorder caused by postzygotic activating mutations of the *GNAS1* gene, encoding the alpha subunit of the stimulatory G protein. The syndrome is characterized by the triad of polyostotic fibrous dysplasia, café-au-lait macules, and endocrine hyperactivity, classically causing precocious puberty. There is no relation between RB1 mutations and McCune-Albright syndrome. Ewing sarcoma (answer B), while clinically sharing many similarities with osteosarcoma, has not been linked to RB1 mutations. Paget disease (answer D) is an important risk factor for the development of osteosarcoma in adults but is not related to RB1 mutations. Langerhans cell histiocytosis and adenocarcinoma of the colon are also not related to RB1 mutations (answers E and F).

2. A 16-year-old female is referred to an orthopedic oncologist after a biopsy of a distal femur metaphyseal tumor is confirmed to be an osteosarcoma. The tumor is contained to the medial metaphysis. Which treatment regimen is considered the standard of care for this patient's tumor?
   A. Above-the-knee amputation
   B. Neoadjuvant radiation therapy followed by limb-salvaging resection
   C. Radiation therapy
   D. Chemotherapy
   E. Limb-salvaging resection
   F. Neoadjuvant chemotherapy, limb-salvaging resection, followed by adjuvant chemotherapy

Answer: F

Learning Objective: Discuss treatment options for osteosarcoma

Explanation: The standard of care for resectable osteosarcomas is neoadjuvant chemotherapy, limb-salvaging resection, followed by adjuvant chemotherapy (Answer F). Overall survival is equal between limb salvage and amputation, with increased morbidity associated with amputation (Answer A). Osteosarcomas are radioresistant (Answers B and C). Chemotherapy and limb salvage surgery should always be used in combination to shrink the tumor size before curettage (Answers D and E).

3. A 17-year-old male presents to your office complaining of right knee pain after track practice. Plain radiographs of the affected limb demonstrate a pathologic fracture through the metaphysis of the distal femur with an associated bone mass. The patient's mother was diagnosed with breast cancer at age 35, and the patient is a known carrier of a germline mutation in the TP53 gene. What would you most likely expect to find on a biopsy of the patient's tumor?
   A. Monotonous small round blue cells with high nuclei-to-cytoplasm ratio
   B. Multicystic inoculations of expansile vascular tissue
   C. Metastatic intraductal breast tissue
   D. Tumor cells with high nuclear-to-cytoplasmic ratio in a lacey osteoid matrix
   E. Enlarged chondrocytes with plump multinucleated lacunae

Answer: D

Learning Objective: Explain the histologic hallmarks of osteosarcoma and the various subtypes

Explanation: The patient described has Li-Fraumeni Syndrome (LFS), which predisposes the patient to the development of osteosarcoma, among other tumors. Conventional osteosarcoma is described histologically as tumor cells with high nuclear-to-cytoplasmic ratio in a lacey osteoid matrix (Answer D). Ewing sarcoma is not associated with LFS and is characteristically composed of small round blue cells on histology (Answer A). Multicystic inoculations of expansile vascular tissue describe an aneurysmal bone cyst (Answer B). While breast cancer is associated with LFS, it is almost exclusively found in women with the germline mutation, making it much less likely (Answer C). A tumor of chondrocytic origin is more consistent with a chondrosarcoma and is not associated with LFS (Answer E).

References

1. Canadian Sport for Life. Long-term athlete development 2.1. Balyi & Way; 2005. p. 30.
2. Bedrosian I, Somerfield M, Achatz M, Boughey J, Curigliano G, Friedman S, Kohlmann W, Kurian A, Laronga C, Lynce F, Norquist B, Plichta J, Rodriguez P, Shah P, Tischkowitz M, Wood M, Yadav S, Yao K, Robson M. Germline testing in patients with breast cancer: ASCO–Society of Surgical Oncology guideline. J Clin Oncol. 2024;42(5):584–604. https://doi.org/10.1200/JCO.23.02225.
3. Meyers PA, Gorlick R. Osteosarcoma. Pediatr Clin N Am. 1997;44:973–89.
4. Messerschmitt PJ, Garcia RM, Abdul-Karim FW, Greenfield EM, Getty PJ. Osteosarcoma. J Am Acad Orthop Surg. 2009;17(8):515–27.
5. Scully SP, Ghert MA, Zurakowski D, Thompson RC, Gebhardt MC. Pathologic fracture in osteosarcoma: prognostic importance and treatment implications. J Bone Joint Surg Am. 2002;84:49–57.
6. Ottaviani G, Jaffe N. The epidemiology of osteosarcoma. Cancer Treat Res. 2009;152:3–13. https://doi.org/10.1007/978-1-4419-0284-9_1.
7. Papagelopoulos PJ, Galanis EC, Vlastou C, Nikiforidis PA, Vlamis JA, Boscainos PJ, Fragiadakis EG, Stamos KG, Pantazopoulos T, Sim FH. Current concepts in the evaluation and treatment of osteosarcoma. Orthopedics. 2000;23(8):858–67; quiz 868–9. https://doi.org/10.3928/0147-7447-20000801-11.
8. UpToDate. https://www.uptodate.com/contents/osteosarcoma-epidemiology-pathology-clinical-presentation-and-diagnosis?search=osteosarcoma&source=search_result&selectedTitle=1~132&usage_type=default&display_rank=1#H12. Accessed 21 May 2024.
9. Sajadi KR, Heck RK, Neel MD, Rao BN, Daw N, Rodriguez-Galindo C, Hoffer FA, Stacy GS, Peabody TD, Simon MA. The incidence and prognosis of osteosarcoma skip metastases. Clin Orthop Relat Res. 2004;426:92–6. https://doi.org/10.1097/01.blo.0000141493.52166.69.
10. Panicek DM, Gatsonis C, Rosenthal DI, Seeger LL, Huvos AG, Moore SG, Caudry DJ, Palmer WE, McNeil BJ. CT and MR imaging in the local staging of primary malignant musculoskeletal neoplasms: report of the radiology diagnostic oncology

group. Radiology. 1997;202(1):237–46. https://doi.org/10.1148/radiology.202.1.8988217.
11. Kesselring FO, Penn W. Radiological aspects of 'classic' primary osteosarcoma: value of some radiological investigations: a review. Diagn Imaging. 1982;51(2):78–92.
12. Link MP, Goorin AM, Horowitz M, et al. Adjuvant chemotherapy of highgrade osteosarcoma of the extremity: updated results of the multi-institutional osteosarcoma study. Clin Orthop Relat Res. 1991;270:8–14.
13. Bacci G, Longhi A, Versari M, Mercuri M, Briccoli A, Picci P. Prognostic factors for osteosarcoma of the extremity treated with neoadjuvant chemotherapy: 15-year experience in 789 patients treated at a single institution. Cancer. 2006;106:1154–61.
14. Gibbs CP Jr, Weber K, Scarborough MT. Malignant bone tumors. Instr Course Lect. 2002;51:413–28.
15. Herzog CE. Overview of sarcomas in the adolescent and young adult population. J Pediatr Hematol Oncol. 2005;27:215–8.
16. Green DM. Diagnosis and management of malignant solid tumors in infants and children. Boston: Martinus Nijhoff Publishing; 1985.
17. Grier HE. The Ewing family of tumors. Ewing's sarcoma and primitive neuroectodermal tumors. Pediatr Clin N Am. 1997;44(4):991–1004. https://doi.org/10.1016/s0031-3955(05)70541-1.
18. Reinus WR, Gilula LA. IESS committee: radiology of Ewing's sarcoma: intergroup Ewing's sarcoma study. Radiographics. 1984;4:929–44.
19. Maheshwari AV, Cheng EY. Ewing sarcoma family of tumors. Am Acad Orthop Surg. 2010;18(2):94–107.
20. Brien EW, Mirra JM, Kerr R. Benign and malignant cartilage tumors of bone and joint: their anatomic and theoretical basis with an emphasis on radiology, pathology and clinical biology. I. The intramedullary cartilage tumors. Skeletal Radiol. 1997;26(6):325–53. https://doi.org/10.1007/s002560050246.
21. Xu H, Nugent D, Monforte HL, Binitie OT, Ding Y, Letson GD, Cheong D, Niu X. Chondroblastoma of bone in the extremities: a multicenter retrospective study. J Bone Joint Surg Am. 2015;97(11):925–31. https://doi.org/10.2106/JBJS.N.00992.
22. Aboulafia AJ, Kennon RE, Jelinek JS. Begnign bone tumors of childhood. J Am Acad Orthop Surg. 1999;7(6):377–88. https://doi.org/10.5435/00124635-199911000-00004.
23. Amary F, Mahar AM, Horvai AE, Bredella MA. Osteoblastoma. In: Who classification of tumours. Soft tissue and bone tumours. 5th ed. Lyons: International Agency for Research on Cancer; 2022. https://tumourclassification.iarc.who.int/home. Accessed 22 May 2024.
24. Copley L, Dormans JP. Benign pediatric bone tumors. Evaluation and treatment. Pediatr Clin N Am. 1996;43(4):949–66. https://doi.org/10.1016/s0031-3955(05)70444-2.
25. Greenspan A. Benign bone-forming lesions: osteoma, osteoid osteoma, and osteoblastoma. Clinical, imaging, pathologic, and differential considerations. Skeletal Radiol. 1993;22(7):485–500. https://doi.org/10.1007/BF00209095.
26. Athanasou NA, Bansal M, Forsyth R, et al. Giant cell tumour of bone. In: Fletcher CDM, Bridge JA, Hogendoorn P, Mertens F, editors. WHO classification of tumours of soft tissue and bone. 4th ed. Geneva: IARC; 2013. p. 321.
27. Foster CE, Taylor M, Schallert EK, Rosenfeld S, King KY. Brodie abscess in children: a 10-year single institution retrospective review. Pediatr Infect Dis J. 2019;38(2):e32–4. https://doi.org/10.1097/INF.0000000000002062.
28. Rapp TB, Ward JP, Alaia MJ. Aneurysmal bone cyst. J Am Acad Orthop Surg. 2012;20(4):233–41. https://doi.org/10.5435/JAAOS-20-04-233.
29. Carrle D, Bielack SS. Current strategies of chemotherapy in osteosarcoma. Int Orthop. 2006;30:445–51.
30. Bielack SS, Kempf-Bielack B, Delling G, et al. Prognostic factors in high-grade osteosarcoma of the extremities or trunk: an analysis of 1,702 patients treated on neoadjuvant cooperative osteosarcoma study group protocols. J Clin Oncol. 2002;20:776–90.
31. Meyers PA, Schwartz CL, Krailo M, et al. Osteosarcoma: the addition of muramyl tripeptide to chemotherapy improves overall survival: a report from the children's oncology group. J Clin Oncol. 2008;26:633–8.
32. Ferrari S, Smeland S, Mercuri M, et al. Neoadjuvant chemotherapy with highdose ifosfamide, high-dose methotrexate, cisplatin, and doxorubicin for patients with localized osteosarcoma of the extremity: a joint study by the Italian and Scandinavian Sarcoma Groups. J Clin Oncol. 2005;23:8845–52.
33. Grimer RJ. Surgical options for children with osteosarcoma. Lancet Oncol. 2005;6:85–92.
34. Smith J, Heelan RT, Huvos AG, et al. Radiographic changes in primary osteogenic sarcoma following intensive chemotherapy: radiological-pathological correlation in 63 patients. Radiology. 1982;143:355–60.
35. Hosalkar HS, Dormans JP. Limb sparing surgery for pediatric musculoskeletal tumors. Pediatr Blood Cancer. 2004;42:295–310.
36. Longhi A, Errani C, De Paolis M, Mercuri M, Bacci G. Primary bone osteosarcoma in the pediatric age: state of the art. Cancer Treat Rev. 2006;32:423–36.
37. Bacci G, Ferrari S, Bertoni F, et al. Histologic response of high-grade nonmetastatic osteosarcoma of the extremity to chemotherapy. Clin Orthop Relat Res. 2001;386:186–96.
38. Kager L, Zoubek A, Pötschger U, et al. Primary metastatic osteosarcoma: presentation and outcome of patients treated on neoadjuvant Cooperative

Osteosarcoma Study Group protocols. J Clin Oncol. 2003;21:2011–8.
39. Simon MA, Aschliman MA, Thomas N, Mankin HJ. Limb-salvage treatment versus amputation for osteosarcoma of the distal end of the femur. J Bone Joint Surg Am. 1986;68:1331–7.
40. Rougraff BT, Simon MA, Kneisl JS, Greenberg DB, Mankin HJ. Limb salvage compared with amputation for osteosarcoma of the distal end of the femur: a long-term oncological, functional, and quality-of-life study. J Bone Joint Surg Am. 1994;76:649–56.
41. Nichter LS, Menendez LR. Reconstructive considerations for limb salvage surgery. Orthop Clin North Am. 1993;24:511–21.
42. Fuchs B, Kotajarvi BR, Kaufman KR, Sim FH. Functional outcome of patients with rotationplasty about the knee. Clin Orthop Relat Res. 2003;415:52–8.
43. Horner MJ, Ries LAG, Krapcho M, et al. SEER cancer statistics review, 1975–2006. Bethesda: National Cancer Institute. Available at: http://seer.cancer.gov/csr/1975_2006. Accessed 15 May 2009.
44. Hayden JB, Hoang BH. Osteosarcoma: basic science and clinical implications. Orthop Clin North Am. 2006;37:1–7.
45. Howlader N, Noone AM, Krapcho M, et al., editors. SEER cancer statistics review, 1975–2018. Bethesda: National Cancer Institute; 2021. Based on November 2020 SEER data submission, posted to the SEER web site, . https://seer.cancer.gov/csr/1975_2018/. Accessed 17 Apr 2021.
46. Mirabello L, Troisi RJ, Savage SA. Osteosarcoma incidence and survival rates from 1973 to 2004: data from the surveillance, epidemiology, and end results program. Cancer. 2009;115(7):1531–43. https://doi.org/10.1002/cncr.24121. PMID: 19197972; PMCID: PMC2813207.
47. Kumar R, Kumar M, Malhotra K, Patel S. Primary osteosarcoma in the elderly revisited: current concepts in diagnosis and treatment. Curr Oncol Rep. 2018;20(2):13. https://doi.org/10.1007/s11912-018-0658-1.
48. Cole S, Gianferante DM, Zhu B, Mirabello L. Osteosarcoma: a surveillance, epidemiology, and end results program-based analysis from 1975 to 2017. Cancer. 2022;128(11):2107–18. https://doi.org/10.1002/cncr.34163. Epub 2022 Feb 28. PMID: 35226758.
49. Ward ZJ, Yeh JM, Bhakta N, Frazier AL, Atun R. Estimating the total incidence of global childhood cancer: a simulation-based analysis. Lancet Oncol. 2019;20(4):483–93. https://doi.org/10.1016/S1470-2045(18)30909-4. Epub 2019 Feb 26. PMID: 30824204.
50. Klein MJ, Siegal GP. Osteosarcoma: anatomic and histologic variants. Am J Clin Pathol. 2006;125:555–81.
51. Fletcher CD, Unni KK, Mertens F, editors. World Health Organization classification of Tumours: pathology and genetics of Tumours of soft tissue and bone. Lyon: IARC Press; 2002. p. 227–232, 264–85.
52. Mervak TR, Unni KK, Pritchard DJ, McLeod RA. Telangiectatic osteosarcoma. Clin Orthop Relat Res. 1991;270:135–9.
53. Murphey MD. Wan Jaovisidha S, Temple HT, Gannon FH, Jelinek JS, Malawer MM: Telangiectatic osteosarcoma: radiologic-pathologic comparison. Radiology. 2003;229:545–53.
54. Andresen KJ, Sundaram M, Unni KK, Sim FH. Imaging features of low-grade central osteosarcoma of the long bones and pelvis. Skeletal Radiol. 2004;33:373–9.
55. Nakajima H, Sim FH, Bond JR, Unni KK. Small cell osteosarcoma of bone: review of 72 cases. Cancer. 1997;79:2095–106.
56. Temple HT, Scully SP, O'Keefe RJ, Katapurum S, Mankin HJ. Clinical outcome of 38 patients with juxtacortical osteosarcoma. Clin Orthop Relat Res. 2000;373:208–17.
57. Rose PS, Dickey ID, Wenger DE, Unni KK, Sim FH. Periosteal osteosarcoma: long-term outcome and risk of late recurrence. Clin Orthop Relat Res. 2006;453:314–7.
58. Okada K, Unni KK, Swee RG, Sim FH. High grade surface osteosarcoma: a clinicopathologic study of 46 cases. Cancer. 1999;85:1044–54.
59. Wang LL, Gannavarapu A, Kozinetz CA, Levy ML, Lewis RA, Chintagumpala MM, Ruiz-Maldanado R, Contreras-Ruiz J, Cunniff C, Erickson RP, Lev D, Rogers M, Zackai EH, Plon SE. Association between osteosarcoma and deleterious mutations in the RECQL4 gene in Rothmund-Thomson syndrome. J Natl Cancer Inst. 2003;95(9):669–74. https://doi.org/10.1093/jnci/95.9.669.
60. Wang LL. Biology of osteogenic sarcoma. Cancer J. 2005;11:294–305.
61. Brady MS, Gaynor JJ, Brennan MF. Radiation-associated sarcoma of bone and soft tissue. Arch Surg. 1992;127(12):1379–85. https://doi.org/10.1001/archsurg.1992.01420120013002.
62. Newton WA Jr, Meadows AT, Shimada H, Bunin GR, Vawter GF. Bone sarcomas as second malignant neoplasms following childhood cancer. Cancer. 1991;67(1):193–201. https://doi.org/10.1002/1097-0142(19910101)67:1<193::aid-cncr2820670132>3.0.co;2-b. PMID: 1985716.
63. Tucker MA, D'Angio GJ, Boice JD Jr, Strong LC, Li FP, Stovall M, Stone BJ, Green DM, Lombardi F, Newton W, et al. Bone sarcomas linked to radiotherapy and chemotherapy in children. N Engl J Med. 1987;317(10):588–93. https://doi.org/10.1056/NEJM198709033171002. PMID: 3475572.

64. Henderson TO, Rajaraman P, Stovall M, Constine LS, Olive A, Smith SA, Mertens A, Meadows A, Neglia JP, Hammond S, Whitton J, Inskip PD, Robison LL, Diller L. Risk factors associated with secondary sarcomas in childhood cancer survivors: a report from the childhood cancer survivor study. Int J Radiat Oncol Biol Phys. 2012;84(1):224–30. https://doi.org/10.1016/j.ijrobp.2011.11.022. Epub 2012 Jul 14. PMID: 22795729; PMCID: PMC3423483.
65. Grimer RJ, Cannon SR, Taminiau AM, Bielack S, Kempf-Bielack B, Windhager R, Dominkus M, Saeter G, Bauer H, Meller I, Szendroi M, Folleras G, San-Julian M, van der Eijken J. Osteosarcoma over the age of forty. Eur J Cancer. 2003;39(2):157–63. https://doi.org/10.1016/s0959-8049(02)00478-1.
66. Hadjipavlou A, Lander P, Srolovitz H, Enker IP. Malignant transformation in Paget disease of bone. Cancer. 1992;70(12):2802–8. https://doi.org/10.1002/1097-0142(19921215)70:12<2802::aid-cncr2820701213>3.0.co;2-n. PMID: 1451058.
67. Nellissery MJ, Padalecki SS, Brkanac Z, Singer FR, Roodman GD, Unni KK, Leach RJ, Hansen MF. Evidence for a novel osteosarcoma tumor-suppressor gene in the chromosome 18 region genetically linked with Paget disease of bone. Am J Hum Genet. 1998;63(3):817–24. https://doi.org/10.1086/302019. PMID: 9718349; PMCID: PMC1377407.
68. Mankin HJ, Hornicek FJ. Paget's sarcoma: a historical and outcome review. Clin Orthop Relat Res. 2005;438:97–102. https://doi.org/10.1097/01.blo.0000180053.99840.27.

Part III

Cardiovascular

6 Chronic Fatigue

Leeann Qubain

Learning Objectives

1. Explain the mechanism behind altered fluid balance in cardiogenic shock.
2. Explain the cause of hypotension in heart failure. Discuss the cardio-renal mechanisms that come into play as the patient deteriorates.
3. Describe the signs and symptoms of cardiogenic shock.
4. Discuss common treatments for cardiogenic shock.
5. Describe risk factors for developing chronic heart failure.
6. Discuss treatments for chronic heart failure including their mechanism of action, main side effects, and effect on target organs.
7. Describe the emotional and societal impact of heart failure.

Chief Complaint

Easily tired with activity and a hard time breathing for the last two years.

Prompt: Given only this information, what systems are you considering for your differential diagnosis? List 5 systems and give at least 1 example from each.

L. Qubain (✉)
Banner University Medical Center-Phoenix,
Phoenix, AZ, USA
e-mail: leeannqubain@arizona.edu

There is a large differential diagnosis that will be outlined later in the case. At this point, the students should cover all these major categories with at least one example.

Brief Diff Dx:

- Vascular: pulmonary embolism
- Infectious: upper respiratory infection, pneumonia, endocarditis
- Neoplastic: lung cancer
- Degenerative: COPD, congestive heart failure (CHF)
- Idiopathic: noncardiogenic pulmonary edema (ARDS)
- Congenital: congenital heart defect, cystic fibrosis, alpha-1 antitrypsin deficiency
- Autoimmune/allergy: asthma, transfusion-related acute lung injury (TRALI)
- Traumatic: pneumothorax
- Endocrine/environment: high altitude

History of Present Illness

Mark Doe is a 65-year-old retired man with social history of current tobacco use and alcohol overuse, who presents to the Emergency Department with complaints of feeling tired with activity and a hard time breathing over the last two years. He was playing baseball on a warm day with his family while attending a summer picnic and after hitting the baseball, he ran to first base and felt

C. A. Standley (ed.), *Biomedical Science and Clinical Foundations*,
https://doi.org/10.1007/978-3-031-98353-5_6

short of breath and fatigued, started wheezing, and had difficulty concentrating. He reports that he is not very active at baseline. The patient cannot remember the last time he went to the doctor.

Past Medical History

Patient has a history of hypertension but admits he does not take any medications daily.

Prompt: Is this a concern?

Yes, this will be of importance, since hypertension can be a risk factor for heart failure and since this patient is not followed by a PCP regularly, it can be inferred it is not managed.

Medications

No daily medications

Allergies

No known drug allergies

Immunizations

Up-to-date childhood immunizations. No flu shot since he was 35 years old.

Social History

White. Lives alone in apartment. Retired, minimal activity at baseline. Positive one question alcohol screen and 60 pack year tobacco history.

Family History

Father: Heart attack at 70 years old. Deceased. Mother: Diabetes diagnosed at 55 years old. Alive.

Prompt: Does he have any modifiable risk factors?

Yes, tobacco and alcohol use are modifiable risk factors.

Review of Systems

- General: +5 lb weight gain. No fevers or chills.
- Hematopoietic: No history of anemia.
- HEENT: No rhinorrhea or cough. No epistaxis.
- Respiratory: + Dyspnea. No hemoptysis
- Cardiovascular: + chest pain, + lightheadedness. + Orthopnea, decreased activity tolerance. + Paroxysmal nocturnal dyspnea.
- GI: No nausea, vomiting, diarrhea, or constipation
- GU: +Remote h/o STI, treated with antibiotics.
- All other ROS negative.

Prompt: How have these data modified your problem list and preliminary diagnosis?

- No weight loss or hemoptysis, less likely COPD
- No fever, less likely infection
- No abdominal distention/pain, less likely GI abnormality

Really nothing has been totally ruled out.

Physical Examination

VITALS

Temp: 97.4 F
Ht: 5’9”
Wt: 240 lbs
BP: 145/95 mmHg
HR: 120 bpm
RR: 30 breaths/min
O_2sat: 93%

Prompt: How do his vitals look?

His BMI is 35.4, which is in the obesity range. His O_2 sat is low. Tachycardia with elevated BP = compensated shock, if BP drops, ominous sign = uncompensated shock, need resuscitation to be prompt and aggressive!

Physical Examination (Continued)

General: Alert and conversant. Patient appears fatigued. Mild shortness of breath.
Neck: + JVD
Respiratory: Crackles and rales at the base of bilateral lungs.
CV: Tachycardic. Normal S1, S2. Positive S3. No S4, murmurs, or rubs. Laterally displaced PMI. + Hepatojugular reflux
Extremities: 2+ edema of bilateral lower extremities. Capillary refill 5 seconds.

Prompt: What can you determine from the physical exam?

The patient's S3 is an abnormal heart sound indicative of a low-frequency, brief vibration occurring in early diastole at the end of the rapid diastolic ventricular filling. The laterally displaced PMI is indicative of left ventricular hypertrophy. A capillary refill of 5 seconds is abnormal. Anything longer than 3 seconds is considered abnormal. The hepatojugular reflux: jugular venous congestion induced by exerting manual pressure over the patient's liver → ↑ right heart volume overload → inability of the right heart to pump additional blood → visible jugular venous distention that persists for several seconds. The positive breath sounds are significant for the presence of fluid or mucous in the airways overload. *Significance of these findings is the presence of fluid overload likely indicating the diagnosis of something cardiogenic.*

Prompt: *Has your problem list and/or preliminary diagnosis changed based on the physical exam?*

Cannot have a certain diagnosis yet. Some differential diagnoses are more or less likely. More likely includes congestive heart failure, chronic obstructive pulmonary disease, or pulmonary fibrosis. Less likely is infection considering lack of fever or chills. Important to keep in mind that the patient's history notes a progressively worsening shortness of breath. As always, monitoring the patient's vitals and hemodynamic status is most important.

Prompt: *What labs/imaging would you want to order and how do they help you determine the diagnosis?*

Always keep in mind that you want to rule out life-threatening conditions and ensure patient is hemodynamically stable. Tests to order include:

CBC, blood culture
UA, urine culture (not totally necessary but could be considered because of the patient's slight confusion)
CMP (patient presented with mild confusion and fluid overload, important to evaluate electrolytes and kidney function)
Chest radiograph (to evaluate for obstructive abdominal process)
Troponin
BNP
Need immediate EKG and troponin to help rule out MI
Other labs to be considered: TSH, fasting lipid studies, inflammatory markers, HbA1c

Diagnostic Studies

Chest X-ray was normal. Airway clear. No pleural effusion or infiltrates. Normal heart size.

Comprehensive metabolic panel (CMP)

	Patient	Normal Range
Glucose, random	130 mg/dL	64–100 mg/dL
BUN	6 mg/dL	5–12 mg/dL
Creatinine	1.9 mg/dL	0.3–1.0 mg/dL
Sodium	132 mmol/L	135–145 mmol/L
Protein, total	6.5 g/dL	6.0–8.0 g/dL
Albumin	4.2 g/dL	3.5–5.0 g/dL
Bilirubin, total	0.8 mg/dL	< 1.20 mg/dL
ALT	26 U/L	0–35 U/L
AST	27 U/L	0–35 U/L

Prompt: *What can you determine from the CMP?*

Glucose is elevated, maybe underlying, undiagnosed diabetes mellitus that could be further explored. Importantly, creatinine is elevated, and sodium is low. Creatinine is elevated because of the hypoperfusion of the kidneys that leads to low GFR and elevates creatinine. Sodium is low because of the fluid retention due to congestive heart failure and that also could contribute to the confusion the patient reported in the HPI.

Blood Culture

Pending

Complete Blood Count

	Patient	Normal value
Hemoglobin	10.8	12.6–14.4
WBC	4.7	4.5–11 × 10^3/microL
Platelets	250	150–44 × 10^3/microL

Other Tests:

	Patient	Normal value
BNP	1200 pg/mL	<400 pg/mL
Troponin I	0 ng/mL	0–0.04 ng/mL

EKG

Sinus tachycardia, normal rhythm. No other abnormalities and no signs of arrhythmia.

Prompt: *Has your problem list and/or preliminary diagnosis changed?*

Given the labs, students should be able to recognize the low likelihood of myocardial infarction from the normal EKG and negative troponin. In addition, pneumonia is less likely given normal white count and normal chest X-ray. They should continue to work through their differential but recognize this is a cardiovascular abnormality and particularly fluid status is pertinent.

Prompt: *Are there other tests you are considering at this point?*

Given the fluid overload and suspicion for heart failure, a diagnosis would need to be made with an echocardiogram. Transthoracic echocardiogram to evaluate ejection fraction and structural abnormalities.

New Development

After the patient is admitted for management, he suddenly complains of worsening chest pain, begins to breathe more rapidly, and becomes diaphoretic. On examination, his pulse is weak, and his hands are cold and pale. Blood pressure is 80/40 mmHg and HR is 130 bpm. He has not urinated at all in the last 13 hours.

Prompt: *What is the reason for the change in vitals?*

The patient is now hypotensive and no longer able to compensate. Students should recognize that the patient is in shock. Given the information they have and the clues that the patient's hands are cold and pale, either distributive shock or cardiogenic shock should come to mind. This patient had heart failure that led to cardiogenic shock.

Prompt: *What is the treatment plan for somebody who comes in with an acute episode like this patient?*

Provide supportive care
Elevate the patient's head
Provide respiratory support for signs of fluid overload
Administer ionotropic therapy to maintain perfusion
Consider diuretics
Since this patient is hemodynamically unstable, prioritize respiratory support and consider ionotropics.

End of Case

Answers to Learning Objectives

1. **Explain the mechanism behind altered fluid balance in cardiogenic shock.**

Key Points:

Cardiogenic shock is caused by decreased cardiac output (CO).

Decreased CO leads to release of catecholamines and increases vasoconstriction.

Renin-angiotensin-aldosterone system (RAAS) is activated by increased myocardial oxygen demand.

Increased RAAS leads to further fluid retention and leads to pulmonary edema.

Underlying causes of heart dysfunction cause a decrease in cardiac contractility and/or stroke volume that leads to a decrease in cardiac output. This leads to compensation measures by the release of catecholamines and the decreased perfusion of the kidneys triggers the renin-angiotensin-aldosterone system (RAAS) to therefore increase fluid retention. Increased perfusion volume leads to increased heart filling and preload. This leads to stronger contractions of the heart, consistent with Frank-Starling mechanisms. [1]

Catecholamines and RAAS work together to increase vasoconstriction and retention of sodium and water. In addition, blood is shunted to the brain and vital organs, leading to insufficient perfusion of the peripheral organs [1]. Meanwhile, pulmonary circulation becomes congested due to hydrostatic pressure and leads to pulmonary edema.

Long-term fluid retention can lead to fluid leaking into the tissues and specifically fluid buildup in the lungs, causing congestion. Blood backs up into the pulmonary veins and increases pressure in the pulmonary artery which leads to pulmonary edema (congestion) because there is fluid in the alveoli. This slows the exchange of oxygen for disposed carbon dioxide and leads to symptoms of dyspnea, orthopnea, and crackles or rales on examination [2]. Due to the increased pressure, the capillaries can rupture and leak blood into the alveoli, which is then removed by macrophages. These macrophages are known as hemosiderin macrophages (aka “heart failure cells”) [2, 3].

2. **Explain the cause of hypotension in heart failure. Discuss the cardio-renal mechanisms that come into play as the patient deteriorates.**

Key Points:

Heart failure leads to decreased perfusion of the kidneys.

Decreased kidney perfusion activates RAAS system.

RAAS increases fluid retention which puts further stress on the heart.

There are three main compensations to maintain cardiac output when stroke volume is reduced [4]:

- Increased adrenergic activity that increases heart rate, blood pressure, and ventricular contractility
- Increase RAAS: increases angiotensin II
  - Increased peripheral vasoconstriction and therefore systemic blood pressure which then increases afterload
  - Increased vasoconstriction of efferent arterials then increases intraglomerular pressure and thus, GFR is maintained
  - Increase aldosterone secretion which increases renal sodium and water resorption and thus increases preload
- BNP secretion
  - Ventricular myocyte released in response to ventricular filling and stretching
  - Works on intracellular smooth muscle cGMP to increase vasodilation causing hypotension and decreased pulmonary capillary wedge pressure

3. **Describe the signs and symptoms of cardiogenic shock.**

Key Points:

- Main signs and symptoms of cardiogenic shock are those of chronic heart failure.
- Cardiogenic shock leads to a decrease in cardiac output but an increase in preload and afterload.

Cardiogenic shock can be caused by the inability of the heart to pump. This can be secondary to a myocardial infarction leading to wall ischemia and weakened contractions. A subtype of cardiogenic shock is obstructive shock, which is caused by reasons that restrict the heart from pumping, such as fluid in the pericardial sack, that leads to constriction of the heart muscles [5]. This leads to reduced blood flow and therefore cool and clammy extremities. Clinical features of cardiogenic shock are those of heart failure. In cardiogenic shock, cardiac output decreases while estimated preload and afterload increase [6].

Heart failure leads to decreased perfusion of the kidneys, which triggers the renin-angiotensin-aldosterone system (RAAS), and therefore increases fluid retention. Increased perfusion volume leads to increased heart filling and preload. This leads to stronger contractions of the heart, consistent with Frank-Starling mechanisms [5].

This long-term fluid retention can lead to fluid leaking into the tissues and specifically fluid buildup in the lungs causing congestion. Blood backs up into the pulmonary veins and increases pressure in the pulmonary artery and leads to pulmonary edema (congestion) because there is fluid in the alveoli. This slows the exchange of oxygen for disposed carbon dioxide and leads to symptoms of dyspnea, orthopnea, and crackles or rales on examination. Due to the increased pressure, the capillaries can rupture and leak blood into the alveoli which is then removed by macrophages. These macrophages are known as hemosiderin macrophages (aka "heart failure cells").

In addition, cardiogenic shock leads to hypoperfusion which can present as weakness, fatigue, altered mental status, and signs of poor peripheral perfusion (i.e., cold, clammy skin, peripheral cyanosis, and skin mottling). Blood pressure may be low, normal, or elevated, and should be interpreted in relation to patient's baseline blood pressure [6].

4. **Discuss common treatments for cardiogenic shock.**

Hemodynamically Stable Patients

- Treatment depends on the classification of acute heart failure
  - There are four types of acute heart failure [1, 7]:
    - Warm and dry
    - Cold and dry
    - Warm and wet
    - Cold and wet
- Evidence of congestion (wet and warm)
  - Respiratory support (positioning, supplemental oxygen)
  - Start diuretic therapy
    - Diuretic naïve patients should be started on IV furosemide or bumetanide
    - Adjust dosage every 6 hours after reassessment of fluid status
  - Consider vasodilators if the patient has refractory acute heart failure with high-dose loop diuretics, flash pulmonary edema, or hypertensive emergency
    - Options for vasodilators include IV nitroglycerin or sodium nitroprusside
    - Can consider nesiritide if nitroglycerin is contraindicated
- Monitor treatment by measuring renal function and electrolytes. Replete electrolytes as needed

Hemodynamically Unstable

- Variable presentation
- Hypertensive emergency: HTN (SBP >180) with flash pulmonary edema and hypoxemic respiratory failure
- SBP <90 or signs of end-organ hypoperfusion (mottling, cold skin, pale, cyanosis)
- *(As was our patient when they entered cardiogenic shock)*
- Prioritize respiratory support
- Consider inotropic support

5. **Describe risk factors for developing chronic heart failure** [8].
   - *Coronary artery disease:* A common cause of heart failure, due to an occlusion of arteries by fatty buildup and reduced perfusion of heart muscle.

- *Hypertension (high blood pressure):* Increases afterload causing the left ventricle to work harder to push blood to the aorta. This extra exertion by the left ventricle can make the heart muscle weak and ineffective.
- *Valvular issues:* Can force the heart to work harder and therefore place strain on the heart and weaken contractions.
- *Cardiomyopathy:* Damage to the heart muscle. Can have many causes including genetics, diseases, infections, alcohol, and drugs.
- *Myocarditis*: Inflammation of the heart muscle that can lead to left-sided heart failure.
- *Heart arrhythmias:* May increase work for the heart due to increased heart rate. However, bradycardia can also lead to heart failure.
- *Comorbidities:* Diabetes mellitus, HIV, hyperthyroidism, hypothyroidism, hemochromatosis (iron buildup), or amyloidosis (protein buildup).
- *Medications:* Diabetes drugs (i.e., rosiglitazone and pioglitazone) increase rate of heart failure. Possible connection with NSAIDs.
- *Sleep apnea:* Lower than normal amounts of oxygen to the heart leads to weakening of the heart muscles.
- *Modifiable factors:* Obesity, alcohol, tobacco use.

6. **Discuss treatments for chronic heart failure including their mechanism of action, important side effects, and effect on target organs.**

Medications:

Aimed at improving blood flow. Two main classes are angiotensin-converting enzyme (ACE) inhibitors to dilate blood vessels and diuretics to reduce fluid buildup [7].

- Angiotensin-converting enzyme (ACE) inhibitors block conversion of angiotensin I to angiotensin II, which in effect lowers peripheral resistance and increases venous capacity. A main side effect of ACE inhibitors is a chronic cough.
- Angiotensin II receptor blockers (ARBs) block the action of angiotensin II by prohibiting binding to its receptor on smooth muscles in the walls of blood vessels. This leads to dilation of blood vessels and reduction in blood pressure. A main side effect of ARBs is hyperkalemia.
- Angiotensin-receptor neprilysin inhibitors (ARNIs) combine a neprilysin inhibitor and ARB and are sold as sacubitril/valsartan. Sacubitrilat inhibits the enzyme neprilysin that degrades BNP. As a result, BNP levels increase and act to further dilate vessels and stimulate sodium excretion to reduce extracellular fluid. A main side effect of ARNI is hyperkalemia and hypotension.
- Beta blockers: Reduce heart rate and lower blood pressure. A main side effect of beta blockers is bradycardia and hypotension.
- Calcium channel blockers (CCB) reduce heart rate similar to beta blockers and are used if heart failure is not managed fully with beta blockers. The main side effects of CCBs are flushing and arrhythmia.
- Aldosterone receptor antagonists: Directly inhibit effects of aldosterone to help lower blood pressure and reduce congestion. The main side effects are hyperkalemia and gynecomastia.
- Diuretics help excrete excess fluid and sodium through the kidneys. Side effects include hypotension and worsening gout.

*****Drugs that improve prognosis: Beta blockers, ACEIs, ARNIs, aldosterone antagonists, hydralazine with nitrate, and SGLT2 inhibitors.*

**** *Diuretics and digoxin are used to improve symptoms and reduce the number of hospitalizations.*

Medication regimen depends on the stage of heart failure [7]:

- Stage A:
  - Heart failure medications are not recommended
  - Treat risk factors
- Stage B:
  - ACEIs for every patient with heart failure with reduced ejection fraction. Should monitor blood pressure, renal function, and potassium 1-2 weeks after initiation.
  - ARBs for patients who cannot tolerate ACEIs (i.e., dry cough). Monitor blood pressure, renal function, and potassium 1-2 weeks after initiation.
  - Beta blockers can be added on once a patient is stable on ACEIs. Should be avoided in patients with decompensated cardiac failure. Assess for symptoms of worsening heart failure or bradycardia.
- Stage C: Additions:
  - Aldosterone antagonists should be used in all patients with heart failure with reduced ejection fraction, NYHA class II-IV symptoms, and LVEF <35%. Monitor for hyperkalemia.
  - Use loop diuretics and thiazide diuretics to treat volume overload. Check electrolytes regularly.
  - Isosorbide dinitrate and hydralazine are for patients who cannot tolerate ACEIs or ARBs. Monitor for hypotension.
  - ARNIs are for persistent heart failure despite first-line drugs. Monitor for hypotension and measure blood tests for hyperkalemia.
  - SGLT-2 inhibitors are useful for patients with heart failure with reduced ejection fraction and NYHA class II-IV symptoms in combination with first-line drugs. Check for hypotension and monitor GFR.
- Stage D: At this stage, additional measures including invasive interventions or change in focus to palliative care are applicable.
  - Consider continuous IV inotropic support as bridge to heart transplant.

Cardiac Resynchronization Therapy:

Heart failure can lead to irritation of the heart cells which ultimately causes a heart arrhythmia that worsens the patient's symptoms and the situation. Cardiac resynchronization therapy helps encourage the ventricles to pump at the same time and eventually could improve cardiac output.

Ventricular assist devices (VAD):

Can help assist the heart pump blood.

Heart Transplant:

A treatment option for end-stage heart failure where other treatments have failed.

7. **Describe the emotional and societal impact of heart failure.**
   - Incidence: 6.2 million adults in the United States have heart failure [8].
   - Heart failure costs were an estimated $30.7 billion in 2012. Includes cost of health care services, medicines to treat heart failure, and missed days of work [8].
   - Heart disease deaths vary by sex, race, and ethnicity [8]:
     - Leading cause of death for people of most racial and ethnic groups in the United States, including African American, American Indian, Alaska Native, and Hispanic women.
     - Increased incidence in men>women.
   - Death varies by geography [8]:
     - Highest death rates: Mississippi, Louisiana, Arkansas, Oklahoma, Texas, Kentucky, Tennessee, Indiana, Illinois, and Wisconsin. Pockets of high-rate counties also were found in Oregon, Utah, Montana, South Dakota, and Nebraska.

Exam Questions

1. A 65-year-old retired man presents to clinic with complaints of feeling tired with activity and a hard time breathing over the last two years. His symptoms were worsened when he played baseball on a warm day with his family while attending a summer picnic. After hitting

a baseball, he ran to first base and felt short of breath, fatigued, had difficulty concentrating, and started wheezing. He reports that he is not very active at baseline. The patient cannot remember the last time he went to the doctor. He reports tobacco and alcohol use. On physical exam, his blood pressure is 145/85, heart rate 130, oxygen saturation 93%. Cardiac exam shows a displaced apical heartbeat, 2+ pitting edema, and rales in bilateral lung bases. Laboratory results are most likely to reveal which of the following?

(a) Elevated sodium levels
(b) Polycythemia
(c) Normal creatinine
(d) Elevated troponin
(e) Elevated BNP

Answer: E

Objective: LO #3. Describe the signs and symptoms of cardiogenic shock, including a differential diagnosis list for each. Explain factors that could make each diagnosis more or less likely.

Explanation: An elevated BNP has a high predictive index in patients with heart failure as this patient appears to have in the presentation. Brain natriuretic peptide (BNP) is a ventricular myocyte hormone released in response to increased ventricular filling and stretching. It functions on smooth muscle cGMP to cause vasodilation and leads to hypotension and decreased pulmonary capillary wedge pressure. A is incorrect: Sodium levels can be normal or decreased due to fluid overload and dilution. Hyponatremia can indicate a poor prognosis. B is incorrect: Anemia can be a trigger of CHF as the heart would need to increase work by increasing cardiac output to compensate and increase oxygen delivery to cells. C is incorrect: Glomerular filtration rate decreases due to hypoperfusion which causes an increase in serum creatinine and BUN. D is incorrect: Troponin levels are variable with heart failure. It could be elevated due to heart damage from long-standing heart failure or myocardial infarction. However, it is possible not to have any heart damage with heart failure and patients with heart failure could then present with a normal troponin.

2. A 62-year-old man comes to the clinic because of worsening shortness of breath and fatigue over the last two years. He smoked two packs of cigarettes per day for the last 30 years. Physical exam shows positive jugular venous distention, positive hepatojugular reflux, and bilateral lower extremity edema. The patient was started on an initial medication. At the patient's yearly visit, he reported a persistent cough that started 1 week ago. What is the next course of action?
   (a) Continue the patient's current regimen as this is likely unrelated.
   (b) Immediately discontinue medication without a new regimen as the patient is doing well.
   (c) Discontinue current regimen and start a new medication.
   (d) Observe the patient and re-evaluate in 6 weeks.

Answer: C

Objective: LO #6: Discuss treatments for chronic heart failure including their mechanism of action, important side effects, and effect on target organs.

Explanation: The patient was most likely started on an ACE inhibitor as the first line for heart failure. The cough is most likely a side effect of the ACE inhibitor that causes a buildup of bradykinin which results in a symptomatic cough. This adverse effect can start at any time and is not limited to starting with initiation of the ACE inhibitor. If patients are experiencing this side effect, they should be immediately started on a new regimen.

3. A 70-year-old-woman came into the clinic with 5 days of worsening shortness of breath and increased fatigue with activity. Last year she was able to walk 15 minutes, but now can only walk for 5 minutes before she must stop to catch her breath. On initial presentation, the patient's blood pressure is 145/85 with a heart rate of 80. On physical exam, she has rales and crackles in bilateral lungs and pitting edema in bilateral lower extremities. Ejection fraction measured 45%. She and her provider decided to start her on a medication that inhib-

its production of angiotensin II. Which of the following medications was the patient started on?
(a) Ramipril
(b) Valsartan
(c) Losartan
(d) Aliskiren

Answer: A

Objective: LO #6: Discuss treatments for chronic heart failure including their mechanism of action and effect on target organs.

Explanation: An Angiotensin-converting enzyme (ACE, "-pril") inhibitor is the most likely choice as the patient has elevated blood pressure and reduced ejection fraction. ACE inhibitors provide a survival benefit (though the mechanisms are poorly understood) in patients with heart failure with reduced ejection fraction. By inhibiting ACE, the medication decreases the production of angiotensin II and its downstream effects. B is incorrect: Angiotensin-receptor blockers (ARBs, "-sartans") are used as second-line treatment if ACE inhibitors are not tolerated. In addition, ARBs work directly to block the receptor for angiotensin, but do not block the production of angiotensin II. C is incorrect: Angiotensin-receptor blockers (ARBs, "-sartans") are used as second-line treatment if ACE inhibitors are not tolerated. In addition, ARBs work directly to block the receptor for angiotensin, but do not block the production of angiotensin II. D is incorrect: This is a direct renin inhibitor that is opted for when ACE inhibitors and ARBs are not tolerated. This results in an accumulation of angiotensin II and renin as they are produced but renin cannot initiate downstream effects as the receptor is blocked.

References

1. Konstam MA, Kramer DG, Patel AR, Maron MS, Udelson JE. Left ventricular remodeling in heart failure: current concepts in clinical significance and assessment. JACC Cardiovasc Imaging. 2011;4(1):98–108.
2. Cronmiller JR, Keyes DA, Vest JJ. Mark's failing heart: three blood volume regulating hormone systems. National Center for Case Study Teaching in Science; 2020.
3. Osmosis. (Producer). n.d. Congestive heart failure. Running time: 14:27 min. http://www.osmosis.org/learn/Congestive_heart_failure (Accessed 12.15.2022).
4. Kiernan MS, Udelson JE, Sarnak M. Cardiorenal syndrome: definition, prevalence, diagnosis, and pathophysiology. 2022. https://www.uptodate.com/contents/cardiorenal-syndromedefinition-prevalence-diagnosis-and pathophysiology?search=heart%20failure&topicRef=113235&source=see_link (Accessed 12.15.2022).
5. Colucci W, Cohn J. Pathophysiology of heart failure with reduced ejection fracture: hemodynamic alterations and remodeling. 2022. https://www.uptodate.com/contents/pathophysiology-of-heart-failure-with-reduced-ejection-fraction-hemodynamic-alterations-and remodeling?sectionName=NORMAL%20LV%20PRESSURE-VOLUME%20RELATIONSHIP&search=cardiogenic%20shock&topicRef=44&anchor=H1568377579&source=see_link#H1568377579 (Accessed 12.15.2022).
6. Colucci W, Dunlay S. Clinical Manifestations and diagnosis of advanced heart failure. 2022. https://www.uptodate.com/contents/clinical-manifestations-and-diagnosis-of-advanced-heart-failure?search=heart%20failure&source=search_result&selectedTitle=1~150&usage_type=default&display_rank=1#H1379588286 (Accessed 12.15.2022).
7. American Heart Association. 2017. Medications used to treat heart failure. [Webpage] https://www.heart.org/en/health-topics/heart-failure/treatment-options-for-heart-failure/ medications-used-to-treat-heart-failure. (Accessed 12.15.2022).
8. Centers for Disease Control and Prevention. 2019. Heart failure. [Webpage] https://www.cdc.gov/heartdisease/heart_failure.htm (Accessed 12.15.2022).

Stomach Pain

7

Joseph Neely

Chief Compliant: "My Stomach hurts"

Encourage students to draw a wide differential for this intentionally vague chief complaint.

Differential diagnosis for "stomach pain" in VINDICATES format as below:

What are the possible etiologies of this pain?

Vascular: Mesenteric ischemia (both acute/chronic), aneurysm (aortic, superior mesenteric artery (SMA), etc.), acute coronary syndrome, ovarian torsion.

Infectious/Inflammatory: Crohn's, ulcerative colitis, gastritis, diverticulitis, gastroesophageal reflux disease (GERD), pelvic inflammatory disease (PID), ascending cholangitis, hepatitis, abdominal abscess, irritable bowel syndrome.

Neoplastic: Obstructive colon cancer, GI fistula from cancerous process.

Degenerative: Gastroparesis from type II diabetes mellitus (DM2) and/or autonomic dysfunction, dysautonomia.

Iatrogenic: Constipation from opioids, gastritis/peptic ulcer disease (PUD) from NSAID use, short gut from intestinal removal surgeries, small bowel obstruction. Urinary retention from histamine blockers.

Congenital: Hirschsprung's, bowel incarceration from hernias, Meckel's diverticulum.

Autoimmune: Celiac, Hashimoto's hypothyroidism causing constipation.

Trauma: Blunt force trauma to the abdomen causing necrosis, abdominal hematoma, splenic laceration, liver laceration, perforated colon/intestines.

Endocrine: Hypothyroidism, Ogilvie's, kidney stone, PCOS, normal or abnormal menses, ectopic pregnancy, endometriosis.

Supratentorial: Malingering, conversion disorder, physical manifestation of anxiety/depression.

What questions would you ask to take a thorough history?

Onset: Suddenly or slowly?

Position/Progression: Which part of your stomach hurts? How has the pain changed over time?

Quality: What type of pain is it? Ache, burn, sharp, tearing? Does the pain spread anywhere else?

Severity: Rate your pain 1–10.

Timing: Does this pain happen at a specific time of day? Does it happen when you are doing anything in particular?

Aggravating Factors: Does anything make the pain worse?

J. Neely (✉)
Internal Medicine, UC Davis Medical Center, Sacramento, CA, USA
e-mail: JLNeely@UCDavis.edu

C. A. Standley (ed.), *Biomedical Science and Clinical Foundations*,
https://doi.org/10.1007/978-3-031-98353-5_7

Alleviating Factors: Does anything make the pain better?
Duration: How long does the pain last for normally?
Associated Symptoms: Is there anything else you notice with this pain?

History of Presenting Illness: Maria Irving is a 54-year-old female with a past medical history of hypertension, diabetes type 2, and mild irritable bowel syndrome who returns for ongoing care at your primary care clinic. She states that she has been feeling well without any specific complaints. Her IBS has been at baseline, managed with dietary supplements. She notes she is having significant family problems lately. She denies any intimate partner violence or signs/symptoms of depression. As you finish your history, she says "It's probably nothing, but when I feel worked up from the stress, my stomach hurts. It's strange, but I don't think it's my IBS since my bowel movements have been normal. It's probably nothing."

Upon further questioning,

She describes low level 4/10 epigastric "discomfort" when she feels stressed, mostly when she is looking over bills or arguing with her family which started 2 months ago. She is unsure if this is getting worse but states it certainly has not been getting better. She notes that she consistently feels this when she is stressed and lying down helps the pain go away. She lives a mostly sedentary lifestyle and eats fast food frequently due to working double time. She has been adherent will all her medications.

How does this change your differential?

Vascular: Chronic mesenteric ischemia, aneurysm (aortic, SMA, etc.), myocardial ischemia, ovarian torsion.
Infectious/Inflammatory: Crohn's, ulcerative colitis, gastritis, diverticulitis, GERD, PID, cholelithiasis, chronic pancreatitis, irritable bowel syndrome.
Neoplastic: Obstructive colon cancer, GI fistula from cancerous process.
Degenerative: Gastroparesis from DM2 and/or autonomic dysfunction, dysautonomia.
Iatrogenic: Constipation from opioids, gastritis/PUD from NSAID use, small bowel obstruction. Urinary retention from histamine blockers.
Congenital: Bowel incarceration from hernias, Meckel's diverticulum.
Autoimmune: Celiac, Hashimoto's hypothyroidism causing constipation.
Trauma: Blunt force trauma to the abdomen causing necrosis, abdominal hematoma, splenic laceration, liver laceration, perforated colon/intestines.
Endocrine: Hypothyroidism, Ogilvie's, kidney stone, PCOS, normal or abnormal menses, ectopic pregnancy, endometriosis.
Supratentorial: Malingering, conversion disorder, physical manifestation of anxiety/depression.

Past Medical History

PMH

Type 2 diabetes x 15 years
Hypertension (HTN) x 17 years
IBS x 20 years

Past Surgical History

Cholecystectomy at age 32 small bowel obstruction (SBO)

OB/GYN History

G4P1112 (4 total pregnancies, 1 at term, 1 preterm, 1 abortion, 2 total living children)
C-section at age 28
No history of sexually transmitted infection (STI), all Pap smears normal
Menopause at age 48

Family History

Father: Passed away last month from car accident. Had HTN, DM2, three-vessel coronary artery bypass graft (3 V CABG), 1xMI at age 40
Mother: Passed away last month from car accident. Had hypothyroidism. Hemorrhagic stroke at age 64
Siblings: 1 older sister, healthy
One younger brother with heart problems and opioid use disorder
One younger sister. Estranged. No known health issues

ProSmpt: Is there any information here that is pushing us toward a leading diagnosis? What in her history seems concerning to you?

Students should identify significant heart history from her father and vascular disease from mother. Advanced points for identifying DM2 and HTN as risk factors for cardiac disease.

Social History

Married to husband of 30 years. Lives at home with husband and 2 kids, ages 25 and 20.

Her parents recently passed away tragically 1 month ago and her siblings have been fighting over inheritance (increased stress which can exacerbate or cause anginal symptoms).

Never smoker, 1 glass of wine a night, denies problematic drinking (daily alcohol use as potential risk factor for CVD disease).

Rare Marijuana use in past year, denies any other illicit/nonprescribed drug abuse.

Mostly sedentary lifestyle. Works as a secretary during the day, maintains her Esty store for knitted mug sweaters in the afternoons (sedentary lifestyle and likely high salt/cholesterol diet as factors contributing to CVD cause of chief complaint).

Medications

Metformin 1000 mg BID
Lisinopril 20 mg QAM
Daily OTC multivitamin OTC
Daily OTC fiber supplements
(Intentionally not taking a statin though would be indicated given this patient's diabetes and likely atherosclerotic cardiovascular disease (ASCVD) score)

Allergies

No known drug allergies

ROS

Gen: +5-pound weight gain over past 5 months attributed to increased fast food intake. No fevers, chills, night sweats.

Heme: No easy bruising, bleeding, lymphadenopathy.

Resp: No cough, sputum production.

CV: No chest pain, palpitations, syncope, lightheadedness.

GI: IBS-C (C = with constipation) symptoms, but at baseline controlled with supplements. No hematochezia, melena, gross changes in bowel habits.

GU: No dysuria, frequency, urgency, hematuria, urgency, flank pain.

Endo: No change in sleeping patterns.

MSK: No pain, tenderness, tenderness in joints.

Neuro: No paresthesias or seizures. Diabetic foot exam without neuropathy.

Stop and Think

What is the chief complaint?

CC: My Stomach hurts

Briefly summarize this patient's relevant history, symptoms, past medical history, family history, and social history.

Mrs. Irving is a 54-year-old female with PMH of DM2, HTN, and IBS who presents with 3/10 epigastric pain exacerbated by emotional distress for last 2 months. This is different from her baseline IBS pain and reports no change in bowel habits. Family history is significant for father having an MI at age 40 and mother having CVA at 64. Social history significant for sedentary lifestyle, mainly fast-food diet, and 5-pound weight gain in past 5 months.

Formulate a differential diagnosis, how does each pertinent positive and negative contribute to your differential?

1. *Stable angina*
   (a) *Intermittent epigastric pain exacerbated by emotional distress (considered an atypical presentation, but a common presentation of angina in women). Alleviated by resting. Hx of DM2 and HTN. FHx significant for vascular pathology (like early MI in father and CVA in mother). Atypical pain from IBS symptoms.*
2. *Cholelithiasis*
   (a) *Intermittent epigastric pain. High fast-food intake. Unclear relationship with food/eating times.*

3. *IBS exacerbation*
   (a) *History of IBS. Recent increase in stress in patients' life. Recent weight gain, high fast-food diet*
4. *Ischemic bowel*
   (a) *Intermittent abdominal pain with vascular risk factors of DM2 and HTN.*
5. *Physical manifestation of anxiety/stress (psychosomatic)*
   (a) *Acute increase in stress in patient's life recently.*

Physical Exam

BP: 125/75, HR: 89, R: 22, SP: 99% on room air, Temp: 98.6 F, BMI: 37.5
Gen: Obese woman sitting in exam room in
HEENT: NC/AT. Conjunctiva clear, sclera anicteric, PERRLA, moist mucous membranes (MMM), turbinates nonedematous. No lymphadenopathy
Pulm: Clear to auscultation bilaterally (CTAB). Breathing nonlabored
CV: Regular rate and rhythm (RRR). Nl S1, S2, s S3, S4. PMI fifth ICS MCL
Abdomen: NT/ND, BS +4, No rebound. Murphy's test negative
GU: Deferred
MSK: No gross deformities
Neuro: Moving all limbs symmetrically
Psych: Normal mood and affect. Admits to stress due to family issues
Extremities/Pulses: No cyanosis, clubbing or edema (CCE). Radial/femoral DP, PT 2+ symmetrical

Stop and Think
How does this physical exam change your differential?

This physical exam is grossly normal other than her obese habitus. This supports a waxing and waning process or a psychiatric process. A normal exam in this case, however, cannot effectively rule in or rule out most of our differential diagnoses. Of note, a negative Murphy's test would make the diagnosis of Cholelithiasis less likely.

What labs, testing, imaging, would you order for this patient?

CBC/CMP: *As a common first-line screening tool looking for anemia, infection, and other bone marrow abnormalities. Liver function test (LFT) assessment to rule out liver damage/hepatitis. ALK Phos to help determine cholelithiasis.*
TSH: *Given her recent weight gain, a TSH would be warranted though this is likely more attributed to her diet and sedentary lifestyle.*
A1C: *Given her diabetes and recent weight gain, we would likely obtain A1C assuming this was not done within the last 3 months.*

Lab Interpretation

CBC: Everything within normal limits. This would be expected in our patient with angina. Effectively rules out infection, anemia, platelet disturbances.
CMP: Everything within normal limits except elevated fasting glucose to 111, compatible with diabetes. Effectively rules out electrolyte abnormalities, acute hepatitis. Normal ALK Phos makes cholelithiasis less likely. Kidney function normal.
TSH: Normal, rules out hypothyroidism as reason for weight gain and potential hypothyroid constipation.
A1C: Elevated to 8.5 compatible with poorly controlled diabetes and patient's recent weight gain from sedentary lifestyle and fast-food intake. Advanced students might recognize this as increased risk for ACS/atherosclerotic disease.

12 Lead EKG

The patient's EKG shows a normal sinus rhythm with rate of 98, normal axis, normal PR/QT/

QRS intervals, without evidence of ST changes. Essentially, a normal EKG of a resting person.

Stop and Think

How do these findings change your differential?

These grossly normal labs should still keep our differential vague, but should make a waxing/waning process more likely. Cholelithiasis should be lower on the differential due to normal ALK Phos.

Is there anything else you would have done?

Abdominal U/S: *Would be a great tool to rule out cholelithiasis. Not all providers offer this in-office, however.*

Abdominal X-Ray: *Not indicated since exam is not concerning for acute abdomen or intestinal perforation.*

Continued Clinical Course

Maria Irving returns to your clinic 4 months later for an urgent appointment. She recently started an exercise routine to lose weight with her friends but has had difficulty keeping up. When she is on the treadmill, she has intense epigastric pain similar to her pain from her last visit. She feels sweaty, short of breath, and general malaise when running. This becomes so intense she must stop exercising and her symptoms go away with 15 minutes of rest. She attributed all of this to being out of shape, but this has not gotten better since starting her exercise regimen 1 week ago.

Stop and Think

How does this new manifestation change your differential?

This new exertional component should prompt students to think of an ischemic cause of her disease, particularly angina. If students are not making this jump, ask "If this were a man who came in complaining of exertional epigastric pain associated with SOB and sweating but is relieved with rest, what would your first thought be?" If this prompt is required, this is a great point to drive home with the students. Anginal symptoms are classically taught as the male variant of chest pain with radiation to the arm; however, angina symptoms can present in many other ways. This particular presentation is a common female anginal symptom and often goes unrecognized [4]. *This should always be considered especially since this patient is a diabetic with poor glucose control. These patients especially have altered pain perception and can present with angina in many atypical patterns.*

What labs, imaging, testing, and referrals does this patient need?

This patient recently had labs done (4 months ago at her normal visit) that were all normal. Given this new symptom, her diagnosis should be fairly clear and labs would not be indicated. CBC/CMP would be expected to return normal in angina. A1c would technically meet indications for recheck due to being 3 months past due, but would not help in her current diagnosis of angina. She does need a stress test and a cardiology referral for stable angina.

Next Steps

Mrs. Irving is diagnosed with stable angina and is instructed to refrain from exercise and given a stat cardiology outpatient referral. Due to high patient volume, the next open appointment is 4 weeks away.

What counseling should you do for Mrs. Irving? Does she meet any indications for medications?

Students should counsel her on refraining from exercise or any activity that causes her epigastric pain (angina) to increase. There would be consideration of giving her Nitro tabs prior to cardiac evaluation, but this is usually done by cardiology after a formal diagnosis of angina is made.

Prompt: What symptoms should you tell Mrs. Irving to look out for to seek emergency medical care?

Students should be able to describe signs/symptoms of a myocardial infarction that should prompt Mrs. Irving to seek emergency care. Specifically, unrelieving epigastric pain accompanied with SOB and sweating that is not going away with rest.

Clinical Course

Mrs. Irving follow-up with her cardiologist who performs stress testing. After 5 minutes of exercising, she reports the same epigastric discomfort as before. EKG during exercise is shows sinus rhythm with left azis deviation, normal PR/QT/QRS intervals, with significant ST elevations in Leads V1-V4 and reciprocal changes in II, III, and aVF. ST depressions in Leads V5 and V6. EKG normalizes after she stops and rests for 5 minutes.

Prompt: Given that the EKG normalizes and she is asymptomatic after 5 minutes, what does this mean?

This is a positive stress test that shows inducible ischemia with exercise. This patient is likely to have coronary artery disease, most likely in her LAD given where her ST elevations are on EKG. The fact that this normalizes after resting means this is not an MI, but rather a significant blockage.

Stop and Think

- *How do you interpret this stress test?*
  - *As above, this is an abnormal stress test concerning for coronary artery obstruction that shows inducible ischemia to the heart.*
- *Is this test compatible with her previous diagnosis?*
  - *This is in line with our diagnosis of stable angina. The true diagnostic/confirmatory test for this would be to perform a cardiac catheterization to evaluate for blockages and potentially place stent if blockage is of high enough grade (typically > 70%).*

Clinical Course

Due to her abnormal stress testing, cardiac catheterization is performed. She is found to have 90% stenosis of her left anterior descending. Her LAD is subsequently stented.

Prompt: Angina/ischemia can be hard to visualize. Can you appreciate how this narrowing causes ischemia downstream?

Though seemingly rudimentary, cardiac catheterization presents a great opportunity to visualiz how CAD actually causes flow disturbances and limitations downstream. A mechanical intervention such as a stent can fix this issue.

Clinical Course Continued

Mrs. Irving eases back into her exercise regimen and no longer has her previous complaints of epigastric pain either with physical exertion or emotional stress. She is counseled by her cardiologist on the importance of a heart-healthy diet and exercise regimen. She is understanding and expresses concern of a potential heart attack in the future. She is determined to make changes to her lifestyle as well as medical management to prevent worsening coronary artery disease.

Prompt: What risk factors did Mrs. Irving have to develop her condition? What can she do currently to help decrease her risk in the future?

Developing: FHx, DM2, HTN, sedentary lifestyle, fast food diet.
Preventing: Diet/exercise, medication adherence, no smoking.

Social Determinants of Health

Was Mrs. Irving's presentation typical or atypical for female angina?

Epigastric pain that worsens with activity or emotional distress is a recognized classic form of angina in females.

Think about what the "classic" angina picture is for you.

This is likely left-sided crushing chest pressure with radiation to the arm associated with SOB and diaphoresis.

Who typically present like this?

Typically, males. Females have a wider range of presenting symptoms for angina. Recognition of this is crucial to closing the disparities of male/female acute coronary syndrome disparities.

End of Case

Learning Objective Explanations

1. Describe the pathophysiology of atherosclerosis, specifically pertaining to the coronary arteries. Include the specific risk factors this patient has.
    - Atherosclerosis is a chronic condition of cholesterol deposition in the arteries of the body, most commonly coronary, cerebral, aorta, renal, and other peripheral arteries.
        - These plaques have a fatty center with a fibrous "cap" at the interface between the fatty plaque and the actual blood flow. These plaques build up in the arterial walls below the endothelium.
    - This process begins in childhood as "fatty streaks" and grows over time in line with both modifiable risk factors (diet/exercise/medication) and nonmodifiable risk factors (family history, genetics).
        - Endothelium dysfunction underlies this disease. Inflammatory macrophages come in and lead to a maladaptive response and cause increase in fat production locally that grows plaques. These foamy macrophages build up and become part of the core of the plaque.
    - This patient's risk factors are FHx, DM2, and HTN.
        - FHx is a nonmodifiable risk factor that increases her likelihood of atherosclerotic disease given that her mother and father both had evidence of this (MI in father and CVA in mother).
        - DM2: This patient's diabetes is poorly controlled with an A1C of 8.5%. Diabetes represents an endocrine disease, but systemic elevations in sugars lead to an increase in glycated proteins (hence A1c). These proteins are proinflammatory and accelerate atherosclerosis by promoting plaque deposition and destabilizing fibrous plaques.
        - HTN: Though this patient's HTN is controlled, HTN accelerates atherosclerotic disease by increasing arterial shear forces at turbulent zones (usually where plaques form). Increased wall stress from this higher pressure also contributes to accelerated plaque deposition.
        - Obesity: Increased adiposity increases proinflammatory cytokines that accelerate atherosclerosis by increasing local inflammation similar to the mechanism of diabetes.
        - Alcohol Use: Alcohol has mixed data but chronic alcohol users have been shown to have accelerated atherosclerotic disease due to the inhibitions of fatty acid metabolism of alcohol likely promoting plaque growth.
        - Postmenopausal status. Estrogen is a protective factor against MI and plaque formation. This patient being postmenopausal means she has diminished estrogen and therefore an increase in MI risk and increase in pro-plaque forming factors.
2. Compare and contrast the physiology of angina vs. an MI from plaque rupture. Describe the mechanisms that factor into plaque stability and how the coagulation cascade plays a role in this.

   Angina: Pain (multiple manifestations) from cardiac ischemia due to decreased blood flow usually from a partially obstructive plaque. Angina represents a stable plaque that physically and partially obstructs blood flow downstream, therefore limiting the oxygen delivery downstream of the heart. The heart is an incredibly metabolically active muscle (constantly beating without breaks) that requires a lot of oxygen to maintain contractions and cell membrane potentials.

Patients with a stable plaque will have angina that starts with the same level of exertion (i.e., walking 2 blocks, but never before).

Patients with a growing plaque will note the classic symptoms of earlier onset of their anginal symptoms. This is because the plaque is growing and is further obstructing blood flow, further limiting downstream oxygen delivery. Factors that contribute to plaque growth are the same as discussed above, lack of exercise/healthy diet, proinflammatory conditions. The key is that the fibrous plaque remains stable here and there is no acute event of complete blockage. The plaque can remain stable indefinitely, but if it continues to grow, it will eventually occlude the entire artery causing an MI.

Patients with sudden plaque rupture. When a plaque's fibrous cap becomes unstable and ruptures, it exposes the blood to the fatty core which is extremely thrombogenic. This immediately triggers the coagulation cascade and platelet aggregation resulting in an occlusive plaque that obstructs the entire lumen. This is how a 30% obstructive plaque that would not have any angina/symptoms associated with it can become a life-threatening MI very quickly due to plaque fibrous cap instability. This mechanism underlies why not everyone who has an MI has anginal symptoms leading up to it.

Plaque stability: This is similar to the points above that affect plaque growth. Rapid plaque growth is associated with fibrous cap instability. This is largely multifactorial and is highly affected by genetics and local inflammation. This patient's increased wall stress from HTN, local inflammation from DM2, and her postmenopausal status all negatively affect plaque stability.

3. What are the most common manifestations of angina? List these for both men and women. Describe the major differences.

   Emphasis that the predominant symptoms are the male-based systems and how this can affect the early identification, diagnosis, and treatment of angina and underlying coronary artery disease in women.

   Women have a wider range of anginal symptoms that mainly include upper abdominal pain as well as more constellation of symptoms (i.e., abdominal pain and shortness of breath vs. just chest pain).

4. Coronary artery disease and its main symptom of angina represent a spectrum of disease. Discuss the classification of stable angina, unstable angina, and acute myocardial infarction based on patient symptoms and lab tests.

   Stable Angina: Patient has reproducible anginal pain (any symptom including or combination of chest pain/abdominal pain, nausea, lightheadedness, shortness of breath) with specific exertional requirements without EKG findings concerning for ischemia (ST depression/elevation). This pain/symptom recedes with rest.

   Unstable Angina: Patient has anginal pain symptoms that are not relieved with rest with an EKG without ST segment changes. Troponins in this case will be positive indicating myocardial ischemia and cellular death.

   Acute Myocardial Infarction: Patient will have anginal symptoms with evidence of ST changes on EKG (ST elevations for STEMI or depression for NSTEMI). Troponins for this will be positive, indicating myocardial ischemia and cellular death.

5. Discuss the treatments for stable angina, unstable angina, and acute myocardial infarction for both medical and procedural interventions. What are the indications for each?

   Stable angina represents symptomatic coronary artery disease. This is treated outpatient as this is a chronic condition. Lifestyle modifications should be emphasized to reduce plaque progression over time and reduce likelihood of acute rupture. A heart-healthy diet (low fat/salt) is recommended and exercise within the patient's tolerance is advised depending on progression/severity of disease. Stable angina is a primary indication for use of a statin medication as well as titration of blood pressure to an appropriate level based on patient's age and tolerance. The use of aspirin 81 mg daily has been historically used, but has been called into question on grounds of efficacy as of lately. Current indications show benefit in diabetics as well as those with known/proven CAD. Oral/sublingual nitrates are given to patients as symptomatic relief of their chest pain as well.

Unstable Angina represents an acute episode of angina, likely brought on by plaque rupture forming a thrombus. Reminder that this is anginal symptoms without EKG changes, but a positive troponin indicating myocardial damage. This is treated similar to an NSTEMI based mainly on medications to reduce oxygen demand by the heart including beta-blockers and afterload reduction (i.e., blood pressure control) if indicated.

Acute myocardial infarction represents a complete blockage of a coronary artery causing myocardial death. This can manifest in a number of ways, but most commonly with severe, nonrelieving anginal symptoms, ST changes on EKG, and positive troponins. The management of this can vary depending on the artery blocked/side of the heart that is affected, but can include sublingual aspirin to prevent further thrombus formation, nitrates to relieve cardiac congestion and vasodilate coronary arteries, and beta-blockers to reduce myocardial ischemia from decreased chronotropy/inotropy. Definitive management is done in the cardiac catheterization lab to visualize blockage and stent the artery if possible. Post-MI care is then mainly supportive, with indications for dual antiplatelet (aspirin and antiplatelet medication) therapy to prevent stent thrombosis, high-intensity statin therapy to reduce plaque progression, blood pressure management, and cardiology follow-up.

6. Discuss the disease burden of coronary artery disease by sex.
   - The number one cause of death in the United States is cardiovascular disease [4].
     - This is true when counting separately for men and women individually.
     - Slightly higher in males, but still number one cause of deaths in females [5].
7. Summarize the disparities in health care specifically for coronary heart disease for females. Briefly discuss these issues.

   Due to the wider variation in anginal symptoms that women have, they are less likely to be diagnosed, diagnosed, or receive care for cardiovascular disease. This is seen in both inpatient and outpatient settings.

   This undertreatment and missed diagnostic criteria are also seen in critical setting. Women have been shown to have a higher hospital mortality for acute coronary syndrome due to delayed diagnosis and delayed intervention.

   Even with correct diagnosis and acute management, females are less likely to receive guideline-directed medical therapy as compared to their male counterparts.

   Optional side note, these disparities widened even further for females of non-white ethnicities.

   Many of these disparities are founded on the fact that the majority of historic cardiovascular research was conducted on a mostly male population, which is why much of the literature describes classic male anginal symptoms, but the wider female presentation of angina is left by the wayside.

Exam Questions

1. A 38-year-old previously healthy female is found unresponsive on a popular hiking route that is known to be very strenuous. She is rushed to the emergency room and unfortu-

nately pronounced dead. She had no known health issues despite seeing the physician regularly and did not take any medications. Her partner denies her ever complaining of chest pain, palpitations, lightheadedness, syncope, or any other exertional symptoms as she frequently ran half marathons without issue. Autopsy reveals a massive myocardial infarction as a cause of death. Which of the following most likely represents the pathophysiology that resulted in this patient's death?

A. An unruptured atherosclerotic plaque in a coronary artery that has slowly been growing until it completely occluded the artery.
B. A ruptured atherosclerotic plaque that has 30% of coronary artery lumen obstructed with fatty material and the remaining 70% occluded by a large thrombus.
C. Multiple unruptured atherosclerotic plaques in the LAD, RCA, and Ramus coronary arteries but none greater than 30% stenosis.
D. All coronary vessels examined would not have any atherosclerotic plaques due to her highly active lifestyle.

Answer: B

Learning objective: Compare and contrast the physiology of blood in angina vs an MI from plaque rupture. Describe the mechanisms that factor into plaque stability and how the coagulation cascade plays a role in this.

Explanation: This patient's history of no anginal symptoms despite a highly active lifestyle who suffers a sudden cardiac death from and MI is classic for an unstable plaque rupture causing an acute massive thrombosis in a major coronary artery causing death. These MIs are usually not preceded with any anginal symptoms as the plaques themselves are not large enough to cause a significant flow blockage, but the thrombus formed by the plaque rupture completely blocks off the artery causing massive MI. Option A is unlikely as slowly progressing plaques like these will cause anginal symptoms before completely closing off the artery. Symptoms would be expected at approximately 70% occlusion, but would certainly be present with higher grade blockage over time. This patient had no risk factors or signs/symptoms concerning for angina especially given her highly active lifestyle. C is incorrect as while this patient may have subclinical atherosclerotic disease in her coronary arteries, this situation would not account for her lethal MI. Obstructions of less than 70% are usually asymptomatic. Unruptured low-grade multivessel disease such as this would not be expected to cause a myocardial ischemia. D is incorrect as atherosclerotic plaques such as fatty streaks have been observed on autopsy of completely healthy children. Fatty streaks and minimal blockages are likely to be observed in even healthy people who are highly active such as this patient. Plaque stability and growth is determined most by modifiable and non-modifiable factors, but the presence of atherosclerotic plaques is ubiquitous. Also, this finding would not explain the patient's massive and lethal heart attack.

2. A 62-year-old man presents to the emergency department with chest discomfort. After a detailed evaluation, he is diagnosed with unstable angina. Which of the following profiles would fit this diagnosis?

Option	Anginal symptom	EKG changes	Troponins	Complete occlusion on cath
A	Negative	Negative	Negative	Negative
B	Positive	Negative	Negative	Negative
C	Positive	Positive	Negative	Negative
D	Positive	Positive	Positive	Negative
E	Positive	Positive	Positive	Positive

Answer: D

Learning Objective: Discuss the classification of stable angina, unstable angina, and acute myocardial infarction based on patient symptoms and lab tests.

Explanation: Row D indicates unstable angina with is shown by anginal symptoms and EKG/lab findings consistent with myocardial ischemia/damage. Unstable angina represents non-complete occlusion of a coronary artery and can be appear similar to a Non-ST elevation myocardial infarction. Because of this, a complete occlusion on cardiac cath would not be expected for unstable angina. Row A represents a patient at baseline without any symptoms. This is not compatible with unstable angina. Row B represents a patient who has stable angina as indicated by the presence of anginal symptoms but without any EKG changes or troponins indicating cardiac damage. Row C also represents a patient with stable angina as would be found during an exercise stress test indicating myocardial ischemia with EKG changes. However, the troponins are negative indicating stable angina due to the absence of myocardial damage/ischemia. Row E represents a STEMI as these are typically complete occlusions of major coronary arteries causing transmural infarction of the myocardium. These are often visualized as complete occlusions of cardiac cath.

3. Which of the following scenarios is most concerning for anginal pain in a 52-year-old female with past medical history of Type II diabetes mellitus, hypertension, and hyperlipidemia?
   A. Lightheadedness and shortness of breath after running 0.5 miles. Patient notes this used to occur at the 1 mile mark but has slowly started sooner.
   B. Sudden episodes of lightheadedness and vision narrowing after standing up quickly from a seated position that lasts for 10 seconds.
   C. Sudden episodes of diaphoresis and lightheadedness that last for 10 minutes and are relieved with movement/exertion.
   D. A sharp left-sided chest pain worsened with inspiration that started 2 weeks ago after getting over a cold.

Answer: A

Learning objective: What are the most common manifestations of angina? List these for both men and women. Describe the major differences.

Explanation: This is a non-classical anginal symptom that can be seen in women and men. Particularly those who are diabetic. The main concerning feature for this is the exertional nature of the pain as well as the quicker time to onset that she notes which may indicating a growing coronary plaque. B is incorrect as these symptoms are most consistent with transient orthostatic hypotension from standing too quickly. This is commonly seen in the elderly as well as those who are diabetic due to neuropathy that can blunt vascular reflexes that protect from this transient hypotension. While these symptoms can be seen as anginal symptoms, the nature of these symptoms lacks the exertional component and appear to self-relieve quickly which would be uncharacteristic of angina. C is incorrect as while these symptoms can also be seen as anginal symptoms, the characteristic of being relieved with movement/exertion is the opposite of what would be expected of angina. Since the nature of angina is myocardial ischemia, anything that would increase myocardial demand such as exercise or exertion, should cause the pain to worsen, not improve. Due to this, this scenario is highly unlikely to be anginal in nature. D is incorrect as the nature of this pain comes off as pleuritic especially given that the pain worsens with inspiration. The further history that this pain started after recovering from a recent cold makes this a classic case of pleurisy and not angina. Though this case of left-sided chest pain initially could be concerning for a classical angina presentation, the nature and characteristics of the pain make it less likely. Sharp pain is a less common form of angina as most angina is described as a pressure sensation and should not fluctuate with respirations.

Works Cited

1. Centers for Disease Control and Prevention. FASTSTATS – leading causes of death. Centers for Disease Control and Prevention. 2024, May 2. https://www.cdc.gov/nchs/fastats/leading-causes-of-death.htm.
2. Centers for Disease Control and Prevention. Lower your risk for the number 1 killer of women. Centers for Disease Control and Prevention. 2024a, February 22. https://www.cdc.gov/healthequity/features/heart-disease/index.html#:~:text=about%20alcohol%20use.-,Heart%20disease%20is%20the%20leading%20cause%20of%20death%20for%20women,some%20form%20of%20heart%20disease.
3. Angina in women can be different than men. www.heart.org. 2024, January 30. https://www.heart.org/en/health-topics/heart-attack/angina-chest-pain/angina-in-women-can-be-different-than-men
4. Gulati M. Yentl's bikini: sex differences in STEMI. J Am Heart Assoc. 2019;8:e012873. https://www.ncbi.nlm.nih.gov/pmc/articles/PMC6585326/
5. Hemingway H, Langenberg C, Damant J, Frost C, Pyörälä K, Barrett-Connor E. Prevalence of angina in women versus men: a systematic review and meta-analysis of international variations across 31 countries. Circulation. 2008;117(12):1526–36. https://doi.org/10.1161/CIRCULATIONAHA.107.720953.

Part IV

Respiratory

8 Irritating Cough

Cynthia A. Standley

Learning Objectives

1. Differentiate key characteristics of asthma in relation to other common obstructive pulmonary disorders, including anatomic lesion site, major pathologic changes, etiology, and signs/symptoms.
2. Explain the underlying pathogenesis of atopic asthma (inflammatory process, cells, and mediators involved), and compare the airway in atopic asthma to a normal bronchus.
3. Explain normal pulmonary function testing, including defining the measurements made (FEV1, FVC, FEV1/FVC) and briefly explaining how they are determined. Discuss how a bronchodilator affects these variables.
4. Compare and contrast obstructive lung disorders with restrictive lung disorders using pulmonary function testing. Which one does the patient have?
5. Categorize and describe the various treatments for asthma, including rescue vs. maintenance medication and the goals of asthma treatment.
6. Describe an asthma exacerbation and how to recognize life-threatening signs. Can children outgrow asthma?
7. Identify indications for and the efficacy of influenza and pneumococcal vaccines in people with asthma. Discuss how poor living, working, and environmental conditions can contribute to respiratory tract disease.

Chief Complaint:
"My cough is really bothering me and keeping me up at night."

Prompt: *What is the differential for cough in adults? In children?*

In adults, common causes of cough include angiotensin-converting enzyme inhibitor use, asthma, gastroesophageal reflux disease (GERD) and upper airway cough syndrome [1]. Less common causes include chronic bronchitis and irritants such as cigarette smoke. Rare causes to consider are aspiration, arteriovenous malformation, persistent pneumonia, and psychogenic cough.

In children, common causes include asthma, GERD, and respiratory tract infection. Less common causes include foreign body aspiration, pertussis, or post-infectious cough. Rare causes to consider are congenital abnormalities, or cystic fibrosis.

History of Present Illness
Jordan Johnson is a 19-year-old female who reports she has had a cough off and on since moving to Arizona a year ago. She says that it comes and goes, but it tends to be worse at night, and the

C. A. Standley (✉)
Department of Bioethics and Medical Humanism, University of Arizona College of Medicine-Phoenix, Phoenix, AZ, USA
e-mail: cstand@arizona.edu

C. A. Standley (ed.), *Biomedical Science and Clinical Foundations*,
https://doi.org/10.1007/978-3-031-98353-5_8

last month it has been happening every couple of nights. She says she never coughs anything up. She gets especially wheezy whenever she goes running outside, but when she runs inside, she is fine. She says it gets hard to breathe when she does anything physical, but even inside sometimes she gets short of breath with physical activity. She usually catches her breath after about 30 minutes. This happens about 3–4 times a week.

Prompt: *What does 'wheezy' mean? Are there different kinds of breath sounds?*

- Abnormal breath soundsAsthmaabnormal breath sounds indicate underlying conditions. Most common types of abnormal breath sounds include:
- Rales. Small clicking, bubbling, or rattling sounds in the lungs. They are heard when a person breathes in (inhales). They are believed to occur when air opens closed air spaces. Rales can be further described as moist, dry, fine, or coarse
- Rhonchi. Sounds that resemble snoring. They occur when air is blocked or air flow becomes rough through the large airways.
- Stridor. Wheeze-like sound heard when a person breathes. Usually, it is due to a blockage of airflow in the windpipe (trachea) or in the back of the throat.
- Wheezing. High-pitched sounds produced by narrowed airways Wheezing and other abnormal sounds can sometimes be heard without a stethoscope.

There can also be abnormal patterns to breathing rate:

- Bradypnea**:** an abnormally slow rate of respiration
- Apnea**:** the absence of respirations, typically lasting more than 15 second
- Cheyne–Stokes: a cyclical pattern of breathing that includes a progression of increased rate and depth of respirations followed by periods of apnea

History of Present Illness (continued)
Jordan reports she has not had this shortness of breath or coughing previously. She tried some over-the-counter allergy medications, but this has not helped.

Prompt: *What are some examples of over-the-counter allergy medications?*

Over-the-counter (OTC) medications are widely used to manage allergy symptoms. These medications fall into several categories [2]:

- Antihistamines such as cetirizine (Zyrtec®), fexofenadine (Allegra®), levocetirizine (Xyzal®), and loratadine (Claritin®) are taken by mouth. Brompheniramine (Dimetapp®), chlorpheniramine (Chlor-Trimeton®), clemastine (Tavist®), and diphenhydramine (Benadryl®) can induce drowsiness.
- Decongestants such as pseudoephedrine (Sudafed® tablets or liquid), phenylephrine (Neo-Synephrine®) and oxymetazoline (Afrin®) nasal sprays
- Some Visine® eye drops
- Combination medications such as cetirizine and pseudoephedrine (Zyrtec-D®), fexofenadine and pseudoephedrine (Allegra-D®), diphenhydramine and pseudoephedrine (Benadry® 1 Allergy and Sinus), loratadine and pseudoephedrine (Claritin-D®), and pseudoephedrine/triprolidine (Actifed®) for nasal allergies; and naphazoline/pheniramine (Naphcon A®) for allergic conjunctivitis
- Nasal corticosteroids: budesonide (Rhinocort® Allergy), fluticasone (Flonase® Allergy Relief), and triamcinolone (Nasacort® Allergy 24HR)
- Other over the counter products include salt-water solution, or saline containing no active drug ingredient, available as a nasal spray to relieve mild congestion, loosen mucus, and prevent crusting.
- Artificial tears, which also contain no active drug, are available to treat itchy, watery, and red eyes.
- Humidifier

She denies any fatigue, chest pain, lightheadedness, or palpitations. She has not been afebrile. She does not have any chest pain or burning sensations after eating.

She also denies ever smoking. She has not had any new pets.

Past Medical History (PMH)
Seasonal allergies

Prompt: *Is this specific to an allergen or general?*

In Arizona, these could be related to ragweed, tumbleweeds, Bermuda grass, juniper trees, mesquite trees, olive trees. More recently, the rapid growth of the invasive weed stinknet, also known as globe chamomile, can trigger allergic reactions.

Past Surgical History (PSH)
Appendectomy, age 15

Medications
Claritin® (loratadine) daily for allergies

Allergies
No known drug allergies

Family History
Mother: Hypertension, hyperlipidemia, seasonal allergies
Father: atopic dermatitis
No other family history of heart disease, diabetes, or cancer.

Social History
First-year community college student
Lives at home with parents and siblings
Denies ever using alcohol, tobacco, or illicit drugs

Prompt: *How could you ask this patient about vaping?*

As vaping is prevalent among teenagers in the United States and is considered a public health concern, it would be appropriate to ask the patient about her experience with it. Most teens believe e-cigarettes contain only water and flavoring. Thus, it would be a good time to educate her that e-cigarettes do contain nicotine. Vaping can cause chronic cough and can lead to other lung conditions. Point out the dangers of vaping without judgement and let them know you are concerned about their health.

Prompt: *What is significant about the family history?*
Personal or family history of atopy—A strong family history of asthma and allergies or a personal history of atopic diseases such as atopic dermatitis, seasonal allergic rhinitis and conjunctivitis, favors a diagnosis of asthma in a patient with suggestive symptoms [3].

Review of Systems (ROS):
Gen: no fever, no chills, no weight changes
Skin: dry spots on knees and elbows, acne, no skin changes, lesions
Head: no headache, head trauma
Eyes: no blurred vision, no pain, no glasses
Ears: no tinnitus, pain, or discharge
Nose: occasional runny nose, no epistaxis, obstruction
Throat: no pharyngitis, dysphagia
Chest: *see HPI*
GI: no nausea, vomiting, diarrhea, constipation, changes in bowel movements, or hematochezia
GU: no dysuria, polyuria, or frequency
MSK: no muscle or joint tenderness, no history of injury
Neuro: no syncope, paresthesia, or coordination issues
Endo: no hair changes, no facial or hand swelling, no changes in appetite
Psych: no mood changes, sleep issues, or increased sadness

Prompt: *What can you determine from the ROS?*

The dry spots on her knees and elbows could suggest atopic dermatitis. She has some postnasal drip but no bloody noses. There is no inflammation of the pharynx that could cause sore throat and she has no difficulty swallowing. It is a relatively normal ROS except as mentioned in HPI, although looks like she has evidence of allergies and possible link to atopic dermatitis.

Prompt: *What diagnoses should be considered now?*

Asthma, allergies, upper airway cough syndrome

Prompt: *What physical examination findings and ancillary studies (laboratory tests, imaging studies, etc.) can be used to distinguish the hypotheses given?*

Check labs for any signs of infection; pulmonary function tests, check breath sounds, CT image of sinuses.

Physical Examination

Vitals: P: 68 bpm R: 15 breaths/min T: 98.6° F BP: 110/80 mmHg O_2: 98%

General: Well-developed/well-nourished (WD/WN) female, alert and conversant, no acute distress (NAD)

HEENT: Normocephalic/atraumatic, sclera anicteric, conjunctiva clear, PERRLA (pupils equal, round, and reactive to light and accommodation), turbinates erythematous, no nasal polyps, no sinus tenderness,

Neck: no LAD (lymphadenopathy)

Lungs: CTAB (clear to auscultation bilateral)

CV: RRR (regular rate, rhythm) Normal S1, S2; no S3, S4; no murmur, rub, or gallop

Extremities: no CCE (clubbing, cyanosis, edema)

Pulses: 2+ bilaterally

Prompt: *Could the patient still have asthma if lungs are clear on auscultation?*

The presence or absence of wheezing on physical examination is a poor predictor of the severity of airflow obstruction in asthma. Wheezing may be heard in patients with mild, moderate, or severe airway narrowing, while widespread airway narrowing may be present in individuals without wheezing. Thus, the presence of wheezing alerts one to the likely presence of airway narrowing, but not its severity [3].

Prompt: *What Tests/Studies would you like to order? Does she need an X-ray?*

She most likely does not need a chest Xray. The chest radiograph is almost always normal in patients with asthma. However, many clinicians obtain a chest radiograph for new-onset moderate-to-severe asthma in adults over age 40 to exclude the occasional alternative diagnosis that may mimic asthma. In contrast, chest radiographs are routinely recommended when evaluating severe or "difficult-to-control" asthma and when co-morbid conditions exist. [3]

She also does not need blood work currently. May consider allergy testing. While allergy tests are not useful for the diagnosis of asthma, they can be helpful to confirm sensitivity to suspected allergic triggers of respiratory symptoms and to guide on-going management of asthma.

Peak Flow Meter

500 L/min

Prompt: *What is this and why is it used?*

A peak flow meter is a portable, handheld device that is used to measure how well air moves out of the lungs. It works by measuring how fast air moves out of the lungs after inhaling fully and then exhaling forcefully. It measures peak expiratory flow (PEF) rate, and by keeping track of the PEF, it provides an indication of whether asthma conditions are controlled or worsening. Peak Expiratory Flow Predictions vary with age, height, and sex. This is close to the predicted value for an 18-year-old female at 65 inches in height [4].

Pulmonary Function Testing

Spirometry, including Post-Bronchodilator Values (Table 8.1).

Table 8.1 Patient's Spirometry Results

Pre-Bronchodilator				Post-Bronchodilator		
	Predicted	Measured	% Predicted	Measured	% Predicted	% Change
FVC	4.85 L	4.10 L	84.5%	4.51 L	93%	8.5%
FEV_1	4.05 L	2.81 L	69.4%	3.28 L	79%	9.6%
FEV_1/FVC %	83.5%	68.5%		72.7%		

FVC Forced vital capacity, *FEV_1* Forced expiratory volume in 1 second

Prompt: *How do these test results help you to refine your hypothesis?*

A reduced ratio of FEV1 /FVC indicates obstruction to the flow of air from the lungs, whereas a reduced FVC with a normal FEV1 / FVC ratio suggests a restrictive pattern. The severity of abnormal spirometric measurements is evaluated by comparison of the patient's results with reference values based on age, height, sex, and race. The FEV_1 being 69.4% of predicted suggests a moderate airflow obstruction based on the 2005 ATS/ERS guide for severity of obstruction [5]. The fact that her spirometry results improve significantly after a bronchodilator was administered (post-bronchodilation), indicates that she likely has airway obstruction, which is often seen in conditions like asthma. This indicates her airways are narrowing and can be opened up with medication like an inhaler; this is considered a positive bronchodilator response and can help diagnose asthma or assess the effectiveness of asthma treatment.

Prompt: *What is the best diagnostic choice for this patient? How does this relate to the initial chief complaint?*

The best diagnostic choice is asthma. The results of her spirometry signify variable expiratory airflow limitation testing before and after use of a bronchodilator, and alternative diagnoses have been excluded. The most common type of asthma is atopic asthma, a type I IgE-mediated hypersensitivity reaction triggered by environmental allergens [6].

This patient's chief complaint was cough. People with airflow limitation, cough because the narrowed airways in their lungs trap mucus, irritating the cough receptors and triggering a cough reflex, which is the body's attempt to clear the airways and remove the excess mucus buildup.

Prompt: *What is the next step in management?*

- Albuterol inhaler 2 puffs prior to exercise, or as needed
- Return to clinic if symptoms do not resolve or worsen

Plan

This patient was diagnosed with atopic asthma. She was prescribed an albuterol inhaler and instructed to use 2 puffs prior to exercise or as needed. She is to follow up with the clinic in 2 weeks.

Prompt: *How much is too much (use of albuterol)?*

The dosage should not exceed 12 puffs within 24 hours. The "Rule of Two" is a guideline that indicates that well-controlled asthmatics should use their rescue inhaler no more than two times per week (excluding pre-exercise use) [7].

Prompt: *What should she use for her dry skin?*

With her atopic dermatitis, she could use any of the following to reduce irritation:

- Lotions/moisturizers with lanolin, aloe, petrolatum
- Antihistamines and pain relievers (Benadryl®, Claritin®)
- Topical hydrocortisone
- Medicated shampoos (ketoconazole)

Two Week Follow Up

When Jordan follows up in your office 2 weeks later, she reports she has been able to manage her asthma by using an albuterol inhaler prior to exercise and as needed.

She is told to return to the clinic if symptoms do not resolve or worsen.

The Case Continues

You have been seeing Jordan off and on for the past 2 years to refill her albuterol inhaler and prescribe birth control. It's been a few months since you last saw her. Today she presents with the following complaint:

"1-week history of cough and sore throat."

Prompt: *What are the most common causes of pharyngitis?*

Viral causes of pharyngitis account for 50% of cases, the most common ones being rhinovirus, adenovirus, influenza A and B, Epstein-Barr virus (mononucleosis), coronavirus (including COVID-19), and herpes simplex virus [8]. The most common bacterial infection is Group A streptococci, which causes 5% to 36% of cases of acute pharyngitis.

History of Present Illness
Jordan is a 21-year-old female with 1-week history of cough, sore throat, and difficulty breathing.

Jordan reports she has had this cough for 7 days and that it is not getting better. When the cough started, she was having a runny nose and nasal congestion, with a sore throat. She reports she had a swollen lymph node, but it has since gone away. Her throat no longer hurts, and her nose has stopped running, but she still feels congested. She also reports that she felt febrile for a couple of days, but not anymore. Her cough is productive sometimes, but not always. The only medication she takes is her albuterol as needed.

Jordan has been having difficulty breathing, which is significantly interfering with her normal activities. She has been using her albuterol inhaler every few hours for the last week and waking up short of breath every night.

Prior to the onset of these new symptoms, she was using her inhaler about 3 days a week, in addition to use prior to exercise, and woke up about 3 nights a month, but has only had minor limitations with her regular activities.

She denies chest pain, hemoptysis, fever or chills currently, nausea, vomiting, or diarrhea.

She has no other complaints at this time, except she would like another Depo-Provera® shot.

Prompt: *What does the frequency of her albuterol use tell you?*

The increased use of her inhaler outside of pre-exercise use has dramatically increased and this is a concern.

More than 2 puffs twice a week = uncontrolled. If more than one inhaler is used in a year, it means a better 'controller' or prevention program is needed.

Additional History
Largely unchanged from before except:

Social History
Recently returned from living in California with her boyfriend for the summer
Tobacco: denies
Alcohol: 1–2 drinks on weekends
Drug use: denies

Review of Systems
Diffusely normal except as noted in HPI

Physical Examination (II)
Vitals: P: 65 bpm R: 18 breaths/min T: 98.4° F BP: 115/75 mmHg O2: 96%
Gen: WD/WN female, alert and conversant, NAD
HEENT: NC/AT, sclera anicteric, conjunctiva clear, PERRLA, no sinus tenderness, erythematous throat, exudate, +erythematous turbinates
Neck: no tenderness, no LAD
Lungs: widespread, variably high-pitched wheezes, louder on expiration
CVA: RRR nl S1, S2; no S3, S4; no murmur, rub, or gallop
Extremities: no CCE
Pulses: 2+ bilaterally

Labs
Peak Flow: 250 L/min (normal = 500 L/min)
Peak Flow after Albuterol Treatment: 350 L/min

Prompt: *What do you think is going on?*

Asthma Exacerbation, likely viral etiology, now resolving

Prompt: *What should be done next?*

Treat her exacerbation and consider longer term treatment

Plan
Jordan is diagnosed with an asthma exacerbation, likely of viral etiology, now resolving. Her treatment plan is as follows:

- Xopenex HFA® via nebulizer, 3 or 4 times a day, once every 6 to 8 hours for 5–7 days
- Prednisone dose pack

Return to office in 2 weeks to discuss a long-term treatment plan for asthma.

End of Case

Answers to Learning Objectives

1. **Differentiate key characteristics of asthma in relation to other common obstructive pulmonary disorders, including anatomic lesion site, major pathologic changes, etiology, and signs/symptoms.**

   Expiratory airflow obstruction may be caused by a variety of conditions (Table 8.2) [9]. They are distinguished by distinct anatomic lesions and hence different mechanisms for airflow obstruction.

2. **Explain the underlying pathogenesis of atopic asthma (inflammatory process, cells, and mediators involved), and compare the airway in atopic asthma to a normal bronchus.**

Atopic asthma is the most common type of asthma. It is a classic example of type I IgE-mediated hypersensitivity reaction. The disease usually begins in childhood and is triggered by environmental allergens, such as dust, pollen, roach or animal dander, and foods. A positive family history of asthma is common, and a skin test with the offending antigen in these patients results in an immediate wheal-and-flare reaction. Atopic asthma may also be diagnosed based on evidence of allergen sensitization by serum radioallergosorbent tests, which identify the presence of IgE specific for a panel of allergens.

Asthma is a chronic inflammatory disorder of the airways that causes recurrent episodes of wheezing, breathlessness, chest tightness, and cough, particularly at night and/or in the early morning. These symptoms are usually associated with widespread but variable bronchoconstriction and airflow limitation that is at least partly reversible, either spontaneously or with treatment. Some of the stimuli that trigger attacks in patients would have little or no effect on subjects with normal airways. Many cells play a role in the inflammatory response, in particular lymphocytes, eosinophils, mast cells, macrophages, neutrophils, and epithelial cells.

The major etiologic factors in atopic asthma are a genetic predisposition to type I hypersensitivity ("atopy") and exposure to environmental triggers. In the airways, the initial sensitization to inhaled allergens stimulates induction of T helper 2 (Th2) cells, a type of white blood cell. Th2 cells secrete cytokines that promote allergic inflammation and stimulate B cells to produce IgE and other antibodies. These cytokines include

Table 8.2 Comparison of common obstructive pulmonary disorders

	Asthma	Chronic Bronchitis	Emphysema	Bronchiectasis
Anatomic Lesion Site	Bronchi	Bronchi	Alveoli and terminal bronchioles	Bronchi and bronchioles
Major Pathological Changes	Smooth muscle hypertrophy, mucus hypersecretion, inflammation	Mucus gland hyperplasia, airway inflammation	Alveolar wall destruction, loss of elastic recoil	Airway dilation, wall thickening, mucus buildup
Etiology	Allergens, infections, irritants, genetic factors	Smoking, air pollution, recurrent infections	Smoking, alpha-1 antitrypsin deficiency	Recurrent infections, congenital conditions (cystic fibrosis)
Signs/ Symptoms	Wheezing, episodic dyspnea, cough, reversible airflow limitation	Chronic productive cough, cyanosis, wheezing	Dyspnea, barrel chest, pursed-lip breathing	Chronic cough, purulent sputum, hemoptysis

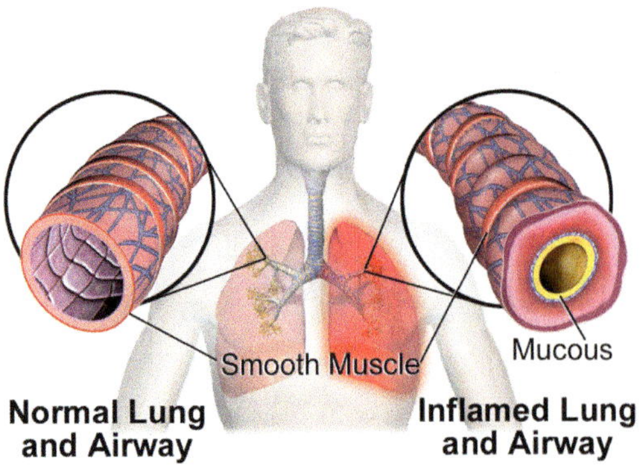

Fig. 8.1 Comparison of normal lung and airway with that of an inflamed lung and airway. (From Blausen.com staff (2014). "Medical gallery of Blausen Medical 2014". WikiJournal of Medicine 1 (2), licensed under CC BY 3.0) *(*https://commons.wikimedia.org/wiki/File:Blausen_0620_Lungs_NormalvsInflamedAirway.png*))*

- IL-4, which stimulates the production of IgE;
- IL-5, which activates locally recruited eosinophils; and
- IL-13, which stimulates mucus secretion from bronchial submucosal glands and also promotes IgE production by B cells.

Figure 8.1 compares a normal lung to that of an inflamed lung. Note the accumulation of mucus in the bronchial lumen of the inflamed airway resulting from an increase in the number of mucus-secreting goblet cells in the mucosa and hypertrophy of submucosal glands. In addition, there is intense chronic inflammation and airway restriction due to recruitment of eosinophils, macrophages, and other inflammatory cells. The basement membrane underlying the mucosal epithelium is thickened, and there is hypertrophy and hyperplasia of smooth muscle cells.

3. **Explain normal pulmonary function testing including defining the measurements made (FEV1, FVC, FEV1/FVC) and briefly explaining how they are determined. Discuss how a bronchodilator affects these variables.**

Pulmonary function tests (PFTs) are used to evaluate lung function by measuring airflow and lung volumes [5]. They include spirometry, lung volume tests, and exercise tests. The primary measurements obtained from spirometry include

- Forced Expiratory Volume in one second (FEV1). This is the volume of air exhaled in the first second of a dynamic expiratory maneuver, expressed in liters. The value reflects the degree of airway obstruction. FEV1 is a function of lung size, elasticity of the lungs, and airway diameter (airway resistance).
- Forced Vital Capacity (FVC). This is the total volume of air that can be forcibly exhaled after a maximal inhalation, expressed in liters.
- FEV1/FVC ratio. This is reflective of the proportion of FVC expelled in the first second, expressed as a percentage. In a normal lung, FEV_1 is $\approx 80\%$ of FVC.

To obtain these measurements, a patient takes a deep breath and exhales forcibly into a spirometer. The device records airflow and volume over time, generating a flow-volume curve. A bronchodilator is administered to assess reversibility of any airway obstruction that is present. In asthma, FEV1 typically increases by $\geq 12\%$ and ≥ 200 ml following administration of a bronchodilator, confirming reversible airway obstruction. In a patient with chronic obstructive pulmonary disease, the response to a bronchodilator is often limited or absent.

The FEV_1 is the most important spirometric variable for assessment of the severity of airflow obstruction. In patients with asthma, the FEV_1 declines in direct and linear proportion with clinical worsening of airway obstruction, and it increases with successful treatment of airway obstruction. The FEV_1/FVC ratio is the most important parameter for detecting airflow limitation in diseases like asthma and chronic obstructive pulmonary disease (COPD). However, once it has been determined that a patient has airway obstruction, the FEV_1/FVC ratio is not useful for gauging severity of disease, since the FVC also tends to decrease with increasing obstruction. The FEV_1, not the FEV_1/FVC ratio, should be used to monitor patients with asthma or COPD [3].

4. **Compare and contrast obstructive lung disorders with restrictive lung disorders using pulmonary function testing. Which one does the patient have?**

Based on pulmonary function tests, pulmonary diseases can be classified into two categories:

- Obstructive diseases, characterized by an increase in resistance to airflow due to partial or complete obstruction at any level, from the trachea and larger bronchi to the terminal and respiratory bronchioles, or
- Restrictive diseases, characterized by reduced expansion of lung parenchyma and decreased total lung capacity.

Spirometry is a fundamental tool in evaluating pulmonary function, aiding in the differentiation between obstructive and restrictive lung diseases. Table 8.3 outlines characteristic spirometric patterns associated with these conditions [10]. In obstructive lung diseases, the hallmark is a reduced FEV_1/FVC ratio, reflecting difficulty in expelling air from the lungs. Conversely, restrictive lung diseases are characterized by a proportional reduction in both FEV_1 and FVC, resulting in a normal or elevated FEV_1/FVC ratio. The patient in this case clearly has an obstructive lung disease.

Table 8.3 Characteristic Patterns of Obstructive and Restrictive Lung Disease as Measured by Spirometry

Parameter	Obstructive Lung Disease	Restrictive Lung Disease
FEV1	Decreased	Decreased
FVC	Normal or decreased	Decreased
FEV1/FVC ratio	Decreased (typically <70%)	Normal or Increased
Interpretation	Indicates airflow limitation due to airway obstruction (e.g., asthma, COPD)	Suggests reduced lung volumes due to parenchymal or extrapulmonary restriction (e.g., pulmonary fibrosis, chest wall disorders)

FEV1—forced expiratory volume; FVC—forced vital capacity

Some tips to keep in mind when evaluating spirometry results are:

- If the FEV_1/FVC ratio is normal and the FEV_1 is greater than 80 percent of predicted, then the spirometry is normal.
- If the FEV_1/FVC is reduced and the FEV_1 is >80 percent predicted, spirometry may be normal; this finding may be due to a prolonged exhalation phase leading to overestimation of the FVC.
- If the FEV_1/FVC ratio is normal, but the FVC is mildly reduced (70 to 80 percent of predicted), the cause may be abdominal obesity or poor technique.
- If the FEV_1/FVC ratio is normal, but the FVC is below 80 percent of predicted, consider referring the patient to a pulmonary function laboratory for measurement of lung volumes and diffusing capacity (DLCO) to assess for a possible restrictive ventilatory defect (e.g., interstitial lung disease or respiratory muscle weakness).
- FEV_1 decreases with age, so the lower limit of normal should be used to detect airway obstruction rather than the absolute value of FEV_1/FVC.

5. **Categorize and describe the various treatments for asthma, including rescue vs. maintenance medication and the goals of asthma treatment.**

Asthma management involves a combination of rescue and maintenance medications, each serving distinct roles in controlling symptoms and preventing exacerbations [11].

Rescue Medications

Also known as quick-relief medications, these are used to provide rapid alleviation of acute asthma symptoms or to prevent exercise-induced bronchoconstriction.

- Short-Acting Beta$_2$-Agonists (SABAs): These bronchodilators, such as albuterol, act quickly to relax airway smooth muscles, easing breathing during an asthma attack. They are typically administered via inhalers and are effective within minutes.
- Anticholinergics: Medications like ipratropium serve as alternative or adjunctive therapy to SABAs, particularly in emergency settings. They work by inhibiting muscarinic receptors and reducing the intrinsic vagal tone of the airway, leading to bronchodilation.
- Systemic Corticosteroids: Oral or intravenous corticosteroids are used as adjuncts to SABAs for severe exacerbations to reduce airway inflammation. Due to potential side effects, they are not intended for long-term use.

Maintenance Medications

These long-term control medications are taken daily to manage chronic symptoms and prevent asthma attacks by addressing underlying inflammation and hyperresponsiveness.

- Inhaled Corticosteroids (ICS): Considered the most effective long-term therapy, ICS reduce airway inflammation and hyperreactivity. Examples include beclometasone, budesonide, and fluticasone.
- Long-Acting Beta$_2$-Agonists (LABAs): Used in combination with ICS, LABAs like formoterol and salmeterol provide prolonged bronchodilation (at least 12 hours after a single dose), aiding in symptom control. Monotherapy with LABAs is not recommended due to safety concerns.
- Leukotriene Receptor Antagonists (LTRAs): Oral medications such as montelukast block leukotrienes, which are inflammatory mediators, thus helping to prevent asthma symptoms.
- Long-Acting Muscarinic Antagonists (LAMAs): Agents like tiotropium provide additional bronchodilation and are used as add-on therapy in certain cases.
- Biologic Therapies: Targeted treatments such as omalizumab (anti-IgE) and mepolizumab (anti-IL-5) are used for severe asthma with specific phenotypes, aiming to reduce exacerbations and improve control.

Non-Pharmacologic Treatments

- Avoidance
  - Wipe floor with damp cloth, mite-proof mattress covers, regularly wash bedding with high heat, and change air filters routinely
- Special breathing techniques
  - Relaxing effects
  - Calm and controlled breathing during asthma attacks
  - Yoga
  - "Pursed-lips" breathing
- Regular exercise
  - Improves performance of heart and lungs
  - Research has shown long-term symptom reduction
  - Some evidence that interval training can prevent exercise-induced asthma
    High-energy exercise alternated with periods of rest
  - Warm up, keep rescue medication handy, or use reliever medication before exercise
- Smoking cessation

The goal of asthma therapy is to effectively manage asthma symptoms, prevent asthma attacks, maintain near-normal lung function, and minimize the interference of asthma on daily activities by controlling symptoms and reducing the risk of future exacerbations, all while minimizing adverse effects from medications used to treat it [11]. The expert panel recommends that the goal of asthma therapy is to maintain control of asthma with the least amount of medication and hence minimal risk for adverse effects.

Key aspects of asthma therapy goals include:

- Symptom control: Preventing chronic symptoms like wheezing, coughing, chest tightness, and breathlessness by keeping symptoms under control
- Preventing asthma attacks: Avoiding exacerbations and minimizing the need for emergency room (ER) visits or hospitalizations by managing triggers and using appropriate medications
- Preserving lung function: Maintaining optimal lung capacity and function
- Maintaining normal activity levels: Allowing individuals to participate in daily activities such as work, school, and exercise without limitations
- In frequent use of rescue medications: Use of SABA for quick relief of symptoms (≤2 days a week)

6. **Describe an asthma exacerbation and how to recognize life-threatening signs. Can children outgrow asthma?**

Asthma exacerbations are acute episodes of progressively worsening shortness of breath, cough, wheezing, and chest tightness, or some combination of these symptoms. Exacerbations are characterized by decreases in expiratory airflow that can be determined by spirometry. Milder exacerbations may be managed at home, while more serious exacerbations may require an urgent care visit, an ER visit, or a hospital admission. The most severe exacerbations require admission to the intensive care unit (ICU) for optimal monitoring and treatment.

The classic acute asthma attack lasts up to several hours. Symptoms of chest tightness, dyspnea, wheezing, and cough with or without sputum production can persist at a low level constantly. In severe cases, symptoms can persist for days or weeks. Under these conditions, airflow obstruction might be so extreme as to cause severe cyanosis and even death. With appropriate therapy to relieve the attacks, most individuals with asthma can maintain a productive life.

Life-threatening signs of an asthma attack to watch for include:

- Severe shortness of breath: struggling to breathe, can't catch breath, can't speak or eat
- Cyanosis: bluish skin or lips
- Decreased alertness: severe drowsiness, confusion
- Rapid worsening of symptoms: rescue medication is no longer helping
- Inability to breathe while lying down
- Sweating
- Tachycardia

If any of these occur, 911 should be called, or the patient should be taken to the ER.

Can children outgrow asthma? The majority of opinion suggests no. Asthma is a lifelong disease. While some children experience a reduction or absence of symptoms as they grow older, this does not equate to a complete cure. Studies indicate that approximately 50% of children with asthma may see their symptoms diminish or disappear during adolescence; however, these symptoms can return in adulthood [12]. Children who had asthma as children and no longer have it as teens may just be in remission. Without a long-term epidemiological study of young asthmatics in the U.S., it is impossible to determine who might go into remission. Children may become asymptomatic, but the chronic changes in their lungs most likely don't go away.

There are several theories that attempt to explain why asthma symptoms may diminish or disappear after childhood [13]. One theory has to do with lung maturation. As children grow, so do the airways in their lungs, potentially reducing airway hyperresponsiveness. Boys, in particular, often show improvement, possibly due to changes in airway size and responsiveness. The immune system also matures, leading to a shift away from the Th2-dominant inflammatory response characteristic of atopic asthma, and some children develop immune tolerance to allergens. Additionally, some children experience fewer asthma symptoms as they grow older due to changes in their environment. Moving away from allergens such as pet dander, dust mites, or tobacco smoke may lead to symptom improvement. Even if symptoms disappear, many former childhood asthmatics remain at risk for recurrence in adulthood, especially with triggers like viral infections or occupational exposures.

7. **Identify indications for and the efficacy of influenza and pneumococcal vaccines in people with asthma. Discuss how poor living, working, and environmental conditions can contribute to respiratory tract disea**se.

For persons with asthma, influenza vaccination has been shown to prevent 59–78% of asthma attacks leading to emergency visits and/or hospitalizations [14]. Thus, for persons with asthma, vaccination may be effective in both reducing influenza infection and asthma attacks.

Pneumococcal disease can be very serious in persons with asthma. Corticosteroids, a common asthma medicine, may also increase risk for pneumonia because they suppress the immune system. Health care providers suggest that those with asthma also get the vaccine for pneumococcal disease [15].

Poor living, working, and environmental conditions can significantly contribute to respiratory tract disease by exposing individuals to irritants like air pollution, dust, mold, chemicals, and allergens, which can inflame the airways, damage lung tissue, and increase susceptibility to infections, particularly in poorly ventilated spaces, leading to conditions like asthma, COPD, and allergic rhinitis; this is especially concerning in areas with high levels of overcrowding and limited access to clean air and sanitation. Exposure to air pollution puts people at risk for lung cancer, heart attacks, stroke, and, in extreme cases, premature death. Occupational and environmental lung diseases are caused by the inhalation of chemical irritants, allergens, or toxins in work or home environments. Excessive use of potent disinfectants and cleaning agents can release volatile organic compounds (VOCs) into the air, which may cause respiratory issues. Most diseases are caused by repeated, long-term exposure, but even a one-time or indirect contact with a hazardous agent can result in lung diseases with lasting effects [16].

Ways to mitigate these environmental factors include improving indoor air quality by enhancing airflow, using air purifiers with HEPA filters, and minimizing exposure to toxic cleaning products by choosing alternatives such as hydrogen peroxide and vinegar. Choose to stay indoors during air pollution alert days.

Acknowledgement The case scenario was provided by Bryan K. Hendrikson, M.D.

Exam Questions

1. A 28-year-old male presents with chronic cough and shortness of breath on exertion. It is worse at night and when he spends time outside. He reports he used an inhaler when he was a kid, but it stopped sometime in high school. He also has a history of seasonal allergies and atopic dermatitis. Which of the following would you expect upon pulmonary function testing with spirometry in comparison to normal?
   A. FVC decreased, FEV1 decreased, and FEV1/FVC increased
   B. FVC normal, FEV1 normal, FEV1/FVC normal
   C. FVC normal, FEV1 decreased, FEV1/FVC decreased
   D. FVC decreased, FEV1 normal, FEV1/FVC decreased

   Answer: C

   Learning Objective: #4 Compare and contrast obstructive lung disorders with restrictive lung disorders using pulmonary function testing. Which one does the patient have?

   Explanation: This patient most likely is having a recurrence of childhood asthma. As there is airflow limitation due to airway obstruction in asthma, while FVC can remain normal, FEV1 decreases, and thus, the ratio of FEV1/FVC also decreases. A is incorrect, as these are the results for someone with restrictive lung disease. B is incorrect, as this is for a patient without any lung disease. While it is possible for FVC and FEV1/FVC to be normal early in obstructive disease, it is unlikely for obstructive disease to have anything but a decreased FEV1. D is incorrect, as this is an unlikely scenario in results of spirometry.

2. A 15-year-old boy is diagnosed with atopic asthma and is prescribed a maintenance inhaler for asthma control. Which of the following is the purpose of the corticosteroid in the patient's maintenance inhaler?
   A. Reduce bronchoconstriction
   B. Reduce inflammation of bronchial walls
   C. Inhibit leukotriene signaling

Answer: B

Learning Objective: #5 Categorize and describe the various treatments for asthma, including rescue vs. maintenance medication and the goals of asthma treatment

Explanation: Corticosteroids target the inflammatory processes in asthma, leading to long-term prevention of symptoms. A is incorrect, as rescue inhalers, such as albuterol, are primarily beta-agonists, which reduce bronchoconstriction but have no effect on inflammation. C is not the best answer, as while corticosteroids can inhibit leukotriene production in some cases, they don't always block the release of leukotrienes. Newer drugs such as montelukast target leukotriene signaling specifically.

3. An 8-year-old girl recently diagnosed with asthma is prescribed a quick-relief medication to relax her bronchial smooth muscle for immediate relief during an asthma attack. Which of the following is the mechanism of action of the most likely prescribed medication?
   A. Activation of sympathetic beta 2 adrenergic receptors
   B. Inhibition of sympathetic cholinergic receptors
   C. Activation of parasympathetic muscarinic receptors
   D. Activation of alpha-adrenergic receptors
   E. Inhibition of beta 2 adrenergic receptors

Answer: A

Learning Objective: #5 Categorize and describe the various treatments for asthma, including rescue vs. maintenance medication and the goals of asthma treatment

Explanation: Bronchodilators, such as albuterol, are short-acting beta$_2$-agonists (SABAs). They act quickly to relax airway smooth muscle by stimulating beta 2 adrenergic receptors, easing breathing during an asthma attack. They are typically administered via inhalers and are effective within minutes. B is incorrect, as, unlike the parasympathetic system, the sympathetic cholinergic system does not play a major role in regulating airway tone in most situations and would not be related to the patient's most likely prescribed medication. C is incorrect, as activation of parasympathetic muscarinic receptors causes bronchoconstriction and increased mucus secretion, opposite the desired therapeutic effect. D is incorrect, as activation of alpha-adrenergic receptors in the lungs primarily causes bronchoconstriction by contracting the smooth muscle in the airways, essentially narrowing the airway passages and making it harder to breathe; this effect is mainly due to the activation of alpha-1 adrenergic receptors in the pulmonary vasculature, which can also contribute to increased blood pressure in the lungs. E is incorrect, as this would cause bronchoconstriction, the opposite of the desired effect.

References

1. Benich JJ, Carek PJ. Evaluation of the patient with chronic cough. Am Fam Physician. 2011;84(8):887–92.
2. deShazo RD, Kemp SF Pharmacotherapy of allergic rhinitis. UpToDate. 2024. Retrieved from www.uptodate.com.
3. Lange-Vaidya N. Asthma in adolescents and adults: evaluation and diagnosis. UpToDate. 2024. Retrieved from www.uptodate.com.

4. Hankinson JL. Estimated/Expected Peak Expiratory Flow(PeakFlow). MDCalc. 2025. Retrieved from www.mdcalc.com (https://www.mdcalc.com/calc/790/estimated-expected-peak-expiratory-flow-peak-flow).
5. Stanojevic S, Kaminsky DA, Miller MR, et al. ERS/ATS technical standard on interpretive strategies for routine lung function tests. Eur Respir J. 2022;60(1):2101499. https://doi.org/10.1183/13993003.01499-2021.
6. Akar-Ghibril N, Casale T, Custovic A, Phipatanakul W. Allergic endotypes and phenotypes of asthma. J Allergy Clin Immunol Pract. 2020;8(2):429–40. https://doi.org/10.1016/j.jaip.2019.11.008. Erratum in: J Allergy Clin Immunol Pract 2020 May;8(5):1779.
7. Millard M, Hart M, Barnes S. Validation of rules of two™ as a paradigm for assessing asthma control. Proc (Bayl Univ Med Cent). 2014;27(2):79–82.
8. Wolford RW, Goyal A, Belgam Syed SY, et al. Pharyngitis. [Updated 2023 May 1]. In: StatPearls. Retrieved from: https://www.ncbi.nlm.nih.gov/books/NBK519550/
9. Global Initiative for Chronic Obstructive Lung Disease. Global strategy for the diagnosis, management, and prevention of chronic obstructive pulmonary disease: 2023 report. 2023. https://goldcopd.org.
10. Pellegrino R, Viegi G, Brusasco V, et al. Interpretative strategies for lung function tests. Eur Respir J. 2005;26(5):948–68.
11. Cloutier MM, et al. Focused updates to the asthma management guidelines: a report from the national asthma education and prevention program coordinating committee expert panel working group. J Allergy Clin Immunol. 2020;146(6):1217–70.
12. Ross KR, et al. Severe asthma during childhood and adolescence: a longitudinal study. J Allergy Clin Immunol. 2020 Jan;145(1):140–6.
13. Koefoed HJL, Vonk JM, Koppelman GH. Predicting the course of asthma from childhood until early adulthood. Curr Opin Allergy Clin Immunol. 2022;22(2):115–22.
14. Vasileiou E, et al. Effectiveness of influenza vaccines in asthma: a systematic review and meta-analysis. Clin Infect Dis. 2017;65(8):1388–95.
15. CDC; Advisory Committee on Immunization Practices. Updated recommendations for prevention of invasive pneumococcal disease among adults using the 23-valent pneumococcal polysaccharide vaccine (PPSV23). MMWR Morb Mortal Wkly Rep. 2010;59:1102–6.
16. Holden KA, Lee AR, Hawcutt DB, Sinha IP. The impact of poor housing and indoor air quality on respiratory health in children. Breathe (Sheff). 2023;19(2):230058.

9 Painful Breathing

Kelby Schaeffler

Learning Objectives

1. Explain the anatomy and physiology of pleuritic chest pain and explore a broad differential diagnosis.
2. Describe the clinical approach to the diagnosis of suspected pulmonary embolism.
3. Briefly discuss the clinical presentation and findings in the different forms of histoplasmosis (acute, chronic, and disseminated), as well as the treatment approach for these different clinical scenarios.
4. Compare and contrast the geographical distribution, carriers/disease vectors, and main clinical features of the systemic respiratory fungi (histoplasmosis, blastomycosis, coccidiomycosis, and paracoccidioidomycosis).
5. Define sepsis and explain the criteria for diagnosing a patient with sepsis. Did our patient meet these criteria? Does the absence of signs such as leukocytosis and fever rule out infectious processes?

Chief Complaint: "It hurts to breathe"

Prompt: Based on this patient's chief complaint, what differential diagnoses can you think of?

K. Schaeffler (✉)
Emergency Physician, University of Arizona College of Medicine Phoenix, Phoenix, AZ, USA

The differential diagnosis for pleuritic chest pain is broad and clinicians should prioritize evaluating the most critical causes first [1].

- Cardiac
  - Pericarditis
  - Myocardial infarction (not typically pleuritic pain but must be considered)
- Vascular
  - Pulmonary embolism (most common cause of pleuritic chest pain in the ED)
- Pulmonary
  - Pneumothorax
  - Infectious
    - Bacterial pneumonia
    - Viral (adenovirus, coxsackieviruses, cytomegalovirus, EBV, mumps, influenza, parainfluenza, RSV)
    - TB pleuritis
    - Fungal pneumonia (histoplasmosis, blastomycosis, coccidiomycosis, cryptococcus)
  - Inflammatory
    - Reactive eosinophilic pleuritis
    - Sarcoidosis
  - Exposure
    - Asbestosis
    - Some medications known to cause pleural disease: amiodarone, bleomycin, bromocriptine, cyclophosphamide, methotrexate, minoxidil (would not expect students to know these)

C. A. Standley (ed.), *Biomedical Science and Clinical Foundations*,
https://doi.org/10.1007/978-3-031-98353-5_9

- Genetic
  - Familial Mediterranean fever
- Hematologic/Oncologic
  - Malignancy
  - Sickle cell disease
- Rheumatologic
  - Lupus pleuritis
  - Rheumatoid pleuritis
  - Sjogren's syndrome

History of Present Illness: A 26-year-old previously healthy African American woman presents to the emergency department with a 1-week history of worsening pleuritic chest pain. She recalls the development of a dull, substernal ache beginning several days after a 5-hour flight home from Puerto Rico, where she spent 3 weeks hiking in national parks and exploring several caves. She now describes a constant ache in the middle of her chest that feels sharp with deep inspiration or coughing. She has not taken any medication for the pain. She does report a mild dry cough, feeling mildly short of breath, headache, fatigue, and subjective fever. She denies hemoptysis, weight loss, night sweats, leg swelling, or diarrhea. No changes in appetite or urination. No history of blood clots, no personal or family history of coagulopathy, and no history of cancer.

Past Medical History: None

Medications: Combination estrogen/progesterone OCP (started 10 months ago).

Prompt: Is her use of OCP a concern?

Risk of VTE in current users of OCP's decreases with duration of use and decreasing estrogen use [2].

Allergies: None

Surgical History: None

Social History:

Monogamous relationship with male partner

Lifetime nonsmoker but is exposed to second-hand smoke by boyfriend

Drinks 1–2 alcoholic beverages per week. Denies drug use.

Has no pets

Family History: Mother has rheumatoid arthritis

Review of Systems: Negative except as noted in the HPI

Prompt: What parts of the patient's history are especially relevant to the chief complaint?

- Young age and lack of medical history or other risk factors make ACS less likely.
- OCPs and history of recent flight are risk factors for pulmonary embolism.
- Description of the chest pain as pleuritic, gradual, and progressive, with shortness of breath making PE, inflammatory, or infectious etiologies more likely.
- Cough and subjective fever are concerning for infection, although both could be present with PE.
- Recent travel to tropical climates, as well as hiking/cave exploring make many infectious diseases possible (such as histoplasmosis, rabies, leptospirosis, tick-borne diseases, Lyme disease, and others).
- Absence of rash is reassuring for some infectious diseases such as Lyme disease.

Prompt: Review your key hypotheses

- Pulmonary embolism, bronchitis, bacterial pneumonia, fungal pneumonia

Prompt: What physical exam findings may help you differentiate the causes of the patient's symptoms?

- Vital signs: fever could point towards infection, tachycardia and/or hypotension could suggest infection or PE
- Lung sounds: look for presence of coarse breath sounds, focal findings such as egophony/bronchophony and dullness to percussion

may suggest focal pneumonia, compare breath sounds bilaterally
- Chest wall: is the substernal pain reproducible with palpation?
- Inspect skin for rashes/lesions/bites
- Unilateral lower extremity edema/erythema/warmth would be concerning for DVT/PE

Physical Exam

Vital signs: BP 100/60, P 105, RR 18, O2 98% on RA, T 38.2 °C.

Gen: Well-developed, well-nourished, alert, and conversant, in no acute distress.

HEENT: Normocephalic, atraumatic. PERRLA, EOMI, MM moist, oropharynx without erythema or exudates.

Neck: Supple, no LAD.

Chest: No tenderness to palpation. Symmetric expansion. Lungs clear to auscultation bilaterally. No wheezes, rhonchi, or rales.

CV: Mildly tachycardic, normal S1, S2, s S3, S4, murmurs or rubs. JVP 5 cm H20.

Abdomen: Soft, nontender, nondistended.

Extremities: FROM in all joints, no joint swelling, no edema, no tenderness, no warmth. 2+ symmetric DP, PT, and radial pulses.

Skin: Warm, dry, normal capillary refill, no rashes.

Neuro: A&O x4, no focal weakness.

Psych: Normal behavior and mentation.

Prompt: Anything concerning in the physical exam?

Borderline low blood pressure and mild tachycardia should raise suspicion for sepsis, hemodynamic instability from large PE, etc. Temperature may be elevated due to infection, and a low-grade fever can be seen in PE.

Prompt: What initial tests would you like to order?

- EKG
- CXR (looking for consolidations, pleural effusion, interstitial edema, bronchial thickening, wedge infarct, etc.)
- CBC, CMP
- D-dimer
- Blood cultures
- Urine pregnancy test

Prompt: Review algorithm for work-up of suspected pulmonary embolism.

The **Pulmonary Embolism Rule-Out Criteria (PERC) rule** [3] can be used when pre-test probability gestalt is low. If all eight criteria of the PERC rule are negative, there is a < 2% chance of PE and no further work-up may be indicated.

- Age < 50
- HR >100
- O2 sat on room air <95%
- Unilateral leg swelling
- Hemoptysis
- Recent surgery or trauma (<4 weeks ago requiring general anesthesia)
- Prior PE or DVT
- Hormone use (OCP's, hormone replacement, or estrogenic hormone use)

The patient's score is addressed in learning objective #2.

If one or more of the PERC criteria are positive, and history and physical suggest possible PE, you may use the Well's Score (Table 9.1) to further risk stratify patients and provide an estimate pre-test probability of PE, which can guide next steps in testing [4]. The patient's score is addressed in learning objective #2.

Laboratory and Imaging Findings

A complete blood count (CBC) and complete metabolic panel (CMP) are shown in Tables 9.2 and 9.3, respectively.

EKG: Sinus tachycardia, rate of 102 beats per minute. Normal axis, normal intervals. No ST elevations or depressions, no T wave inversions.

Chest X-Ray: Patchy right upper lobe infiltrate, enlargement of right hilar lymph nodes

D-dimer: 583 ng/mL (reference range < 500 ng/mL)

Table 9.1 Wells score criteria

Criteria	Absent	Present
Clinical signs and symptoms of DVT	No (0)	Yes (+3)
PE is #1 diagnosis or equally likely	No (0)	Yes (+3)
Heart rate > 100	No (0)	Yes (+1.5)
Immobilization at least 3 days OR surgery in the previous 4 weeks	No (0)	Yes (+1.5)
Previous, objectively diagnosed PE or DVT	No (0)	Yes (+1.5)
Hemoptysis	No (0)	Yes (+1)
Malignancy with treatment within 6 months or palliative	No (0)	Yes (+1)

0–1 points: Low risk, 1.3% incidence of PE. Consider D-dimer
2–6 points: Intermediate risk, 16.2% incidence of PE. Consider D-dimer or CTA
7+ points: High risk, 37.5% incidence of PE. Order CTA, D-dimer not recommended

Table 9.2 CBC

Component (units)	Patient	Normal range
White blood count ($\times 10^6$/L)	7500	4000–10,000
Hemoglobin (g/dL0	13.1	11.5–16.4
Hematocrit (%)	38.5	36.0–48.0
Platelets ($\times 10^6$/L)	244,000	150,000–450,000

Table 9.3 CMP

Component (units)	Patient	Normal range
Na (mEq/L)	139	136–145
K (mEq/L)	3.6	3.4–5.0
Bicarb (mEq/L)	19	22–31
Cl (mEq/L)	101	98–107
BUN (mg/dL)	6	6–23
Cr (mg/dL)	0.6	0.5–1.2
Glucose (mg/dL)	85	70–100
AST (IU/L)	15	10–50
ALT (IU/L)	11	10–50
Alk Phos (units/L)	65	35–130
T bili (mg/dL)	0.7	0.1–1.0

CTA chest (Ordered after D-dimer resulted positive): No defects in pulmonary arterial filling. The mediastinal windows show hilar and mediastinal lymphadenopathy in both lungs, findings that suggest a reactive process. The lung windows show diffuse ground-glass nodules, with trace bilateral pleural effusions. No pneumothorax, no consolidations.

Prompt: Review your top differential diagnoses at this point.

- Atypical bacterial pneumonia
- Fungal pneumonia (Atypical bacterial or fungal pathogens can cause multifocal ground-glass nodules, mediastinal lymphadenopathy, and pleural effusions. Fungal or atypical bacterial infections should be considered, given this patient's fever and recent travel to Puerto Rico; a more detailed history of exposures may help to ascertain possible pathogens.)
- May consider sarcoidosis (Young, African-American female with new-onset chest pain, shortness of breath, pulmonary nodules, and mediastinal lymphadenopathy. Although sarcoidosis is most often accompanied by extrapulmonary features when patients present acutely. Lofgren's syndrome is the classic acute presentation of sarcoidosis—triad of hilar lymphadenopathy, arthralgias, and erythema nodosum)

Hospital Admission:
The patient was admitted to the hospital for further workup. She continued to have a temperature as high as 38.3 °C. The patient was treated empirically with levofloxacin for presumed pneumonia.

Blood, urine, and sputum cultures: No growth to date

HIV serologic testing negative

Upon further questioning of the patient about potential exposures, you discover that during her recent travel to Puerto Rico, the caves she visited were densely populated by bats and their droppings (guano) covered the cave floors.

Prompt: Given the labs and imaging findings and this further history, what is now your key hypothesis?

- Histoplasmosis (especially given the bat guano exposure)

Prompt: What further testing might you do to confirm this diagnosis?

- Urine and serum antigen testing for histoplasma
- Biopsy of mediastinal/hilar lymph nodes
- Bronchoalveolar lavage with bacterial and fungal cultures

Results of Additional Testing:
Biopsy specimens of the R mediastinal and hilar lymph nodes were obtained via endobronchial ultrasound-guided fine-needle aspiration. Preliminary histologic analysis revealed a few yeast forms, which suggested the possibility of fungal infection.

Bronchoalveolar lavage was also performed, and samples were sent for bacterial and fungal acid-fast staining and culture.

Histopathological Analysis:
Necrotizing granulomatous inflammation and a few yeast forms were observed that were consistent with a finding of histoplasmosis. Staining for acid-fast bacilli and gram-positive species was negative.

Prompt: What are the next steps in management?

- Infectious disease consultation.
- Option 1: Defer antifungal therapy. Most acute cases of histoplasmosis are self-limited. The patient is immunocompetent, the disease is not disseminated and not life-threatening.
- Option 2: Start Itraconazole (6–12-week course).
- If this patient were immunocompromised or if the disease was severe and life-threatening, treatment would be amphotericin B

Management and Outcome:
The patient was initially treated conservatively, without antimicrobial therapy, and was discharged with NSAIDs and a short course of oxycodone for pain, after which her symptoms abated somewhat. Serologic tests for histoplasmosis were negative, as were tests for antigens in urine and serum samples. Several weeks later, fungal cultures of the mediastinal lymph-node aspirates grew *H. capsulatum*.

Her fevers resolved, but pleuritic CP persisted over the ensuing 3 weeks, at which point treatment with Itraconazole was started. After a 12-week course of treatment, the respiratory symptoms and pain resolved completely. The results of liver function tests were unremarkable throughout the course of treatment.

End of Case

Learning Objective Answers

1. **Explain the anatomy and physiology of pleuritic chest pain and explore a broad differential diagnosis.**

Pleuritic chest pain is a sudden, intense, sharp/stabbing/burning pain in the chest with inhalation or exhalation and can be exacerbated by coughing, sneezing, or laughing.

The visceral pleura is innervated by the vagus nerve and sympathetic fibers and does have pain-sensing fibers. The parietal pleura has somatic nerves and therefore senses pain due to trauma or irritation. Parietal pleura at the periphery of the rib cage and lateral diaphragm is innervated by intercostal nerves and therefore causes pain localized in the cutaneous distribution of those nerves. The phrenic nerve innervates the central diaphragm and irritation here can cause pain radiating to the ipsilateral neck/shoulder.

Differential Diagnosis for Pleuritic Chest Pain:
*PE, MI, pericarditis, aortic dissection, pneumonia, and pneumothorax are six life-threatening conditions that must be considered initially.

*Pulmonary embolism is the most common serious cause, found in 5–21% of patients who present to an ED with pleuritic chest pain (AAFP)

- Cardiac
  - Pericarditis
  - Myocardial infarction (not typically pleuritic pain but must be considered)
- Vascular
  - Pulmonary embolism (most common cause of pleuritic chest pain in the ED)
- Pulmonary
  - Pneumothorax
  - Infectious
    Bacterial pneumonia
    Viral (adenovirus, coxsackieviruses, cytomegalovirus, EBV, mumps, influenza, parainfluenza, RSV)
    TB pleuritis
    Fungal pneumonia (histoplasmosis, blastomycosis, coccidiomycosis, cryptococcus)
  - Inflammatory
    Reactive eosinophilic pleuritis
    Sarcoidosis
  - Exposure
    Asbestosis
    Some medications known to cause pleural disease: amiodarone, bleomycin, bromocriptine, cyclophosphamide, methotrexate, minoxidil (would not expect students to know these)
  - Genetic
    Familial Mediterranean fever
  - Hematologic/Oncologic
    Malignancy
    Sickle cell disease
  - Rheumatologic
    Lupus pleuritis
    Rheumatoid pleuritis
    Sjogren's syndrome

2. **Describe the clinical approach to the diagnosis and management of suspected pulmonary embolism.**

In the case of suspected PE in a patient without hemodynamic instability, first assess the clinical probability of PE. If the probability of PE is low, intermediate, or unlikely, perform a D-dimer test. If this is negative, no treatment is needed. If this is positive, perform a CTPA. If PE is confirmed, proceed to treatment. If negative, no treatment is needed. If there is high clinical probability of a PE, proceed right to a CTPA. If negative, no treatment is needed, although further investigation may be warranted. If PE is confirmed, proceed to treatment.

Calculate a Well's score for the patient [4].

The patient's results are denoted in the parentheses for each of the Well's score criteria:

1. Clinical signs and symptoms of DVT (leg swelling, pain with palpation) → 0 points (no signs of DVT)
2. PE is the most likely diagnosis → 3 points (PE is a leading consideration based on history)
3. Heart rate > 100 bpm → 1.5 points (HR = 105)
4. Immobilization (≥3 days) or surgery in the past 4 weeks → 0 points (recent travel but not immobilization)
5. Previous history of DVT/PE → 0 points (no history)
6. Hemoptysis → 0 points (none reported)
7. Active cancer (treatment within 6 months, or palliative care) → 0 points (no cancer)

Total Well's score for this patient: 4.5 points

Interpretation of the Well's score: *<2 points:* low-risk (1.3% incidence of PE) - consider D-dimer or use PERC criteria (below) to rule-out PE

2–6 points: intermediate-risk (16.2% incidence of PE)—consider D-dimer or CTA

7+ points: high-risk (37.5% incidence of PE)—order CTA. D-dimer not recommended

The patient falls in the intermediate risk category.

PERC (PE-Rule Out Criteria) [3]: If all criteria present in low-risk patient, PE can be ruled out.

This patient's answer to each of the criteria is denoted by the arrows:

1. Age ≥ 50 → No
2. HR ≥ 100 → Yes
3. Oxygen saturation < 95% → No
4. Unilateral leg swelling → No

5. Hemoptysis → No
6. Recent surgery/trauma (past 4 weeks) → No
7. Prior history of PE/DVT → No
8. Hormone use (OCP, HRT, etc.) → Yes

This patient fails PERC due to HR ≥ 100 and OCP use → PE cannot be ruled out without further testing.

If the patient is hemodynamically *unstable* → bedside Echo → if presence of RV dysfunction, treat for PE (consider anticoagulation vs. thrombolysis vs. embolectomy)

3. **Discuss the clinical presentation and findings in the different forms of Histoplasmosis (acute, chronic, and disseminated), as well as treatment approach for the different clinical scenarios.**

Like the other systemic fungi, histoplasma is asymptomatic/subclinical in most people [5]. Histoplasmosis can be acute or chronic, and in immunocompromised patients, the disease can become disseminated (Table 9.4).

Treatment approach: [5, 6]

In most instances, acute histoplasmosis is self-limiting in immunocompetent patients and requires no definitive antifungal therapy.

Local and mild infections → azole drugs.

Disseminated, chronic cavitary, and acute forms are treated with itraconazole for 1 year if they are NOT life-threatening.

Life-threatening disease or an immunocompromised host → amphotericin B (a nasty drug with lots of side effects, which is why it is reserved for only potentially life-threatening infections).

4. **Compare and contrast the geographical distribution, carriers/disease vectors, and main clinical features of the systemic respiratory fungi (histoplasmosis, blastomycosis, coccidiomycosis, and paracoccidioidomycosis).**

A comparison of fungal infections of the lungs is presented in Table 9.5.

5. **Define sepsis and explain the criteria for diagnosing a patient with sepsis. Did our patient meet these criteria? Does the absence of signs such as leukocytosis and fever rule out infectious process?**

Sepsis is defined as life-threatening organ dysfunction caused by a dysregulated host response to infection [9].

The guidelines for the diagnosis of sepsis have evolved over time, and still several criteria are used for diagnosis and early identification of sepsis. In general, it is important to understand the meaning of the SIRS criteria, and how to use the qSOFA index to identify patients likely to develop sepsis.

Table 9.4 Categorization of histoplasmosis and the clinical and radiographic findings

Disease form	Clinical features	Radiographic findings
Acute	After incubation period of 2 weeks, fevers, dyspnea, pleurisy, and cough present Inflammatory arthralgias	Ground-glass nodules in lungs Unilateral mediastinal or hilar adenopathy Mediastinal granulomas Pleural effusions (rare)
Chronic	Productive cough, fever, night sweats, weight loss Formation of esophageal or bronchial fistulas (rare)	Fibrocavitary lesions in upper lobes of lungs Calcified hilar and mediastinal lymph nodes Mediastinal granulomas Formation of histoplasmomas (rare)
Disseminated	Anemia, leukopenia, transaminitis, adrenal insufficiency Seen in immunocompromised patients	Calcified lesions in lungs, liver, spleen, GI tract, bone marrow, skin, and CNS

Table 9.5 Comparison of systemic respiratory fungal infections [7, 8]

	Histoplasmosis	Blastomycosis	Coccidiomycosis	Paracoccidioidomycosis
Geographical distribution	Mississippi and Ohio River Valleys, Central America	Great Lakes and Ohio River Valley	California and Southwestern US	Latin America
Spore origin	Bird or bat droppings (cave spelunking, farmers with chicken coops)	Dust	Dust (especially during dust storms, near construction sites, following earthquakes)	Dust
Transmission	Spores inhaled into lungs and digested by macrophages	Spores inhaled into lungs then replicates through single broad-based budding	Spores inhaled into lungs and forms spherules of endospores in the lungs, eventually rupturing and spreading through lungs and possibly rest of the body	Spores inhaled into lungs
Types of fungus	Dimorphic (mold in the cold, yeast in the heat)	Dimorphic (mold in the cold, yeast in the heat)	Dimorphic (mold in the cold, but spherule of endospores in the body/heat)	Dimorphic (mold in the cold, yeast in the heat)
Diagnosis	Rapid urine or serum antigen test KOH prep of tissue sample (sputum or biopsy) showing macrophages filled with histoplasma Serology (Ab titers)	KOH prep (round yeast with single broad-based bud) Urine antigen test Serology (Ab titers)	Clinical diagnosis KOH prep of sputum Serology (Ab titers)	Clinical diagnosis KOH prep Serology (Ab titers)
Size compared to RBC	Much smaller than RBS (10–100's of histoplasma in each macrophage)	About the same size as RBC	Larger than RBC	Much larger than RBC
Clinical presentation	Subclinical/Asymptomatic in most people Can cause granuloma formation and pneumonia if granulomas calcify, can cause chronic pulmonary issues that can mimic TB	Subclinical/Asymptomatic in most people Can cause acute fungal pneumonia	Subclinical/Asymptomatic in most people Can present as self-limited acute pneumonia with fever, sweats, arthralgias Lasts several weeks	Acute pneumonia Lymphadenopathy (especially cervical)
Extrapulmonary findings	Erythema nodosum	Skin ulcers Osteomyelitis	Arthralgias Erythema nodosum	Upper respiratory symptoms Muscosal ulcers in mouth Lymphadenopathy
Chest X-ray findings	Hilar/mediastinal lymphadenopathy Focal consolidations	Patchy alveolar infiltrates May also see cavitary lesions	Unremarkable in majority of patients Can show lung nodules or cavities or both	Granulomas

(continued)

Table 9.5 (continued)

	Histoplasmosis	Blastomycosis	Coccidiomycosis	Paracoccidioidomycosis
Features in dissemination	Hepatosplenomegaly with calcifications	Skin ulcers Osteomyelitis	Skin ulcers Osteomyelitis Meningitis	More severe infection seen in immunocompormised but infection is not disseminated
Treatment	Local and mild infections: Azole's Systemic infections: Amphotericin B	Local and mild infections: Azole's Systemic infections: Amphotericin B	Local and mild infections: Azole's Systemic infections: Amphotericin B	Mild infections: Azole's Severe infections: Amphotericin B

SIRS (Systemic Inflammatory Response Syndrome) Criteria [9]

- Body temperature > 38 °C or < 36 °C.
- Heart rate > 90 beats per minute.
- Tachypnea manifested by a respiratory rate >20 breaths per minute or a $PaCO_2$ of <32 mmHg.
- White blood count >12,000/mm^3 or <4000/mm^3, or the presence of >10% immature neutrophils.

≥2 SIRS criteria meet definition of "Systemic Inflammatory Response Syndrome"

SIRS + source of infection = sepsis criteria

Sepsis + organ dysfunction, hypotension or hypoperfusion (lactate ≥4) = severe sepsis

Severe sepsis with hypotension, despite adequate fluid resuscitation = septic shock

Evidence of ≥2 organs failing = MODS (Multiple Organ Dysfunction Syndrome)

More recently, the term "severe sepsis" has been eliminated.

A potential problem with the SIRS criteria: many hospitalized patients, including those who never develop an infection, technically meet SIRS criteria. After exercising, a healthy person will even meet SIRS criteria for example. Additionally, patients with sepsis may even be SIRS-negative.

So, the SOFA scoring system was developed and is more predictive of in-hospital mortality from sepsis (Table 9.6) [9]. The qSOFA ("quick SOFA) is an abbreviated version of this score, more practical for quick and easy identification of patients potentially at risk of dying from sepsis.

Table 9.6 Quick sequential organ failure assessment (qSOFA) score

Criteria	Points
Respiratory rate ≥ 22	1
Change in mental status	1
Systolic blood pressure ≤ 100 mmHg	1

A qSOFA score of ≥2 points indicates organ dysfunction and a greater likelihood of prolonged ICU stay or in-hospital mortality.

OUR PATIENT: Our patient *did* meet SIRS criteria (pulse >90, temp >38 °C) and with a known source of infection, we could technically have diagnosed her with sepsis. However, her qSOFA score was zero. She was appropriately started on broad-spectrum antibiotics initially; however, once fungal pneumonia was identified these were discontinued and she was safely discharged home on antifungal medication. Given her overall clinical picture, mild symptoms, focal findings, and lack of disseminated infection, and immunocompetent status, I do not think we would say this patient was really "septic." This highlights some of the difficulties in the diagnosis of sepsis and the lack of a reliable definition of sepsis.

*Note on our patient's normal WBC count:

Leukocytosis is associated with infection; however, a normal WBC count does *not* rule out infection. A significant percentage of patients with blood-culture-proven bacteremia have normal temperature and normal WBC count upon presentation. Bandemia ("left shift" caused by rapid production of young neutrophils) may be a useful clue in identifying occult bacteremia in these patients. Signs such as fever and leukocytosis may appear later in the course of an infection, particularly in elderly populations. Temperature can be masked by medication, chilled IV fluids, etc. Patients may have a normal WBC count due to poor host immune response or due to mild or localized infection.

Important point: do not rule out a likely diagnosis just because common signs or symptoms are absent. Seigel TA et al. Inadequacy of temperature and white blood cell count in predicting bacteremia in patients with suspected infection. *J Emerg Med* 2012 Mar; 42:254.

Exam Questions

1. A 30-year-old previously healthy male presents to the clinic with 3 weeks of mild dry cough and shortness of breath. He denies fever, sputum production, hemoptysis, rhinorrhea, or congestion. He smoked cigarettes daily for 2 years but quit 5 years ago. He denies any alcohol or drug use. He works as a construction worker in Phoenix, AZ. He has lived in the US his whole life and denies any recent travel. His vital signs are as follows: BP 120/72 mmHg, R 18 breaths/min, P 85 bpm, T 37.1 C. Labs are unremarkable. Chest x-ray shows small right upper lobe consolidation and multiple diffuse nodules. What microbe is the most likely cause of this patient's symptoms?
   A. *Mycobacterium tuberculosis*
   B. *Histoplasma capsulatum*
   C. *Blastomyces dermatitidis*
   D. *Coccidioides immitis*
   E. *Staphylococcus aureus*

Answer: D

Learning Objective #4

Explanation: This patient's mild respiratory symptoms, and the absence of fever or leukocytosis may be consistent with atypical pneumonia or fungal pneumonia. His occupation as a construction worker in Arizona makes coccidioidomycosis more likely (Coccidioides is endemic to the Southwestern United States, and is particularly found in dusty areas such as construction sites). His CXR findings of a focal consolidation with multiple nodules are classic for acute pulmonary coccidiomycosis.

A is incorrect because this patient is at low risk for TB, and although the nodules seen on CXR could be consistent with TB, this is not the most likely answer.

B is incorrect because the *Histoplasma* is endemic to the Mississippi and Ohio River Valleys and Central America and is therefore less likely.

C is incorrect because *Blastomyces* is endemic to the Great Lakes and Ohio River Valley and is therefore less likely.

E is incorrect because although the consolidation on CXR could be bacterial, the nodular pattern is more consistent with fungal infection.

2. A 52-year-old HIV-positive male presents to the emergency department with 2 weeks of dry cough, fevers, and fatigue. His most recent CD4 count 3 months ago was 200 and he is not currently on antiretroviral therapy. His vital signs are as follows: BP 140/86 mmHg, P 92 bpm, R 20 breaths/min, T 38.6 °C. On physical exam, heart sounds are normal, and mild coarse rhonchi are heard through bilateral lung fields. You notice several skin ulcers on his arms and legs. CXR shows patchy alveolar infiltrates and several cavitary lesions in both lungs. Sputum sample is sent and KOH prep shows many yeasts with broad-based budding. What is the most appropriate therapy for this patient?
   A. Itraconazole
   B. Amphotericin B
   C. Trimethoprim-Sulfamethoxazole
   D. Terbinafine
   E. Clotrimazole

Answer: B

Learning Objective: #4

Explanation: This patient has disseminated Blastomycosis and is immunocompromised (most recent CD4 count was 200 and without antiretroviral therapy this number is likely lower now). The patchy alveolar infiltrates and cavitary lesions on CXR and yeast with broad-based budding are classic for Blastomycosis. This patient's skin ulcers and immunocompromised status suggest that the infection is disseminated. Disseminated infections with systemic fungi such as *blastomyces* are treated with Amphotericin B.

A is incorrect because Itraconazole is the treatment for local and mild fungal pneumonia in immunocompetent patients. This patient is immunocompromised and his infection is disseminated.

C is incorrect because TMP-SMX is an antibiotic used to treat and prevent Pneumocystis jiroveci Pneumonia (PJP) in AIDS patients, and this patient has a fungal infection. If his CD4 count remains <200 he should be started on TMP-SMX prophylaxis, but this is not the appropriate treatment for his current illness.

D is incorrect because terbinafine is an antifungal medication used to treat dermatophyte fungi and other types of ringworm and is not effective for the systemic fungi.

E is incorrect because clotrimazole is a topical antifungal used to treat dermatophyte fungal infections and candidiasis and is not effective for the systemic fungi.

3. A 32-year-old man comes to the emergency department due to 3 weeks of fever, night sweats, fatigue, cough, and shortness of breath. He has lost 10 lb over this period. The patient was diagnosed with HIV a year ago but is not taking antiretroviral medication. His CD4 count was 80 three months ago. The patient is unemployed and recently moved to Missouri to live with his parents. He does not use tobacco, alcohol, or illicit drugs. Blood pressure is 113/66, pulse 106, temperature 101.3 F. There are small ulcers on the hard palate and multiple enlarged cervical and inguinal lymph nodes. A pulmonary exam reveals scattered lung crackles. The patient's abdomen is soft and nontender, but there is prominent hepatosplenomegaly. Labs show pancytopenia and elevated aminotransferase levels. CXR reveals bilateral reticulonodular opacities with hilar lymphadenopathy. Which of the following is the best next step in the management of this patient?
   A. Bronchoalveolar lavage for *Pneumocystis* infection
   B. Fungal blood cultures
   C. Lymph node biopsy
   D. *Treponema pallidum* enzyme immunoassay
   E. Urine *Histoplasma* antigen

Answer: E

Learning Objective: #3 and 4

Explanation: This patient most likely has disseminated *Histoplasma capsulatum* infection, given his immunocompromised status. Patients with CD4 count <100 are far more likely to develop progressive disseminated histoplasmosis. The patient's fever, weight loss, respiratory symptoms, mucocutaneous lesions, lymphadenopathy, and hepatosplenomegaly are the classic presentation of disseminated histoplasmosis. Diagnosis is confirmed most rapidly with serum or urine *Histoplasma* antigen immunoassay (sensitivity >95%).

A is incorrect because PCP (*Pneumocystis pneumonia)*, although a common opportunistic infection in advanced HIV patients, does not commonly cause lymphadenopathy, hepatosplenomegaly, or pancytopenia.

B is incorrect because although most patients with suspected histoplasmosis receive fungal blood cultures, culture results take 4–6 weeks. Therefore, this is not the correct choice for diagnosis.

C is incorrect because a biopsy of a lymph node is not required to make a diagnosis of histoplasmosis, which is the most likely diagnosis in this case.

D is incorrect because syphilis does not feature pulmonary involvement and pancytopenia.

References

1. Hunter MP, Goldin J, Regunath H. Pleurisy. [Updated 2024 Nov 14]. In: StatPearls [Internet]. Treasure Island (FL): StatPearls Publishing; 2025 Jan-. Available from: https://www.ncbi.nlm.nih.gov/books/NBK558958/.
2. Lidegaard Ø, Edström B, Kreiner S. Oral contraceptives and venous thromboembolism: a five-year national case-control study. Contraception. 2002;65(3):187–96.
3. Freund Y, Cachanado M, Aubry A, et al. PROPER Investigator Group. Effect of the pulmonary embolism rule-out criteria on subsequent thromboembolic events among low-risk emergency department patients: the PROPER randomized clinical trial. JAMA. 2018;319(6):559–66.
4. Lin LW. Wells clinical prediction rule for DVT in primary care. Am Fam Physician. 2006;73(4):709–10.
5. Akram SM, Koirala J. Histoplasmosis. [Updated 2023 Aug 8]. In: StatPearls [Internet]. Treasure Island (FL): StatPearls Publishing; 2025 Jan-. Available from: https://www.ncbi.nlm.nih.gov/books/NBK448185/.
6. Azar MM, Hage CA. Clinical perspectives in the diagnosis and management of histoplasmosis. Clin Chest Med. 2017;38(3):403–15. https://doi.org/10.1016/j.ccm.2017.04.004. Epub 2017 May 17.
7. Smith JA, Kauffman CA. Pulmonary fungal infections. Respirology. 2012;17(6):913–26.
8. Miller AS, Wilmott RW. 31 – The Pulmonary Mycoses. In: Wilmott RW, Deterding R, Li A, Ratjen F, Sly P, Zar HJ, Bush A, editors. Kendig's disorders of the respiratory tract in children (Ninth Edition). Elsevier; 2019. p. 507–527.e3.
9. Singer M, Deutschman CS, Seymour CW, et al. The third international consensus definitions for sepsis and septic shock (Sepsis-3). JAMA. 2016;315(8):801–10.

Short of Breath

10

Cynthia A. Standley

Learning Objectives

1. Review the possible causes of dyspnea based on O_2 content vs. O_2 delivery.
2. Explain the pathophysiology of emphysema, including alveolar destruction and airflow limitation.
3. Describe how this patient was adjusting the work of breathing.
4. Interpret relevant laboratory findings in a patient with emphysema, such as spirometry results and arterial blood gas analysis.
5. Discuss the causes of hypoxemia in this patient and explain why the blood gas data did not change dramatically after oxygen supplementation.
6. List the types of agents that alter bronchiolar smooth muscle tone and explain why bronchodilator therapy was effective in this patient.
7. Explain the importance of self-management strategies, such as breathing exercises and medication adherence.

Chief Complaint

I can't really catch my breath.

C. A. Standley (✉)
Department of Bioethics and Medical Humanism, University of Arizona College of Medicine-Phoenix, Phoenix, AZ, USA
e-mail: cstand@arizona.edu

Prompt: *Construct a broad differential for this chief complaint.*

Dyspnea, or the sensation of breathlessness, has a broad differential encompassing pulmonary, cardiac, hematologic, neuromuscular, metabolic, and psychogenic causes [1]. Below is a categorized differential diagnosis:

Pulmonary causes include

- Obstructive lung disease, such as chronic bronchitis, emphysema, asthma
- Restrictive lung disease, such as pulmonary fibrosis
- Infections such as pneuomoia, bronchitis, tuberculosis
- Pulmonary vascular disease such as pulmonary embolism, pulmonary hypertension
- Pleural disease such as pneumothorax
- Foreign body aspiration

Cardiac causes include

- Heart failure
- Myocardial ischemia/infarction
- Valvular disease
- Cardiomyopathy
- Pericardial disease

Hematological causes include

- Anemia
- Carbon monoxide poisoning
- Methemoglobinemia

C. A. Standley (ed.), *Biomedical Science and Clinical Foundations*,
https://doi.org/10.1007/978-3-031-98353-5_10

Neuromuscular causes include

- Guillain-Barré syndrome
- Myasthenia gravis
- Amyotrophic lateral sclerosis
- Cervical spinal cord injury

Metabolic/Endocrine causes include

- Diabetic ketoacidosis
- Severe metabolic acidosis
- Thyrotoxicosis

Psychogenic causes include

- Panic attack, anxiety

History of Present Illness

A 55-year-old man presents to the clinic with progressive shortness of breath. He indicates that he must sleep sitting up with the aid of several pillows. He's had a mild morning cough and fatigue with activities such as climbing stairs. More recently, he has experienced dyspnea at rest and has lost approximately 10 pounds in the last 2 months. He denies fever, chills, chest pain, palpitations, leg swelling, hemoptysis, or wheezing. No known sick contacts or recent travel. He has a 40 pack-year smoking history but no prior pulmonary diagnosis.

Prompt: *What might be the cause of his 10-pound weight loss?*

His work of breathing, the force required to move the lung and chest wall, is so great. Caloric consumption and oxygen consumption increase as he is expending a lot of energy.

Past Medical History

Hypertension—poorly controlled
Coronary artery disease, history of myocardial infarction 5 years ago
Congestive heart failure—diagnosed 2 years ago
Type 2 Diabetes Mellitus—on oral hypoglycemic agents
Hyperlipidemia

Past Surgical History

Coronary artery bypass graft surgery 5 years ago
Appendectomy in childhood

Medications

Lisinopril 10 mg daily
Metoprolol succinate 50 mg daily
Furosemide 40 mg daily
Atorvastatin 40 mg daily
Metformin 1000 mg twice daily

Allergies

No known drug allergies

Family History

Grandfather had "lung problems," several brothers and sisters have "hay fever."
No other history of pulmonary disease involving the family

Prompt: *What are some pulmonary disorders that are hereditary?*

Cystic fibrosis, alpha-1 antitrypsin deficiency, certain types of asthma, surfactant deficiency.

Social History

40 pack-year smoking history
Denies alcohol and drug use.
No history of exposure to extraordinary environmental pollutants.
President of a local university

Review of Systems

- **General:** Unintentional weight loss (10 lbs in 2 months), fatigue
- **Cardiovascular:** Dyspnea on exertion, orthopnea, no known history of palpitations or syncope
- **Pulmonary:** Chronic morning cough, worsening shortness of breath, no hemoptysis
- **Gastrointestinal:** No nausea, vomiting, or abdominal pain
- **Genitourinary:** No urinary symptoms
- **Neurologic:** No dizziness, headaches, or weakness
- **Musculoskeletal:** No joint pain or swelling

Physical Examination

Vitals: T 98.4 °F (36.9 °C) BP 145/90 mmHg, HR 88 bpm, Resp 22 breaths/min, O_2 Saturation 90% on room air

Weight: 165 lbs, **Height**: 73 inches

General: Thin, frail-looking man in acute respiratory distress, restless

Cardiovascular: Normal S1, S2; S3 sound present; JVD, displaced apical impulse. No murmurs, rubs, gallops, or edema.

Pulmonary: Tachypneic and using pursed-lip breathing. Diminished breath sounds bilaterally, prolonged expiratory phase with wheezes, hyperresonance on percussion.

Extremities: Mild bilateral lower extremity pitting edema, no clubbing or cyanosis

Abdomen: Soft, non-tender, no hepatosplenomegaly or ascites

Prompt: *What is your assessment so far?*

This 55-year-old man with a history of CHF, CAD, and a significant smoking history presents with progressive dyspnea, orthopnea, weight loss, and chronic cough. His thin/cachectic appearance, diminished breath sounds, hyperresonance, and prolonged expiration strongly suggest emphysema.

Prompt: *What tests would you like to order?*

Blood gas analysis, pulmonary function testing (PFTs), EKG, echocardiogram, chest Xray.

Laboratory

Blood Gas Analysis

Arterial blood gases were drawn while the patient was breathing room air (barometric pressure (PB) = 710 mmHg) (Table 10.1).

The patient was then placed on 2 L nasal oxygen per minute (fraction of oxygen in inspired air (FiO_2) = 28%) and sent to the medical intensive care unit for further evaluation. Arterial blood gases were redrawn after the administration of oxygen (Table 10.2).

Prompt: *What's happening?*

He actually got worse! This patient has hypercapnic respiratory failure with worsening CO_2 retention and persistent hypoxemia despite supplemental oxygen. Oxygen reverses hypoxic vasoconstriction, leading to worsened ventilation-perfusion (V/Q) mismatch and further CO_2 retention. High PaO_2 reduces hemoglobin's affinity for CO_2, leading to increased dissolved CO_2 in the blood, contributing to hypercapnia. Lastly, in chronic CO_2 retainers, peripheral chemoreceptors (which respond to low oxygen) become the main stimulus for breathing, rather than the cen-

Table 10.1 Blood gas analysis

Component	Patient	Reference
PaO_2 (mmHg)	39	75–100
SaO_2 (%)	75	≥95
$PaCO_2$ (mmHg)	52	35–45
pH	7.32	7.38–7.44
Hemoglobin (g/dL)	14	14–18

Table 10.2 Blood gas analysis following supplemental oxygen

Component	Patient	Reference
PaO_2 (mmHg)	49	75–100
$PaCO_2$ (mmHg)	60	35–45
pH	7.25	7.38–7.44

tral chemoreceptors in the medulla. Supplemental oxygen reduces this drive, leading to worsening CO_2 retention.

Prompt: *Calculate PAO_2 and A-a gradient using the alveolar gas equation for this patient before and after nasal oxygen. What is the explanation for the high $PaCO_2$?*

$$\text{Alveolar Gas Equation}: PAO_2 = (PB - PH_2O) \times FiO_2 - PaCO_2 / R$$

Where PAO_2 = Alveolar partial pressure of oxygen, PB = barometric pressure, PH_2O = water vapor pressure, FiO_2 = fraction of oxygen in inspired air, $PaCO_2$ = arteriolar partial pressure of carbon dioxide, R = respiratory quotient.

Using standard values for PB, PH_2O, FiO_2, and R, and the patient's value for $PaCO_2$ *before* supplemental oxygen:

$$PAO_2 = (710 - 47) \times 0.21 - 52 / 0.8 = 74\,\text{mmHg}$$

Using standard values for PB, PH_2O, FiO_2, and R, and the patient's value for $PaCO_2$ *after* supplemental oxygen:

$$PAO_2 = (710 - 47) \times 0.28 - 60 / 0.8 = 111\,\text{mmHg}$$

Alveolar oxygen improved following oxygen supplementation. Now calculate the Alveolar-arterial (A-a) gradient using the following equation:

$$\text{A} - \text{a gradient} = PAO_2 - PaO_2$$

Before O_2 supplementation:

$$\text{A} - \text{a gradient} = 74 - 39 = 35\,\text{mmHg}$$

After O_2 supplementation:

$$\text{A} - \text{a gradient} = 111 - 49 = 63\,\text{mmHg}$$

The normal A-a gradient is 5–20 mmHg. Thus, before O_2 supplementation, the patient's A-a gradient was already high, and after O_2 supplementation, it was even higher! The supplemental oxygen is not helping him.

Initial Pulmonary Function Tests

Pulmonary function was assessed via static and dynamic spirometry (Table 10.3).

Prompt: *Interpret the pulmonary function tests.*

The patient's static lung volumes of VC, RV, and TLC are all significantly increased, indicated air trapping in the lungs. His tidal volume is reduced, so he is not moving air as well as he should be. The dynamic pulmonary function test results (FVC, FEV1 and FEV1%) indicate an obstructive disease in his lungs.

Prompt: *What should be done now?*

Consider a bronchodilator. Various inhalers, etc. nebulizer treatment—an atomizer equipped to produce an extremely fine spray of medication for deep penetration into the lungs.

The Case Continues

The patient was placed on nebulizer treatment with albuterol. After treatment, the following arterial blood gases were measured (Table 10.4).

After 24 h of treatment, the patient's lungs were auscultated and it was noted that his

Table 10.3 Pulmonary function tests

Component	Patient	Reference
VC (L)	5.5	4.50
VT (L)	0.35	0.50
RV (L)	3.88	1.20
TLC (L)	9.13	5.70
RV/TLC %	42	20–25%
Rate (breaths/min)	29	12–20
FVC (L)	4.75	4.5
FEV1	1.52	3.6
FEV1%	32	80

VC Vital Capacity, *VT* Tidal Volume, *RV* Residual Volume, *TLC* Total Lung Capacity, *FVC* Forced Vital Capacity, *FEV1* Forced Expiratory Volume in 1 s, *FEV1%* Forced Expiratory Volume in 1 s as a percentage of Forced Vital Capacity

Table 10.4 Blood gas analysis following nebulizer treatment

Component	Patient	Reference
PaO_2 (mmHg)	58	75–100
$PaCO_2$ (mmHg)	42	35–45
pH	7.38	7.38–7.44

wheezes were decreased, he was less restless, and his respiratory rate decreased to 22 breaths/min.

Prompt: *Will supplemental oxygen help him now?*

Yes, now that his $PaCO_2$ has gone down following albuterol, supplemental oxygen may help.

The Case Continues

After a few days in the intensive care unit, the patient was transferred to a medical floor, where he received supplemental oxygen, bronchodilator therapy, counseling on how to stop smoking, and breathing retraining through the use of effective pursed-lip breathing. After 1 week, it was felt that the patient could return home with the use of home oxygen at 2 L/min. A visiting nurse will follow him at home for periodic checkups and consultation.

His orthopnea, JVD, S3 heart sound, and lower extremity edema also raise concern for decompensated heart failure, which could be contributing to his symptoms. Further evaluation with chest X-rays, echocardiograms, BNP levels, and arterial blood gases is warranted to assess the degree of cardiac vs. pulmonary involvement in his dyspnea.

End of Case

Learning Objective Answers

1. **Review the possible causes of dyspnea based on O_2 content vs. O_2 delivery.**

Dyspnea is the medical term for shortness of breath. It is an uncomfortable feeling of not being able to breathe well enough. Dyspnea can be analyzed physiologically based on two key components of oxygen transport [2, 3]:

1. Oxygen Content (CaO_2)—The total amount of oxygen carried in the blood.
2. Oxygen Delivery (DO_2)—The amount of oxygen delivered to tissues per minute.

The oxygen content of blood can be determined by the following equation:

$$CaO_2 = (1.34 \times Hb \times SaO2) + (0.003 \times PaO_2)$$

where Hb = Hemoglobin concentration (g/dL), SaO_2 = Arterial oxygen saturation (%), and PaO_2 = Partial pressure of oxygen in arterial blood (mmHg)

A decrease in CaO_2 can occur due to low PaO_2 (hypoxemia) or low hemoglobin (anemic hypoxia). Hypoxemia can result from hypoventilation, ventilation/perfusion (V/Q) mismatch as in emphysema, right-to-left shunts as in acute respiratory distress syndrome, diffusion impairment, or high altitude. Low hemoglobin can result from iron deficiency or carbon monoxide poisoning

Oxygen delivery depends on cardiac output (CO) and arterial O_2 content, as demonstrated by the following equation:

$$DO_2 = CO \times CaO_2$$

A decrease in DO_2 can be caused by low CO or impaired oxygen extraction. Low CO, causing a stagnant hypoxia, can be seen in heart failure, myocardial infarction, hypovolemia, and shock. Impaired oxygen extraction causing a histotoxic hypoxia can be seen in cyanide poisoning (inhibits mitochondrial electron transport chain) and sepsis (mitochondrial dysfunction, impaired tissue O_2 utilization).

The patient in this case has low PaO2, or O_2 content, and labored breathing. Using the equation $DO_2 = CO \times CaO_2$, low O_2 content leads to decreased O_2 delivery. The patient experiences hypoxia, low PaO_2, and the sensation that they can't breathe.

2. **Explain the pathophysiology of emphysema, including alveolar destruction and airflow limitation.**

Emphysema is a chronic, progressive lung disease characterized by the destruction of alveolar walls and airflow limitation due to loss of elastic recoil and small airway collapse. It is a key component of chronic obstructive pulmonary disease (COPD) and is most commonly caused by cigarette smoking or α1-antitrypsin (AAT) deficiency [4]. Smoking may act to reduce the activity of elastase inhibitors, thus promoting lysosomal elastase released from neutrophils in the lungs to destroy elastin, an important structural protein in the lungs. Smoking can also lead to chronic inflammation of the mucous glands [5].

In emphysema, the walls of the tiny air sacs (alveoli) in the lungs are damaged and eventually break down, resulting in larger, less numerous air spaces instead of many small ones [4]. The emphysema lung shows loss of alveolar walls with consequent destruction of the capillary bed (Fig. 10.1). This destruction of alveolar walls significantly reduces the surface area available for gas exchange (oxygen uptake and carbon dioxide removal). The elastic recoil of the lungs, which helps to expel air during exhalation, is compromised due to the loss of alveolar walls and supporting structures. The loss of elastic recoil makes it difficult to exhale air, leading to airflow limitation. The loss of tethering (i.e., loss of radial traction forces) from alveolar destruction can also lead to airway collapse during exhalation, further restricting airflow. Air becomes trapped in the lungs, leading to hyperinflation (increased lung volume) and further exacerbating airflow limitation.

In summary, emphysema causes airflow limitation through a combination of alveolar destruction, loss of elastic recoil, and airway collapse, leading to reduced gas exchange and increased air trapping in the lungs.

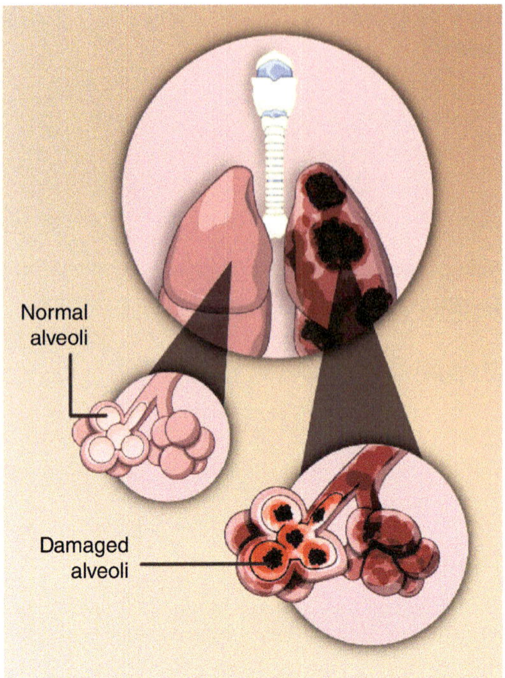

Fig. 10.1 Normal alveoli compared to damaged alveoli. (From https://www.myupchar.com/en via Wikimedia Commons, licensed under CC BY-SA 4.0) <https://creativecommons.org/licenses/by-sa/4.0>, via *Wikimedia Commons*

3. **Describe how this patient was adjusting the work of breathing.**

The work of breathing is the force required to move the lung and chest wall and makes up 33% of resting oxygen consumption. It is composed of elastic and resistance work; elastic work is volume dependent, and resistance work is rate dependent [2]. Emphysema is characterized by increased compliance, decreased radial traction forces, and increased resistance forces due to small airway collapse. In emphysema, the work of breathing can increase dramatically [6]. Because the small airways collapse during expiration, the patient must work harder to exhale, significantly increasing the work of breathing. To compensate, emphysema patients adopt a breathing pattern with lower respiratory rates and higher tidal volumes. This strategy minimizes airway resistance, prevents dynamic airway collapse, and optimizes alveolar ventilation. However, the patient in this case has a respiratory rate of 29 breaths per minute and a tidal volume of 350 mL, suggesting that they are in respiratory distress and unable to maintain the typical compensatory strategy of emphysema (slow, deep breaths). Instead, they have shifted to a rapid, shallow breathing pattern, which indicates increased work of breathing and impending respiratory failure. This patient's rapid, shallow breathing suggests that their respiratory muscles are fatigued, forcing them into an inefficient breathing pattern. This leads to increased dead space ventilation, worsening CO_2 retention (hypercapnia). The caloric consumption and percent of resting oxygen consumption will consequently increase, and these people are often thin.

4. **Explain the significance of the expiratory wheezes and why pursed-lip breathing was beneficial.**

Dynamic airway compression refers to the collapse or narrowing of airways during forced expiration when intrapleural pressure exceeds intra-airway pressure [2, 6]. In healthy individuals, the pressure inside the airway remains higher than the surrounding intrapleural pressure during most of expiration, preventing collapse. However, in emphysema, the loss of alveolar elastic recoil reduces airway support, making the small bronchioles more prone to collapse even at normal expiratory efforts. This causes increased airflow resistance, air trapping, and prolonged expiration. Expiratory wheezing occurs when narrowed or collapsing airways create turbulent airflow. Although wheezing is not a hallmark of pure emphysema, it may be heard in coexisting chronic bronchitis or secretions. In severe emphysema, breath sounds are often diminished rather than wheezy due to poor airflow.

Pursed-lip breathing (PLB) is a compensatory technique used during expiration in order to increase airway pressure (increase resistance at the mouth) and prevent dynamic compression of the airways [2, 6]. PLB helps prevent airway collapse by creating positive end-expiratory pressure (PEEP), keeping the bronchioles open during exhalation. By prolonging exhalation and reducing expiratory flow velocity, PLB reduces dynamic hyperinflation and dyspnea. The fact that this patient is using PLB suggests an attempt to reduce work of breathing, but their high respiratory rate indicates decompensation and impending respiratory muscle fatigue.

5. **Discuss the causes of hypoxemia in this patient and explain why the blood gas data did not change dramatically after oxygen supplementation.**

This patient has a very wide alveolar-arterial (A-a) gradient, which is characteristic of emphysema and results from severe ventilation-perfusion (V/Q) mismatch associated with his hypoxemia [2, 6]. In emphysema, alveolar destruction leads to areas of high V/Q (ventilation without perfusion, dead space) due to loss of capillaries and areas of low V/Q (perfusion without adequate ventilation) due to small airway collapse. Oxygen supplementation improves PaO_2 but not dramatically because it only helps low V/Q areas and cannot restore perfusion to high V/Q (dead space) regions.

CO_2 retention in emphysema results from increasing dead space and ventilatory failure, stemming alveolar destruction [2, 6]. This causes an increase in alveolar dead space, which the patient must then overcome by increasing his minute volume to maintain ventilation. In early disease, patients compensate with an increased minute ventilation, keeping $PaCO_2$ near normal. As lung destruction worsens, alveolar ventilation declines, leading to hypercapnia and worsening respiratory acidosis.

His blood gas data did not change dramatically after O_2 supplementation. One of the main reasons oxygen therapy can worsen CO_2 retention in emphysema patients is related to the Haldane effect: high PaO_2 reduces hemoglobin's affinity for CO_2, increasing dissolved CO_2 in blood [7]. Additionally, oxygen reverses hypoxic vasoconstriction in poorly ventilated alveoli, increasing perfusion to low V/Q regions, worsening CO_2 retention. Lastly, in some patients with chronic hypercapnia, peripheral chemoreceptors drive ventilation. Because these sites are sensitive to a decrease in oxygen (<60 mmHg), oxygen administration may tend to decrease the stimulus for breathing in these patients, resulting in decreased ventilation. The hypoxic drive for breathing is then eliminated.

In summary, the increase in CO_2 after oxygen therapy is mainly due to V/Q redistribution and the Haldane effect, rather than just loss of the hypoxic drive. Clinicians must carefully titrate oxygen to prevent severe hypercapnia, with close monitoring of $PaCO_2$ levels in patients with advanced disease.

6. **List the types of agents that alter bronchiolar smooth muscle tone, and explain why bronchodilator therapy was effective in this patient.**

Bronchodilators increase bronchiolar radius and decrease airway resistance. Since obstructive lung disease, such as emphysema, is characterized by increased resistance work, this is the best medication to treat the disease. In emphysema, airways close too soon as airway resistance is increased. Bronchodilation lessens this resistance, allowing fuller expiration. Table 10.5 shows agents that alter bronchiolar smooth muscle that can be used in the treatment of emphysema [8].

7. **Explain the importance of self-management strategies, such as breathing exercises and medication adherence.**

Both medication and breathing exercises help in the management of emphysema. For individuals with emphysema, breathing exercises like pursed-lip breathing and diaphragmatic breathing can help manage airflow and improve lung function. Purse-lip breathing makes it easier to breathe because the increase in airway pressure created by pursed lips opens the airways [2, 6]. It helps maintain PEEP, reducing dynamic airway collapse and improving airflow. It also slows breathing rate and reduces work of breathing. Additionally, it increases alveolar emptying, minimizing air trapping. Learning how to belly breathe, also known as diaphragmatic breathing, strengthens the diaphragm, promoting more efficient breathing [8]. It also reduces reliance on accessory muscles, decreasing fatigue.

Medication adherence is crucial in emphysema because it directly impacts disease management, reducing exacerbations and hospitalizations and improving overall quality of life [9].

Table 10.5 Agents that alter bronchiolar smooth muscle

Class	Examples	Mechanism of action	Major side effects
Short Acting β_2-Agonists	Albuterol, Levalbuterol	Stimulate β_2-adrenergic receptors and produce bronchodilation via increase in cAMP	Tremor, tachycardia, hypokalemia
Long Acting β_2-Agonists	Salmeterol, Formoterol	Prolonged β_2- receptor activation and sustained bronchodilation	Headache, palpitations, muscle cramps
Short Acting Muscarinic Antagonists	Ipratropium	Block M3 muscarinic receptors and reduce bronchoconstriction	Dry mouth, urinary retention, blurry vision
Long Activiting Muscarinic Antagonists	Tiotropium, Aclidinium	Prolonged M3 receptor blockade and sustained reduction in bronchoconstriction	Dry mouth, constipation, increased glaucoma risk
Methylxanthines	Theophylline	Adenosine receptor blockade; inhibits phosphodiesterase, increases cAMP, and produces bronchodilation	Narrow therapeutic window, arrhythmias, nausea, seizures
Inhaled Corticosteroids	Fluticasone, Budesonide	Inhibit cytokine production and reduce airway inflammation	Oral candidiasis, hoarseness, pneumonia risk

Bronchodilators make it easier to breathe because the vascular smooth muscle relaxes and increases opening of airways. Medications are optimally effective when used as prescribed, and non-adherence can lead to reduced clinical benefit.

For individuals with emphysema, crucial lifestyle modifications include quitting smoking, maintaining a healthy weight, staying physically active, following a balanced diet, and avoiding irritants [8]. Smoking cessation is the most effective intervention to slow disease progression. Other measures for patients with emphysema include slowly adding exercise training to improve endurance and reduce dyspnea. Dietary modifications and nutritional support help prevent weight loss and muscle atrophy. Use of a face mask protects from particles which cause bronchoconstriction via stimulation of irritant receptors in airway submucosa. Staying up to date on vaccinations, including the flu and pneumonia vaccines, can help prevent respiratory infections that can worsen emphysema. Learning stress management techniques can help improve overall well-being. And finally, regular checkups with a healthcare provider are important to monitor and adjust the treatment plan as needed.

Exam Questions

1. A 65-year-old man with emphysema has worsening dyspnea on exertion. Pulmonary function tests show air trapping and hyperinflation. Which of the following mechanisms best explains these findings?
   A. Decreased compliance of alveolar walls
   B. Destruction of alveolar elastic fibers
   C. Increased mucus secretion in small bronchi
   D. Increased airway smooth muscle contractility

Answer: B

Learning Objective: #2 Explain the pathophysiology of emphysema, including alveolar destruction and airflow limitation

Explanation: In emphysema, destruction of elastin fibers leads to loss of elastic recoil → lungs do not empty properly → air trapping; increased lung compliance → hyperinflation and increased total lung capacity; dynamic airway collapse → worsens expiratory airflow obstruction. A is incorrect, as this happens in restrictive lung diseases (e.g., fibrosis). C is incorrect, as this is the hallmark of chronic bronchitis. D is incorrect, as this is seen in asthma, where bronchoconstriction is prominent.

2. A 55-year-old man with a 40-pack-year smoking history presents to the clinic with progressive shortness of breath and a chronic cough. Pulmonary function testing is ordered to assess his lung function. One of the measured parameters is forced expiratory volume in 1 s (FEV_1). Which of the following best defines this parameter?
   A. The total volume of air that a person can forcefully expel after a full inhalation.
   B. The volume of trapped air in the lung after complete and forceful expiration.
   C. The mean airflow rate during the first second of exhalation.
   D. The volume of air that a person can forcefully expel in 1 s after a full inhalation.

Answer: D

Learning Objective: #4 Interpret relevant laboratory findings in a patient with emphysema, such as spirometry results and arterial blood gas analysis.

Explanation: FEV_1 is a key pulmonary function test measurement that quantifies the volume of air exhaled in the first second of a forced expiratory maneuver. It is critical in diagnosing obstructive lung diseases (e.g., emphysema, chronic bronchitis, asthma) and restrictive lung diseases (e.g., pulmonary fibrosis). In obstructive lung disease, FEV_1 is markedly reduced due to airway collapse and increased resistance. A is incorrect as this describes forced vital capacity (FVC), which is the total volume of air exhaled after a maximal inhalation. B is incorrect, as this describes residual volume (RV), which is the amount of air that remains in the lungs even after maximal expiration. C is incorrect, as this describes forced expiratory flow (FEF 25–75%), which is a measure of mid-expiratory flow rate and reflects small airway function rather than FEV_1.

3. A 60-year-old man with a 40-pack-year smoking history presents with progressive dyspnea and chronic cough. He is diagnosed with emphysema, which is characterized by ventilation-perfusion (V/Q) mismatch. In a lung region where the V/Q ratio decreases, which of the following changes in alveolar gas composition is expected?
   A. Higher PO_2 and higher PCO_2
   B. Lower PO_2 and lower PCO_2
   C. Higher PO_2 and lower PCO_2
   D. Lower PO_2 and higher PCO_2
   E. Lower PO_2 and unchanged PCO_2

Answer: D

Learning Objective: #5 Discuss the causes of hypoxemia in this patient and explain why the blood gas data did not change dramatically after oxygen supplementation.

Explanation: The V/Q ratio represents the balance between ventilation (V) and perfusion (Q) in a given lung region. If the V/Q ratio decreases, it means that ventilation is reduced relative to perfusion. Decreased ventilation results in less oxygen delivery to the alveoli, leading to lower alveolar PO_2. Impaired CO_2 removal due to reduced ventilation causes PCO_2 to rise in the alveoli. A is incorrect, as an increase in both PO_2 and PCO_2 is physiologically unlikely. Areas with higher PO_2 generally have lower PCO_2 due to efficient gas exchange. B is incorrect, as while PO_2 does decrease, PCO_2 does not decrease. If ventilation is reduced, CO_2 accumulates rather than being cleared. C is incorrect, as this scenario occurs in high V/Q regions (e.g., areas with dead space ventilation, such as in pulmonary embolism), where ventilation exceeds perfusion. E is incorrect, as inadequate ventilation leads to both lower PO_2 and higher PCO_2, so PCO_2 would not remain unchanged.

References

1. McGee S. Evidence-based physical diagnosis. 4th ed. Elsevier; 2017.
2. West JB. Respiratory physiology: the essentials. 11th ed. Lippincott Williams & Wilkins; 2020.
3. Hall JE, Guyton AC. Guyton and Hall textbook of medical physiology. 14th ed. Elsevier; 2020.
4. Agustí A, Hogg JC. Update on the pathogenesis of chronic obstructive pulmonary disease. N Engl J Med. 2019;381(13):1248–56.
5. Famutimi OG, Adebiyi VG, Akinmolu BG, et al. Trypsin, chymotrypsin and elastase in health and disease. Futur J Pharm Sci. 2024;10:126.
6. Marini JJ, Wheeler AP. Critical care medicine: the essentials and more. 6th ed. Lippincott Williams & Wilkins; 2022.
7. Abdo WF, Heunks LM. Oxygen-induced hypercapnia in COPD: myths and facts. Crit Care. 2012;16(5):323.
8. Global Initiative for Chronic Obstructive Lung Disease (GOLD) Report 2024. Global strategy for the diagnosis, management, and prevention of chronic obstructive pulmonary disease. Available at: www.goldcopd.org.
9. Restrepo RD, Alvarez MT, Wittnebel LD, Sorenson H, Wettstein R, Vines DL, Sikkema-Ortiz J, Gardner DD, Wilkins RL. Medication adherence issues in patients treated for COPD. Int J Chron Obstruct Pulmon Dis. 2008;3(3):371–84.

Part V

Renal/Acid Base

11 Inability to Urinate

Abel De Castro

Learning Objectives

1. Describe the anatomic components of the urinary system, placing special emphasis on the microscopic structures in the nephron and their function, as well as the gross structures involved in the passage of urine.
2. Compare and contrast the different etiologies of renal failure, focusing on the physiologic basis for the injury of the kidneys and pertinent lab findings involved with each etiology. Identify which one each patient has.
3. Discuss the diagnosis of acute renal injury. Develop a clinical approach to a patient presenting with "dark urine" or oliguria/anuria and explain a diagnostic schema for renal failure.
4. Discuss the treatment approach for each etiology of renal failure.
5. Discuss epidemiology and prognosis of renal failure, including a discussion on certain barriers to care involving patients with acute kidney disease.

A. De Castro (✉)
Internal Medicine – Pediatrics, UT Southwestern, Dallas, TX, USA
e-mail: abel.decastro@utsouthwestern.edu

Case

Patient A

CC: "Patient stopped peeing"

The patient is a 22-year-old male who initially presented to the hospital following a motor vehicle accident (MVA) in which he was an unrestrained passenger. He had a significant abdominal wound and lost approximately 1.5 L of blood in the field. When he was brought to the emergency department (ED), a massive transfusion protocol was initiated as he continued to hemorrhage. After 10 units of whole blood were administered and the source of the bleeding was stopped, he was stabilized and admitted to the intensive care unit (ICU). Three days later, the patient's nurse notifies them that the patient has stopped peeing completely in the last 24 hours.

Prompt: Why would the patient have stopped peeing?

He had a very significant hypovolemic episode. However, at this point, it is unclear if he could have been developing an infectious cause, had trauma shearing of his urinary tract, or if there was deeper kidney damage.

Prompt: Are there other symptoms or findings that would help us narrow our differential?

We do not know enough if the patient has any other symptoms. He is critically ill, so it may be

C. A. Standley (ed.), *Biomedical Science and Clinical Foundations*,
https://doi.org/10.1007/978-3-031-98353-5_11

challenging to acquire any acute changes since his admission.

Past Medical History (Obtained from EMR)

The patient is a healthy 22-year-old. No medical history other than childhood asthma

Medications

Does not take any medications, but occasionally takes the OTC pain medications. He takes a daily multivitamin and creatine for bodybuilding.

Allergies

Iodine contrast

Social History

Does not smoke. Drinks beer occasionally with his friends. Does not take any recreational drugs. Is a college senior in marketing. Lives with his family in Arizona.

High Risk Behaviors/Habits

None

Family History

Denies any history of diabetes, heart disease, or kidney disease. Remote history of HTN

Prompt: Does anything in the history help with your differential?

There is nothing particularly noteworthy in his history. It is interesting to note that creatine is a bodybuilding supplement that is often frowned upon in the medical community. Creatine is a very well researched and studied supplement that, when taken properly and with adequate hydration, is not linked to renal damage [1].

Review of Systems Unable to provide due to intubated and sedated status

Physical Examination

- General Appearance—asleep, comfortable, intubated
- Vital Signs—Blood pressure 105/60 mmHg, respiration 18 breaths per minute, pulse 47 beats per minute, temperature: 97.8 °F (36.5 °C)
- Skin—numerous abrasions
- HEENT—a few lacerations, but otherwise normal dentition. Moist mucous membranes
- Neck—no thyromegaly or lymphadenopathy. No JVD or carotid bruits
- Chest/Lungs—CTA. Appropriate air movement bilaterally and in the bases. Mechanical ventilation appreciated
- Heart—RRR nl s1 s2 s s3 s4
- Abdomen—soft, non-distended
- Genital/Rectal—Foley inserted with 50 mL over last 24 hours
- Extremities—weak pulse noted in all 4 extremities
- Musculoskeletal—no loss of muscle tone
- Neurological—DTRs normal. Otherwise, unable to complete

Prompt: Is there anything from the ROS and PE that helps with your differential? What kinds of labs are you interested in ordering?

Noteworthy are the hemodynamics for this patient. He has a very weak pulse, and his blood pressure is on the softer side. Because of the concern for anuria and likely new AKI, it will be appropriate to get renal function labs, BUN, UA. Depending on what those find, it may be important to get secondary imaging. However, given this patient's allergy history, a CT w contrast would best be avoided.

Laboratory

- CBC within normal limits
- CMP demonstrated elevated potassium 5.5 mEq/L, up from 3.5 mEq/L; Cr rising from 0.8 mg/dL on admission to 2.0 mg/dL on day 3 of admission. HCO_3 is 18 mEq/L, down from 28 mEq/L on admission. BUN 75 mg/dL
- Urine electrolytes demonstrate elevated fractional excretion of sodium (FeNa)
- UA negative for nitrites and leukocyte esterase. Positive for muddy brown casts

Prompt: What else would you like to order?

Patient had a CBC demonstrating improved anemia with a hemoglobin of 10.1 g/dL. His potassium was elevated to 5.5 mEq/L and his creatinine was increasing from 0.8 mg/dL on admission to 5.5 mg/dL on day 3 of hospitalization. His BUN: Creatinine ratio was greater than 20. Urine electrolytes demonstrated FeNa consistent with prerenal AKI. His urinalysis was also positive for muddy brown casts.

This patient's renal labs are consistent with a prerenal AKI, so any further CT imaging or contrast is not necessary. However, an IVC ultrasound demonstrating IVC collapsibility will further confirm the diagnosis of hypovolemic AKI.

Imaging—contrast Computed tomography (CT) not done due to allergy and due to diagnosed AKI. IVC ultrasound demonstrating collapsible IVC

Treatment

Fluid resuscitation

Follow-Up

Patient gradually woke up and returned to baseline neurologic functionality.

Resolution

After immediate recognition of new AKI in this patient, manifested as anuria, acute rise in creatinine, and numerous electrolyte abnormalities, he was promptly started on continuous renal replacement while in the ICU. Over the next few days, he had a return of his renal function and started to urinate on his own. He was able to come off renal replacement therapy, was transferred to the floor, and eventually was discharged home.

Patient B

CC: "I stopped peeing, and now I have a headache"

Patient is a 33-year-old female with systemic lupus erythematosus (SLE) currently undergoing pulse-dose steroid therapy. She was diagnosed 5 years ago with lupus and has been seeing a rheumatologist since her diagnosis. She noted that a few days before the clinic visit, she had some darkening of her urine.

She didn't think much of it and figured that she just wasn't drinking enough water. Until 1 day ago, she noted that she hadn't been peeing that much over the last 24 hours. In addition, she started to have a persistent headache that was unchanged and not triggered by anything. She has not been wanting to take NSAIDs as per recommendation from her rheumatologist. She presents to the clinic today because she is concerned about her symptoms.

Prompt: Why would the patient have stopped peeing?

This patient's history is very different from our previous one. She has an underlying medical problem that is known to have renal involvement. Given her additional headache, it is concerning for complications related to her lupus.

Prompt: Are there other symptoms or findings that would help us narrow our differential?

At this point it is important to rule out any other toxins, obstructions, infections that may also be contributing and we want to address the headache appropriately.

Past Medical History

As above—SLE. No other renal history. No surgeries, HTN, DM

Medications Prednisone, hydroxychloroquine, previously on mycophenolate

Allergies None

Social History Married, lives with her husband, and has 2 healthy teenage boys. RN, BSN

High risk behaviors/habits Does not smoke, drinks 1 glass of red wine a night, no recreational drug use

Family History Type 1 DM in mother and Graves disease in her maternal grandmother

Prompt: Does anything in the history help with our differential?

She has a significant medication list, but none of these medications are known to be particularly nephrotoxic. However, they do help us see the severity of her symptoms, at least in the past. She also has a significant autoimmune family history, which is fitting given her presentation.

Review of Systems

- General—denies any fever, chills, or weight loss. Overall feels well except for the headache and is concerned about her urination
- Skin—+red rash on her face, but no bruising, skin lesions, or hair loss
- Hematopoietic—nothing of note
- HEENT—denies any change in vision or hearing
- Respiratory—denies SOB and cough
- Cardiovascular—denies palpitations or chest pain
- GI—has mild abdominal pain. Denies nausea and vomiting
- GU—+Anuria, dark urine. Denies dysuria, urinary frequency
- Endocrine—denies any change in voice or changes in tolerance to heat or cold
- Musculoskeletal—admits to mild back pain but denies other myalgia. Has chronic joint pain
- Neurological—has a headache, but denies syncope, tremor, or ataxia

Physical Examination

- General Appearance—alert and oriented × 3. Well-nourished, in mild discomfort
- Vital Signs—Blood pressure 150/100 mmHg, respiration 16 breaths per minute, pulse 75 beats per minute, temperature: 98.7 °F (37 °C)
- Skin—erythematous malar rash present on her face. Otherwise, normal hair distribution, no skin lesions or ecchymoses
- HEENT—extraocular muscles intact (EOMI), anicteric. moist mucous membranes (MMM)
- Neck—No cervical lymphadenopathy. No carotid bruits noted
- Chest/Lungs—CTA bilaterally. No accessory muscle use. Good airflow equally and in bases
- Heart—RRR. No murmurs, rubs, or gallops
- Abdomen—soft, non-tender, and non-distended. No palpable masses
- Genital/Rectal—not examined
- Extremities—mild 1+ pitting edema noted in all 4 extremities. Otherwise, pulses 2+ symmetrical
- Musculoskeletal—Non-tender, no muscle loss or atrophy
- Neurological*—no focal neurological deficits. CN II-XII grossly intact

Prompt: Is there anything from the ROS and PE that helps with our differential?

Her urinary symptoms in conjunction with her headache are concerning, but it is helpful to know the timing for all of her symptoms and it helps us narrow it against a hyperacute toxicity syndrome or even an infection. She has some of the findings consistent with SLE, which suggests that her disease may not be adequately controlled. Given the fact that she has hypertension as well, we still have to consider the possibility of renal artery stenosis. The abdominal bruits finding is specific but is at times very difficult to note on exam.

Laboratory

- CBC within normal limits (wnl)
- CMP with Cr 2.4 mg/dL, up from 0.9 mg/dL last year
- UA with proteinuria, hematuria, and RBC casts. Neg leukocyte esterase (LE) and nitrites. Proteinuria more than 1.0 g/g in urine protein:CR ratio: proteinuria

Prompt: What else would you like to order?

Given what we previously said, it would be helpful to have renal dopplers and CT angiography to rule out renal artery stenosis. A biopsy can also be done to confirm the diagnosis, but if other etiologies have been ruled out, this diagnosis can be made clinically.

Imaging

- Normal renal Doppler (Fig. 11.1) and MR angiography (Fig. 11.2)
- Kidney biopsy performed demonstrating complex-mediated glomerulonephritis

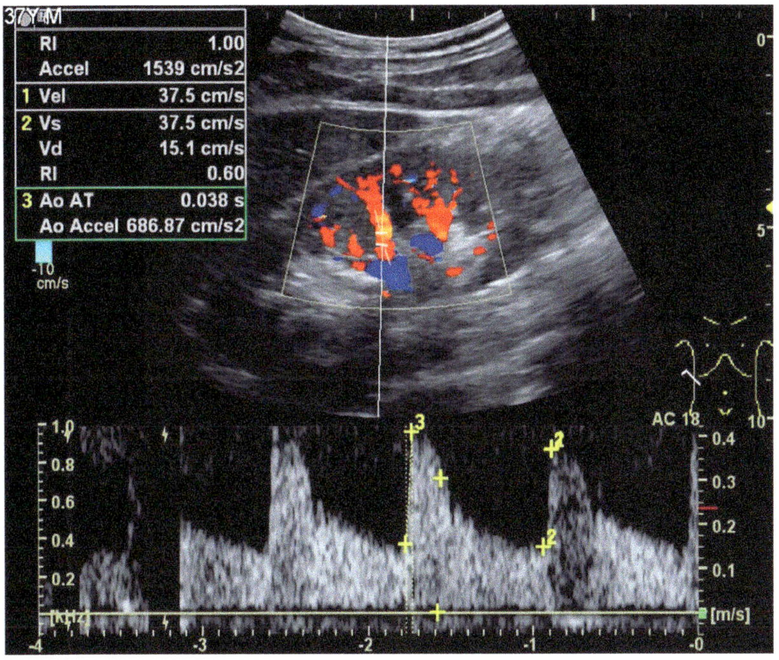

Fig. 11.1 Doppler ultrasound (US) of a normal adult kidney with the estimation of the systolic velocity (Vs), the diastolic velocity (Vd), acceleration time (AoAT), systolic acceleration (Ao Accel), and resistive index (RI). Red and blue colors in the color box represent flow toward and away from the transducer, respectively. The spectrogram below the B-mode image shows flow velocity (m/s) against time (s) obtained within the range gate. The small flash icons on the spectrogram represent initiation of the flow measurement. (From Kristoffer Lindskov Hansen, Michael Bachmann Nielsen and Caroline Ewertsen, licenced under CC BY 4.0). https://commons.wikimedia.org/wiki/File:Doppler_ultrasound_of_systolic_velocity_%28Vs%29,_diastolic_velocity_%28Vd%29,_acceleration_time_%28AoAT%29,_systolic_acceleration_%28Ao_Accel%29_and_resistive_index_%28RI%29_of_normal_kidney.jpg

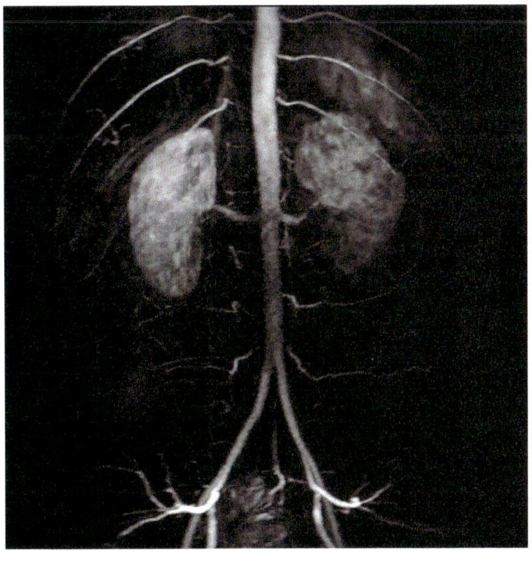

Fig. 11.2 Contrast enhanced MRA of the abdominal aorta and kidneys. (From Frank Gaillard, licensed under CC BY-SA 3.0.). https://commons.wikimedia.org/wiki/File:Abdominal_aorta.jpg

Treatment

- Induction therapy with IV methylprednisolone, restarting mycophenolate. Six weeks later, maintained on oral prednisone and mycophenolate

Follow-Up

- Seen in the clinic, and urinary symptoms resolved

Resolution

Her lupus flare and glomerulonephritis were quickly diagnosed after renal biopsy, and she was restarted on induction therapy with IV steroids, and she was restarted on mycophenolate as an adjunct to her regimen. Six weeks later, she was maintained on oral prednisone and mycophenolate, and by her next clinic visit, her urinary symptoms and headache had resolved.

Patient C

CC: "I stopped peeing, doc"

Patient is a 70-year-old male with history of granulomatosis with polyangiitis (GPA), previously treated with medications, who started developing urinary symptoms over the past 6 months. He mentions that he initially had some darker urine attributed to not drinking enough water. 3 days ago, he says he stopped being able to pee, and that no matter how hard he pushed, nothing or very little would come out. He gradually noticed that he had to wake up in the middle of the night to urinate multiple times and gradually more often. He also felt as though whenever he would urinate, the stream would not be as strong, and he had the sense that he wasn't urinating the full amount he could. He also often felt like he needed to pee very badly out of nowhere. Otherwise, he hasn't had any other major complaints.

Prompt: What aspects to this patient's history are important in our differential?

Given this patient's history and gradual worsening of his symptoms over a long period of time, the highest priority on the differential is something neoplastic in nature. Be less concerned for something happening acutely at this point. However, it could be a recurrence of his GPA. Hypovolemia also seems very unlikely given his over stable condition at this point.

Past Medical History GPA, well managed, diagnosed 30 years ago. Has been in remission for 5 yrs

Medications Previously on cyclophosphamide

Allergies Shellfish, anaphylaxis

Social History Retired veteran. Lives with his wife in a senior living facility. Enjoys going on walks for 30 min every day. Owns a dog

High risk behaviors/habits 20 pk yr history. Drinks 2 beers a day

Family History Lung cancer in his dad after smoking significantly. Mom died of a heart attack at age 84

Prompt: Does anything in the history help with our differential?

He is elderly, had significant tobacco use history, and cyclophosphamide use is also a risk factor for developing bladder carcinoma.

Review of Systems

- General—+20 lb. unintentional weight loss over 6 months. Denies any fever or chills. Overall, it feels well
- Skin—no bruising, skin lesions, or hair loss
- HEENT—denies any change in vision or hearing
- Respiratory—denies SOB and cough
- Cardiovascular—denies palpitations or chest pain
- GI—has mild abdominal pain. Denies nausea and vomiting
- GU—+Anuria, dark urine. Denies dysuria, urinary frequency
- Endocrine—denies any change in voice or changes in tolerance to heat or cold
- Musculoskeletal—denies any joint pain or swelling
- Neurological—denies headache, syncope, tremor, or ataxia

Physical Examination

- General Appearance—Alert and oriented. No acute distress.
- Vital Signs—Blood pressure: 127/85 mmHg. Breathing: 16 breaths per minute. Pulse: 73 beats per minute. Temperature: 99.1 °F (37.3 °C)
- Skin—normal hair distribution, no skin lesions or ecchymoses.
- HEENT—EOMI, anicteric. MMM.
- Neck—No cervical lymphadenopathy. No carotid bruits noted
- Chest/Lungs—CTA bilaterally. No accessory muscle use. Good airflow equally and in bases

- Heart—RRR. No murmurs, rubs, or gallops
- Abdomen—soft, non-tender, and mildly distended. No palpable masses
- Genital/Rectal—not examined
- Extremities—mild 1+ pitting edema noted in all 4 extremities. Otherwise, pulses 2+ symmetrical
- Musculoskeletal—Non-tender, no muscle loss or atrophy
- Neurological*—no focal neurological deficits. CN II-XII grossly intact

Prompt: Is there anything from the ROS and PE that helps with our differential?

He has a significant weight loss in addition to his urinary symptoms, which is concerning even more for a neoplastic process. The fact that his physical exam and ROS are otherwise benign makes suggests that his current situation is not due to worsening or remission of his GPA. And in conjunction with the chronicity of his symptoms, a mass is highest among the differential. Because it is rare to have a neoplasm causing an intrinsic or prerenal AKI, an obstructive pattern in his labs would be expected, and should send him for imaging to confirm the diagnosis.

Laboratory

- CBC wnl
- CMP with Cr 4.0 mg/dL, up from 0.8 mg/dL last year.
- UA with hematuria, 4 RBCs per HPF. Neg LE and nitrites.

Prompt: Anything else you would like to order?

At this point, would request imaging to visualize the obstruction seen in his labs. He has gross hematuria, but hematuria by itself is not cause for obstructive symptoms. It would be important also to assess for metastasis in order to grade and stage his tumor.

Imaging

CT urography demonstrating bilateral hydronephrosis and large bladder mass impinging on the bladder neck

CTA/P w/o contrast performed, and bone scan done to measure for metastasis, which comes back negative

Patient C Patient had a normal CBC, but his creatinine increased from 0.8 mg/dL to 4.0 mg/dL in the last year. His urinalysis contained hematuria with 4 red blood cells per high-power field but was negative for leukocyte esterase and nitrites. His presentation was concerning for malignancy, and so CT urography was obtained, demonstrating bilateral hydronephrosis with a large bladder mass impinging on his bladder neck. A PET scan was obtained to evaluate metastasis but was negative.

Treatment Diagnosed with non-muscle invasive bladder carcinoma (Fig. 11.3) and treated with TURBT

Follow-up Follow-up in clinic 6 weeks later, well healed and improved urinary symptoms

Resolution

After imaging, he had a subsequent biopsy and further imaging to characterize the mass visual-

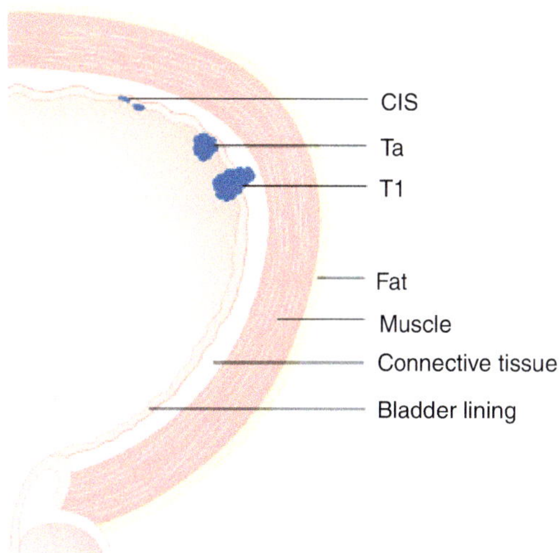

Fig. 11.3 Diagram showing early stage bladder cancer. (From Cancer Research UK uploader, licensed by CC BY-SA 4.0). https://commons.wikimedia.org/wiki/File:Diagram_showing_early_stage_bladder_cancer_CRUK_442.svg

ized on his CT. He was diagnosed with a non-muscle invasive bladder carcinoma and treated with transurethral resection of his tumor. He did not need any adjunctive chemotherapy or radiotherapy and remained cancer-free. He attended his frequent oncology outpatient appointments, and a few months later presented to the primary care clinic with many of his symptoms resolved and his weight returning to his baseline.

Learning Objective Answers

1. **Describe the anatomic components of the urinary system, placing special emphasis on the microscopic structures in the nephron and their function, as well as the gross structures involved in the passage of urine.**

A nephron consists of a renal tubule and a glomerulus. The glomerulus is a tuft of capillaries formed by the afferent arteriole and drained by the efferent arteriole. The glomerulus is housed within Bowman's capsule, where filtration begins.

Filtration occurs through a barrier composed of fenestrated capillary endothelium with pores 70–90 nm in diameter, the glomerular basement membrane, and podocytes with filtration slits approximately 25 nm wide. These structures work together to allow selective passage of substances based on size and charge.

The nephron is divided into several segments, each with specific functions. The proximal convoluted tubule (PCT) has a brush border of microvilli for absorption. The loop of Henle consists of a descending limb made of thin, permeable cells and an ascending limb composed of thick cells with many mitochondria. Cortical nephrons have short loops, while juxtamedullary nephrons have long loops. The distal convoluted tubule (DCT) begins at the macula densa and has fewer microvilli than the PCT. Collecting ducts, formed by the coalescence of distal tubules, are composed of principal cells involved in sodium and water reabsorption and intercalated cells responsible for acid secretion.

The juxtaglomerular apparatus, located at the end of the thick ascending limb of the loop of Henle near the glomerulus, includes the macula densa, extraglomerular cells, and renin-secreting granular cells. This apparatus plays a critical role in regulating filtration and blood pressure.

The nephron's blood supply is crucial for its function. Afferent arterioles branch from interlobular arteries to form glomerular capillaries. Efferent arterioles drain the glomerulus, forming peritubular capillaries and, in juxtamedullary nephrons, the vasa recta. This renal capillary network supports filtration and reabsorption processes, ensuring the nephron's efficient operation in maintaining homeostasis [2].

Blood enters the kidneys through the renal arteries, which branch into smaller arterioles, forming the glomeruli in the renal cortex. Within the glomeruli, blood is filtered, and the filtrate passes into Bowman's capsule and space. From Bowman's capsule, the filtrate enters the PCT, where significant reabsorption of water, ions, and nutrients occurs. The filtrate then moves into the loop of Henle, which plays a crucial role in concentrating the urine by creating a gradient of increasing osmolarity.

After passing through the loop of Henle, the filtrate enters the DCT, where further reabsorption and secretion occur, fine-tuning the composition of the urine. The filtrate then flows into the collecting ducts. These ducts gather urine from multiple nephrons and transport it through the renal medulla to the minor calyces. From the minor calyces, urine drains into the major calyces and then into the renal pelvis. The renal pelvis funnels the urine into the ureter, which carries it to the bladder for storage.

When the bladder reaches its capacity, urine is expelled through the urethra during the process of urination. This sequential flow ensures that blood is efficiently filtered, and waste products are excreted from the body as urine [3].

2. **Compare and contrast the different etiologies of renal failure, focusing on the physiologic basis for the injury of the kidneys and pertinent lab findings involved with**

each etiology. Identify which one each patient has.

Acute kidney injury is defined by any of the following criteria: an increase in serum creatinine by 0.3 mg/dL (26.5 μmol/L) or more within 48 hours; an increase in serum creatinine to 1.5 times or more from the baseline, which is known or presumed to have occurred within the prior 7 days; or a urine volume of less than 0.5 mL/kg/h for 6 hours [4]. These criteria are designed to identify AKI promptly, allowing for early intervention and management to prevent further kidney damage and associated complications. Causes of AKI can further be stratified based on anatomically where they are happening in relation to the kidney, namely, prerenal azotemia, intrinsic renal parenchymal disease, and postrenal obstructions [5].

Prerenal Azotemia

Prerenal azotemia, as the name suggests, is the acute rise of BUN or creatinine due to insufficient blood flow into the kidneys to allow for proper glomerular filtration. Prerenal azotemia is primarily linked to hypovolemia, decreased cardiac output, and medications like NSAIDs and angiotensin II inhibitors that disrupt renal vascular responses. It is characterized by reversible kidney function impairment without parenchymal damage, though prolonged prerenal azotemia can lead to acute tubular necrosis (ATN). Normal glomerular filtration rate (GFR) relies on renal blood flow and the balance of renal arteriole resistances. Hypovolemia—*as is seen in Patient A* requiring multiple units of blood—and reduced cardiac output trigger compensatory mechanisms, such as renal vasoconstriction and salt and water reabsorption, mediated by agents like angiotensin II, norepinephrine, and vasopressin, to maintain blood pressure and perfusion.

To sustain GFR, the kidneys employ mechanisms like afferent arteriole dilation via a concerted effort of numerous players, including the juxtaglomerular apparatus (JGA), leading to increased production of vasodilators in response to low perfusion pressure. However, these mechanisms have limits, particularly when systolic blood pressure drops below 80 mmHg. The patient in the vignette had a blood pressure that qualified as hypovolemic shock and was therefore too low to allow for physiologic compensation. Factors like atherosclerosis, hypertension, age, and chronic kidney disease (CKD) can impair autoregulatory responses, increasing the risk of prerenal azotemia. Medications such as NSAIDs and ACE inhibitors or ARBs can further compromise these compensatory processes, especially in patients with renal artery stenosis [5].

Intrinsic Renal AKI

The most common causes of intrinsic AKI are sepsis, ischemia, and nephrotoxins, with prerenal azotemia often progressing to tubular injury. While AKI is frequently attributed to "ATN," it is rarely confirmed on biopsy, and factors like *inflammation (as is the case for Patient B)*, apoptosis, and altered perfusion may play significant roles [5].

(a) Sepsis Associated AKI

In the United States, AKI complicates more than 50% of severe sepsis cases, significantly increasing mortality risk. This is also a major contributor to AKI in the developing world. Pathophysiology involves factors like inflammation, mitochondrial dysfunction, and interstitial edema, beyond just tubular injury. Hemodynamic effects of sepsis, including arterial vasodilation and renal vasoconstriction, reduce GFR and cause endothelial damage, leading to tubular cell injury.

(b) Ischemia-Associated AKI

Healthy kidneys receive an uneven amount of cardiac output for their size. The renal medulla is one of the most hypoxic regions and is highly susceptible to ischemic damage due to its blood vessel architecture and high metabolic activity. Ischemia and mitochondrial dysfunction, along with leukocyte-endothelial interactions, contribute to renal tubular injury, with persistent preglomerular vasoconstriction and factors like tubuloglomerular feedback and necrotic debris further reducing GFR. The 22-year-old in the vignette likely suffered an ischemia-associated AKI while he was in hypovolemic shock and subsequently developed anuria as a result.

(c) Nephrotoxin-associated AKI

As was mentioned above, the kidneys have high blood perfusion and concentration of filtered substances, making them highly at risk to nephrotoxic agents. Nephrotoxic injury can be caused by various pharmacologic compounds, endogenous substances, and environmental exposures, affecting structures like the tubules, interstitium, vasculature, and collecting system. Risk factors for nephrotoxicity include older age, CKD, and prerenal azotemia.

Iodinated contrast agents used in imaging can cause "contrast nephropathy," especially in patients with CKD or diabetic nephropathy. Antibiotics such as vancomycin, aminoglycosides, and amphotericin B are associated with AKI through mechanisms like tubular injury and necrosis. Chemotherapeutic agents such as cisplatin and carboplatin cause nephrotoxicity, often mitigated by intensive hydration regimens.

Toxic ingestions, including ethylene glycol and diethylene glycol, can cause AKI through direct tubular injury and obstruction. Endogenous toxins like myoglobin, hemoglobin, uric acid, and myeloma light chains also contribute to AKI, with mechanisms involving intrarenal vasoconstriction, direct tubular toxicity, and mechanical obstruction of the nephron lumen [5].

Postrenal AKI

Postrenal AKI occurs when urine flow is acutely obstructed, leading to increased retrograde hydrostatic pressure and interference with glomerular filtration. This obstruction can result from functional or structural issues anywhere from the renal pelvis to the urethra, *as is the case with Patient C having a prostate causing obstruction.* Common causes of postrenal AKI include bladder neck obstruction from prostate disease, neurogenic bladder, or anticholinergic drugs, as well as obstructed Foley catheters. Other lower tract obstructions can be due to blood clots, calculi, and urethral strictures, while ureteral obstructions can result from intraluminal issues, wall infiltration, or external compression [5].

3. **Discuss the diagnosis of acute renal injury. Develop a clinical approach to a patient presenting with "dark urine" or oliguria/anuria and explain a diagnostic schema for renal failure**

Accurate diagnosis of acute kidney injury (AKI) relies on clinical context, detailed history, and physical examination. Changes in urinary frequency, such as polyuria, hematuria, nocturia, and urgency, as well as new-onset hypertension and worsening edema in dependent areas, are frequently observed. Nonspecific symptoms like nausea, vomiting, and malaise may be present, and in some cases, specific symptoms such as ipsilateral flank pain due to obstructing nephrolithiasis occur [6]. Prerenal azotemia is suspected with symptoms like vomiting, diarrhea, and use of specific medications, along with physical signs such as orthostatic hypotension and dry mucous membranes. Postrenal AKI considerations include a history of prostatic disease or nephrolithiasis, with symptoms like colicky flank pain or urinary frequency.

Medication review is crucial, as nephrotoxic drugs and dose adjustments are common in AKI, and a kidney biopsy may be necessary for diagnosing interstitial nephritis. Systemic features such as palpable purpura or a history of autoimmune disease can indicate systemic vasculitis or lupus-related AKI, and pregnancy may suggest preeclampsia as a contributor [7].

When evaluating patients referred for AKI or any renal complaint, it is important to obtain a thorough history. Conditions like congestive heart failure, liver disease, and nephrotic syndrome can reduce renal blood flow, while vascular diseases suggest renal artery issues [4]. Any previous diagnosis of kidney disease and documentation of blood urea nitrogen (BUN) and serum creatinine values, a history of asymptomatic urinary abnormalities, and changes in urinary frequency, urgency, or character ought to be included. Information on diabetes, including its duration, severity, and any end-organ damage, as well as a history of hypertension and cardiac issues, should be gathered [5]. Previous exposure to nephrotoxic medications, adverse reactions to renin-angiotensin-aldosterone system blocking agents, and recent gastrointestinal endoscopic procedures requiring bowel cleansing are also relevant. Exposure to contrast-requiring procedures, recent systemic infections or intercurrent illnesses, and a family history of kidney disease or renal replacement therapy are crucial details. Additionally, a history of autoimmune diseases, recent changes in medication doses, new medications, and the use of over-the-counter medications or herbal supplements should be documented [5].

In advanced kidney disease, patients often exhibit nonspecific signs and symptoms initially detectable by increased serum creatinine levels. Common symptoms include loss of appetite, easy fatigability, generalized weakness, involuntary weight changes, mental alterations such as lethargy and difficulty concentrating, nausea, vomiting, dyspepsia, a metallic taste, generalized itching, seizures, difficulty breathing, edema, intractable hiccups, frothy urine, decreased sexual interest, and restless legs. Physical signs include elevated blood pressure, pallor due to anemia, volume overload (evidenced by jugular venous distention, peripheral and pulmonary edema, and anasarca), pericarditis (friction rub), and neurological signs like asterixis and myoclonus (uremic encephalopathy).

A bedside diagnostic test that suggests underlying diabetic nephropathy is funduscopy. This test is useful because the vascular similarities between the retina and kidneys correlate with the microvascular complications seen in diabetes mellitus. Patients with type 2 diabetes and proliferative retinopathy often exhibit kidney involvement, such as microalbuminuria or overt proteinuria. Therefore, it is recommended that all diabetic patients with proliferative retinopathy undergo kidney function evaluation, including testing for microalbuminuria. However, the absence of retinopathy does not rule out diabetic nephropathy [7].

Patients with renal failure may exhibit abnormal blood laboratory results such as elevated BUN and serum creatinine, decreased estimated glomerular filtration rate (eGFR), or abnormal serum electrolyte values. Asymptomatic urinary abnormalities like microscopic hematuria, proteinuria, or microalbuminuria are also common [8].

1. Urinalysis

   Urine volume, specific gravity, and sediment each have a role in characterizing an AKI. Urine volume is generally not a reliable indicator for distinguishing various forms and causes of acute kidney injury (AKI). While anuria might suggest complete urinary tract obstruction, it can also occur in other etiologies of AKI, such as renal artery occlusion, severe proliferative glomerulonephritis, vasculitis, or bilateral cortical necrosis. Conversely, patients with partial urinary tract obstruction may exhibit polyuria due to secondary impairment of urine-concentrating mechanisms. This complexity underscores the need for a thorough assessment beyond just urine volume to accurately diagnose the underlying cause of AKI. Measured urine specific gravity can provide valuable clues; values above 1.015 to 1.020 are often associated with prerenal AKI, whereas a value of 1.010 is characteristic of ATN. Sediment should be inspected for cells, casts, and crystals. In prerenal AKI, the urine sediment is typically bland but may contain transparent hyaline casts. Postrenal AKI may also present with a bland sediment, though hematuria is common with intraluminal obstructions. Renal tubular epithelial cells, epithelial cell casts, and muddy brown granular casts are characteristic of ischemic or nephrotoxic ATN, often accompanied by microscopic hematuria and mild tubular proteinuria.

Various other urinary findings can further help differentiate between AKI types. Hematuria on dipstick assessment can result from various conditions, including urologic trauma, urologic disease, interstitial nephritis, acute glomerulonephritis, atheroembolic disease, and renal infarction. Pigment nephropathy may also have hematuria, but mainly when blood is strongly positive in the setting of few or no red blood cells on microscopic examination. Red blood cell casts typically indicate acute glomerular disease but may rarely be seen in acute interstitial nephritis (AIN). Dysmorphic RBCs are more common in glomerular injury. White blood cell casts and nonpigmented granular casts suggest interstitial nephritis, while broad granular casts are indicative of CKD. Eosinophiluria, common in drug-induced allergic interstitial nephritis, lacks sensitivity and specificity for AIN diagnosis. Specific crystal types, such as uric acid and oxalate crystals, can indicate specific conditions like acute urate nephropathy or ethylene glycol toxicity. Proteinuria patterns also provide diagnostic clues, with increased excretion reflecting tubular injury or glomerular damage, and heavy proteinuria often associated with allergic interstitial nephritis triggered by NSAIDs. Analyzing urine biochemical parameters, such as fractional excretion of sodium (FE Na) and urea (FE urea), can help differentiate prerenal AKI from intrinsic AKI, though these indices have limitations, particularly in patients on diuretics or with certain underlying conditions [8].

2. Basic Metabolic Panel

   AKI presents with distinct patterns in serum creatinine (SCr) changes depending on the underlying cause. Prerenal azotemia typically causes SCr increases that normalize with improved hemodynamic status, whereas its effect on BUN is much more significant, leading to a ratio >20:1. This is due to enhanced tubular reabsorption of filtered urea in prerenal states [4, 7]. Contrast nephropathy results in a parallel increase of both SCr and BUN within 24–48 hours, peaking at 3–5 days (maintaining a ratio of 10:1), and resolving by 5–7 days. Epithelial cell toxins like aminoglycosides are delayed in their effects on SCr increases, occurring 3–5 days to 2 weeks post-exposure. Additionally, AKI often leads to electrolyte abnormalities like hyperkalemia, hyperphosphatemia, and hypocalcemia. And the basic metabolic panel can also provide insight as to the cause of the AKI. Increased anion gaps suggest ethylene glycol poisoning, while low anion gaps may indicate multiple myeloma [5, 8].

3. Complete Blood Count

   Diagnostic clues from a complete blood count include anemia, which is common and multifactorial in AKI. Peripheral eosinophilia may indicate interstitial nephritis or vasculitis, while severe anemia without bleeding points to hemolysis, multiple myeloma, or thrombotic microangiopathy (TMA). TMA is characterized by thrombocytopenia, schistocytes, elevated lactate dehydrogenase, and low haptoglobin, with further testing for ADAMTS13 and Shiga toxin necessary for thrombotic thrombocytopenic purpura (TTP) or hemolytic uremic syndrome (HUS) diagnosis [5].

Imaging Studies

Imaging of the abdomen is helpful in addition to laboratory testing in determining the cause of AKI. Post-void residual volumes exceeding 100 to 150 mL can indicate bladder outlet obstruction. While plain films may reveal calcium-containing stones, renal ultrasonography is the preferred screening test, providing insights into cortical thickness, medullary density, collecting system integrity, and kidney size. CT can visualize the kidneys and collecting system, but contrast use should be avoided in AKI patients. Unenhanced CT scans are effective for detecting obstructing ureteral stones. Ultrasonography and

CT have largely replaced intravenous pyelography, which is now rarely used in AKI evaluation.

Cystoscopic retrograde or percutaneous anterograde pyelography can precisely localize obstructions and facilitate therapeutic interventions like ureteral stenting or nephrostomy. Magnetic resonance angiography (MRA) is useful for detecting renal artery stenosis but is generally contraindicated in AKI patients due to the risk of nephrogenic systemic fibrosis associated with gadolinium-based contrast. Doppler ultrasonography and spiral CT are also helpful in suspected vascular obstructions, but contrast angiography remains the gold standard for definitive diagnosis [8].

Other Diagnostic Modalities

1. Kidney Biopsy

   When the cause of acute kidney injury (AKI) remains unclear after clinical, laboratory, and radiologic evaluations, a kidney biopsy should be considered. This procedure can provide definitive diagnostic and prognostic information for both acute and CKD. It is particularly useful when other diagnoses like glomerulonephritis, vasculitis, interstitial nephritis, myeloma kidney, HUS, TTP, and allograft dysfunction are suspected. Although kidney biopsy carries a risk of severe bleeding, especially in patients with thrombocytopenia or coagulopathy, the valuable diagnostic and prognostic information it provides often outweighs the risks [4].
2. Novel Biomarkers

   Novel biomarkers for kidney injury, such as serum cystatin C, NGAL, KIM-1, IL-18, L-FABP, TIMP-2, and IGFBP7, are being evaluated for early AKI detection, differential diagnosis, and prognosis. Although not yet widely available for routine clinical use, these biomarkers show promise in providing earlier diagnoses and distinguishing between prerenal and intrinsic AKI. For example, cystatin C, a 13-kDa protein, changes more rapidly than serum creatinine in response to kidney function changes, making it a potential early marker for tubular injury [7]

4. **Discuss the treatment approach for each etiology of renal failure**

General Principles of Management

The management of AKI varies significantly depending on its underlying cause and clinical presentation. For certain forms of AKI, such as ATN, there is no specific pharmacologic therapy to stop renal damage, so treatment focuses on prevention, supportive care for fluid and electrolyte imbalances, and mitigating uremic complications. In severe cases, renal replacement therapy (RRT) may be necessary. The primary goals are to prevent mortality, promote kidney function recovery, and reduce the risk of chronic kidney disease (CKD) [8].

Volume Management Prerenal AKI, often reversible by restoring renal perfusion, requires early recognition and treatment of conditions causing extracellular fluid loss using isotonic crystalloid solutions, which are preferred over isotonic saline due to reduced adverse kidney events. Volume overload in AKI, exacerbated by excessive IV fluids or enteral nutrition, can lead to severe complications like hypertension, edema, and pulmonary edema, with potential cardiac issues such as arrhythmias and myocardial infarction.

Potassium Homeostasis Hyperkalemia, a common and dangerous complication of AKI due to impaired potassium excretion, dietary intake, and cell injury, can cause ECG abnormalities and cardiac arrhythmias, requiring urgent treatment with intravenous calcium, insulin and glucose, and potassium removal methods. Hypokalemia, though rare in AKI, is managed by replacing potassium deficits and correcting underlying causes, with oral potassium chloride as the main treatment and intravenous administration for severe cases.

Other Electrolyte Derangements Hyperphosphatemia in AKI is managed with phosphate binders, while symptomatic hypocalcemia is treated with calcium gluconate or calcium chloride, and ionized calcium levels should be monitored in hypoalbuminemia. Hypermagnesemia is addressed by discontinuing magnesium-containing antacids, and asymptomatic hyperuricemia is common, though very high levels may indicate acute urate nephropathy.

Acid-Base Homeostasis Metabolic acidosis, common in AKI due to acid retention, is treated when severe (pH < 7.20 and serum bicarbonate <15 mmol/L) with sodium bicarbonate, while avoiding overcorrection to prevent metabolic alkalosis and other complications. Metabolic alkalosis, though less common, can result from excessive correction of acidosis, diuretic overuse, or gastric acid loss.

Malnutrition In AKI, particularly with multisystem organ failure, adequate nutrition is critical to prevent protein energy wasting and complications like starvation ketoacidosis, with Kidney Disease Improving Global Outcomes (KDIGO) guidelines recommending 20–30 kcal/kg per day and protein intake tailored to AKI severity and treatment modality. Overnutrition should be avoided to prevent worsening azotemia.

Anemia Anemia in AKI, often multifactorial, is not typically responsive to erythropoiesis-stimulating agents, requiring treatments like desmopressin or dialysis for severe uremic bleeding and gastrointestinal prophylaxis with proton pump inhibitors or H2 blockers. Venous thromboembolism prophylaxis should consider the clinical setting, avoiding certain anticoagulants in severe AKI due to unpredictable pharmacokinetics.

Heart Failure AKI management in heart failure varies with the clinical context, involving withholding diuretics and cautious volume replacement for diuresis-induced AKI and intensified diuretic therapy for acute decompensated heart failure. Additional treatments may include inotropes, vasodilators, mechanical support, and possibly extracorporeal ultrafiltration, though its efficacy remains debated.

Liver Failure and Hepatorenal Syndrome Differentiating volume-responsive prerenal AKI from hepatorenal syndrome (HRS) in liver failure involves volume expansion with hyperoncotic albumin for prerenal AKI, while HRS treatment focuses on liver transplantation and vasoconstrictor therapy with albumin. Transjugular invasive treatment for portal hypertension (TIPS) has largely replaced peritoneovenous shunting for better ascites control and reduced HRS incidence.

Postrenal AKI Management of postrenal AKI involves relieving urinary tract obstructions using bladder catheters, percutaneous nephrostomy tubes, or ureteral stents, followed by IV fluid replacement for persistent diuresis and subsequent urologic evaluation to address the underlying cause.

Renal Replacement Therapies

Dialysis is indicated for acute kidney injury (AKI) when medical management fails to control volume overload, hyperkalemia, acidosis, certain toxic ingestions, and severe uremic complications such as encephalopathy or pericardial effusion. While delaying dialysis can lead to preventable complications, starting it too early may expose patients to unnecessary risks, including infections and procedural complications. Randomized controlled trials have not shown a survival benefit from early initiation of dialysis, and many nephrologists start dialysis empirically when BUN levels exceed 100 mg/dL in patients without signs of kidney recovery. Dialysis options include peritoneal dialysis and various forms of hemodialysis, with hemodialysis being the most common. Hemodialysis can be intermittent or continuous, with vascular access typically through the femoral, internal jugular, or subclavian veins, and is associated with complications like hypotension, especially in critically ill patients [5].

5. **Discuss epidemiology and prognosis of renal failure, including a discussion on certain barriers to care involving patients with acute kidney disease**

In developed countries, AKI is a significant concern in hospitalized patients, with a systematic review of 312 cohort studies (49 million patients) revealing that 1 in 5 adults and 1 in 3 children hospitalized with acute illness develop AKI. In a large US population study, the incidence of non-renal replacement therapy (RRT)-requiring AKI was 384.1 per 100,000 person-years, and RRT-requiring AKI was 24.4 per 100,000 person-years. Between 1996 and 2003, the incidences of these conditions increased significantly, with non-RRT-requiring AKI rising by 38% and RRT-requiring AKI by 33%. AKI is most common among elderly, male, and Black patients. In ICUs, the incidence of AKI was 5.7%, with severe cases requiring RRT. Subacute kidney injury, affecting about 1% of hospitalized patients, is linked to increased hospital mortality [9].

In developing countries, the epidemiology of AKI is less well-documented due to limited, low-quality data often derived from small, single-center studies. Despite these challenges, AKI is increasingly recognized as a major contributor to morbidity, mortality, and economic loss. Extremes of age, comorbid diseases (such as CKD, diabetes, hypertension, cardiovascular diseases, chronic liver disease, and chronic obstructive pulmonary disease), and conditions like sepsis significantly increase the risk of AKI. Fluid resuscitation methods, particularly the use of synthetic colloids compared to crystalloids, have been shown to elevate the risk of AKI and RRT use, especially in septic patients. Fluid overload is also associated with adverse renal outcomes and higher mortality in critically ill patients [8].

Acute kidney injury (AKI) significantly increases the risk of both in-hospital and long-term mortality, extends hospital stays, and raises healthcare costs. It also heightens the risk of subsequent cardiovascular events, though the mechanisms are not fully understood. While prerenal and postrenal azotemia generally have better prognoses, severe intrinsic AKI, even when requiring dialysis, can see kidney recovery. However, survivors of severe AKI are at high risk for progressive CKD, with up to 10% potentially developing end-stage kidney disease (ESKD) requiring long-term dialysis or transplantation. AKI and CKD are interrelated, with each condition increasing the risk of developing the other; thus, measuring albuminuria post-AKI can help predict kidney disease progression, and nephrologist-led post-discharge care is recommended for secondary prevention [4].

Exam Questions

1. A 70-year-old male with history of granulomatosis with polyangiitis presents with a 3-day history of anuria. He mentions that he was previously on a medication for his vasculitis for more than 10 years but has not taken the medication for 20 years. He said his pee had also been darker for the past 6 months, but he did not know why. He also has a 30 pk yr history but does not drink. What is likely to be found in this patient?
   A. 3 g of protein in his urine
   B. Muddy brown casts
   C. Bladder neck outflow obstruction
   D. Drop in creatinine

Answer: C

Explanation: This patient likely has an outflow obstruction leading to anuria; hence, C is the correct answer. His history of GPA treatment, likely cyclophosphamide, coupled with his smoking history and age, puts him at the highest risk for developing a bladder carcinoma. A is incorrect, as this finding is indicative of nephrotic syndrome, which is not what this particular patient has. B is incorrect, as this finding is indicative of ATN, and nothing in this patient's history reflects a toxic or ischemic event. D is incorrect, as a drop in creatinine is antithetical to an AKI, as this patient will likely experience a bump in his creatinine.

2. A 22-year-old male presents on his third day of ICU stay with new anuria. He initially presented to the ED as a trauma, having lost multiple liters of blood, requiring the massive transfusion protocol to be initiated. He was initially presenting with a BP of 80/30 mmHg and an HR of 145 bpm. After receiving 3 units of blood and aggressive fluid resuscitation, he was stabilized, intubated, and admitted to the ICU. Currently, his vitals have normalized. His labs demonstrate a rise in creatinine from 0.9 mg/dL on admission to 3.4 mg/dL. He has not been given any antibiotics or any other medications other than opioids for pain. He remains afebrile. Which of the following would be most similar to his etiology of AKI?
   A. Nephrolithiasis of his right ureter
   B. Sepsis
   C. Post-infections glomerulonephritis
   D. Tacrolimus toxicity

Answer: B

Explanation: This patient's AKI is caused by hypovolemia and shock due to his significant loss of blood in the field. This would be categorized as a prerenal AKI, which is in the same category as something like sepsis. Although this is due to widespread vasodilation as opposed to low circulating volume, the effect is ultimately the same. A is incorrect, as this choice would lead to a postrenal obstructive AKI, which is different than what the patient is experiencing. C is incorrect, as this choice would lead to an intrinsic renal AKI, likely due to the deposition of immune complexes within the glomerulus, which is a different etiology from that of hypovolemia. D is incorrect, as this choice, like choice C, would lead to an intrinsic renal AKI due to the chemical damage of the nephron structures.

3. A 10-year-old boy is brought to the clinic by his parents because of fatigue and painful urination for the past 2 weeks. His parents report that he has also had a weak urine stream and often strains to initiate urination. On physical examination, the child appears fatigued, and his bladder is palpable above the pubic symphysis. His vital signs are within normal limits, but there is mild periorbital edema. A urine dipstick test is positive for blood and protein, and a bladder ultrasound reveals significant post-void residual volume. Laboratory tests reveal the following:
   - Blood urea nitrogen (BUN): 60 mg/dL (normal: 7–20 mg/dL)
   - Serum creatinine: 3.0 mg/dL (normal: 0.5–1.0 mg/dL)
   - Serum sodium: 135 mEq/L
   - Urine output: decreased to 0.3 mL/kg/hour

   Which of the following is the most likely underlying cause of this patient's acute kidney injury?
   A. Acute tubular necrosis (ATN)
   B. Urethral stricture
   C. Minimal change disease
   D. Hypovolemia from dehydration
   E. Post-infectious glomerulonephritis

Answer: B

Explanation: This child presents with clinical signs and symptoms suggestive of a urinary outflow obstruction. A urethral stricture can cause obstructive AKI by leading to significant urinary retention, elevated intravesical pressure, and subsequent damage to the upper urinary tract. The palpable bladder, weak urinary stream, and significant post-void residual volume strongly point to a lower urinary tract obstruction, which impairs normal urine flow and results in obstructive AKI. A is incorrect because this patient's symptoms and signs, such as painful urination, bladder distension, and significant post-void residual volume, are not characteristic of ATN. Additionally, there are no risk factors for ischemic or nephrotoxic injury in this patient's history. C is incorrect because the edema in nephrotic syndrome is typically generalized and severe, not mild and periorbital as seen in this patient. Furthermore, nephrotic syndrome does not explain the urinary symptoms or evidence of bladder outlet obstruction seen in this case. D is incorrect because this child does not have signs of dehydration (e.g., dry mucous membranes, tachycardia), and the palpable bladder with a weak urinary stream indicates a problem related to urinary retention rather than decreased perfusion to the kidneys. E is incorrect because while the periorbital edema and hematuria could fit this picture, the condition does not explain the painful urination, bladder distension, or obstructive symptoms. The key findings in this case—urinary retention and a palpable bladder—are inconsistent with glomerulonephritis.

References

1. Hall M, Manetta E, Tupper K. Creatine supplementation: an update. Curr Sports Med Rep. 2021;20(7):338–44. https://doi.org/10.1249/JSR.0000000000000863. PMID: 34234088.
2. Barrett KE, Barman SM, Brooks HL, Yuan JJ. eds. Renal function & micturition. In: Ganong's review of medical physiology, 26e. McGraw-Hill Education; 2019. Accessed 05 Aug 2024. https://accessmedicine.mhmedical.com/content.aspx?bookid=2525&sectionid=204297900.
3. Chung KW, Chung HM. Gross anatomy. Philadelphia: Lippincott Williams & Wilkins; 2012.
4. Kellum JA, Lameire N, for the KDIGO AKI Guideline Work Group. Diagnosis, evaluation, and management of acute kidney injury: a KDIGO summary (Part 1). Crit Care. 2013;17(3):204.
5. Waikar SS, Bonventre JV. Acute kidney injury. In: Loscalzo J, Fauci A, Kasper D, Hauser S, Longo D, Jameson J, editors. Harrison's principles of internal medicine, 21e. McGraw-Hill Education; 2022. Accessed 30 July 2024.
6. Remuzzi G, Perico N, Remuzzi G. Acute kidney injury: diagnostic approaches and controversies. Clin J Am Soc Nephrol. 2019;14:335–43.
7. Lerma EV, Sparks MA, Nissenson AR, editors. Nephrology secrets. 4th ed. Elsevier; 2018.
8. Weisbord SD, Palevsky PM. Prevention and management of acute kidney injury. In: Brenner BM, Rector FC, editors. Brenner and Rector's the kidney. 10th ed. Philadelphia: Elsevier; 2016. p. 940–977.e15.
9. Mehta RL, Cerdá J, Burdmann EA, et al. International society of nephrology's initiative for acute kidney injury (AKI): a human rights case for nephrology. Nat Rev Nephrol. 2015;11(10):687–97. https://doi.org/10.1038/nrneph.2015.28.

Face Swelling

12

Sandeep Dhadvai

Learning Objectives

1. Illustrate the components of the glomerular filtration barrier and describe their function.
2. Explain the general pathophysiology behind nephrotic syndrome, in particular the cause of proteinuria and minimal change disease.
3. Describe how irregularities in calcium labs are affected by serum albumin. Explain the different states in which calcium exists in the body, the equation for calcium correction, and how to correct our patient's calcium based on their serum albumin.
4. Describe the typical clinical presentation and laboratory findings expected in pediatric nephrotic syndrome.
5. Differentiate the pathology and imaging (light microscopy, electron microscopy, and immunofluorescence) among the various types of pediatric nephrotic syndrome.
6. Describe the management of minimal change disease in a child and the steps necessary when a patient becomes refractory to the initial treatment regimen.
7. Discuss side effects of long-term corticosteroid therapy.
8. Describe some of the consequences and sequelae of nephrotic syndrome, with a focus on the pediatric population.
9. Discuss the incidence, prevalence, and epidemiology of nephrotic syndrome in both adult and pediatric patients.

S. Dhadvai (✉)
Department of General Pediatrics & Adolescent Medicine, University of North Carolina School of Medicine, Chapel Hill, NC, USA
e-mail: Sandeep_Dhadvai@med.unc.edu

Case Presentation

Chief Complaint

Face swelling in a 6-year-old male

Prompt: *Using on this information, build a differential using VINDICATE to guide you.*

Encourage the students to build a differential using VINDICATES as a guide. (Push them to think about the physiological causes behind decreased capillary oncotic pressure vs. increased capillary permeability)

V—Vascular (Angioma, heart failure, nephrotic syndrome, liver vascular obstruction)
I—Infectious (SEPSIS!, Sinusitis, abscess, dental infection)
N—Neoplastic (rhabdomyosarcoma, Ewing Sarcoma)
D—Degenerative
I—Iatrogenic/ingestion (malnutrition, medications—CCB, vasodilatory agents)

C. A. Standley (ed.), *Biomedical Science and Clinical Foundations*,
https://doi.org/10.1007/978-3-031-98353-5_12

C—Congenital (nasal dermoid, nasal glioma, epidermal cyst, hereditary angioedema,
A—Autoimmune/Allergy (anaphylaxis, JIA)
T—Traumatic (traumatic injury)
E—Endocrine/metabolic (protein-losing enteropathy)

Prompt: *What do you want to ask the mother of the patient?*

Suggested Questions:

- How long as the swelling been going on (acute, subacute, chronic)?
- Any other specific trauma or inciting event (new medication, insect sting, preceding illness)?
- Is there swelling in any other part of the body?
- Is the patient on any medications?
- Are they fully up to date with immunizations?
- Has anything like this ever happened before?

History of Presenting Illness (HPI)

A previously healthy 6-year-old male presents to your primary care office with his mother with new-onset facial puffiness and swelling. His mother noticed the swelling starting 3 days ago and says that it has been getting worse. She says that throughout the day, the facial puffiness seems to be worst in the morning and better at the end of the day; however, she has been noticing more overall puffiness each day since the symptoms began. Other than being a little more fatigued than normal, he is doing otherwise well.

His sister and he both had a "bad cold" that resolved 2 weeks ago.

Prompt: *What would you ask in Cheif Complaint-SPECIFIC review of systems. Why would you ask those questions? What are you trying to rule out and why?*

Questions to ask in a specific review of symptoms (and what you are trying to rule out):

- Were there any new exposures to foods and any history of food allergy? (Evaluate for anaphylaxis)
- Any difficulty breathing, vomiting, sleepiness, lethargy, hives? (Evaluate for anaphylaxis)
- Any precipitating trauma, insect bite? (Evaluate local swelling reaction)
- Any swelling in other parts of the body? (Evaluate for generalized edema rather than localized edema)
- Fever? (Evaluate for infectious etiology)
- Chest pain, dyspnea, progressive fatigue? (Evaluate for CHF)
- Joint swelling/pain (Evaluate for arthritis)
- Change in quality, color of urine? (Evaluate for nephrotic syndrome)

HPI Cont

No fevers, chills, nausea, vomiting, dental pain, cough, respiratory distress, dyspnea, traumatic inciting event, exposure to new foods/injury/medication, swelling of the neck specifically, abdominal pain, sinus pain, joint pain, or weakness. Patient has a normal diet for his age.

Positive recent URI, face and extremity swelling, and mild fatigue as per HPI.

No family history of vascular disorders or kidney disorders other than a father with hypertension.

Past Medical History

Normal spontaneous vaginal delivery (NSVD), normal development. Born at 38w. Had a few ear infections as a child.

Past Surgical History

Circumcision at birth

Allergies

None

Medications

None

Family History

Father with hypertension, mother with type 2 diabetes mellitus

Social History

Lives at home with mother, father, healthy older sibling (8-year-old girl), pet dog, and new pet kitten. He just finished his first year of kindergarten and is well-liked by his teacher and peers. No concerns with developmental milestones.

Immunizations Up to date

ROS Negative except as per HPI.

Physical Exam

Vitals: T 37.1 °C, HR 115 bpm, RR 21 breaths/min, BP 111/68 mmHg, O_2 sat: 96% on room air. Height and weight are both 50th%ile.

Gen: alert and cooperative, in mild distress and fussy

Skin: no rashes, erythema, or ecchymosis

HEENT: moderate periorbital edema, sclera anicteric, conjunctiva clear, tympanic membrane clear with normal light reflex, throat non-edematous, mucous membranes dry with cracked lips.

CV: Tachycardic, but regular rhythm, without murmurs or rubs.

Lung: CTAB, no wheezes, crackles, or rhonchi

Abdomen: soft, non-tender, non-distended, without masses or shifting dullness. No HSM

Genital: normal male genitalia, no scrotal edema

Extremities: Dorsal surfaces of hands and feet have 1+ pitting edema. Cap refill in 3 seconds. 2+ pulses radial, DP, and PT.

Prompt: *Review the physical exam and point out pertinent positive physical exam findings. Focus especially on blood pressure and heart rate in this situation. Why is this patient tachycardic?*

Did the students mention the blood pressure—if they don't, use it as a good teaching point for blood pressure in pediatric patients. While this blood pressure might be normal for an adult, this patient is in the 95th percentile for systolic and 90th percentile for diastolic blood pressure based on the 2017 revised American Academy of Pediatrics (AAP) practice guidelines for Hypertension [1]. Use this as a teaching point for how "normal" vital signs need to be taken within the context of the patient at hand. Table 12.1 categorizes blood pressure according to ages and stages.

Table 12.1 2017 AAP Definitions of BP Categories and Stages

Children Aged 1 to less than 13	Children Aged 13 to 18
Normal BP is <90%ile	Normal BP is less than 120/80 mm Hg
Elevated BP is 90%ile to less than 95%ile o3 120/80 mm Hg to less than 95%ile (whichever is lower)	Elevated BP is 120/<80 to 129/<80 mm Hg
Stage 1 HTN is 95%ile to 95%ile + 12 mm Hg or 130/80 to 139/89 mm Hg (whichever is lower)	Stage 1 HTN is 130/80 to 139/89 mm Hg
Stage 2 HTN is 95%ile + 12 mm Hg or 140/90 mm Hg or greater (whichever is lower)	Stage 2 HTN is 140/90 mm Hg or higher

For our patient (6-year-old male 50%ile height) refer to AAP BP %ile definition tables for children aged 1–13 years old

Prompt: *What does it mean that the patient also has edema in his extremities in addition to his face? How does diffuse edema change the differential from edema only in the face? What has become more or less likely with all the components of the history and physical now available?*

Generalized edema has a very different differential to localized edema/facial edema. Insect bites, cellulitis, anaphylaxis, local trauma, abscess, mass (benign or not) all become less high on the differential whereas causes such as nephrotic syndrome, congestive heart failure, juvenile idiopathic arthritis, and malnutrition, causes that lead to generalized edema, become much higher on the differential despite being less common overall (especially in pediatric patients)

Prompt: *What workup do you want to initiate for this patient? What labs/imaging do you want to do? Name the tests and imaging and explain why they are important. How will they help to complement the findings from the history and physical to arrive at a diagnosis and treat the patient appropriately?*

Labs to order:

CBC, CMP, Urinalysis, Lipid Panel
NO IMAGING/BIOPSY needed at this time unless there is suspicion of pleural effusion or ascites.

Laboratory Data

A complete blood count (CBC) and comprehensive metabolic panel (CMP) are shown below in Tables 12.2 and 12.3, respectively. Urinalysis is shown in Table 12.4, and a lipid panel is shown in Table 12.5.

Prompt: *Interpret the CBC*
Labs are normal.

Prompt: *Interpret the CMP*
Calcium and albumin are abnormal. What do you think about this and why do you think this might happen? A learning objective later will be why calcium is low in this patient and how to correct for calcium based on albumin.

Table 12.2 CBC with Differential/Platelet

	Patient	Reference
WBC (×10³/μL)	5.7	4.0–10.5
RBC (×10⁶/μL)	5.27	4.10–5.60
Hemoglobin (g/dL)	15.4	12/5–17.0
Hematocrit (%)	44.1	36.0–50.0
MCV (fL)	84	80–98
MCH (pg)	29.2	27–34
MCHC (g/dL)	34.9	32–36
RDW (%)	13.7	11.7–15.0
Platelets (x10³/μL)	268	140–415
Neutrophils (%)	47	40–74
Lymphocytes (%)	46	14–46
Monocytes (%)	6	4–13
Eosinophils (%)	1	0–7
Basophils (%)	0	0–3
Neutrophils (Absolute) (×10³/μL)	2.6	1.8–7.8
Lymphocytes (Absolute) (×10³/μL)	2.6	0.7–4.5
Monocytes (Absolute) (×10³/μL)	0.4	0.1–1.0
Eosinophils (Absolute) (×10³/μL)	0.1	0.0–0.4
Basophils (Absolute) (×10³/μL)	0.0	0.0–0.2
Immature Granulocytes (%)	0	0–1
Immature Granulocytes (Absolute) (×10³/μL)	0.0	0.0–0.1

Prompt: *Interpret the urinalysis*
Specific gravity is slightly increased, appearance/color indicative of concentrated urine, and there is significant protein in the urine without frank blood, RBCs, with negative leukocyte esterase and nitrites.

Prompt: *Interpret the lipid panel.*
LDL is significantly elevated; triglycerides are slightly elevated.

Table 12.3 CMP

Test	Patient	Reference
Glucose (mg/dL)	90	65–99
BUN (mg/dL)	16	5–26
Creatinine (mg/dL)	0.77	0.7–1.3
eGFR (mL/min/1.73)	>60	>59
Sodium (mmol/L)	137	1,350,145
Potassium (mmol/L)	4.4	3.5–5.2
Chloride (mmol/L)	101	97–108
Carbon Dioxide, Total (mmol/L)	23	20–32
Calcium (mg/dL)	6.7	8.7–10.2
Protein, Total (g/dL)	7.6	6–8.5
Albumin (g/dL)	1.5	3.5–5.5
Bilirubin (mg/dL)	0.8	0–1.2
Alkaline Phosphatase (IU/L)	65	25–150
AST (IU/L)	15	0–40
ALT (IU/L)	12	0–55

Table 12.4 Urinalysis

Component	Patient	Reference
Color	Dark Yellow	Yellow
Appearance	Hazy	Clear
pH	6.0	5.0–8.0
Specific Gravity	1.030	1.005–1.029
Protein	4+	Negative
Nitrite	Negative	Negative
Leukocyte esterase	Negative	Negative
RBC	4	0–5/HPF
WBC	3	0–3/HPF
Glucose	Negative	Negative
Urobilinogen	<2.0	<2.0 mg/dL

Table 12.5 Lipid Panel

Component	Patient	Reference
Total Cholesterol (mg/dL)	350	150–200
HDL (mg/dL)	65	>40
LDL (mg/dL)	265	<130
VLDL (mg/dL)	18	<0
Triglycerides (mg/dL)	180	<150

Prompt: *Summarize the important lab findings.*
Significant labs include:
Urinalysis: 4+ protein, spec gravity 1.030
Chemistry: Calcium 6.7 mg/dL, serum albumin 1.5 g/dL, cholesterol 350 mg/dL

Prompt: *What is the diagnosis? What should the treatment plan be? Is there anything we didn't get that you want to order that you think will help aid in the care of this patient?*

Minimal Change Disease is the correct diagnosis. No other tests are necessary at this time as Minimal Change Disease can be treated empirically, especially at the first symptomatic exacerbation of the disease. If there are further complications, new symptoms that suggest another nephrotic etiology, new information that comes up about the patient (maybe they thought they got Hepatitis B immunization, but they didn't) or frequent exacerbations in the future, renal biopsy and further analysis may be indicated.

The Curious Case of the Kidney... Continued...

The patient is treated with a dose of 20 mg per day of oral prednisone for 6 weeks with a follow-up appointment in 4 weeks. A taper would then begin. The patient's family was told to come back if the swelling did not improve or the child's symptoms worsened.

The patient's edema began to improve quickly, and by the time the child was seen for follow-up there were no present medical concerns.

Prompt: *What advice should the pediatrician give regarding diagnosis of Minimal Change Disease? What complications do the pediatrician and parents need to be aware of in this child?*

The most important advice centers around helping the parents to understand the diagnosis. Minimal Change Disease is the most common cause of *kidney disease* **in** children, characterized by significant protein loss in urine due to changes in the kidney's filtration system. The exact cause is unknown, but it is thought to be immune mediated. Provide information on treatment and management strategies, including dietary modifications (low sodium diet, watching protein intake) and maintaining fluid balance. Complications that parents need to be aware of are *increased infection risk* due to *protein loss* (which includes protective antibodies) and steroid use. Parents should also be aware of the possibility of relapses often triggered by infections.

End of Case

Learning Objective Answers

1. **Illustrate the components of the glomerular filtration barrier and describe their function.**

The kidneys have the job of forming a protein-free filtrate. Critical substances such as sodium cannot be excreted unless they are first filtered. The renal corpuscle is the initial blood-filtering component of the nephron. It consists of two structures, a glomerulus and a Bowman's capsule. Figure 12.1c shows an illustration of the filtration barrier. The barrier consists of 3 layers [2]. The first is the capillary endothelium, composed of pores in the endothelium. This barrier is primarily to the cellular elements of blood. The second barrier layer is the basement membrane. The basement membrane is a barrier to plasma proteins. It is the most significant barrier to filtration because it does not permit the filtration of plasma proteins. The basement membrane is lined by negatively charged polyanions, and they repel anions. Anions tend to be plasma proteins, and plasma proteins tend to be large. The third layer is the capsular epithelial cells. This is also a barrier to plasma proteins. It is composed of podocytes, or foot processes, that extend from the epithelial cells. The foot processes line up along the basement membrane. Between the foot processes are little diaphragms called filtration slits. The slits are the pathways for filtration. Filtrate will flow from plasma through the endothelial pores, across the basement membrane, and through the filtration slits.

Certain diseases cause renal corpuscles to become "leaky" by reducing the negative charge

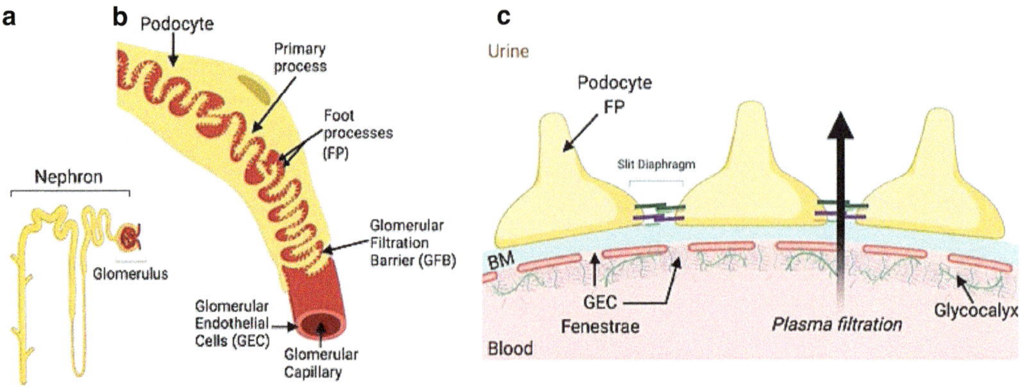

Fig. 12.1 Illustration of a nephron (**a**), a glomerular capillary (**b**), and a cross-section of the glomerular filtration barrier (**c**). Plasma filtrate flows from the blood through the pores of the glomerular endothelial cells (GEC), across the basement membrane (BM), between the foot processes (FP) of the epithelial podocytes, and through the slit diaphragms into Bowman's capsule to become the first part of the urine. *Kerstin Ebefors, Emelie Lassén, Nanditha Anandakrishnan, Evren U Azeloglu, Ilse S Daehn, CC BY 4.0* <https://creativecommons.org/licenses/by/4.0>, via *Wikimedia Commons*

in the membrane, allowing proteins to pass. The endothelium acts as a barrier only to cells. The basement membrane is an important barrier to proteins. The podocytes are responsible for the final filtration of proteins and macromolecules.

2. **Explain the general pathophysiology behind nephrotic syndrome, in particular the cause of proteinuria and minimal change disease.**

Nephrotic syndrome is a kidney disorder characterized by massive proteinuria (>3.5 g/day in adults or >40 mg/m^2/hour in children), hypoalbuminemia, hyperlipidemia, and edema. The hallmark of nephrotic syndrome is proteinuria, which occurs due to disruption of the glomerular filtration barrier [3]. The glomerular filtration barrier serves to maintain size- and charge-selective permeability, preventing protein loss under normal conditions. Proteinuria can result from *damage or dysfunction* in any of the three components of the glomerular filtration barrier. In minimal change disease, the most common cause of nephrotic syndrome in children, there is a loss of anionic charge that is not accompanied by any structural damage or change to the glomerular filtration unit observed by light microscopy. However, electron microscopy demonstrates epithelial podocyte effacement, a key pathological feature [4].

3. **Describe how irregularities in calcium labs are affected by serum albumin. Explain the different states in which calcium exists in the body, the equation for calcium correction, and how to correct our patient's calcium based on their serum albumin.**

Calcium in serum is bound to proteins, principally albumin. As a result, total serum calcium concentrations in patients with low or high serum albumin levels may not accurately reflect the physiologically important ionized (or free) calcium concentration. As an example, in patients with hypoalbuminemia (as may occur in patients with acute or chronic illness, volume overload, or malnutrition), total serum calcium concentration may be low when serum ionized calcium is normal. This phenomenon is called pseudohypocalcemia. The serum total calcium concentration falls approximately 0.8 mg/dL for every 1 g/dL reduction in the serum albumin concentration [5]. Thus, in patients with hypoalbuminemia or hyperalbuminemia, the measured serum calcium concentration should be corrected for the abnormality in albumin or for standard units. Patients with normal corrected serum calcium concentrations do not have true hypocalcemia and therefore do not require treatment for hypocalcemia.

The total serum calcium concentration consists of three fractions: [6]

1. Approximately 15% is bound to multiple organic and inorganic anions such as sulfate, phosphate, lactate, and citrate.
2. Approximately 40% is bound to albumin in a ratio of 0.8 mg/dL (0.2 mmol/L or 0.4 mEq/L) of calcium per 1.0 g/dL (10 g/L) of albumin.
3. The remaining 45% circulates as physiologically active ionized (or free) calcium. The ionized serum calcium concentration is tightly regulated by parathyroid hormone (PTH) and vitamin D and can be modified by a variety of factors.

The wide range in the normal total serum calcium concentration is probably due to variations in the serum concentration of albumin among normal healthy individuals and, occasionally, to variations in the state of hydration that can alter the serum albumin concentration.

Thus, measurement of the total serum calcium concentration alone is sometimes misleading, since this parameter can change without affecting the concentration of ionized calcium. In addition, the ionized fraction can change without an alteration in the total serum calcium concentration.

To correct calcium, use the equation: [7]

$$\text{Corrected Calcium} = 0.8 \times (\text{normal albumin} - \text{patient's albumin}) + \text{serum calcium}$$

Since 40% of calcium is normally bound to albumin, normal albumin = 4.

So, for this patient, Corrected Ca = 0.8 × (4–1.5) + 6.7 = 8.7, which is in the normal range.

4. **Describe the typical clinical presentation and laboratory findings expected in pediatric nephrotic syndrome.**

Childhood idiopathic nephrotic syndrome is characterized by a set of signs and symptoms resulting from increased glomerular permeability to plasma proteins [8]. The typical presentation generally presents with edema and often occurs after an inciting event, such as an upper respiratory infection or an insect bite. Initially, periorbital edema is noted, especially in the morning, and is often misdiagnosed as a manifestation of allergy. The edema progresses to dependent edema and thus, over the day, periorbital edema decreases while edema, of the lower extremities increases.

With the marked increase in extracellular fluid volume, patients experience rapid weight gain due to fluid accumulation. Some children with nephrotic syndrome, primarily those with minimal change disease, present with or develop signs of a decrease in effective circulating volume, such as increased heart rate, reduced urine output, and peripheral vasoconstriction. Patients can become fatigued and irritable with general malaise.

Laboratory findings include

- Proteinuria due to damaged glomerular filtration barrier
- Hypoalbuminemia due to protein loss
- Hyperlipidemia as a compensatory response to low oncotic pressure
- Hypertriglyceridemia
- Hyponatremia
- Hypocalcemia

5. **Differentiate the pathology and imaging (light microscopy, electron microscopy, and immunofluorescence) among the various types of pediatric nephrotic syndrome.**

Table 12.6 Pathological and Imaging Differences Among Pediatric Nephrotic Syndrome

Feature	Minimal Change Disease	Focal Segmental Glomerulosclerosis	Membranous Nephropathy
Pathogenesis	T-cell dysfunction leading to podocyte injury and foot process effacement	Podocyte injury with segmental glomerular scarring	Subepithelial immune complex deposition, leading to GBM thickening
Light Microscopy	Normal glomeruli	Focal and segmental sclerosis of some glomeruli, hyalinosis	Diffuse capillary and GBM thickening without hypercellularity
Electron Microscopy	Diffuse podocyte foot process effacement	Podocyte foot process effacement, focal collagenous sclerosis	Subepithelial electron-dense deposits, "spike and dome" pattern on GBM
Immunofluorescence	Negative (no immune deposits)	Usually negative, or focal IgM and C3 deposits in sclerotic areas	Granular IgG and C3 deposits along the GBM

GBM Glomerular basement membrane, *IgM* Immunoglobulin M, *IgG* Immunoglobulin G, *C3* Complement component 3

The various types of pediatric nephrotic syndrome include focal segmental glomerulosclerosis, membranous nephropathy, and minimal change disease. Table 12.6 shows the pathological and imaging differences among them [9].

6. **Describe the management of minimal change disease in a child and the steps necessary when a patient becomes refractory to the initial treatment regimen.**

The first-line treatment for minimal change disease in children is a course of oral prednisone, as most cases are steroid-responsive [8]. The patient is started on oral prednisone at a dose of 60 mg/m^2 per day (maximum of 60 mg/day). When proteinuria disappears, prednisone is continued at the same daily dose for 30 days, followed by alternate-day therapy (at the same dose). Alternate-day therapy is tapered over a 1–2-month period. Remission is defined as resolution of proteinuria for 3 consecutive days.

Additional management involves supportive care [10]. Dietary modifications consist of a low-sodium diet to manage edema. Diuretics can be used in the case of severe edema with symptomatic fluid overload. Vaccination for pneumococcal and varicella should be up to date (before immunosuppressive therapy begins). Prophylactic antibiotics can be considered if the patient is on long-term immunosuppression.

Most children with idiopathic nephrotic syndrome will respond to steroid therapy. Approximately 90% of responding patients attain complete remission within the first 4 weeks of steroid therapy, and the remaining 10% respond after an additional 2–4 weeks of steroid therapy.

If a child fails to respond to initial steroid therapy or experiences frequent relapses (≥2 relapses in 6 months or ≥ 4 in 12 months), additional therapies are considered. Treatment with a non-steroidal agent (levamisole or mycophenolate mofetil) should be started to maintain remission while reducing steroid dosing and toxicity.

Alternative options include the use of a 12-week course of cyclophosphamide in patients with frequently relapsing nephrotic syndrome, but the long-term remission rate is much lower and does not warrant the significant potential toxicity. Patients are at an increased risk of bone marrow suppression, gonadal toxicity, and increased infection risk.

Although cyclosporine is effective in inducing or maintaining remission in patients with frequently relapsing or steroid-dependent nephrotic syndrome, sustained remission requires prolonged treatment and increases the risk of nephrotoxicity. It may be best to use cyclosporine only in patients who fail to maintain remission after a course of mycophenolate mofetil or cyclophosphamide without a significant steroid dose.

Our patient in this case should have steroids initially. NO diuretics are needed due to signs of dehydration and hypovolemia.

7. **Discuss the Side Effects of Long-term Corticosteroid Therapy**

Corticosteroids, such as prednisone, are the first-line treatment for many pediatric conditions, including minimal change disease. However, prolonged use can lead to significant adverse effects, particularly in growing children [8].

Steroid side effects include the following:

- Growth suppression, delayed puberty
- Hyperglycemia, insulin resistance
- Decreased bone density, muscle weakness
- Moon face, truncal obesity
- Increased infection risk, poor wound healing
- Hypertension, dyslipidemia
- Peptic ulcers, gastritis
- Skin thinning, easy bruising
- Mood swings

Treatment with steroids can disrupt hormone balance, leading to increased androgen levels, which stimulate hair growth on the face and body, a symptom commonly known as hirsutism.

Strategies to minimize side effects of steroids in children include: [11]

- Alternate-day therapy with steroid treatment to help reduce adrenal suppression and growth impairment
- Supplementation with calcium and vitamin D to protect the bones
- Regular tracking of height and weight
- Stay up to date on immunizations
- Infection prevention
- Regular screening of glucose and blood pressure to detect metabolic changes

8. **Describe some of the consequences and sequelae of nephrotic syndrome, with a focus on the pediatric population.**

Pediatric *nephrotic syndrome* can lead to several complications due to *massive protein loss, immune dysfunction, and metabolic disturbances* [12, 13]. These consequences can affect multiple organ systems and influence long-term health outcomes. Infections and venous thrombosis are the two most significant consequences of nephrotic syndrome for the patient (especially pediatric) throughout life. *Loss of immunoglobulins (IgG)* in urine and steroid-induced immunosuppression account for the increased risk of infections. Loss of coagulation cascade regulators, increased hepatic production of procoagulant factors, thrombocytosis, and platelet aggregation account for the risk of thromboembolism. Other complications include hypotension and acute kidney injury due to hypovolemia; pleural effusion due to sodium retention and hypoalbuminemia; and dyslipidemia due to increased LDL, total cholesterol, and triglycerides as the liver overproduces lipoproteins in response to low oncotic pressure. Chronic steroid use, vitamin D deficiency, and metabolic acidosis can lead to growth suppression and metabolic bone disease. As the pediatric patient grows older, steroid toxicity and renal impairment (chronic kidney disease) will become more problematic.

9. **Discuss the incidence, prevalence, and epidemiology of nephrotic syndrome in both adult and pediatric patients.**

Nephrotic syndrome affects both *children and adults*, with variations in *incidence, prevalence, and histological subtypes* based on age, ethnicity, and geographic region (Table 12.7) [14]. It is most common in school age and adolescence, with minimal change disease being the most seen histopathology of childhood nephrotic syndrome (~70–90% of cases) [15]. Primary nephrotic syndrome is more common in younger children, particularly in those less than 6 years of age. Eighty percent of patients with MCD and 50% of patients with FSGS presented before 6 years of age. There is an increased incidence of nephrotic syndrome in family members when compared with the general population [16]. In affected siblings, nephrotic syndrome usually presents at the same age with the same histopathology and outcome.

Table 12.7 Incidence and Prevalence of Nephrotic Syndrome

Population	Incidence	Prevalence	Notes
Pediatric	1.15–16.9 per 100,000 children per year	~16 per 100,000 children	Highest incidence in South Asia; most cases are MCD
Adult	3.5 per 100,000 adults per year	~27 per 100,000 adults	More common in males; FSGS and MN predominate
Global Variation	Higher in Asian, Middle Eastern, and African populations	Lower in Europe and North America	Possibly due to genetic and environmental factors

MCD Minimal Change Disease, *FSGS* Focal Segmental Glomerulosclerosis, *MN* Membranous Nephropathy

Nephrotic syndrome is less common in adults [16]. Minimal change disease accounts for 10–15% of cases of primary nephrotic syndrome in adults. In adults, the disease is usually secondary (it is caused by another disease or drug). Risk factors include older age, diabetes, obesity, and autoimmune disorders, such as lupus. Additionally, secondary causes for minimal change disease may be related to:

- Allergic reactions
- Use of certain painkillers called non-steroidal anti-inflammatory drugs (NSAIDs)
- Tumors
- Infections caused by a virus

Exam Questions

1. A 6-year-old boy is brought to a physician with a 2-week history of diffuse, worsening edema. He has an unremarkable medical history and is not taking any medications. He had a small cold 1 month ago but has since recovered. His vital signs are as follows: T 38 °C, BP 110/71 mm Hg, HR 90 bpm, RR 17 breaths/min. On physical exam he has facial edema and edema of all extremities with +2 pitting. His lab findings show electrolytes within normal limits, a total protein of 5.2 g/dl, and a serum albumin of 1.8. Urinalysis shows 4+ proteinuria without any RBCs in the urine. What is the next step in managing this patient?
   A. Start IV albumin immediately.
   B. Establish 2 large-bore IVs and begin treating with fluids.
   C. Get an ultrasound of the kidneys before deciding on a medical regimen.
   D. Start prednisone.
   E. Biopsy and access via microscopy.
   F. Start a calcineurin inhibitor like cyclosporine.
   G. List the patient for elective kidney transplantation.

   Answer: D

   Learning Objective #8. Describe some of the consequences and sequelae of nephrotic syndrome, with a focus on the pediatric population.

   Explanation: The most likely diagnosis for this patient is minimal change disease based on presentation, patient age, gender, symptoms, and epidemiology. 1st line treatment is prednisone WITHOUT biopsy or other invasive measures.
2. A 6-year-old boy is brought to a physician with a 2-week history of diffuse, worsening edema. He has been in the hospital for this problem 3 times in his life, usually once or twice a year. He is not currently on any medication. He had a small cold 1 month ago but has since recovered. His vital signs are as follows: T 38 °C, BP 110/71 mm Hg, HR 90 bpm, RR 17 breaths/min. On physical exam he has facial edema and edema of all extremities with +2 pitting. Since the problem has not resolved, a renal biopsy was done. What is the defining pathologic feature of his condition that would be seen on microscopy?
   A. Effacement of the FP, segmental sclerosis, and hyalinosis on light microscopy
   B. Effacement of the FP on electron microscopy and normal light microscopy
   C. Effacement of the FP on electron microscopy and glomerular thickening on light microscopy

D. Normal electron microscopy and normal light microscopy
E. Normal electron microscopy and segmental sclerosis and hyalinosis on light microscopy
F. A spike and dome appearance on electron microscopy and diffuse capillary and GBM thickening on light microscopy

Answer: B

Learning objective #5. Differentiate the pathology and imaging (light microscopy, electron microscopy, and immunofluorescence) among the various types of pediatric nephrotic syndrome.

Explanation: The most likely diagnosis for this patient is minimal change disease based on presentation. Effacement of the FP on electron microscopy while having normal light microscopy is the hallmark combination of pathologic features seen in minimal change disease. (A) would be found in focal segmental glomerulosclerosis; (C) has electron microscopic findings that would be seen in focal segmental glomerulosclerosis and light microscopy findings of membranous nephropathy; (D) is normal; (E) has electron microscopy findings that would be found in a normal kidney and light microscopy findings that would be seen in focal segmental glomerulosclerosis; and (F) would be found in membranous nephropathy.

3. A 16-year-old male patient presents to your pediatrics office. He has a history of minimal change disease that was first diagnosed when he was 4 years old and has been on long-term corticosteroid treatment. He has been hospitalized for frequent exacerbations since then. When you see your patient in the office, he has very apparent fat accumulation in the face and central obesity. What else might you expect to find in this patient?

A. Hypoglycemia
B. Hearing loss
C. Excessive daytime sleepiness
D. Hirsutism
E. Tall stature for age

Answer: D

Learning Objective #7. Discuss side effects of long-term corticosteroid therapy.

Explanation: Prolonged steroid use can lead to significant adverse effects, such as moon face and truncal obesity, as seen in this patient. Treatment with steroids can disrupt hormone balance, leading to increased androgen levels, which stimulates increased hair growth known as hirsutism. A is incorrect, as hyperglycemia can occur with steroid treatment, not hypoglycemia; B is incorrect—while hearing loss can be a side effect of long-term steroid treatment, it's not a guaranteed outcome, and the severity and type of hearing loss can vary. C is incorrect, as corticosteroids do not usually cause sleepiness. E is incorrect, as long-term steroid treatment causes growth suppression rather than tall stature.

References

1. Flynn JT, et al. Clinical practice guideline for screening and management of high blood pressure in children and adolescents. Pediatrics. 2017;140(3):e20171904.
2. Ebefors K, Lassén E, Anandakrishnan N, Azeloglu EU, Daehn IS. Modeling the glomerular filtration barrier and intercellular crosstalk. Front Physiol. 2021;12:689083.
3. Tryggvason K, Wartiovaara J. Molecular basis of glomerular permselectivity. Kidney Int. 2001;59(5):1732–41.
4. Reiser J, Altintas MM. Podocytes. N Engl J Med. 2016;375(22):2095–106.
5. Goyal A, Anastasopoulou C, Ngu M, et al. Hypocalcemia. [Updated 2023 Oct 15]. In: StatPearls [Internet]. Treasure Island: StatPearls Publishing; 2025. Available from: https://www.ncbi.nlm.nih.gov/books/NBK430912/.
6. Yu E, Sharma S. Physiology, calcium. [Updated 2023 Aug 14]. In: StatPearls [Internet]. Treasure Island: StatPearls Publishing; 2025. Available from: https://www.ncbi.nlm.nih.gov/books/NBK482128/.
7. Parent X, Spielmann C, Hanser AM. "Corrected" calcium: calcium status underestimation in non-hypoalbuminemic patients and in hypercalcemic patients. Ann Biol Clin (Paris). 2009;67(4):411–8.
8. Rodriguez-Ballestas E, Reid-Adam J. Nephrotic syndrome. Pediatr Rev. 2022;43(2):87–99.
9. Lennon R, Stuart HM, Bierzynska A. Molecular genetics and the nephrotic syndrome: what have we learned so far? Front Pediatr. 2019;7:81.

10. Gipson DS, Trautmann A, Mendley SR, et al. Management of childhood nephrotic syndrome. Clin J Am Soc Nephrol. 2021;16(8):1318–28.
11. Weaver DJ, Swinford RD. Glucocorticoid toxicity in pediatric patients: strategies for monitoring and management. Pediatr Nephrol. 2020;35(5):813–25.
12. Trautmann A, Vivarelli M, Samuel S, et al. IPNA clinical practice recommendations for the diagnosis and management of children with steroid-resistant nephrotic syndrome. Pediatr Nephrol. 2020;35(8):1529–61.
13. Kerlin BA, Ayoob R, Smoyer WE. Epidemiology and pathophysiology of nephrotic syndrome-associated thromboembolic disease. Clin J Am Soc Nephrol. 2012;7(3):513–20.
14. Eddy AA, Symons JM. Nephrotic syndrome in childhood. Lancet. 2003;362(9384):629–39.
15. Primack WA, Chevalier RL, Friedman A, Lemley KV, Norwood VF, Schwartz GJ, Silverstein D, Kaskel F. The first randomized controlled trial in pediatric nephrology: the history of the International Study of Kidney Disease in Children (ISKDC). Pediatr Nephrol. 2023;38(12):3947–54.
16. Tapia C, Bashir K. Nephrotic syndrome [Updated 2023 May 29]. In: StatPearls [Internet]. Treasure Island: StatPearls Publishing; 2025. Available from: https://www.ncbi.nlm.nih.gov/books/NBK470444/.

13 Vomiting Teenager

Jennifer Kirkpatrick

Case Learning Objectives

1. Describe the pathophysiology of diabetic ketoacidosis (DKA) and how it results in associated laboratory and clinical findings.
2. Review the concept of the anion gap to aid in identifying the etiology of metabolic acidosis and discuss differential diagnoses for elevated and normal anion gap acidosis.
3. Discuss a simple, stepwise approach to identify acid-base disturbances.
4. Describe the clinical presentation of an individual presenting in DKA.
5. Describe the epidemiology and prognosis of patients presenting with DKA.
6. List the diagnostic criteria for DKA.
7. Outline the treatment for DKA.
8. Recognize cerebral edema as the most serious complication of DKA and discuss management.

Patient Megan Brooks

Chief complaint "My daughter has been throwing up since last night and now isn't acting quite right"

History of present illness

A 14-year-old female was brought into your pediatric emergency department by her mother with complaints of vomiting and abdominal pain for the past 2 days. There is no known fever. She was assumed to have picked up a stomach bug from one of her friends. She noted feeling thirsty, so her mother has been giving her sports drinks at home. She appeared to be more tired over the past few days and reported feeling weak this morning, so she was allowed to stay home from school; however, upon returning from work this afternoon, her mother noticed she appeared to be lethargic. Her mother relays that due to work and Megan spending more time with her friends recently, she is unsure if Megan had any other symptoms. She does report that her clothes appear to be fitting more loosely recently but thought she may have been dieting due to peer pressure.

Facilitators should ask students what they find notable in this HPI and what further questions they would ask, which would include obtaining a prior medical, surgical, and family history. Allergies and medication lists should be ascertained. Students should note the vomiting, abdominal pain, lethargy, and absence of fever

J. Kirkpatrick (✉)
Department of Emergency Medicine, The Permanente Medical Group, Sacramento, CA, USA
e-mail: Jennifer.t.kirkpatrick@kp.org

C. A. Standley (ed.), *Biomedical Science and Clinical Foundations*,
https://doi.org/10.1007/978-3-031-98353-5_13

Allergies: No known drug allergies
Medications: None
Past medical history: No past medical history. Immunizations are up-to-date. Last menstrual period was about 2 weeks ago.
Past surgical history: None
Social history: Sophomore in high school. No recent travel. Lives at home with mother.
Family history: Mother has a history of hypertension. Father is estranged, family history unknown

Gastrointestinal: +nausea, + vomiting, + abdominal pain. No constipation or diarrhea. No melena, hematochezia, or hematemesis.
Genitourinary: No dysuria or hematuria
Musculoskeletal: No joint pain or myalgias
Skin: No rashes
Endocrine: +polydipsia, +polyuria
Neurologic: +lethargy, no focal weakness, seizure, and speech changes

What are some of your differential diagnoses thus far? Gastroenteritis, pregnancy (given age and gender), viral illness, appendicitis, cholecystitis, diabetic ketoacidosis (DKA), ovarian torsion, ingestions/intoxication, urinary tract infection, dehydration, electrolyte/metabolic disturbance.

What ROS questions do you want to ask, and what specific areas do you want to focus on in the physical exam?

Students should ask about stool consistency and habits, including hematochezia or melena, appetite changes, blood or bile in emesis, urinary frequency or dysuria, polydipsia or polyuria, and presence of constitutional symptoms.

Physical exam areas to assess: Although a head-to-toe assessment should be performed, students should pay particular attention to the general appearance, abdominal exam, check for signs of dehydration from vomiting (assessment of mucous membranes, skin turgor, capillary refill, and pulses), and a thorough neurologic exam due to the mother's report of lethargy.

Review of systems—*elicited by mother*
General: No fever or chills. +Weight loss
Head, ears, eyes, nose, throat: No headache. No vision changes. No ear pain or hearing issues.
Neck: No neck pain or swelling
Cardiac: No chest pain or syncope.
Respiratory: No cough or shortness of breath

Physical examination
Height: 5′4″ Weight: 105 lb
Vital signs: T: 37 °C, HR: 120 bpm, BP: 100/66 mm Hg, RR: 26, SpO2: 99%
General: ill-appearing female, somnolent. Knows her name but not oriented to place or time.
Head: Normocephalic/atraumatic
Ears: Tympanic membranes clear. Normal external exam.
Eyes: PERRL. EOMI. Conjunctiva normal.
Nose: Normal turbinates. Nares patent.
Throat: Mucous membranes dry. No pharyngeal edema or exudates. Fruity breath odor on exhalation
Neck: Supple without thyromegaly. No rigidity.
Cardiac: Tachycardic, regular. No murmur, rub or gallop
Pulmonary: Tachypneic, taking deep breaths. Lungs clear to auscultation bilaterally.
Abdomen: Soft, non-distended. Moderate diffuse tenderness to palpation without rebound or guarding. Bowel sounds normal.
Extremities: No edema. Extremities cool to touch.
Skin: Capillary refill >3 seconds. Poor skin turgor.
Neuro: Somnolent, uncooperative for formal neurologic texting; however, no focal deficits noted

What is notable in the physical exam? How has your differential diagnosis changed? What tests do you want to order?

Students should note that the patient is clearly volume depleted. She is tachycardic, her blood pressure is borderline low, her capillary refill time is delayed, mucous membranes are dry, and skin turgor is poor. Her abdominal exam is abnormal but nonspecific. Her somnolence, orientation to only self, and lack of cooperation in neurologic exam should be concerning.

They may put together that she has DKA based on her Kussmaul breathing, fruity breath odor, abdominal tenderness, and dehydration. DKA should now be high on the differential.

Tests to order: CBC, BMP, fingerstick glucose, urinalysis or urine dip, serum osmolality, ABG or VBG, urine pregnancy test

Students should be reminded that in a female of child-bearing age, it is important to exclude pregnancy, as patients may not always be forthright with sexual history, especially in the emergency setting.

Initial labs

Point-of-care testing:

Urine pregnancy test: negative
Fingerstick glucose: Too high to read.
Urine dipstick: +++ ketones, +++ glucose

Bloodwork:

--------CBC---------

Component	Patient	Units	Reference
WBC	12.0	K/ul	4.0–10.5
Hb	14.2	g/dl	12.5–17.0
Hct	42.5%	%	36.0–50.0
MCH	31.5	pg	27.0–34.0
PLT	190	K/ul	150–450

--------BMP---------

Component	Patient	Units	Reference
Na+	130	mEq/L	135–145
K+	4.6	mEq/L	3.5–5.1
Cl–	97	mEq/L	98–110
CO2	11	mEq/L	20–32
Glu	592	mg/dL	65–99
BUN	40	mg/dL	6–24
Creat	1.4	mg/dL	0.76–1.24

Serum osmolality: 316 mOsm 285–295 mOsm

What do you make of the laboratory findings?

Students should note slightly decreased Na^+, extremely elevated glucose, and decreased Cl^- and CO_2. Have them interpret a BUN/Cr ratio of >20 and ask them the significance (dehydration or prerenal azotemia). They should recognize that the patient has a decreased bicarbonate (represented by CO_2 in the BMP) and that the anion gap is elevated at 22. They should also note large glucose and ketones in the urine.

ABG result

Component: Patient Value	Reference
pH: 7.05	7.35–7.45
PCO_2: 28 mm/Hg	35–45 mm Hg
PO_2: 98 mm/Hg	80–100 mm/Hg
HCO_3-: 12 mEq/L	22–26 mEq/L
O_2 sat: 98%	95–100%
B.E. –17	–2 to +2 mEq/L

Have students interpret the ABG

Since the pH is <7.35, there is acidemia. As the HCO_3 is low, this is a metabolic acidosis. Using Winter's formula, students can confirm that there is appropriate respiratory compensation:

$$PCO_2 = 1.5 \times HCO_3^- + 8 + / - 2$$

Ask the students to determine what would happen if the patient were to become more somnolent and how they expect the ABG to change.

They should note that there would be CO_2 retention, which would lead to a worsening of the acidosis (increase the PCO_2 –> increase in H+ –> decrease in pH as per Le Chatelier's Principle)

$$H_2O + CO_2 \langle - \rangle H_2CO_3 \langle - \rangle H^+ + HCO_3^-$$

What is the diagnosis? Diabetic ketoacidosis (DKA)

What is the treatment? Crystalloid IV fluids (0.9% NaCl) bolus for dehydration, insulin, potassium, and maintenance IVF infusion. As glucose levels fall, the patient will also counterintuitively need dextrose supplementation to prevent hypoglycemia.

Ask students why they would give K+ in the setting of seemingly normal levels. Despite the "normal" K+, there is a total body depletion of potassium. Potassium is lost in the urinary system via osmotic diuresis. Due to acidemia, H^+ ions are shifted intracellularly in exchange for K^+ into the plasma; therefore, cellular potassium levels are low.

What complications should you be aware of? Insulin administration without potassium repletion can lead to fatal arrhythmias, as insulin will shift potassium out of the plasma and into the intracellular space. Cerebral edema is a feared complication of DKA, and its association with rapid fluid overcorrection is controversial. Insulin administration may precipitate hypoglycemia if overcorrection of blood glucose occurs without dextrose supplementation.

The patient is started on IV fluids and an insulin drip. The ICU resident physician is paged to admit the patient for further management of her DKA. She agrees with your management and will see the patient shortly. You go on to see other patients in the emergency department as it is a busy day.

A few hours later, Megan's nurse tells you she is complaining of a headache, so you order some acetaminophen and tell her you will come for reassessment as soon as you can. As you are examining an infant, Megan's nurse calls out to you that she is seizing. You rush over to her room, give IV lorazepam, intubate the patient, and rush her off to the CT scanner.

Ask the students what the significance of the headache was and have them interpret CT scan

The headache was an early sign the patient was beginning to develop cerebral edema. The seizure is a result of the edema. CT shows diffuse cerebral edema with severely narrowed lateral ventricles to the point of complete effacement, effacement of the sulci, and obliteration of the perimesencephalic cisterns (Fig. 13.1a, b).

Reference: https://onlinelibrary.wiley.com/doi/10.1155/2018/5043752

Recognizing cerebral edema on CT scan, you administer mannitol and elevate the head of her bed. The ICU team arrives, and the patient is transported upstairs.

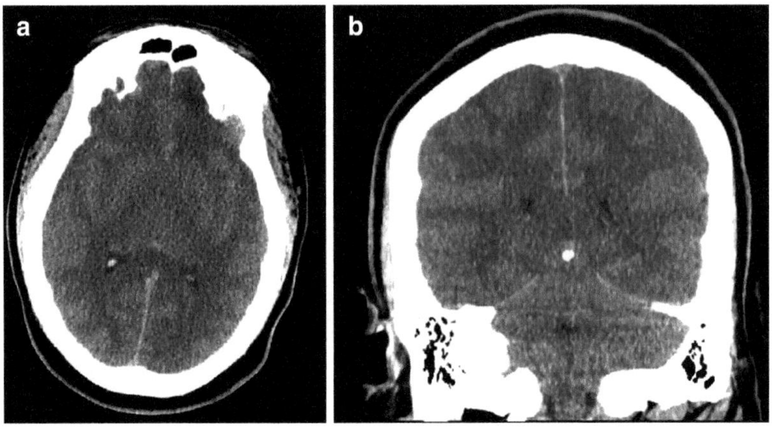

Fig. 13.1 Axial cut (**a**) and coronal cut (**b**) of a noncontrast CT of the head

One week later, the patient returns to her neurologic baseline, is set up with a pediatric endocrinologist for follow-up, and is sent home with insulin and teaching from a diabetes nurse on how to administer self-injections.

Learning Objectives

1. **Describe the pathophysiology of diabetic ketoacidosis (DKA) and how it results in associated laboratory and clinical findings**

In normal physiologic conditions, postprandial increases in blood glucose stimulate the release of insulin, which in turn promotes glucose uptake into cells and glycogen formation in the liver and inhibits gluconeogenesis [1, 2]. In diabetic ketoacidosis, there is a decrease in insulin action, either through an absolute or relative deficiency, coupled with an increase in the action of counterregulatory hormones [2–4].

The majority of DKA is attributed to type 1 diabetes mellitus [5], wherein autoimmune destruction of pancreatic β cells leads to deficient insulin production [1]. Impaired insulin action results in decreased cellular uptake of glucose in the body, primarily in the skeletal muscle, which results in hyperglycemia. The release of catecholamines, such as epinephrine, leads to a blockade of residual insulin action and stimulates the release of glucagon [1]. Increased glucagon activity, along with insulin deficiency, leads to glycogenolysis and gluconeogenesis, further exacerbating hyperglycemia. Hyperglycemia overwhelms the glucose reabsorption ability of the kidneys, resulting in osmotic diuresis, resulting in volume depletion and dehydration.

The imbalance of insulin and glucagon activity also stimulates the activity of lipase to break down adipose stores and generate free fatty acids, which ultimately become converted to ketone bodies [1]. Two important ketone bodies produced in DKA are β-hydroxybutyrate and acetoacetate [2, 4]. Since synthesis occurs more rapidly than tissue utilization can occur, there is a resultant ketonemia and ketonuria. Ketone bodies in the plasma also further worsen the dehydration seen in DKA by contributing to osmotic diuresis and leading to nausea/vomiting. The dissociation of ketone bodies in the blood leads to an increase in plasma hydrogen ion concentration, resulting in a metabolic acidosis. The characteristic fruity odor observed in DKA results from excess acetone production through the conversion of acetoacetate.

Electrolyte disturbances occur in patients with DKA, most notably, total body potassium losses. As plasma H+ ions increase in states of metabolic acidosis, cells attempt to compensate for this acidemia by pumping H+ intracellularly in exchange for a shift of K+ extracellularly [6]. Extracellular K+ is then lost in the urine because of osmotic diuresis. Increased osmolytes in the serum also draw water into the extracellular space, resulting in a dilutional hyponatremia. Na+ is also lost with osmotic diuresis.

2. **Review the concept of the anion gap to aid in identifying the etiology of metabolic acidosis and discuss differential diagnoses for elevated and normal anion gap acidosis**

Fluids in the body, such as plasma, are electrically neutral. To maintain this electroneutrality, there must be an equal proportion of positive and negative ions. [Na+] is the typical cation measured in the plasma, while [Cl^-] and [HCO_3^-] are the measured anions [7]. When you subtract ([Cl^-] + [HCO_3^-]) from [Na^+] in the plasma, there is an apparent difference or "gap," which is comprised of unmeasured anions, largely owing to negatively charged plasma proteins (Fig. 13.2a). Under normal physiologic conditions, the anion gap is typically between 4 and 12 mEq/L.

$$\text{Aniongap} = [\text{Na}+] - ([\text{Cl}^-]\text{and}[\text{HCO}_3^-])$$

In conditions that result in metabolic acidosis, the plasma [HCO_3^-] drop is either accompanied by an increase in unmeasured anions (Fig. 13.2b) or an increase in [Cl^-]

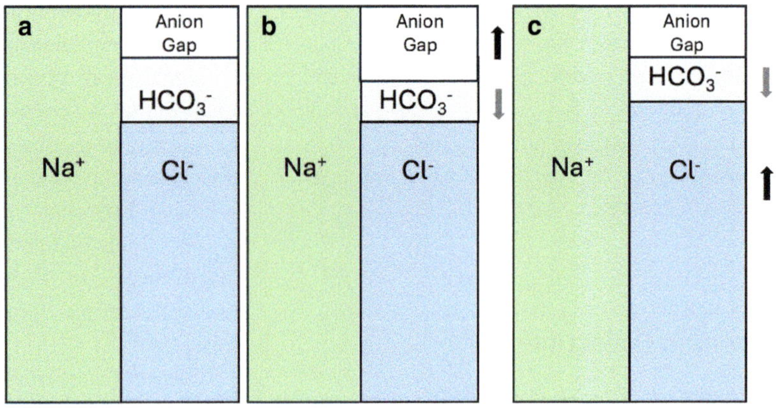

Fig. 13.2 Plasma anion gap in **a**. Normal physiologic states **b**. High Anion Gap Metabolic Acidosis **c**. Normal or non-anion gap metabolic acidosis

(Fig. 13.2c) in maintaining electroneutrality. These are referred to as high anion gap metabolic acidosis and normal (non) anion gap metabolic acidosis, respectively.

Calculating the anion gap helps to narrow the causes leading to a metabolic acidosis and further helps generate a differential diagnosis.

High anion gap metabolic acidosis (HAGMA):

Organic acids dissociate to form unmeasured anions, such as ketone bodies, lactate, and salicylate, which accumulate and lead to an increase in the anion gap [7]. A common mnemonic used to recall causes of HAGMA is "MUDPILES":

M-methanol
U-uremia
D-DKA
P-Propylene glycol
Iron or Isoniazid
L-Lactic acidosis
E-Ethylene glycol
S-Salicylates

Normal (non) anion gap metabolic acidosis [NAGMA]

When there is no accumulation of organic acids, the apparent anion gap is in the usual range, and an increase in plasma [Cl^-] occurs to offset the decrease in [HCO_3^-] [7]. This is referred to as a normal or non-anion gap metabolic acidosis or hyperchloremic metabolic acidosis. NAGMA causes can be remembered by the mnemonic "HARD UP":

H-Hyperalimentation or total parenteral nutrition (TPN)
Acetazolamide or other carbonic anhydrase inhibitors
R-Renal tubular acidosis
D-Diarrhea or diuretic
U-Ureteroenteric fistula
P-Pancreaticoduodenal fistula

3. Discuss a simple, stepwise approach to identify acid-base disturbances

Step 1: Identify if there is acidosis vs. alkalosis

$$\text{Acidosis} = \text{pH}\langle 7.35, \text{Alkalosis} = \text{pH}\rangle 7.45$$

Step 2: Identify whether condition is primarily due to a metabolic or respiratory process

	Acidosis	Alkalosis
Metabolic	↓ HCO_3^-	↑ HCO_3^-
Respiratory	↑ CO_2	↓ CO_2

Step 3: If a metabolic acidosis is present, determine whether the anion gap is elevated or within normal range

$$\text{Aniongap} = [\text{Na}+] - \left(\left[\text{Cl}^-\right] \text{and} \left[\text{HCO}_3^-\right]\right)$$

After calculating the anion gap, attention can be given to generating a differential diagnosis for AGMA vs. NAGMA

Step 4: Is there appropriate compensation?

When a metabolic disturbance is present, the body attempts to offset the change with respiratory compensation. Winter's formula can be used to determine if the expected CO_2 matches what is measured.

$$pCO_2 = 1.5 \times HCO_3^- + 8 + / - 2$$

If the expected pCO_2 is higher than predicted, there is a concomitant respiratory acidosis. If pCO_2 is lower than predicted, there is a concomitant respiratory alkalosis.

Clinical Sciences Learning Objectives

4. **Describe the clinical presentation of an individual presenting in DKA**

History A variety of symptoms are seen in DKA and are often nonspecific. Polyuria and polydipsia are common early symptoms. Constitutional symptoms include weakness and fatigue, and in those with an undiagnosed history of type 1 diabetes, there is often a report of recent weight loss. Gastrointestinal (GI) complaints, such as nausea, vomiting, decreased appetite, and generalized abdominal pain, may be present due to DKA itself or from concomitant processes. The reason for GI symptoms in DKA is incompletely understood; however, proposed mechanisms include mesenteric ischemia secondary to hypovolemia, impaired gastrointestinal motility from hyperglycemia, distention of the hepatic capsule [8], and ketone-mediated activation of the vomiting center in the medulla oblongata (chemoreceptor trigger zone) [9]. Sensorium in those with DKA can range from normal level of alertness to somnolence, confusion, and coma. A variety of symptoms specific to intercurrent illness can be seen at time of presentation in DKA; for example, fever secondary to infectious processes, chest pain in those with myocardial infarction, or focal neurologic symptoms in those with stroke.

Physical examination Patients with DKA are generally ill-appearing. Findings of hypovolemia are common in DKA and can include tachycardia, poor skin turgor, dry mucous membranes, weak or thready pulses, poor capillary refill, and hypotension. Kussmaul (deep, rapid) respirations and a fruity breath odor are due to metabolic acidosis and ketosis. Abdominal tenderness is a common finding in DKA and can mimic acute abdomen. Level of consciousness can range from alert and conversant to confused or obtunded.

5. **Describe the epidemiology and prognosis of patients presenting with DKA**

Epidemiology Most children presenting with DKA have underlying T1DM; however, a minority will occur in those with T2DM [10]. Up to 40% of children with T1DM present in DKA at the time of diagnosis [11]. Risk factors for DKA at initial presentation in T1DM include young age (especially those under the age of 2), children belonging to ethnic minority groups, and those coming from socioeconomic disadvantage [12, 13]. In patients with an established diagnosis of diabetes, infection, poor healthcare access, and medication omission (either through access, noncompliance, or equipment failure) increase the risk of developing DKA [12].

Prognosis

Before insulin was discovered, the mortality of DKA was 100%. In the United States and other similarly developed countries, the mortality of DKA is <0.5% [13]; however, it is increased in developing countries. With early and appropriate treatment, the prognosis of recovery from DKA is generally great. Poor prognostic signs at time of admission include hypothermia, oliguria, deep coma, extremes of age, and hypotension [4, 10]. In children with DKA, cerebral edema is the leading cause of mortality [14]; however, in adults, death occurs more often due to concomitant infection or precipitating illness, and in the elderly.

6. **List the diagnostic criteria for DKA**

There are slight differences in criteria used in the diagnosis of adult DKA; however, the following is commonly accepted [4]:

Blood glucose >250 mg/dL
Arterial pH < 7.3
Bicarbonate <15 mEq/L
Moderate ketonemia or ketonuria

In children, the International Society for Pediatric and Adolescent Diabetes (ISPAD) criteria [15] are:

Blood glucose >200 mg/dl
Venous pH < 7.3 or bicarbonate <18 mEq/L
Ketonemia or moderate or large ketonuria.

7. **Discuss the treatment for DKA**

The first step in DKA treatment is recognition that it is an endocrine emergency, and management should be initiated promptly. As in all emergency presentations, the first assessment should be a primary survey of ABCs (airway, breathing, circulation), and appropriate timely interventions should be taken to address any issues discovered. Simultaneously, patients should quickly have IV access established, a full set of vital signs obtained, and be placed on continuous cardiorespiratory monitoring. The key areas of DKA treatment are listed below:

IV fluids IV fluid bolus should be given with isotonic fluids as soon as IV access is established. Children with DKA are usually 5–10% dehydrated and should be given 10 cc/kg for initial bolus, with evaluation for ongoing signs of poor perfusion to determine the need for additional bolus [16]. Maintenance IV fluids are then started with the goal of correcting fluid deficit over a duration of between 36 and 48 hours [16]. In adults, fluid deficit could be up to 10–15% of body weight [10], and fluid administration is given to reverse shock/hypovolemia. In patients without cardiac or renal impairment, IV fluid bolus is typically given at 15–20 cc/kg in the first hour [4, 10]. Patients with heart failure or end-stage renal disease should have fluids carefully tailored according to their volume status, with special attention to avoiding fluid overload.

Insulin

Insulin therapy should be initiated after volume resuscitation and return of serum potassium level. In children, IV insulin is typically given at a rate of 0.05–0.1 units/kg/hr [16]. As insulin increases activity of Na^+/K^+-ATPase, initiation of therapy will drive potassium into cells and lead to decreased plasma potassium [17]. Generally, insulin is given until the anion gap normalizes and the patient can tolerate an oral diet. Note that hyperglycemia will typically resolve before the acidemia, but insulin must be continued to resolve the acidosis. Dextrose-containing fluids are given along with insulin once glucose levels fall to 300 mg/dL in children to prevent hypoglycemia while awaiting closure of the anion gap. Historically, regular IV insulin therapy has been used to treat both children and adults with DKA; however, subcutaneous insulin has been increasing in popularity for the treatment of mild-to-moderate adult DKA as it allows for decreased hospital resource utilization without any increase in adverse patient events [18].

Potassium replacement Total body potassium depletion occurs in large part due to osmotic diuresis; however, initial levels may appear normal due to decreased insulin activity and acidosis, both of which cause an extracellular shift of potassium. In patients with measured hypokalemia, total body potassium is severely low and must be repleted before insulin administration to avoid fatal arrhythmia. It is recommended to obtain an EKG on initial evaluation of suspected DKA cases to assess for cardiac effects related to hypo/hyperkalemia.

In children, 40 mEq/L K+ containing fluids are administered once serum K+ is <5 mEq/L [16].

Bicarbonate Historically, sodium bicarbonate therapy has been controversial in the treatment of severe DKA. It has been associated with an increased risk of cerebral edema [19] and is generally not recommended except in rare circumstances. It is typically reserved for treating life-threatening hyperkalemia, severe acidosis (pH < 6.9), or peri-arrest situations [12].

Treatment of intercurrent/precipitating illness As infection or illness is a common precipitating factor for DKA, clinicians should be vigilant in identifying and treating conditions presenting concurrently with DKA. Leukocytosis is a common laboratory finding in DKA; however, levels >25,000/μL or bands >10% are suggestive of infection [20] and should prompt further investigation.

Recognition and treatment for DKA-associated cerebral edema are discussed separately below.

8. **Recognize cerebral edema as the most serious complication of DKA and discuss management**

Cerebral edema is the most devastating complication of DKA and is the leading cause of diabetes-associated death in children [2, 19]. It is rarely seen in adults with DKA. Clinically apparent cerebral edema is present in up to 1% [19] of children undergoing treatment for DKA and carries a mortality rate of 20–25% [2]. Among survivors, roughly a quarter have permanent neurologic disability [19]. Signs/symptoms of cerebral edema can be seen at time of presentation or evolve during treatment and include headache, nausea, vomiting, altered mental status, focal neurologic symptoms, posturing, hypertension, bradycardia, combativeness, and seizure.

The underlying mechanism for cerebral edema in DKA is not currently well understood. It was initially thought that rapid fluid correction led to a decrease in serum osmolality, creating an osmotic gradient and shifting fluid into the brain; however, recent evidence, including a multicenter study, failed to demonstrate a difference in neurologic outcomes with different rates and sodium content of infusions [21]. Children presenting with severe DKA appear to be at the highest risk, particularly those with severe acidosis, hypocapnia, and elevated BUN levels at presentation [19, 22]. The use of bicarbonate therapy is also associated with the development of cerebral injury [19].

Patients undergoing treatment for DKA should be closely monitored for the development of cerebral edema. Those with suspected cerebral edema should be promptly treated, as it carries a high risk for mortality and morbidity. Initial management should be focused on addressing the ABCs and administering a hyperosmolar agent. Typically, IV mannitol at 0.5–1 g/kg is given over 10–15 minutes [15]; however, hypertonic (3%) saline may also be used.

Exam Questions

1. A 65-year-old female is brought in by ambulance to your emergency department complaining of cough and shortness of breath. Initial ABG shows a pH of 7.25, PCO_2 of 70, HCO_3 29, PO_2 70. What is the primary underlying etiology of the acid-base disturbance?
   A. Metabolic acidosis
   B. Metabolic alkalosis
   C. Respiratory acidosis
   D. Respiratory alkalosis

   Answer: C

   Learning Objective: #2

   Explanation: The patient has an acute respiratory acidosis. The pH is acidemic, the pCO_2 is markedly elevated (indicating hypoventilation), and the small rise in HCO_3^- reflects early renal compensation, consistent with an acute process. The other options are excluded because metabolic causes require low HCO_3^-, respiratory alkalosis requires low pCO_2, and chronic respiratory acidosis would show a much higher HCO_3.

2. A 13-year-old male with T1DM presents to the pediatric emergency department with nausea, vomiting, weakness, sleepiness, and weight loss. On exam, he exhibits rapid, deep breathing, a fruity breath odor, and diffuse

tenderness to abdominal palpation. All of the following are typically used in the treatment of his condition except which of the following?
A. Potassium
B. Insulin
C. IV fluids
D. Bicarbonate

Answer: D
Learning Objective: #7
Explanation: Bicarbonate is generally not used in DKA because it can cause paradoxical CNS acidosis, hypokalemia, and worsened outcomes. It's reserved only for severe, life-threatening acidosis. A is incorrect as potassium is needed since total body potassium is depleted in DKA (from osmotic diuresis) and insulin therapy drives potassium into cells, chi can cause hypokalemia if not replaced. B is incorrect as insulin is absolutely essential in DKA treatment. C is incorrect as IV fluids are considered first-line therapy.

3. Before initiating insulin treatment for DKA, which laboratory value must be known to prevent the precipitation of a fatal arrhythmia?
A. Sodium
B. Potassium
C. Chloride
D. Creatinine

Answer: B
Learning Objective: #7
Explanation: Insulin therapy without knowing K^+ level is dangerous. If $K^+ < 3.3$ mEq/L, replace potassium before giving insulin. A is incorrect as while sodium is affected by hyperglycemia (pseudohyponatremia), correcting it is not an immediate arrhythmia risk. It is important for fluid management, but not the life-threatening concern before insulin. C is incorrect as chloride may be altered in metabolic acidosis but does not directly impact arrhythmia risk with insulin therapy. D is incorrect as while creatinine is important for assessing renal function, fluid management, and drug dosing, it is not the critical factor that determines immediate arrhythmia risk when starting insulin.

4. DKA at first presentation in T1DM patients occurs in roughly in what percent?
A. 1%
B. 5%
C. 40%
D. 90%

Answer: C
Learning Objective: #5
Explanation: Around 1/3 to 2/5 (or 40%) of patients with new T1DM present in DKA. A is incorrect as 1% is far too low and underestimates the real frequency. B is incorrect as this is still much lower than actual rates. D is incorrect as this is much too high. While common, most T1DM cases are not diagnosed during DKA.

References

1. Kumar V, Abbas AK, Aster JC. Robbins & Cotran pathologic basis of disease. 10th ed. Elsevier - Health Science; 2021.
2. Wolfsdorf J, Glaser N, Sperling MA. Diabetic ketoacidosis in infants, children, and adolescents: a consensus statement from the American Diabetes Association. Diabetes Care. 2006;29(5):1150–9.
3. Calimag APP, Chlebek S, Lerma EV, Chaiban JT. Diabetic ketoacidosis. Disease-a-Month [Internet]. 2022;69(3):101418.
4. Kitabchi AE, Umpierrez GE, Miles JM, Fisher JN. Hyperglycemic crises in adult patients with diabetes. Diabetes Care. 2009;32(7):1335–43.
5. Benoit SR, Zhang Y, Geiss LS, Gregg EW, Albright A. Trends in diabetic ketoacidosis hospitalizations and in-hospital mortality — United States, 2000–2014. MMWR Morb Mortal Wkly Rep [Internet]. 2018;67(12):362–5.
6. Aronson PS, Giebisch G. Effects of pH on potassium: new explanations for old observations. J Am Soc Nephrol [Internet]. 2011;22(11):1981–9.
7. Costanzo LS. Physiology : cases and problems. Philadelphia: Wolters Kluwer Health/Lippincott Williams & Wilkins; 2009.
8. Tavares Bello C, Franco Gago M, Fernandes F, Oliveira MM. Abdominal pain in diabetic ketoacidosis: beyond the obvious. J Endocrinol Metabol. 2018;8(2–3):43–6.

9. Takai T, Okada Y, Takebe R, Nakamura T. Vomiting and hyperkalemia are novel clues for emergency room diagnosis of type 1 diabetic ketoacidosis: a retrospective comparison between diabetes types. Diabetol Int. 2021;13(1):272–9.
10. Lizzo JM, Goyal A, Gupta V. Adult diabetic ketoacidosis [Internet]. PubMed. Treasure Island: StatPearls Publishing; 2023. Available from: https://www.ncbi.nlm.nih.gov/books/NBK560723/
11. Jensen ET, Stafford JM, Saydah S, D'Agostino RB, Dolan LM, Lawrence JM, et al. Increase in prevalence of diabetic ketoacidosis at diagnosis among youth with type 1 diabetes: the SEARCH for Diabetes in Youth Study. Diabetes Care. 2021;44(7):1573–8.
12. EL-Mohandes N, Huecker M. Pediatric diabetic ketoacidosis [Internet]. PubMed. Treasure Island: StatPearls Publishing; 2020. Available from: https://www.ncbi.nlm.nih.gov/books/NBK470282/
13. Klingensmith GJ, Tamborlane WV, Wood J, Haller MJ, Silverstein J, Cengiz E, et al. Diabetic ketoacidosis at diabetes onset: still an all too common threat in youth. J Pediatr [Internet]. 2013;162(2):330–334.e1.
14. Scibilia J, Finegold D, Dorman J, Becker D, Drash A. Why do children with diabetes die? Acta Endocrinol. 1986;113(4_Suppl):S326–33.
15. Glaser N, Fritsch M, Priyambada L, Rewers A, Cherubini V, Estrada S, et al. ISPAD Clinical Practice Consensus Guidelines 2022: diabetic ketoacidosis and hyperglycemic hyperosmolar state. Pediatr Diabetes. 2022;23(7):835–56.
16. Tzimenatos L, Nigrovic LE. Managing diabetic ketoacidosis in children. Ann Emerg Med. 2021;78(3):340–5.
17. Sweeney G, Niu W, Canfield VA, Levenson R, Klip A. Insulin increases plasma membrane content and reduces phosphorylation of Na^{+}-K^{+}pump α_1-subunit in HEK-293 cells. Am J Physiol Cell Physiol. 2001;281(6):C1797–803.
18. Rao P, Jiang S, Kipnis P, Patel DM, Katsnelson S, Madani S, et al. Evaluation of outcomes following hospital-wide implementation of a subcutaneous insulin protocol for diabetic ketoacidosis. JAMA Network Open [Internet]. 2022;5(4):e226417.
19. Glaser N, Barnett P, McCaslin I, Nelson D, Trainor J, Louie J, et al. Risk factors for cerebral edema in children with diabetic ketoacidosis. N Engl J Med. 2001;344(4):264–9.
20. Slovis CM, Mork VGC, Slovis RJ, Bain RP. Diabetic ketoacidosis and infection: leukocyte count and differential as early predictors of serious infection. Am J Emerg Med. 1987;5(1):1–5.
21. Kuppermann N, Ghetti S, Schunk JE, Stoner MJ, Rewers A, McManemy JK, et al. Clinical trial of fluid infusion rates for pediatric diabetic ketoacidosis. N Engl J Med. 2018;378(24):2275–87.
22. Marcin JP, Glaser N, Barnett P, McCaslin I, Nelson D, Trainor J, et al. Factors associated with adverse outcomes in children with diabetic ketoacidosis-related cerebral edema. J Pediatr. 2002;141(6):793–7.

Part VI

GI

14 Unrelenting Diarrhea

Jeffrey Kyaw Wang

Learning Objectives

1. Describe the microbiology for Shiga-toxin hemolytic uremic syndrome (HUS), including nomenclature, serotypes, and Shiga toxin types.
2. Summarize the pathogenesis and mechanism of Shiga-toxin HUS; include how the pathogenesis can lead to the classic symptoms and findings in Shiga-toxin HUS.
3. Define the various definitions of diarrhea, delineating acute vs. chronic and the different forms of diarrhea. Create a broad differential for acute diarrhea for non-infectious etiologies and infectious etiologies.
4. List the common pathogens in acute diarrhea and describe its classic presentation and symptoms. Also summarize the appropriate workup to differentiate between common pathogens.
5. Describe the clinical presentation of HUS.
6. Summarize the general management for STEC infections and Shiga-toxin HUS.
7. What is the epidemiology of Shiga-toxin HUS in regard to both the pediatric and adult populations? What are the different common modes of transmission for STEC infections?

J. K. Wang (✉)
Kaiser Permanente, San Leandro, CA, USA
e-mail: jeffrey.x.wang@kp.org

Chief Complaint

You are an intern on your inpatient wards when your senior resident sends you down to the ED to admit a new patient. He gives you the following basic information:

Monica Brown is a 62-year-old female who presents with 5 days of diarrhea.

History of Present Illness

Mrs. Brown is a theoretical 62-year-old white female with a history of hypothyroidism who presents with 5 days of bloody diarrhea associated with lower abdominal pain. She notes that she had just recently returned from a 5-day hiking trip in Brazil about 7 days prior to arrival. On this hiking trip, she drank unfiltered stream water and cooked store-bought hamburgers for meals. Two days after her trip, she developed diarrhea that was initially non-bloody and progressed to bloody and mucousy diarrhea by the second day. She states that she is still having diarrhea multiple times per day without signs of improvement. She denies any alleviating or aggravating factors. Not recently sick and no recent antibiotic use. One other hiking partner has since developed bloody diarrhea since their return. She notes that this is the first time she has had bloody diarrhea.

C. A. Standley (ed.), *Biomedical Science and Clinical Foundations*,
https://doi.org/10.1007/978-3-031-98353-5_14

Prompt: *What is your broad differential for this chief complaint? What history questions would you like to ask to help you narrow your differential?*

- Broad DDX can include:
  - Gastroenteritis: viral, bacterial
  - Other infectious: protozoal, amoebic, diverticulitis
  - Inflammatory bowel disease
  - Irritable bowel syndrome
  - Mesenteric ischemia
  - Hyperthyroidism
  - Neuroendocrine tumors: VIPoma, gastrinoma, carcinoid tumors
  - Medication effect
  - Laxative abuse
- A history is the critical first step in diagnosis. It is important to understand exactly what patients mean when they say they have diarrhea. Stool volume, frequency, and consistency can help categorize the diarrhea. A travel history is essential; travel to the tropics vastly expands the list of diagnostic possibilities, but in no way rules out common causes. Family or close contacts who are similarly sick could indicate a food-borne gastroenteritis or another infectious cause of diarrhea. A thorough medical, surgical and social history can further narrow your differential and is essential in this case. It is important to consider both infectious and non-infectious etiologies in the work-up of acute diarrhea.

Review of Systems

Significant for abdominal pain, bloody diarrhea, and prolonged epistaxis, but otherwise negative.

Past Medical History

Significant for hypothyroidism diagnosed at age 29.

Past Surgical History

Cholecystectomy at age 33.

Allergies

No known allergies.

Medications

Levothyroxine 75 mcg daily, dose recently increased from 2 weeks prior.

Family History

Crohn's disease (mother), recurrent diverticulitis (father).

Social History

Moderate alcohol use (2 beers after work daily) and current tobacco use (1 pack per day smoker since age 22), but no other illicit or recreational drugs.

Prompt: *How has your differential changed with the history of present illness along with the patient's past medical, surgical, family and social histories? What microbes could be responsible?*

- Exposure to beef, progression from non-bloody to bloody diarrhea → STEC, shiga-toxin HUS
- Drinking unfiltered stream water → possible giardia (protozoal) infection, though less likely associated with bloody diarrhea
- Recent travel to Brazil → traveler's diarrhea (ETEC), Entamoeba histolytica
- Recent medication change → possible adverse med effect from levothyroxine
- Family history of IBD and recurrent diverticulitis → must consider these diagnoses
- No recent antibiotic use → CDiff or other abx-related infection less likely

Physical Examination

Vitals

General: alert and conversant, appearing fatigued but in NAD
Skin: warm and dry; multiple small bruises noted over R arm
Eyes: conjunctiva clear, sclera anicteric; pupils equal, round, and reactive to light
Neck: without lymphadenopathy or thyromegaly
Nose: turbinates non-edematous; dried blood in nares
Mouth: mucous membranes moist without erythema or lesions
Chest: clear to auscultation bilaterally; normal respiratory effort
Cardiac: regular rate and rhythm without murmurs, rubs, or gallops
GI: no jaundice; +BS 4X, lower abdomen mildly tender to palpation; no hepatosplenomegaly
Neuro: no focal deficits; A&O X3; CN II—XII intact; DTR: biceps, triceps, patellar 2+ bilaterally; 5/5 motor strength in UE/LE; sensation intact
Extremities: warm to touch; 2+ pedal pulses bilaterally; no pedal edema

T: 37.0C	(ref 36.5–37.5)
BP: 130/75	(ref 90–130 / 55–80)
P: 75 bpm	(ref 60–100)
R: 14 breaths/min	(reference 12–20)
Wt: 140	Ht: 5′3″

Prompt: *Do any of the objective findings change your differential at this time? What work-up would you like to pursue at this time?*

- *CBC/CMP/TSH* → look for leukocytosis, metabolic derangements
- *Enteric panel* → bacterial etiologies (E coli, C Diff, Campylobacter, Shigella, etc.)
- *Viral panel* → Norovirus, Rotavirus
- *Stool Ova & Parasite* → Giardia, Entameoba histolytica, Cryptosporodium

Not done in this patient but can consider:

- *CT abdomen* → if high suspicion for diverticulitis or other intra-abdominal processes
- *Colonoscopy* → if high suspicion for IBD or non-infectious etiology
- *KUB radiograph* → can detect free air or perforations

Laboratory Data

CBC + Peripheral Smear

Component	Patient	Reference
WBC	10.9	4.0—11.0 k/mm^3
Hgb	8.5	12—15.5 g/dL
Hct	25.3%	37—48%
MCV	94	78—100 fL
Platelet Count	82	130—400 × 10^3/mm^3
Schistocytes	1+	None
LDH	398	140—280 U/L
Haptoglobin	<9	30—200 mg/dL

Component	Patient	Reference
Sodium	139	135—147 mEq/L
Potassium	4.4	3.5—5.0 mEq/L
Bicarbonate	25	24—28 mEq/L
Chloride	104	95—105 mEq/L
BUN	97	8—18 mg/dL
Creatinine	3.82	0.6—1.2 mg/dL
Glucose	104	70—100 mg/dL
AST	32	8—33 U/L
ALT	22	4—36 U/L
Alk Phosp	45	20—130 U/L
Total Bilirubin	0.9	0.1—1.2 mg/dL
Lipase	36	23—85 U/L

Prompt: *How would you interpret the patient's objective data?*

- Normocytic anemia with schistocytes is seen, along with elevated LDH and low haptoglobin—all indicative of a hemolytic process.
- Combined with the thrombocytopenia, AKI and the patient's recent history of bloody diarrhea, this is pointing to HUS (hemolytic uremic syndrome).

- HUS is much rarer in the adult population and therefore, all other causes must still be ruled out.
- Stool studies with gram stain, cultures, enteric panel, O&P should all still be performed to further narrow the differential.

Stool studies: enteric panel, norovirus, rotavirus, stool O&P

- Fecal Leukocytes: positive
- Norovirus: negative
- Rotavirus: negative
- C Diff Ag: negative
- C Diff toxin A/B: negative
- Campylobacter coli/jejuni: negative
- Salmonella sp.: negative
- E coli O157 gene: positive
- Shiga toxin 1 gene: positive
- Shiga toxin 2 gene: positive
- Stool Ova & Parasites:
- Giardia: negative
- Entameoba histolytica: negative
- Cryptosporodium: negative

Patient was immediately started on aggressive IV fluid resuscitation with isotonic saline. On Day 2 of hospital admission, the patient required a 2 U transfusion of RBC after her Hgb dropped to 6.3. The patient continued to improve with supportive care and IV fluids, with renal function improving toward baseline by Day 4. The patient was discharged safely to home on Day 5 without further complications.

End of Case

Learning Objective Answers

1. **Describe the microbiology for Shiga-toxin HUS, discussing basic nomenclature, the most commonly isolated serotypes, and Shiga toxin types.**

Nomenclature [1–5]

- STEC → E. coli that produces Shiga toxins; also known as verotoxigenic E. coli (VTEC) or enterohemorrhagic E. coli (EHEC)

Serotypes [1–5]

- *E. coli* strains and lineages are classified by their O and H antigens.
- O antigen is defined serologically and determined by the repeating polysaccharide chains that are part of the lipopolysaccharide (LPS) embedded in the outer leaflet of the outer membrane. The H antigen is defined serologically by the antigenic specificity of the bacterial flagellum.
- *E. coli* O157:H7 → most commonly isolated STEC serotype worldwide.
  - This serotype does not ferment *sorbitol* when grown on agar plates containing sorbitol as a carbon source.
- A number of other *E. coli* serotypes produce Shiga toxin ("non-O157:H7 STEC"). These non-O157:H7 STEC have been identified less frequently because few possess a phenotype as distinctive as the inability to ferment sorbitol on agar plates. Newer diagnostic microbiology technology increasingly detects non-O157:H7 STEC infections, and knowledge of the illnesses they cause is growing. These STEC are associated with a broader spectrum of illness than *E. coli* O157:H7 and are usually less severe.
- *E. coli* O157:H7 remains, nevertheless, the leading serotype of STEC recovered worldwide, and, in general, causes more severe disease than non-O157:H7 STEC, as discussed elsewhere.

Shiga toxin type [1–5]

STEC infections fall into two clinically relevant categories:

- Infections caused by *E. coli* that contain a gene encoding Shiga toxin 2 (with or without a gene encoding Shiga toxin 1).
  - STEC that contain the gene encoding Shiga toxin 2 are often associated with bloody diarrhea and can cause HUS independent of serogroup. Hence, bloody diarrhea is a reasonable surrogate indicator of the presence of an STEC that contains a gene encoding Shiga toxin 2.

- Infections caused by *E. coli* that contain a gene encoding Shiga toxin 1 but do not contain a gene encoding Shiga toxin 2.
  - These do not typically cause bloody diarrhea or HUS. Some non-O157:H7 STEC that contain a gene encoding Shiga toxin 1 can cause bloody diarrhea even if the Shiga toxin T2 gene is absent, but these pathogens are relatively rare.
- Almost all *E. coli* O157:H7 contain a gene encoding Shiga toxin 2 (~2/3 of this serotype also contain a gene encoding Shiga toxin 1). All *E. coli* O157:H7 isolated from humans should be assumed to possess a gene encoding Shiga toxin 2 and be highly pathogenic.

2. **Summarize the pathogenesis and mechanism of Shiga-toxin HUS; include how the pathogenesis can lead to the classic symptoms and findings in Shiga-toxin HUS.**

Toxin production [2–5]

- The cardinal virulence trait of STEC is their ability to produce Shiga toxins.
- Systemic host injury is the consequence of toxemia, as STEC rarely invade extraintestinal sites or the bloodstream.
- Shiga toxin 2 is more potent and much more frequently associated with severe human disease than Shiga toxin 1. Host injury is likely the consequence of systemic toxin-mediated microangiopathic injury.
- Non-O157:H7 STEC contain, by definition, genes encoding Shiga toxin 1 and/or 2 and a variable set of virulence factors, some of which are shared with E. coli O157:H7. However, from a clinical standpoint, the only relevant issue is whether Shiga toxin 2 is present.
- Other virulence factors include:
  - E. coli O157:H7 possesses a gene encoding intimin, which is located on the locus of enterocyte effacement and is the principal adhesin of E. coli O157:H7
  - The E. coli O157:H7 genome also encodes other adherence factors and the enterohemorrhagic E. coli (EHEC)-hemolysin (a pore-forming toxin encoded on a large plasmid termed pO157).
  - E. coli O157:H7 also form outer membrane vesicles that deliver virulence factors to host cells.

Hemolytic uremic syndrome [2–5]

- Toxin-mediated microangiopathic injury leads to a prothrombotic state in the human host, manifest by the formation of intravascular microthrombi.
- The prothrombotic abnormalities consist of elevated circulating activity of plasminogen activator-inhibitor type 1; elevated concentrations of circulating d-dimers, prothrombin activation fragment 1 + 2, platelet activating factor, sheared Von Willebrand Factor, and chemokine ligand stromal cell-derived factor-1; and dysregulated angiopoietin 1 and 2.
- Intravascular microthrombi, if extensive, can cause acute kidney injury by critically occluding afferent renal vessels. The working hypothesis is that the prothrombotic state that exists at the time of presentation with an infection caused by a high-risk STEC precedes and can lead to the HUS, a complication that develops in approximately 15–20% of E. coli O157:H7-infected children.

3. **Define the various definitions of diarrhea, delineating acute vs. chronic and the different forms of diarrhea. Create a broad differential for acute diarrhea for non-infectious etiologies.**

The following definitions have been suggested according to the duration of symptoms: [6–9]

- Acute—14 days or fewer in duration
- Persistent diarrhea—more than 14 but fewer than 30 days in duration
- Chronic—more than 30 days in duration

Diarrhea can be: [6–9]

- Watery
  - More likely small bowel in origin with large volume, associated often with bloating, cramping, and gas.
- Inflammatory (fevers, bloody, or mucousy)
  - More likely large bowel in origin, associated with fevers, bloody or mucousy stools
  - Visibly bloody stools should raise suspicion for STEC/E. coli O157:H7

Non-infectious etiologies [6–9]

- Drug adverse effects
- Laxative abuse
- Food allergies/intolerances
- Inflammatory bowel disease
- Irritable bowel syndrome
- Ischemic colitis
- Thyrotoxicosis
- Neuroendocrine tumors (VIPoma, carcinoid)

4. **List the common pathogens in acute diarrhea and describe its classic presentation and symptoms. Also summarize the appropriate workup to differentiate between common pathogens.**

Infectious etiologies [6–9]

SEE Table ON NEXT PAGE

Diagnostic workup [6–9]

- *CBC/CMP*—may not reliably differentiate between bacterial etiologies but may point toward complications, metabolic derangements, renal dysfunction, or hypovolemia from acute diarrhea.
- *Fecal leukocytes*—may indicate an inflammatory etiology, though often inaccurate. Peak sensitivity is estimated to be only 70%, and peak specificity is only at 50%.
- *Stool cultures*—routine stool cultures will identify Salmonella, Campylobacter, and Shigella, the three most common causes of bacterial diarrhea in the United States. E. coli O157:H7 can be isolated on sorbitol-MacConkey plates.
- *Multipathogen molecular panels*—can differentiate between bacterial, viral, and parasitic etiologies if found positive. A high degree of clinical correlation is necessary when interpreting results of molecular testing since these assays detect genetic material, which does not always indicate infection with a viable organism. Any positive results should be submitted for confirmatory culture.
- *Stool Ova and Parsites*—Microscopy can identify Giardia, Cryptosporidium, and E. histolytica

Causes of acute infectious diarrhea in adults in resource-rich settings

	Likely pathogens	Mean incubation period	Classic/common food sources	Other epidemiologic clues
Watery diarrhea	Norovirus	24 to 48 hours	Shellfish, prepared foods, vegetables, fruit	▪ Outbreaks in: • Restaurants • Health care facilities • Schools and childcare centers • Cruise ships • Military populations
	Clostridioides (formerly *Clostridium*) *difficile**	N/A	N/A	▪ Antibiotic use ▪ Hospitalization ▪ Cancer chemotherapy ▪ Gastric acid suppression ▪ Inflammatory bowel disease
	Clostridium perfringens	8 to 16 hours	Meat, poultry, gravy, home-canned goods	
	Enterotoxigenic *Escherichia coli*	1 to 3 days	Fecally contaminated food or water	▪ Travel to resource-limited settings
	Other enteric viruses (rotavirus, enteric adenovirus, astrovirus, sapovirus)	10 to 72 hours	Fecally contaminated food or water	▪ Daycare centers ▪ Gastroenteritis in children ▪ Immunocompromised adults
	Giardia lamblia	7 to 14 days	Fecally contaminated food or water	▪ Daycare centers ▪ Swimming pools ▪ Travel, hiking, camping (particularly when there is contact with water in which beavers reside)
	Cryptosporidium parvum	2 to 20 days	Vegetables, fruit, unpasteurized milk	▪ Daycare centers ▪ Swimming pools and recreational water sources ▪ Animal exposure ▪ Chronic diarrhea in advanced HIV infection
	Listeria monocytogenes	1 day (gastroenteritis)	Processed/delicatessen meats, hot dogs, soft cheese, pâtés, and fruit	▪ Pregnancy ▪ Immunocompromising condition ▪ Extremes of age
	Cyclospora cayetanensis	1 to 11 days	Imported berries, herbs	▪ Chronic diarrhea in advanced HIV infection
Inflammatory diarrhea (fever, mucoid or bloody stools)¶	Nontyphoidal *Salmonella*	1 to 3 days	Poultry, eggs, and egg products, fresh produce, meat, fish, unpasteurized milk or juice, nut butters, spices	▪ Animal contact (petting zoos, reptiles, live poultry, other pets) ▪ Travel to resource-limited settings
	Campylobacter spp	1 to 3 days	Poultry, meat, unpasteurized milk	▪ Travel to resource-limited settings ▪ Animal contact (young puppies or kittens, occupational contact)
	Shigella spp	1 to 3 days	Raw vegetables	▪ Daycare centers ▪ Crowded living conditions ▪ Men who have sex with men ▪ Travel to resource-limited settings
	Enterohemorrhagic *E. coli*	1 to 8 days	Ground beef and other meat, fresh produce, unpasteurized milk and juice	▪ Daycare centers ▪ Nursing homes ▪ Extremes of age
	Yersinia spp	4 to 6 days	Pork or pork products, untreated water	▪ Abnormalities of iron metabolism (eg, cirrhosis, hemochromatosis, thalassemia) ▪ Blood transfusion
	Vibrio parahemolyticus	1 to 3 days	Raw seafood and shellfish	▪ Cirrhosis
	Entamoeba histolytica	1 to 3 weeks	Fecally contaminated food or water	▪ Travel to resource-limited settings ▪ Men who have sex with men

* *Clostridioides* (formerly *Clostridium*) *difficile* can also present with inflammatory diarrhea.
¶ Pathogens that are more classically associated with inflammatory diarrhea can also cause watery diarrhea, particularly early in the course of infection.

5. **Describe the clinical presentation of STEC and Shiga-toxin HUS**

STEC Infection [2–4, 10–12]

- Infections with high-risk STEC are characterized by painful diarrhea that becomes bloody, often without persistent fever.
- The course of infection with high-risk STEC follows a patterned sequence of events. We consider the first day of illness to be the first day of diarrhea, although abdominal pain, vomiting, and fever can precede the onset of diarrhea.
- The initially non-bloody diarrhea typically becomes visibly bloody one to 3 days after onset; however, approximately 15–20% of infected patients only experience non-bloody diarrhea.
- Diarrhea generally resolves after about 7 days.
- Other highly prevalent features of E. coli O157:H7 infections include abdominal pain and an acute onset. However, these do not distinguish high-risk STEC infections from bloody diarrhea caused by other pathogens.

Hemolytic uremic syndrome [2–4, 10–12]

- HUS, if it occurs, is a complication of high-risk STEC that is usually established 5–13 days after the onset of diarrhea.
- Characterized and diagnosed by the triad of nonimmune-mediated hemolytic anemia, thrombocytopenia, and acute kidney injury.
  - Hct <30 percent, platelet count <150,000 microL, and serum creatinine greater than the upper limit of normal for age
- The likelihood that a patient infected with E. coli O157:H7 develops HUS varies by age. Fifteen to 20 percent of children younger than 10 years with culture-proven E. coli O157:H7 infection develop HUS. The HUS rate after childhood is difficult to determine with certainty because ascertainment of infection rates might differ between children and adults, and STEC-associated HUS may be misclassified in adults as atypical HUS or thrombotic thrombocytopenic purpura. Nevertheless, although the incidence of diagnosed STEC infection falls markedly during and after adolescence, STEC infections that occur in adults are not categorically more benign than in children.

6. **Summarize the general management for STEC infections and Shiga-toxin HUS.**

Hydration [12, 13]

- For patients with suspected or confirmed high-risk STEC infection, we suggest early and aggressive IV volume expansion with isotonic crystalloid. The main rationale is to reduce the severity of renal injury, particularly anuric renal injury, in patients who develop HUS.
- Meta-analyses and cohort studies have shown that IV fluid administration was associated with a decreased risk of renal replacement therapy and lower rates of anuria (anuric HUS is clinically worse than non-anuric HUS).

Electrolyte management [12, 13]

- Electrolyte disturbances are common, usually due to acute renal insufficiency or failure, including hyperkalemia, hyperphosphatemia, and metabolic acidosis.

Avoid antibiotics and antidiarrheals [12–14]

- We recommend *not treating* confirmed STEC infections (either *E. coli* O157:H7 or non-O157:H7) with antibiotics, based on the association between antibiotics and the development of HUS in patients with STEC infection. We also *do not use* empiric antibiotics in suspected STEC infections, pending microbiologic testing. If STEC is identified in patients in whom antibiotic therapy was initiated empirically, we discontinue it.
- One meta-analysis showed a non-significant trend toward a higher risk of HUS with antibiotic use in STEC infections; however, while the meta-analysis was not significant, multiple individual studies have shown significantly higher incidences of HUS with antibiotic use, both in the pediatric and adult populations.
- Antimotility agents (including opioids) are *not used* due to their association with a higher

risk of HUS and, among those who develop HUS, complicated HUS (e.g., with CNS dysfunction).

Avoid NSAIDs and other nephrotoxic medications [12, 13]

- We avoid the use of aspirin and NSAIDs, as patients with ST-HUS may be at increased risk of bleeding due to thrombocytopenia. NSAIDs and other nephrotoxic meds are avoided also due to the risk of exacerbating ischemic kidney damage/AKI that underlies HUS.

RBC transfusions [12, 13]

- Transfusion is appropriate for severe anemia (e.g., Hgb <7 g/dL) or if they have severe symptoms or signs of end-organ damage (e.g., ACS).

Platelet transfusions [12, 13]

- Transfusion is appropriate when a patient with a platelet count of <50,000/microL requires an invasive procedure or has clinically important bleeding.
- There is no role for routine platelet transfusion without bleeding or anticipated bleeding.

Dialysis [12, 13]

- Dialysis is performed for standard indications including fluid overload unresponsive to diuretics, hyperkalemia refractory to medical therapy, or metabolic acidosis and uremia.

Pain control [12, 13]

- We manage abdominal pain with boluses of isotonic fluid. This is based on our speculation that some of the pain could be related to intestinal ischemia. In particular, we avoid opioids or nonsteroidal anti-inflammatory drugs because of potential risks.

Hypoalbuminemia [12, 13]

- Many STEC-infected patients are hypoalbuminemic. If the patient has peripheral edema or diminishing urine output and the serum albumin concentration is <3 g/dL, we suggest judicious albumin infusions (e.g., 0.5 g/kg once and then repeated several hours later) to draw extracellular fluid into blood vessels and increase circulating blood volume. We do not administer albumin with a diuretic unless there is cardiopulmonary overload.

7. **What is the epidemiology of Shiga-toxin HUS in regard to both the pediatric and adult populations? What are the different common modes of transmission for STEC infections?**

Incidence [15–17]

- In the United States, the incidence of STEC infection was 5.9 per 100,000 persons in 2018, a 26% increase over the incidence from 2015 to 2017. This increase reflects the increasing ability to detect non-O157:H7 STEC. Among the 1570 STEC isolates tested, only 28% belonged to serotype O157:H7.

Affected age groups [15–17]

- STEC infection occurs in patients of all ages. About one-third of *E. coli* O157:H7 infections occur in patients 20–59 years old. However, the greatest burden of HUS occurs in children <5 years of age, followed by adults >60 years old. The median ages of patients infected with non-O157:H7 and O157:H7 STEC are similar.

Transmission [15–17]

- Transmission of STEC is primarily through food and person-to-person or animal contact. In a review of 390 *E. coli* O157:H7 outbreaks in the United States between 2003 and 2012 that included nearly 5000 illnesses, foodborne transmission accounted for 65% of cases, person-to-person contact for 10%, and indirect or direct animal contact for 10%. Water sources accounted for 4% of cases, and the remaining 10% had miscellaneous or unknown sources.

Foodborne [15–17]

- Most STEC infections are transmitted through food. Beef has traditionally been the most common source of foodborne outbreaks, although the proportion of outbreaks associ-

ated with consumption of beef has decreased. Many non-beef food products have also been implicated in STEC outbreaks, including fresh produce (e.g., spinach, lettuce, ready-to-eat salads, fruit, and sprouts), but other uncooked or unpasteurized products, such as raw milk, raw flour, raw dough (both prepackaged and homemade), apple juice, and soy nut butter, have also been linked to outbreaks. Non-beef meats, in particular pork and pork products, have less frequently caused STEC outbreaks.
- The most common reservoir for *E. coli* O157:H7 is the gastrointestinal tract of cattle, and beef is contaminated when the intestinal contents from a colonized animal contaminate the meat during slaughter or processing. Other food items and water can become contaminated when they come in contact with the feces of colonized animals.

Animal contact [15–17]
- STEC outbreaks have been associated with occupational exposure to animals, as well as recreational contact at county fairs, farms, and petting zoos, particularly in association with poor hand hygiene.

Person-to-person [15–17]
- The low infectious dose facilitates person-to-person transmission of *E. coli* O157:H7 infection. The secondary attack rate in outbreaks has ranged from 10 to 22%, particularly among patients in daycare centers and nursing homes. Patients who are ≤9 or ≥ 50 years of age are at increased risk. Hospitalization of STEC-infected patients has been proposed to reduce secondary infections in the community.

Exam Questions

1. An obese 65-year-old female with a history of hypertension and diabetes is admitted with 3 days of bloody diarrhea associated with abdominal pain. She states that she first developed non-bloody diarrhea the day after her weekend backyard barbeque that later progressed to bloody diarrhea 2 days after onset of the initial diarrhea. The patient is hemodynamically stable and non-toxic-appearing. Abdomen is soft and non-distended but tender to palpation diffusely in the lower quadrants. Stool studies are currently pending. While awaiting results, she requests empiric antibiotics for treatment. What is the appropriate antibiotic choice in the treatment of this possible infection?
   A. Antibiotics are not indicated at this time
   B. Ciprofloxacin
   C. Oral Vancomycin
   D. Tinidazole
   E. Metronidazole/Paromomycin

   Answer: A

   Learning Objective: #6 Summarize the general management for STEC infections and Shiga-toxin HUS

   Explanation: Empiric antibiotics are not routinely used in the management of acute diarrhea unless the patient is severely symptomatic. Antibiotics are not used in STEC infections, as they are associated with a higher risk of developing Shiga-toxin HUS. This patient is hemodynamically stable and non-toxic appearing, so empiric antibiotics should not be started at this time. If patients are initially started on empiric antibiotics for acute diarrhea and later found positive for Shiga toxin or positive for *E. coli* O157:H7, antibiotics should be immediately stopped. B is incorrect, as while azithromycin (first line) or fluoroquinolones can be useful antibiotics in traveler's diarrhea, they are not routinely recommended. Antibiotic treatment is reasonable for travelers with severe diarrhea, which is characterized by fever and blood, pus, or mucus in the stool, or for travelers with diarrhea that substantially interferes with the purpose of travel. C is incorrect—patients found positive for C. diff can be treated with oral vancomycin. C. diff diarrhea will be watery and foul-smelling and can be associated with recent antibiotic use, PPIs, and IBD. D is incorrect—patients found positive for Giardia can be treated with tinidazole (first line). Giardia infections result from fecally contaminated water sources, including streams or pools. Diarrhea will typically be watery and non-bloody. E is incorrect—E. histolytica is associated with bloody diarrhea and can be treated with a combination of metronidazole and paromomycin. Infections are typically seen in migrants from and travelers to endemic areas. HIV and male-to-male sex have also been associated with intestinal or extraintestinal amebiasis.

2. A 66-year-old male with a history of recurrent diverticulitis, CKD III presents to the ED with bloody diarrhea, diffuse lower abdominal pain, and fatigue. On admission, he is afebrile, without leukocytosis, but does have a normocytic anemia of Hgb 6.4 with schistocytes seen on peripheral smear, thrombocytopenia 77, and Cr 3.1 (up from baseline of 1.8). Stool studies confirm a bacterial infection that has a known association with undercooked beef. What is the most likely mechanism behind this patient's anemia?
   A. Erythrocyte membrane defects
   B. Autoimmune hemolytic anemia
   C. Microangiopathic hemolytic anemia
   D. Mechanical shearing
   E. Enzyme deficiencies

   Answer: C

   Learning Objective: #2 Summarize the pathogenesis and mechanism of Shiga-toxin HUS; include how the pathogenesis can lead to the classic symptoms and findings in Shiga-toxin HUS

   Explanation: Microangiopathic hemolytic anemias result from intravascular RBC fragmentation that produces schistocytes on the peripheral blood smear. Like other hemolytic anemias, you will also see elevated LDH and reduced haptoglobin. A is incorrect—this is seen in hereditary spherocytosis or hereditary elliptocytosis. Abnormally shaped RBCs will be seen on the peripheral smear with an anemia of variable severity. Chronic hemolysis can lead to gallstones or splenomegaly in either of these diseases. B is incorrect—Shiga-toxin HUS is characterized by a NON-immune-mediated, microangiopathic hemolytic anemia. Autoimmune hemolytic anemias, like other hemolytic anemias, will show elevated LDH and reduced haptoglobin but can be differentiated by a positive direct antiglobulin test (DAT) and further characterized by their thermal reactivity (warm vs. cold). D is incorrect—this is seen in patients with artificial or mechanical heart valves, causing mechanical shearing of RBCs, leading to hemolytic anemia and schistocytes on peripheral smears. E is incorrect—this is seen in G6PD deficiency. Triggered by oxidative stress, hemoglobin becomes denatured and precipitates into erythrocyte inclusions called Heinz bodies; these bodies damage the erythrocyte membrane, resulting in acute intravascular and extravascular hemolysis. Heinz bodies and bite cells are commonly seen in G6PD deficiency.

3. A 28-year-old male with a history of lower back pain and a family history of Crohn's is being admitted for 3 days of fevers and bloody diarrhea, which he has never had before. Additional review of systems was positive for unintended 15 lb weight loss over the last 2 months and irritation/itching of both eyes. He states that he was recently at a potluck with plenty of home-cooked food last week, including hamburgers and chicken skewers, though no one else from the party has been sick. The patient denies any recent travel. The patient is febrile, but otherwise vitals are normal. The patient's abdomen is mildly distended with pain on palpation to the lower quadrants but otherwise appears non-toxic. Which of the following diagnostic workup would be the appropriate next step for this patient?
   A. CT abdomen
   B. Colonoscopy
   C. Enteric bacterial panel
   D. Stool O&P
   E. KUB

   Answer: C

   Learning Objective: #3 Define the various definitions of diarrhea, delineating acute vs. chronic and the different forms of diarrhea. Create a broad differential for acute diarrhea for non-infectious etiologies and infectious etiologies.

   Explanation: The clinical presentation currently points toward IBD as the etiology of this bloody diarrhea; evidence includes the patient's age, lower back pain (possible ankylosing spondylitis), eye involvement, and weight loss. However, we cannot exclude an infectious cause yet. Before jumping to imaging or a colonoscopy, an infectious workup would be initially warranted. The appropriate next step would be to send an enteric bacterial panel. A is incorrect—a CT abdomen can be helpful in ruling out specific etiologies, including hernias, masses, inflammatory changes, and other identifying complications (ischemia, necrosis, perforation). Emergent imaging in this patient is not necessary, as the patient is non-toxic appearing and hemodynamically stable. B is incorrect—colonoscopy with mucosal biopsies would be part of the work-up for IBD. However, this procedure is more invasive and will come after other workups to exclude infectious etiologies. D is incorrect—stool O&P may be warranted if the clinical picture fits; E Histolytica could explain bloody diarrhea and can be detected with stool O&P but nothing in the patients' history suggests that this is the case (no travel history). Giardia and Cryptosporidium can also be detected by stool O&P, but would produce watery diarrhea instead. Infectious rule-out with a bacterial panel would be the appropriate next step for this patient. E is incorrect—a KUB X-ray may be performed to help diagnose the cause of abdominal pain, such as masses, perforations, or obstruction. KUBs can help diagnose kidney and urinary bladder stones, intestinal blockages, perforation of the stomach or intestine, and ingestion of foreign objects.

References

1. GBD 2016 Diarrhoeal Disease Collaborators. Estimates of the global, regional, and national morbidity, mortality, and aetiologies of diarrhoea in 195 countries: a systematic analysis for the Global Burden of Disease Study 2016. Lancet Infect Dis. 2018;18(11):1211–28. https://doi.org/10.1016/S1473-3099(18)30362-1. Epub 2018 Sep 19. PMID: 30243583; PMCID: PMC6202444.
2. Karch H, Bielaszewska M. Sorbitol-fermenting Shiga toxin-producing Escherichia coli O157:H(−) strains: epidemiology, phenotypic and molecular characteristics, and microbiological diagnosis. J Clin Microbiol. 2001;39:2043.
3. Slutsker L, Ries AA, Greene KD, et al. Escherichia coli O157:H7 diarrhea in the United States: clinical and epidemiologic features. Ann Intern Med. 1997;126:505.
4. Tarr PI, Gordon CA, Chandler WL. Shiga-toxin-producing Escherichia coli and haemolytic uraemic syndrome. Lancet. 2005;365:1073.
5. Tesh VL, O'Brien AD. The pathogenic mechanisms of Shiga toxin and the Shiga-like toxins. Mol Microbiol. 1991;5:1817.
6. Shane AL, Mody RK, Crump JA, et al. 2017 Infectious Diseases Society of America clinical practice guidelines for the diagnosis and management of infectious diarrhea. Clin Infect Dis. 2017;65:e45.
7. Riddle MS, DuPont HL, Connor BA. ACG clinical guideline: diagnosis, treatment, and prevention of acute diarrheal infections in adults. Am J Gastroenterol. 2016;111:602.
8. Guerrant RL, Van Gilder T, Steiner TS, et al. Practice guidelines for the management of infectious diarrhea. Clin Infect Dis. 2001;32:331.
9. Thielman NM, Guerrant RL. Clinical practice. Acute infectious diarrhea. N Engl J Med. 2004;350:38.
10. Rohner P, Pittet D, Pepey B, et al. Etiological agents of infectious diarrhea: implications for requests for microbial culture. J Clin Microbiol. 1997;35:1427.
11. Brandt JR, Fouser LS, Watkins SL, et al. Escherichia coli O 157:H7-associated hemolytic-uremic syndrome after ingestion of contaminated hamburgers. J Pediatr. 1994;125:519.
12. Noris M, Remuzzi G. Hemolytic uremic syndrome. J Am Soc Nephrol. 2005;16:1035.
13. Freedman SB, van de Kar NCAJ, Tarr PI. Shiga toxin-producing Escherichia coli and the hemolytic-uremic syndrome. N Engl J Med. 2023;389:1402.
14. Wong CS, Jelacic S, Habeeb RL, et al. The risk of the hemolytic-uremic syndrome after antibiotic treatment of Escherichia coli O157:H7 infections. N Engl J Med. 2000;342:1930.
15. Klein EJ, Stapp JR, Clausen CR, et al. Shiga toxin-producing Escherichia coli in children with diarrhea: a prospective point-of-care study. J Pediatr. 2002;141:172.
16. Davis TK, McKee R, Schnadower D, Tarr PI. Treatment of Shiga toxin-producing Escherichia coli infections. Infect Dis Clin N Am. 2013;27:577.
17. George JN, Nester CM. Syndromes of thrombotic microangiopathy. N Engl J Med. 2014;371:654.

Abdominal Cramping

15

Melanie Schroeder

Learning Objectives

1. Compare and contrast the pathophysiology and presentation of diverticulitis, ischemic colitis, and infectious colitis.
2. Describe the typical microbiology of diverticulitis, including the distinguishing features of the different microbes (Gram stain, shape, special tests, etc.).
3. Consider the broad differential of lower abdominal pain and prioritize those diagnoses which are life- or limb-threatening.
4. List treatment options for acute diverticulitis, including both the short-term (inpatient vs. outpatient) and long-term management strategies. Discuss ways to best counsel this patient on weight loss through diet and exercise changes.
5. Articulate the acute complications of diverticulitis and how they would present in a patient.
6. Summarize important risk factors for diverticulitis and describe the epidemiology of this disease (incidence, prevalence in U.S. and globally).

M. Schroeder (✉)
University of Arizona College of Medicine, Phoenix, AZ, USA

George Washington University Emergency Medicine, Washington, DC, USA
e-mail: mschroeder@gwu.edu

Chief Complaint: "My Stomach Hurts!"

STOP AND THINK: What is your differential diagnosis?

See Table 15.1 *for possible differentials according to the VINDICATES mnemonic, and* Fig. 15.1 *for differentials based on location of abdominal pain.*

STOP AND THINK: What questions do you want to ask this patient?

Onset—Was it abrupt? Gradual?
Position—Where is the pain? (key in narrowing the differential as above)
Progression—Is it changing over time?
Quality—Does it feel stabbing? Burning? Tearing? Dull? Something other descriptor?
Radiation—Does it travel anywhere else?
Severity—On a scale of 1–10 (10 being the worst), how severe is the pain?
Timing/Duration/Frequency—Is the pain intermittent or constant? How long does it last? How often does it occur?
Aggravating/alleviating factors—Is it better or worse with eating? Exertion? Any other triggers or palliating factors?
Associated symptoms—Is it associated with fevers/chills? Nausea/vomiting? Diarrhea? Constipation? Urinary symptoms? Vaginal bleeding or discharge?
Other things—Has it happened before? Any recent or previous abdominal procedures? History of trauma? Sexual history? Alcohol or drug use?

C. A. Standley (ed.), *Biomedical Science and Clinical Foundations*,
https://doi.org/10.1007/978-3-031-98353-5_15

Table 15.1 Differential diagnoses according to body system affected

Vascular	Acute or chronic mesenteric ischemia, abdominal aortic aneurysm rupture, aortic dissection, splenic infarct, radiation from acute coronary syndrome, pulmonary embolism
Infection/ Inflammatory	Cholecystitis, appendicitis, mesenteric lymphadenitis, gastritis, gastroenteritis, GERD, hepatitis, hepatic abscess, cholangitis, biliary colic, splenic abscess, pericarditis, myocarditis, pneumonia, bronchitis, costochondritis, pancreatitis, esophageal spasm, colitis, pyelonephritis, urinary tract infection, tubo-ovarian abscess, pelvic inflammatory disease, STI, psoas abscess, epididymo-orchitis
Neoplastic	Gastric cancer, pancreatic cancer, lung cancer, esophageal cancer, ovarian cancer, colorectal cancer, endometrial cancer, liver cancer, peritoneal carcinomatosis
Drugs/ Degenerative	Epigastric hernia, pill esophagitis, NSAIDs causing gastritis/peptic ulcer disease; gastroparesis secondary to Parkinson's/MS; constipation secondary to opioids
Idiopathic/ Iatrogenic	Post-operative complication (perforation), small bowel obstruction (SBO), large bowel obstruction (LBO), urinary retention
Congenital	Marfan syndrome, indirect inguinal hernia, Meckel's diverticulum
Autoimmune/ Allergy	Ulcerative colitis, Crohn's, gastroparesis secondary to diabetes/scleroderma/hypothyroidism
Trauma	Contusion, pneumothorax, rib fracture, food impaction in lower esophagus, splenic rupture
Endocrine/ Environmental	Ingestions (Tylenol overdose, anticholinergics/opioids causing ileus, heavy metals, etc.), kidney stones, irritable bowel syndrome, black widow spider envenomation
Something else…	Ovarian/testicular torsion, ectopic pregnancy (rupture), ovarian cyst rupture, endometriosis, anxiety

History of Presenting Illness

Mrs. Franco is a 48-year-old female who presents with abdominal pain described as constant cramping and stabbing sensations. Her symptoms came on gradually about 4 days ago and are getting progressively worse. Her pain is worst over her left lower quadrant (LLQ) but occasionally radiates around to her back. Severity is 7/10. She reports subjective fevers (although has not measured her temperature), constipation, and urinary urgency. She had similar symptoms to this about 6 months ago but did not seek treatment.

Past Medical History (PMH):

Hypertension (HTN)
Hyperlipidemia (HLD)
Irritable Bowel Syndrome (IBS)
Prior myocardial infarction (MI) at age 45

Past Surgical History (PSH):

Cholecystectomy at age 36

Tubal ligation at age 40

OB/GYN History:

G3P1112

2 vaginal deliveries without complication

Currently sexually active with men and women

H/o chlamydia in her 20s

Unsure if she went through menopause, irregular vaginal bleeding

Social History (SH):

Patient is an elementary school teacher that lives with her girlfriend.

Smokes ½ pack of cigarettes per day for the past 25 years.

Drinks 1–2 beers every night.

Denies current or past illicit drug use.

Walks around the block 2 nights per week for exercise.

Eats fast food on most days.

Family History (FH):

Grandparents—unknown medical history

Mother—Ovarian cysts

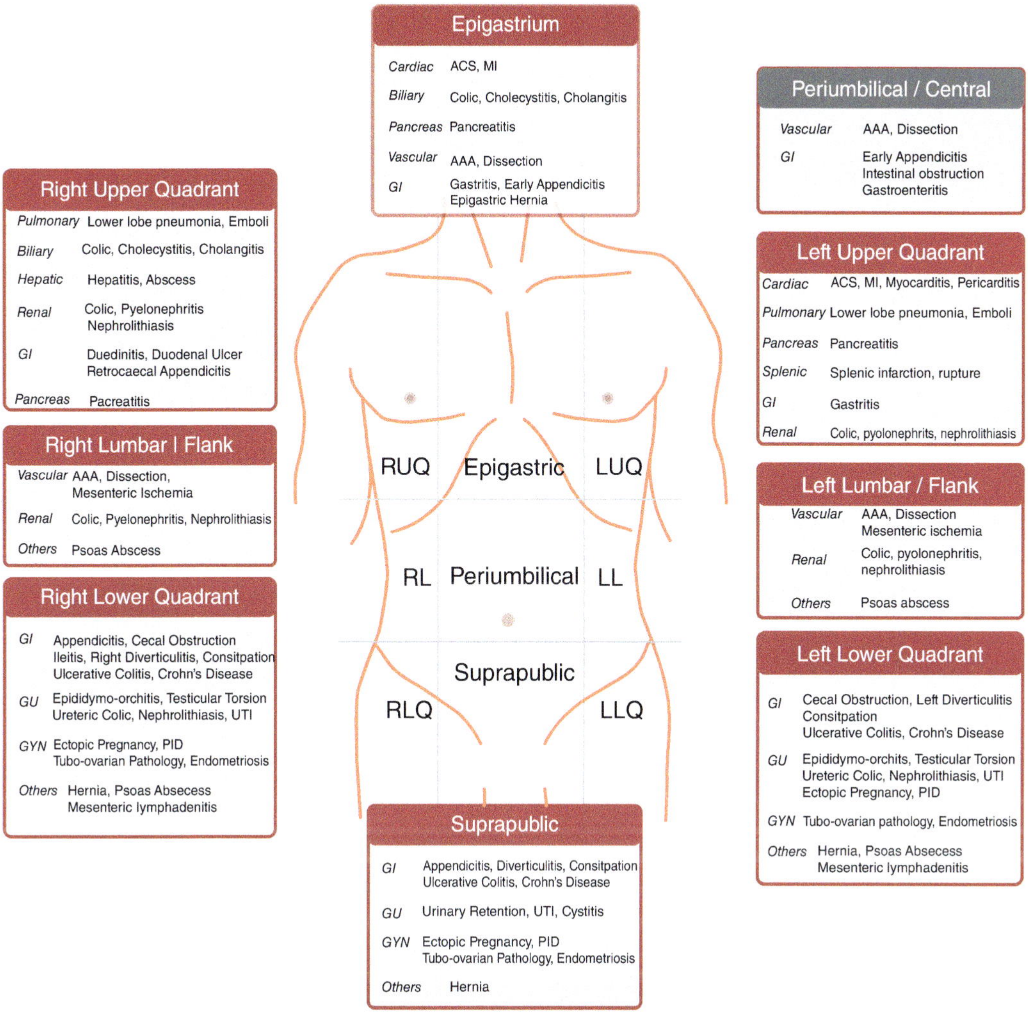

Fig. 15.1 Differential diagnoses according to the location of abdominal pain [1]

Father—Colon cancer at age 70
Daughter, son—healthy

Medications:

Lisinopril 40 mg daily
Atorvastatin 40 mg daily
Ibuprofen 600 mg as needed for arthritic pain

STOP AND THINK: What are the mechanisms of these medications? What are they commonly indicated for?
See Table 15.2 *for a list of medications with their usage* indications.

Allergies

Aspirin—reaction is rash.

Review of Systems (ROS):

General: + subjective fevers, 5 lb. weight gain. No chills, night sweats, or diaphoresis.
Hematologic: No easy bleeding or ecchymosis
Respiratory: No cough, sputum production, dyspnea, or pleuritic chest pain.
Cardiovascular: No chest pain, palpitations, light-headedness, or syncope. Denies dyspnea on exertion.

Table 15.2 Common medications and their mechanisms of action and indications

Lisinopril	*ACE-inhibitor* Inhibits activity of the enzyme ACE which thus decreases plasma angiotensin II and aldosterone and increases renin activity Used for blood pressure management, in acute coronary syndrome, for chronic kidney disease, and in heart failure
Atorvastatin	*Statin* Inhibits the enzyme HMG-CoA reductase thus preventing the conversion of HMG-CoA to mevalonate which decreases cholesterol production in liver Used for hypercholesterolemia, prevention of atherosclerosis
Ibuprofen	*Non-steroidal anti-inflammatory drug (NSAID)* Inhibits the enzyme cyclooxygenase (COX) which prevents the conversion of arachidonic acid into prostacyclins, thomboxanes, and prostaglandins which are involved in the pain and inflammatory process Used in abnormal uterine bleeding, for pain, for fever, in pericarditis, for treatment of acute gout flares, and generally for anti-inflammation

Gastrointestinal: + LLQ abdominal pain, constipation. No reflux, nausea, vomiting, hematemesis, or diarrhea.
Genitourinary: + dysuria, urinary urgency. No frequency, hematuria, or back or flank pain.
Endocrine: No easy fatigue, change in sleeping pattern. No history of thyroid problems.
Musculoskeletal: No pain, tenderness, or swelling of joints or muscles.
Neurologic: No numbness or weakness of extremities, no difficulty speaking or swallowing, no memory impairment.
Other systems: Negative.

STOP AND THINK: What questions would you ask to further quantify the constipation?

- Last bowel movement (BM)? Are you still passing gas?
- Frequency of BM's?
- Consistency of stool?
- Any changes in shape or color?

STOP AND THINK: What symptoms, past medical history, medications, family and social history are relevant to the chief complaint?

- Cramping, stabbing abdominal pain for 4 days that is getting progressively worse
- LLQ pain with radiation to back
- Subjective fevers, constipation, urinary urgency
- Has had these symptoms before but no treatment
- PMH of HTN, HLD, IBS, prior MI
- PSH of cholecystectomy, tubal ligation
- Has a poor diet and limited exercise
- Had chlamydia in 20's, still sexually active without clear evidence of menopause
- Taking frequent NSAIDs for arthritis
- FH of colon cancer in father

STOP AND THINK: What are your key hypotheses?

Differential is still very broad, but given the LLQ location, we can narrow it down to these as most likely:

- Diverticulitis/colitis
- Constipation, IBS
- UTI (cystitis, pyelonephritis)
- Nephrolithiasis
- Pelvic/reproductive pathology

IBD is still possible but less likely given the patient's age and lack of chronic weight loss, fatigue, or hematochezia. She could have a partial bowel obstruction given the pain and constipation, but is less likely without known colon cancer/hernias or exposure to medications that cause decreased GI motility. Obstetric and gynecologic causes still need to be on the radar given the high morbidity and mortality associated with ectopic pregnancy rupture, ovarian torsion, and

PID. Other emergent conditions that can't be missed include mesenteric ischemia, peritonitis, GI perforation. It is also important to consider referred pain from nearby anatomy such as hip pathology, a psoas abscess, left lower lobe pneumonia, or a rectus sheath hematoma.

STOP AND THINK: What physical examination findings and ancillary studies (laboratory tests, imaging studies, etc.) can be used to distinguish the hypotheses given?

Physical Exam: Vital signs, full head-to-toe exam especially including abdominal and cardiovascular

Pending the patient's exam, consider ordering the following:

Laboratory Tests: Complete blood count (CBC), Basic metabolic panel (BMP), Liver function tests (LFTs), Lipase, UA with reflex to culture, Urine pregnancy

Imaging Studies: Consider CT scan with IV +/− oral contrast versus limited abdominal ultrasound (US) versus pelvic US pending on what differential diagnosis is most likely after the physical exam/lab workup and what emergent conditions you cannot miss.

Vital signs:

BP: 100/60, HR: 89, RR: 20, SpO_2: 100% on room air, T: 100.4 °F, Weight: 208 lbs., Height: 66"

Physical Exam:

General appearance: Obese female, alert and conversant, and in pain.

Skin: Warm and dry.

HEENT: Normocephalic atraumatic, pupils equal, round, and reactive to light and accommodation (PERRLA), extraocular motions intact (EOMI). Hearing intact bilaterally; nasal passages clear; oropharynx without exudate or erythema; dentition intact.

Neck/thyroid: Supple with full range of motion. No jugular vein distention. No carotid bruits. No thyromegaly or masses.

Chest/Lungs: Mild respiratory distress. No chest wall tenderness. Clear to auscultation (CTA); breath sounds equal bilaterally. No crackles, rhonchi, or wheezing.

Heart: Regular rate. Normal S1, S2, without S3, S4

Abdomen: Tender over left lower quadrant without rebound or guarding. Non-distended, bowel sounds noted in all 4 quadrants, no hepatosplenomegaly.

Extremities: No clubbing, cyanosis, or edema.

Pulses: Radial, femoral, dorsalis pedis (DP), and posterior tibialis (PT) pulses are 2+ and symmetrical bilaterally; capillary refill <3 seconds.

STOP AND THINK: How do you check capillary refill time?

- It can be measured by pressing on the skin for 5 seconds and noting the time needed for the color to return once the pressure is released.
- Normal is less than 2–3 seconds

Lab Results

CBC:

Laboratory test	Patient value	Reference range
White Blood Cell Count	13 K	4.0–11 K/mm^3
Hemoglobin	13	13.0–18.0 g/dL
Hematocrit	41	40.0–53.0%
Platelets	320	130–450 K /mm^3
MCV	90	80–100 fL
MCHC	32	30–35 g/dL
RDW	15.4	12.1–18.2%

STOP AND THINK: One of your senior residents tells you that this patient also has a left shift—what does this mean physiologically and what does it indicate?

- A left shift means that there is evidence of a predominance of immature neutrophils in the differential including segs, bands, metamyelocytes, myelocytes or even blasts. It is phrased this based off traditional diagrams that show cellular maturation with more immature forms on the left of the diagram differentiating into more mature forms towards the right. It is often associated with bacterial infections [2].

CMP:

Laboratory test	Patient value	Reference range
Sodium	140	135–145 mmol/L
Potassium	4.3	3.5–5.2 mmol/L
BUN	18	8–25 mg/dL
Creatinine	0.9	0.6–1.5 mg/dL
CO2 (bicarbonate)	20	19–31 mmol/L
Chloride	102	96–110 mmol/L
Glucose	125	65–99 mg/dL
AST	39	10–50 IU/L
ALT	23	5–60 IU/L
Alkaline phosphatase	120	40–129 IU/L
Total bilirubin	0.7	0.2–1.3 mg/dL
Albumin	4.5	3.3–4.9 gm/dL

Serum lipase: 70 U/L
bHCG negative
UA

- Light pale in color
- Clear
- pH 5
- Specific gravity 1.020
- Glucose negative
- Ketones negative
- Nitrites negative
- Leukocyte esterase negative
- No blood
- 0 RBCs
- 0 WBCs
- 10 squamous epithelial cells/hpf
- Occasional crystals

Portable abdominal X-ray performed with no free air

STOP AND THINK: How do these test results help you to refine your hypothesis (e.g., what do they confirm or rule out?)

- Likely an infectious or inflammatory process occurring given the leukocytosis with left shift
- Patient is not anemic or thrombocytopenic—less likely an acute hemorrhage such as with ectopic pregnancy rupture, brisk GI bleed
- With a normal lipase and the location of patient's pain, can effectively rule out pancreatitis
- Perforation is also slightly less likely (also given no free air on XR)
- Pt does not have a UTI and unlikely kidney stones given lack of WBC or blood on UA
- No evidence of pregnancy
- Less likely hepatobiliary pathology given the reassuring LFT's

STOP AND THINK: What other tests would you now consider ordering? Defend your rationale for ordering these additional test(s)

- CT abdomen/pelvis with IV and oral contrast to look for a definitive intra-abdominal pathology such as diverticulitis
- Could consider pelvic ultrasound if this was negative to look for ovarian torsion or other reproductive/gynecologic source
- Could also consider limited or right upper quadrant abdominal ultrasound but this is likely lower yield given location of patient's pain and normal liver function tests

CT Scan of Abdomen/Pelvis with IV Contrast

An abdominal CT scan with intravenous contrast is shown in Fig. 15.2.

Results Multiple diverticula associated with signs of acute inflammation of the sigmoid colon, including wall thickening and enhancement, as well as marked stranding of the adjacent fat tissues.

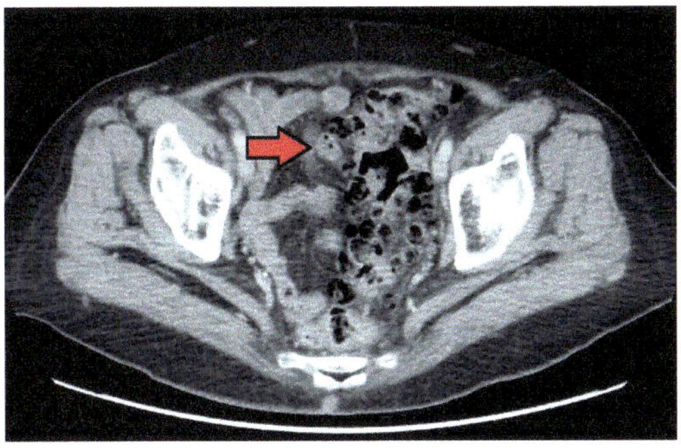

Fig. 15.2 CT Scan of Abdomen/Pelvis with Evidence of Diverticulitis. (From James Heilman, MD, licensed under CC BY-SA 4.0) (https://commons.wikimedia.org/wiki/File:DivertDiseaseMark.png)

STOP AND THINK: What is the diagnosis? Of the differential diagnoses, which were we able to rule out?

- Patient has acute uncomplicated diverticulitis which accounts for all her symptoms
- We were able to rule out abdominal organ perforation, UTI, nephrolithiasis, appendicitis, ectopic pregnancy, pregnancy, pancreatitis, etc.

STOP AND THINK: How does this relate to the patient's initial chief complaint?

- Patient had left lower quadrant pain, constipation, urinary urgency and dysuria which can all commonly occur in diverticulitis, especially given that she had a similar episode previously
- She has many risk factors for this disease include older age, obese BMI, low fiber diet, smoking, NSAID intake

STOP AND THINK: What is the next step in management?

- Risk stratify the patient based on evidence of any complications of diverticulitis, her other comorbidities, age, etc. to determine if she is best suited for outpatient or inpatient management
- With mild cases of uncomplicated diverticulitis, it is best to manage outpatient, often with oral broad spectrum antibiotics, and a diet that is suitable to the patient's symptoms and needs
- Patients will need to follow up with their PCP and a GI specialist to have a colonoscopy done in the subsequent 4–8 weeks after an episode (if they have not had one in the last year) to determine if there is an underlying colorectal cancer or other malignancy

Clinical Course

Patient was diagnosed with uncomplicated diverticulitis and was sent home with oral antibiotics and a clear liquid diet. She will follow up with a GI specialist in 2–3 days and undergo her first colonoscopy next month.

The Case: Abdominal Pain and Diverticulitis

In this case, we explored a presentation of a middle-aged female patient with left lower quadrant pain who was found to have uncomplicated diverticulitis and ultimately discharged home on antibiotics. Let's review the epidemiology, risk factors, pathophysiology, expected microbiology, typical presentation, potential complications, and management of this condition.

Overall, diverticulitis is a common diagnosis that has been increasing in frequency. The incidence of first-time acute diverticulitis in the United States is about 2.9% [3] (learning objective #6). Greater than 50% of adults over the age of 60 in the U.S. have diverticulosis [3]. Of those individuals with diverticulosis, there is anywhere from a 4% up to a 10–25% risk of developing diverticulitis in one's lifetime [4, 5]. It is more common in older adults, and the mean age for presentation with diverticulitis is 63 years old [6]. Nonetheless, roughly 16% of diverticulitis admissions are in those under the age of 45 [7]. In younger individuals less than 50, the diagnosis is more common in men; however, this reverses above the age of 50, and especially above age 70, where there is increased frequency in women [8–10]. The prevalence of hospitalization for diverticulitis in the United States is greatest in white people, relatively similar in African American and Hispanic patients, but lower in those of Asian descent [11].

As mentioned above, older age is a risk factor for diverticulitis. Other risk factors include lack of consumption of dietary fiber, frequent consumption of red meat and fats, limited physical activity, and obese BMI (especially central obesity) [11, 12] (learning objective #6). Interestingly, it was historically thought that nut, corn, popcorn, and grain consumption increased risk of diverticulitis given the theoretical likelihood of these items lodging in diverticulum and causing inflammation. In more recent studies, including a large prospective cohort study, there was an inverse association demonstrated between nut and popcorn consumption and risk of diverticulitis [13]. Other lifestyle factors that increase risk of diverticulosis and thus diverticulitis are smoking and alcohol use. There is up to a 30% increased probability of diverticulosis in patients who smoke and 3x increased likelihood in those who consume alcohol [12]. There are also some medications associated with a higher risk of developing diverticulitis: NSAIDs, acetaminophen, corticosteroids, opioids, and hormone therapy [11, 12, 14–17]. Those with specific genetic syndromes that increase likelihood of forming colonic diverticula are also at higher risk. These include Marfan syndrome, Ehlers-Danlos syndrome, Williams-Beuren syndrome, Coffin-Lowry syndrome, and polycystic kidney disease [11, 12]. All of these involve defects in the extracellular matrix or connective tissue, suggesting that this may be implicated in the pathogenesis of diverticulosis.

The underlying physiology of diverticulitis is not well understood (learning objective #1). It was initially hypothesized that obstruction of diverticula, the sac-like protrusions of the colonic wall that form from increased pressure on weak areas of the colon, caused increased pressure and subsequent perforation [18]. Yet, this obstruction with fecaliths is now presumed to be rarer. Another theory is that increasing intraluminal pressure or congealed digested food particles causes inflammation and local necrosis along with microscopic or macroscopic perforation. This is like the pathogenesis of appendicitis. There are also hypotheses that the development of diverticulitis may be secondary to chronic inflammation and changes in the gut microbiome. Evidence supports these theories: there are elevated circulating inflammatory markers like CRP and IL-6 in patients who develop diverticulitis, and the gut microbiome notably differs in patients with diverticulitis compared to those who have never had it [19–21]. In comparison, ischemic colitis is caused by reduced blood flow to the colon, producing mucosal injury and necrosis without inflammation, whereas infectious colitis arises from microbial invasion and toxin-mediated inflammation of the colonic mucosa.

The inflammation and potential subsequent infection in diverticulitis are due to normal colonic flora being released into the peritoneal cavity (learning objective #2). It is typically polymicrobial, involving both anaerobic and aerobic flora, both gram-positive and gram-negative [22, 23]. The most common anaerobes include Bacteroides fragilis, Fusobacterium spp., Clostridium, and Peptostreptococcus [24]. Other facultative anaerobes implicated include E. coli and Streptococcus. Aerobes, in comparison are far less common. On average, 5 different organisms are found in patients with diverticulitis, and Bacteroides fragilis and E. coli are the species most commonly isolated [23, 25, 26].

Besides diverticulitis, the differential for lower abdominal pain is fairly broad, and includes common etiologies such as constipation/IBS, UTI, nephrolithiasis and pelvic/reproductive pathology (learning objective #3). When patients present with diverticulitis, the most common symptom is constant abdominal pain, particularly in the left lower quadrant, due to involvement of the sigmoid colon [27]. However, in those with redundant inflamed sigmoid colon or right-sided cecal diverticulitis, pain can be in the right lower quadrant or suprapubic area [28–30]. Patients may also have a low-grade fever and change in bowel habits, with constipation reported more frequently than diarrhea [31, 32]. 10–15% of patients also have lower urinary tract symptoms with dysuria, urgency, and frequency secondary to inflamed colon irritating the bladder. More rare findings include palpable tender mass from associated abscess or pericolonic inflammation, hematochezia/occult blood, and hypotension/shock in the setting of perforation and peritonitis [33].

Laboratory evaluation may reveal leukocytosis and elevated CRP, although these tests are not sensitive or specific for diverticulitis [34–37]. Urinalysis may also show sterile pyuria given nearby inflammation. The abdominal CT scan is highly sensitive and specific for making the diagnosis of diverticulitis at 94% and 99%, respectively [38]. Findings include localized bowel wall thickening, increased soft tissue density in pericolonic fat from inflammation, fat stranding, and colonic diverticula [39–41]. High-resolution graded compression ultrasonography and MRI can also diagnose diverticulitis, although they are less commonly done due to operator dependence, availability, and need for expeditious workup [42–44]. It is generally recommended to obtain a CT scan of the abdomen with IV and oral contrast to make the diagnosis and rule out other potential causes of symptoms.

Most cases of diverticulitis are uncomplicated and resolve within about 14 days with treatment [45]. However, about 5 to 12% of patients will go on to develop a complication, usually within 10 days, with obstruction being the most common, followed by abscess, fistula, and perforation [46, 47] (learning objective #5). Obstruction can occur due to narrowing of the colon lumen from inflammation or direct compression from an abscess, as well as from association of a small intestine loop with inflammatory colon mass or from localized irritation causing ileus. In the acute phase, high-grade obstruction is rare. Abscesses occur in about 17% of patients who are hospitalized with diverticulitis [48, 49]. They should be suspected whenever patient's pain or fever doesn't improve after at least 3 days of antibiotics. Fistulas also commonly occur due to inflammation from diverticulitis and most commonly involve the bladder [50]. Although less common and occurring in only 1–2% of patients, perforation is a can't-miss complication with a mortality rate up to 20% [51, 52]. Diverticular hemorrhage is another potential complication. This can occur because the formation of diverticula causes wall weakness, leading to penetrating arteries being separated from the lumen by only thin mucosa. After recurrent injuries and increased wall stress, the artery can rupture into the colon lumen and cause sudden massive rectal bleeding.

Management of diverticulitis depends on the severity of the disease, certain characteristics, and the presence of any complications (learning objective #4). Most can be treated with medical management alone. Indications for inpatient management include complicated diverticulitis or uncomplicated diverticulitis with any of the following findings: SIRS positive/concern for sepsis, intractable pain, age above 70, significant comorbidities, immunosuppression, inability to tolerate oral intake, social/follow-up concerns, or previously failed outpatient treatment [53]. Inpatient management features IV fluids, pain control, and IV antibiotics. Patients are usually given bowel rest and either kept NPO or on a clear liquid diet depending on their clinical status. In general, patients are given IV antibiotics for about 3 to 5 days or until their abdominal tenderness/fever resolves. The regimen must cover gram-negative rods and anaerobes. Refer to Table 15.3 for the recommended IV antibiotic regimen.

Table 15.3 Empiric IV antibiotic regimen for intra-abdominal infection in adults [54, 55]

	Dose
Single-agent regimen	
Ertapenem	1 g IV once daily
Piperacillin-tazobactam (preferred)	3.375 g IV every 6 hours
Combination regimen with metronidazole*	
ONE of the following:	
Cefazolin	1 to 2 g IV every 8 hours
OR	
Cefuroxime	1.5 g IV every 8 hours
OR	
Ceftriaxone	2 g IV once daily
Or	
Cefotaxime	2 g IV every 8 hours
OR	
Ciprofloxacin	400 mg IV every 12 hours or 500 mg PO every 12 hours
OR	
Levofloxacin	750 mg IV or PO once daily
PLUS:	
Metronidazole*	500 mg IV or PO every 8 hours

*For most mild to moderate, uncomplicated infections of the biliary system, the addition of metronidazole is not necessary.

Once abdominal tenderness improves on IV antibiotics, patient can be switched to an oral regimen with either ciprofloxacin and metronidazole or amoxicillin-clavulanic acid for a total of 10 to 14 days. Management differs if there is evidence of diverticulitis complication. For intestinal perforation, emergency surgery is required [56–59]. Of note, this is not required if there is only evidence of a microperforation. For abscesses, one should utilize IV antibiotics, and if there is no resolution with antibiotics, the patient has clinical deterioration, or the abscess is larger than 4 cm, percutaneous drainage is indicated [60]. For those with evidence of diverticulitis with obstruction, it is very difficult to differentiate this from colon cancer on CT; thus, surgery is necessitated. Lastly, if a patient is found to have a fistula, this often also requires surgery, given that diverticular fistulas rarely heal on their own.

For those with uncomplicated diverticulitis, the treatment is usually oral antibiotics for 7 to 10 days. Refer to Table 15.4 for the recommended oral antibiotic regimen.

Table 15.4 Oral antibiotic regimen for adults with acute colonic diverticulitis

	Dose
Single-agent regimen	
Amoxicillin-clavulanate Or Amoxicillin-clavulanate Extended-release	1 tablet [contains 875 mg amoxicillin and 125 mg Clavulanic acid] every 8 hours Or 2 tablets [each tablet contains 1 g amoxicillin and 62.5 mg clavulanic acid] every 12 hours
Moxifloxacin *Reserved for those with Metronidazole or beta lactam allergy	500 mg PO daily
Combination regimen with metronidazole*	
ONE of the following:	
Ciprofloxacin	500 mg PO every 12 hours
OR	
Levofloxacin	750 mg PO daily
OR	
Trimethoprim-Sulfamethoxazole	800 mg—150 mg PO every 12 hours
PLUS:	
Metronidazole*	500 mg PO every 8 hours

*For most mild to moderate, uncomplicated infections of the biliary system, the addition of metronidazole is not necessary.

There is emerging evidence that some patients may not need antibiotics at all. Individuals who lack any of the following characteristics (SIRS criteria/sepsis, severe pain, signs of peritonitis, microperforation, age > 70, significant comorbidities, immunosuppression, intolerance of oral intake, nonadherence with care or unlikelihood to follow-up, or previous failure of outpatient management) can be considered to be treated with liquid diet and pain control alone based on clinician judgment. [Raghavendran, K. (n.d.). Acute colonic diverticulitis: Outpatient management and follow-up. UpToDate. https://www.uptodate.com/contents/acute-colonic-diverticulitis-outpatient-management-and-follow-up#H2041085169]. Patients should be followed up after about 1 week and then weekly thereafter until symptoms resolve. In the long term, it is important that patients undergo colonoscopy within 4–8 weeks of an episode if they have not already had one in the last year to evaluate for colon cancer. If symptoms do not resolve, further treatment may involve elective surgery with sigmoid resection to alleviate symptoms. For those who develop recurrent bouts of diverticulitis or for those at high risk for complications or mortality from further recurrence, surgery is also an option.

As with most things in medicine, an ounce of prevention is worth a pound of cure, and the same thing goes for diverticulitis. Based on the known acquired risk factors, prevention involves exercise, increased fiber and fluids, and smoking cessation [61, 62]. Exercising for 30 minutes per day at least 4 days per week can promote normal bowel function and help decrease luminal pressure on the colon that leads to diverticula. Increased fiber and fluid work by helping the gut absorb more water to soften stool, leading to less pressure on the colonic wall. Observational studies have shown that this may reduce the recurrence of diverticulitis [63, 64]. While these lifestyle changes have been found in studies to reduce the risk of first-time diverticulitis, there remains uncertainty about whether they are equally as helpful in secondary prevention for those who have already had diverticulitis.

In conclusion, diverticulitis is a common cause of abdominal pain, especially in Western countries. In the United States, diverticulitis is associated with about 200,000 hospital admissions and $2.2 billion in healthcare costs yearly. It is important that we recognize patients presenting with this condition and expeditiously evaluate and treat them, just like we did with Mrs. Franco!

Exam Questions

1. A 69-year-old female presents to her family doctor with a 3-day history of left lower quadrant abdominal pain. She also reports diarrhea and mild nausea but is still tolerating PO. On exam, her vitals are T 100.9F HR 80, BP 128/88, RR 16, and SpO2 100% on room air. Abdominal exam is notable for left lower quadrant tenderness to palpation without rebound or guarding. Complete blood count shows a leukocytosis with a left shift. UA was normal. A screening colonoscopy was done last year, which showed diverticulosis. What is the next best step in management?
   A. Urgent colonoscopy
   B. Abdominal CT without contrast
   C. CT angiography of mesenteric vasculature
   D. Laparotomy
   E. Trimethoprim-sulfamethoxazole and metronidazole with a liquid diet

Answer: E

Learning Objective: List treatment options for acute diverticulitis, including both the short-term (inpatient vs. outpatient) and long-term management strategies. Discuss ways to best counsel this patient on weight loss through diet and exercise changes.

Explanation: For the first episode of mild diverticulitis, treatment includes bowel rest, and a liquid diet with close follow-up. Studies have been conflicting regarding the use of broad-spectrum antibiotics, but it is still typical for patients to receive antibiotics such as amoxicillin-clavulanate or combination therapy with TMP-SMX or fluoroquinolones and metronidazole as an outpatient. A is incorrect, as colonoscopy should not be performed in the acute phase of diverticulitis due to the risk of perforation or other complications. Instead, it would be performed 4–6 weeks after the first case of complicated diverticulitis. B is incorrect, as the proper diagnostic study would include intravenous +/- oral contrast. Imaging may not be necessary in a patient with a mild presentation classic for diverticulitis who is still tolerating her diet. She can simply be managed as an outpatient. In diverticulitis, imaging studies are necessitated by the severity of the patient's presentation as well as the concern for other differential diagnoses. C is incorrect. This patient has diverticulitis, not mesenteric ischemia, for which this imaging study would help diagnose. D is incorrect, as acute surgical management such as laparotomy is indicated if evident perforation or ischemia, which would present with peritoneal signs (rebound, guarding, etc.). It may also be indicated if there is evidence of complications on imaging or if a patient has had recurrent episodes of diverticulitis.

2. An elderly man with a history of IBS with a predominant complaint of constipation presents with bright red blood in his stool for 1 day. He denies any straining, abdominal pain, diarrhea, or presyncope. Last colonoscopy was about 15 years ago, and the patient reports he had some "blebs" in his colon. Physical exam is notable for generalized abdominal tenderness, but a rectal exam did not show any perianal fissures or hemorrhoids. Fecal occult blood test is positive. Which class of medications is the strongest pharmacologic risk factor for this patient's disease process?
   A. Non-steroidal anti-inflammatory drugs
   B. Calcium channel blockers
   C. Statins
   D. Selective serotonin reuptake inhibitors
   E. Fiber

Answer: A

Learning Objective: List treatment options for acute diverticulitis, including both the short-term (inpatient vs. outpatient) and long-term management strategies. Discuss ways to best counsel this patient on weight loss through diet and exercise changes.

Explanation: Patients who regularly consume NSAIDs are at a 4.8x increased risk of severe diverticular disease. B is incorrect as this class of medication has actually been associated with a protective effect against diverticular disease and its complications. C is incorrect as this class of medication has actually been associated with a protective effect against diverticular disease and its complications. D is incorrect as this medication is associated with a decreased risk of diverticulitis. E is incorrect as dietary fiber or supplements help prevent diverticulitis and are thus NOT a risk factor.

3. A 63-year-old man presents to his PCP due to changes in his bowel habits, including alternating episodes of diarrhea and constipation over the past several months, with associated cramping abdominal pain. BMI is 34 kg/m^2. Physical examination shows a distended abdomen without focal tenderness, rebound, or guarding. The patient undergoes a colonoscopy which reveals outpouchings of the colonic mucosa and submucosa in the descending colon. Which of the following best describes the pathophysiology of this disease process?
   A. Telescoping of proximal colon into a distal portion
   B. Failure of vitelline duct to involute
   C. Increased intraluminal pressure within the colon
   D. Reduced blood flow at "watershed" areas
   E. Transmural inflammation across colonic mucosal layers

Answer: C

Learning Objective: Compare and contrast the pathophysiology and presentation of diverticulitis, ischemic colitis, and infectious colitis.

Explanation: This is how diverticulosis (and thus diverticulitis) first develops. The increased pressure results in a false diverticulum, which only contains mucosa and submucosa. They usually form at weak areas in the gut, such as near blood vessels. A is incorrect because this describes intussusception, in which some lead point results in peristalsis of proximal into distal colon. While it can present with colicky or cramping abdominal pain, it usually occurs in kids. Additionally, colonoscopy likely would've shown a lead point (tumor, lymphoid hyperplasia, Meckel's diverticulum). B is incorrect because this is the pathophysiology of Meckel's diverticulum, the most common congenital malformation in the GI tract. Patients usually present in childhood with painless bright red blood per rectum, or it is found incidentally with endoscopy. D is incorrect, as this describes ischemic colitis, which would not show outpouchings on colonoscopy but rather segmental bowel wall thickening without inflammation. E is incorrect because this describes Crohn's disease, which can be differentiated from ulcerative colitis by its transmural inflammation. This usually presents in younger patients with low-grade fever, prolonged diarrhea with abdominal pain, weight loss, and generalized fatigue.

References

1. Diaz G. Differential diagnosis according to localization of abdominal pain. 2018. https://www.grepmed.com/images/2886/localization-differential-epigastric-abdominal-quadrants. Accessed 28 June 2024
2. Honda T, Uehara T, Matsumoto G, Arai S, Sugano M. Neutrophil left shift and white blood cell count as markers of bacterial infection. Clin Chim Acta. 2016;457:46–53. https://doi.org/10.1016/j.cca.2016.03.017.
3. Tănase I, Păun S, Stoica B, Negoi I, Gaspar B, Beuran M. Epidemiology of diverticular disease — systematic review of the literature. Chirurgia (Bucharest, Romania : 1990). 2015;110(1):9–14.
4. Hughes LE. Postmortem survey of diverticular disease of the colon. I Diverticulosis and diverticulitis. Gut. 1969;10(5):336–44. https://doi.org/10.1136/gut.10.5.336.
5. Shahedi K, Fuller G, Bolus R, Cohen E, Vu M, Shah R, Agarwal N, Kaneshiro M, Atia M, Sheen V, Kurzbard N, van Oijen MG, Yen L, Hodgkins P, Erder MH, Spiegel B. Long-term risk of acute diverticulitis among patients with incidental diverticulosis found during colonoscopy. Clin Gastroenterol Hepatol. 2013;11(12):1609–13. https://doi.org/10.1016/j.cgh.2013.06.020.
6. Etzioni DA, Mack TM, Beart RW Jr, Kaiser AM. Diverticulitis in the United States: 1998-2005: changing patterns of disease and treatment. Ann Surg. 2009;249(2):210–7. https://doi.org/10.1097/SLA.0b013e3181952888.

7. Nguyen GC, Sam J, Anand N. Epidemiological trends and geographic variation in hospital admissions for diverticulitis in the United States. World J Gastroenterol. 2011;17(12):1600–5. https://doi.org/10.3748/wjg.v17.i12.1600.
8. Wheat CL, Strate LL. Trends in hospitalization for diverticulitis and diverticular bleeding in the United States from 2000 to 2010. Clin Gastroenterol Hepatol. 2016;14(1):96–103.e1. https://doi.org/10.1016/j.cgh.2015.03.030.
9. Acosta JA, Grebenc ML, Doberneck RC, McCarthy JD, Fry DE. Colonic diverticular disease in patients 40 years old or younger. Am Surg. 1992;58(10):605–7.
10. Schauer PR, Ramos R, Ghiatas AA, Sirinek KR. Virulent diverticular disease in young obese men. Am J Surg. 1992;164(5):443–8. https://doi.org/10.1016/s0002-9610(05)81177-8.
11. Strate LL, Morris AM. Epidemiology, pathophysiology, and treatment of diverticulitis. Gastroenterology. 2019;156(5):1282–1298.e1. https://doi.org/10.1053/j.gastro.2018.12.033.
12. Böhm SK. Risk factors for diverticulosis, diverticulitis, diverticular perforation, and bleeding: a plea for more subtle history taking. Viszeralmedizin. 2015;31(2):84–94. https://doi.org/10.1159/000381867.
13. Strate LL, Liu YL, Syngal S, Aldoori WH, Giovannucci EL. Nut, corn, and popcorn consumption and the incidence of diverticular disease. JAMA. 2008;300(8):907–14. https://doi.org/10.1001/jama.300.8.907.
14. Humes DJ, Fleming KM, Spiller RC, West J. Concurrent drug use and the risk of perforated colonic diverticular disease: a population-based case-control study. Gut. 2011;60(2):219–24. https://doi.org/10.1136/gut.2010.217281.
15. Strate LL, Liu YL, Huang ES, Giovannucci EL, Chan AT. Use of aspirin or nonsteroidal anti-inflammatory drugs increases risk for diverticulitis and diverticular bleeding. Gastroenterology. 2011;140(5):1427–33. https://doi.org/10.1053/j.gastro.2011.02.004.
16. Aldoori WH, Giovannucci EL, Rimm EB, Wing AL, Willett WC. Use of acetaminophen and nonsteroidal anti-inflammatory drugs: a prospective study and the risk of symptomatic diverticular disease in men. Arch Fam Med. 1998;7(3):255–60. https://doi.org/10.1001/archfami.7.3.255.
17. Jovani M, Ma W, Joshi AD, Liu PH, Nguyen LH, Cao Y, Tam I, Wu K, Giovannucci EL, Chan AT, Strate LL. Menopausal hormone therapy and risk of diverticulitis. Am J Gastroenterol. 2019;114(2):315–21. https://doi.org/10.14309/ajg.0000000000000054.
18. Rege RV, Nahrwold DL. Diverticular disease. Curr Prob Surg. 1989;26(3):133–89. https://doi.org/10.1016/0011-3840(89)90031-2.
19. Ma W, Jovani M, Nguyen LH, Tabung FK, Song M, Liu PH, Cao Y, Tam I, Wu K, Giovannucci EL, Strate LL, Chan AT. Association between inflammatory diets, circulating markers of inflammation, and risk of diverticulitis. Clin Gastroenterol Hepatol. 2020;18(10):2279–2286.e3. https://doi.org/10.1016/j.cgh.2019.11.011.
20. Daniels L, Budding AE, de Korte N, Eck A, Bogaards JA, Stockmann HB, Consten EC, Savelkoul PH, Boermeester MA. Fecal microbiome analysis as a diagnostic test for diverticulitis. Eur J Clin Microbiol Infect Dis. 2014;33(11):1927–36. https://doi.org/10.1007/s10096-014-2162-3.
21. Barbara G, Scaioli E, Barbaro MR, Biagi E, Laghi L, Cremon C, Marasco G, Colecchia A, Picone G, Salfi N, Capozzi F, Brigidi P, Festi D. Gut microbiota, metabolome and immune signatures in patients with uncomplicated diverticular disease. Gut. 2017;66(7):1252–61. https://doi.org/10.1136/gutjnl-2016-312377.
22. Brook I, Frazier EH. Aerobic and anaerobic microbiology in intra-abdominal infections associated with diverticulitis. J Med Microbiol. 2000;49(9):827–30. https://doi.org/10.1099/0022-1317-49-9-827.
23. Byrnes MC, Mazuski JE. Antimicrobial therapy for acute colonic diverticulitis. Surg Infect. 2009;10(2):143–54. https://doi.org/10.1089/sur.2007.087.
24. Chang GJ, Shelton AA, Welton ML. Large intestine. In: Current surgical diagnosis & treatment. 12th d ed. New York: McGraw Hill; 2006. p. 685–737.
25. Christou NV, Turgeon P, Wassef R, Rotstein O, Bohnen J, Potvin M. Management of intra-abdominal infections. The case for intraoperative cultures and comprehensive broad-spectrum antibiotic coverage. The Canadian Intra-abdominal Infection Study Group. Arch Surg (Chicago, Ill.: 1960). 1996;131(11):1193–201. https://doi.org/10.1001/archsurg.1996.01430230075014.
26. Brook I, Frazier EH. Aerobic and anaerobic microbiology of retroperitoneal abscesses. Clin Infect Dis. 1998;26(4):938–41. https://doi.org/10.1086/513947.
27. Rodkey GV, Welch CE. Changing patterns in the surgical treatment of diverticular disease. Ann Surg. 1984;200(4):466–78. https://doi.org/10.1097/00000658-198410000-00008.
28. Sugihara K, Muto T, Morioka Y, Asano A, Yamamoto T. Diverticular disease of the colon in Japan. A review of 615 cases. Dis Colon Rectum. 1984;27(8):531–7. https://doi.org/10.1007/BF02555517.
29. Markham NI, Li AK. Diverticulitis of the right colon--experience from Hong Kong. Gut. 1992;33(4):547–9. https://doi.org/10.1136/gut.33.4.547.
30. Jacobs DO. Clinical practice. Diverticulitis. N Engl J Med. 2007;357(20):2057–66. https://doi.org/10.1056/NEJMcp073228.
31. Yamada T, Alpers DH, Kaplowitz N, et al. Textbook of gastroenterology. Philadelphia: Lippincott Williams & Wilkins; 2003.
32. Konvolinka CW. Acute diverticulitis under age forty. Am J Surg. 1994;167(6):562–5. https://doi.org/10.1016/0002-9610(94)90098-1.
33. Parks TG. Natural history of diverticular disease of the colon. Clin Gastroenterol. 1975;4(1):53–69.

34. Gallo A, Ianiro G, Montalto M, Cammarota G. The role of biomarkers in diverticular disease. J Clin Gastroenterol. 2016;50(Suppl 1):S26–8. https://doi.org/10.1097/MCG.0000000000000648.
35. Wexner SD, Talamini MA. EAES/SAGES consensus conference on acute diverticulitis: a paradigm shift in the management of acute diverticulitis. Surg Endosc. 2019;33(9):2724–5. https://doi.org/10.1007/s00464-019-06998-2.
36. Ambrosetti P, Robert JH, Witzig JA, Mirescu D, Mathey P, Borst F, Rohner A. Acute left colonic diverticulitis: a prospective analysis of 226 consecutive cases. Surgery. 1994;115(5):546–50.
37. Mäkelä JT, Klintrup K, Rautio T. The role of low CRP values in the prediction of the development of acute diverticulitis. Int J Color Dis. 2016;31(1):23–7. https://doi.org/10.1007/s00384-015-2410-8.
38. Balk EM, Adam GP, Bhuma MR, Konnyu KJ, Saldanha IJ, Beland MD, Shah N. Diagnostic imaging and medical management of acute left-sided colonic diverticulitis : a systematic review. Ann Intern Med. 2022;175(3):379–87. https://doi.org/10.7326/M21-1645.
39. Birnbaum BA, Balthazar EJ. CT of appendicitis and diverticulitis. Radiol Clin North Am. 1994;32(5):885–98.
40. Hulnick DH, Megibow AJ, Balthazar EJ, Naidich DP, Bosniak MA. Computed tomography in the evaluation of diverticulitis. Radiology. 1984;152(2):491–5. https://doi.org/10.1148/radiology.152.2.6739821.
41. Goh V, Halligan S, Taylor SA, Burling D, Bassett P, Bartram CI. Differentiation between diverticulitis and colorectal cancer: quantitative CT perfusion measurements versus morphologic criteria--initial experience. Radiology. 2007;242(2):456–62. https://doi.org/10.1148/radiol.2422051670.
42. Laméris W, van Randen A, Bipat S, Bossuyt PM, Boermeester MA, Stoker J. Graded compression ultrasonography and computed tomography in acute colonic diverticulitis: meta-analysis of test accuracy. Eur Radiol. 2008;18(11):2498–511. https://doi.org/10.1007/s00330-008-1018-6.
43. Heverhagen JT, Sitter H, Zielke A, Klose KJ. Prospective evaluation of the value of magnetic resonance imaging in suspected acute sigmoid diverticulitis. Dis Colon Rectum. 2008;51(12):1810–5. https://doi.org/10.1007/s10350-008-9330-4.
44. Heverhagen JT, Zielke A, Ishaque N, Bohrer T, El-Sheik M, Klose KJ. Acute colonic diverticulitis: visualization in magnetic resonance imaging. Magn Reson Imaging. 2001;19(10):1275–7. https://doi.org/10.1016/s0730-725x(01)00469-6.
45. Daniels L, Ünlü Ç, de Korte N, van Dieren S, Stockmann HB, Vrouenraets BC, Consten EC, van der Hoeven JA, Eijsbouts QA, Faneyte IF, Bemelman WA, Dijkgraaf MG, Boermeester MA, Dutch Diverticular Disease (3D) Collaborative Study Group. Randomized clinical trial of observational versus antibiotic treatment for a first episode of CT-proven uncomplicated acute diverticulitis. Br J Surg. 2017;104(1):52–61. https://doi.org/10.1002/bjs.10309.
46. Rottier SJ, van Dijk ST, Ünlü Ç, van Geloven AAW, Schreurs WH, Boermeester MA. Complicated disease course in initially computed tomography-proven uncomplicated acute diverticulitis. Surg Infect. 2019;20(6):453–9. https://doi.org/10.1089/sur.2018.289.
47. Bharucha AE, Parthasarathy G, Ditah I, Fletcher JG, Ewelukwa O, Pendlimari R, Yawn BP, Melton LJ, Schleck C, Zinsmeister AR. Temporal trends in the incidence and natural history of diverticulitis: a population-based study. Am J Gastroenterol. 2015;110(11):1589–96. https://doi.org/10.1038/ajg.2015.302.
48. Bahadursingh AM, Virgo KS, Kaminski DL, Longo WE. Spectrum of disease and outcome of complicated diverticular disease. Am J Surg. 2003;186(6):696–701. https://doi.org/10.1016/j.amjsurg.2003.08.019.
49. Ambrosetti P, Chautems R, Soravia C, Peiris-Waser N, Terrier F. Long-term outcome of mesocolic and pelvic diverticular abscesses of the left colon: a prospective study of 73 cases. Dis Colon Rectum. 2005;48(4):787–91. https://doi.org/10.1007/s10350-004-0853-z.
50. Woods RJ, Lavery IC, Fazio VW, Jagelman DG, Weakley FL. Internal fistulas in diverticular disease. Dis Colon Rectum. 1988;31(8):591–6. https://doi.org/10.1007/BF02556792.
51. Nagorney DM, Adson MA, Pemberton JH. Sigmoid diverticulitis with perforation and generalized peritonitis. Dis Colon Rectum. 1985;28(2):71–5. https://doi.org/10.1007/BF02552645.
52. Kriwanek S, Armbruster C, Beckerhinn P, Dittrich K. Prognostic factors for survival in colonic perforation. Int J Color Dis. 1994;9(3):158–62. https://doi.org/10.1007/BF00290194.
53. Alonso S, Pera M, Parés D, Pascual M, Gil MJ, Courtier R, Grande L. Outpatient treatment of patients with uncomplicated acute diverticulitis. Colorect Dis. 2010;12(10 Online):e278–82. https://doi.org/10.1111/j.1463-1318.2009.02122.x.
54. Raghavendran K. Acute colonic diverticulitis: triage and inpatient management. In: Connor RF, editor. UpToDate. Wolters Kluwer; 2024. Accessed 28 June 2024.
55. Dichman ML, Rosenstock SJ, Shabanzadeh DM. Antibiotics for uncomplicated diverticulitis. Cochrane Database Syst Rev. 2022;6(6):CD009092. https://doi.org/10.1002/14651858.CD009092.pub3.
56. Krobot K, Yin D, Zhang Q, Sen S, Altendorf-Hofmann A, Scheele J, Sendt W. Effect of inappropriate initial empiric antibiotic therapy on outcome of patients with community-acquired intra-abdominal infections requiring surgery. Eur J Clin Microbiol Infect Dis. 2004;23(9):682–7. https://doi.org/10.1007/s10096-004-1199-0.
57. Morris AM, Regenbogen SE, Hardiman KM, Hendren S. Sigmoid diverticulitis: a systematic review. JAMA.

2014;311(3):287–97. https://doi.org/10.1001/jama.2013.282025.
58. Regenbogen SE, Hardiman KM, Hendren S, Morris AM. Surgery for diverticulitis in the 21st century: a systematic review. JAMA Surg. 2014;149(3):292–303. https://doi.org/10.1001/jamasurg.2013.5477.
59. Stocchi L. Current indications and role of surgery in the management of sigmoid diverticulitis. World J Gastroenterol. 2010;16(7):804–17. https://doi.org/10.3748/wjg.v16.i7.804.
60. Francis NK, Sylla P, Abou-Khalil M, Arolfo S, Berler D, Curtis NJ, Dolejs SC, Garfinkle R, Gorter-Stam M, Hashimoto DA, Hassinger TE, Molenaar CJL, Pucher PH, Schuermans V, Arezzo A, Agresta F, Antoniou SA, Arulampalam T, Boutros M, Bouvy N, et al. EAES and SAGES 2018 consensus conference on acute diverticulitis management: evidence-based recommendations for clinical practice. Surg Endosc. 2019;33(9):2726–41. https://doi.org/10.1007/s00464-019-06882-z.
61. Strate LL, Keeley BR, Cao Y, Wu K, Giovannucci EL, Chan AT. Western dietary pattern increases, and prudent dietary pattern decreases, risk of incident diverticulitis in a prospective cohort study. Gastroenterology. 2017;152(5):1023–1030.e2. https://doi.org/10.1053/j.gastro.2016.12.038.
62. Liu PH, Cao Y, Keeley BR, Tam I, Wu K, Strate LL, Giovannucci EL, Chan AT. Adherence to a healthy lifestyle is associated with a lower risk of diverticulitis among men. Am J Gastroenterol. 2017;112(12):1868–76. https://doi.org/10.1038/ajg.2017.398.
63. Maconi G, Barbara G, Bosetti C, Cuomo R, Annibale B. Treatment of diverticular disease of the colon and prevention of acute diverticulitis: a systematic review. Dis Colon Rectum. 2011;54(10):1326–38. https://doi.org/10.1097/DCR.0b013e318223cb2b.
64. Ünlü C, Daniels L, Vrouenraets BC, Boermeester MA. A systematic review of high-fibre dietary therapy in diverticular disease. Int J Color Dis. 2012;27(4):419–27. https://doi.org/10.1007/s00384-011-1308-3.

16 Painful Nausea

Jessie L. Koljonen

Learning Objectives

1. Describe the physiologic changes during pregnancy that contribute to the increased incidence of gallstone formation.
2. List the incidence and course of gallstone-related disease in pregnancy, and highlight common risk factors for gallstone formation in the general population.
3. Discuss the differential diagnosis of right upper quadrant and epigastric pain in a pregnant woman.
4. Describe two possible mechanisms by which gallstone pancreatitis occurs.
5. Discuss management of gallstone pancreatitis, including timing of cholecystectomy.
6. List the classification of common types of gallstones and their composition.

Chief Complaint

"I am nauseous and have abdominal pain."

- *History of Present Illness*
  - Karen Smith is a 31-year-old female who presents with a 4-day history of constant epigastric pain that she describes as sharp and radiating to her back. She rates the pain as 9/10 in severity.
  - She has noted some associated nausea and diarrhea, but no emesis.
  - She has had similar previous episodes on and off, about three times per year, for about the past 7 years; however, her previous symptoms have never been this severe.
  - Previous workups have been negative.
  - Nobody else at home has similar symptoms, and she does not recall eating anything suspicious.
- *Stop and Think*
  - What is on your differential?
    - Pancreatitis
    - Appendicitis
    - Cholecystitis
    - Gastroenteritis
    - Pregnancy
    - Menstrual cramps
    - Influenza
    - Inflammatory condition—irritable bowel syndrome, inflammatory bowel disease
    - Mesenteric ischemia (vascular cause)
    - Bowel obstruction
    - Kidney stone
    - Neoplasm (less likely, due to acute onset of symptoms)
    - Drug induced
    - Psychiatric

J. L. Koljonen (✉)
Institute for Plastic Surgery, Southern Illinois University School of Medicine, Springfield, IL, USA
e-mail: jkoljonen35@siumed.edu

C. A. Standley (ed.), *Biomedical Science and Clinical Foundations*,
https://doi.org/10.1007/978-3-031-98353-5_16

        - Idiopathic
    - What questions do you want to ask her next?
        - Past medical history, past surgical history, medications, social history (including sexual history, last menstrual period, alcohol use, drug use)
- *Some Important New Information*
    - *"Oh, I forgot to mention—I am currently pregnant. I am about 16 weeks and 5 days along!"*
    - *"This is my first pregnancy; my boyfriend and I are very excited. We don't know the gender yet. We are just hoping for a healthy baby."*
    - *"I went to my OBGYN about 2 weeks ago, and everything has been going well so far; she did not have any concerns."*
    - *"I've had some nausea here and there, but nothing like the nausea and abdominal pain I've been feeling over the last few days."*
    - *"I haven't had any bleeding or anything like that. Just the nausea and belly pain."*
    - *"Is everything going to be okay with the baby? I'm worried."*
- *Stop and Think*
    - How does this change your differential?
        - Sequelae of normal pregnancy:
            - Increased levels of pregnancy/reproductive hormones lead to changes in the biliary system, which can promote gallstone formation.
            - Estrogen and progesterone cause bile to become supersaturated and decrease gallbladder emptying, leading to increased formation of gallstones.
        - At this point, we must also consider pregnancy complications.
            - Placental abruption
                - Though sometimes presents with vaginal bleeding, in some cases, there is a "concealed" or "silent" abruption where bleeding is not apparent and builds up behind the placenta.
            - Placenta accreta, percreta, increta
            - Uterine rupture
                - Less likely as she is only 16 weeks, has not been having active contractions, and has no prior history of uterine surgery that would weaken the uterus for a rupture to occur
            - Miscarriage
- *Patient History*
    - Past Medical History: none
    - Obstetric History: G1P0000
        - G1 = 1 pregnancy
        - P0000 = 0 term deliveries, 0 preterm deliveries, 0 abortions, 0 living children
    - Past Surgical History: none
    - Medications: none
    - Allergies: No known drug allergies
    - Family History:
        - Maternal grand-aunt—throat cancer
    - Social History:
        - Denies current tobacco, alcohol, or drug use
        - Alcohol: 1 beer per week previously, last drink prior to pregnancy
        - Sexually active with one male partner
        - Lives in a rural town near Prescott with boyfriend (the father of the baby). Feels safe at home. Domestic violence screening negative.
            - It is important to always screen pregnant women for domestic violence.
        - Works at a gas station
- *Review of Systems*
    - Gen: +*fatigue*. No fever, chills
    - Head: No headache, vision changes
    - Cardio: No chest pain, palpitations
    - Resp: No shortness of breath
    - Gastrointestinal: +*abdominal pain, nausea, vomiting, diarrhea*. No constipation, melena
    - Genitourinary: No dysuria, hematuria, genital discharge, or vaginal bleeding
    - Neuro: No dizziness
    - Psych: No anxiety, depression
- *Physical Exam*
    - Vital Signs
        - Blood Pressure: 123/70
        - Pulse: 73

    - Temperature: 36.8 °C (Tmax 36.9)
    - Respiratory Rate: 16
    - Oxygen Saturation: 99%
    - Body Mass Index (BMI): 35
      - A major independent risk factor for gallstones is pre-pregnancy obesity.
  - General: well-developed, well-nourished female alert and conversant in no acute distress
  - Head: normocephalic, atraumatic
  - Eyes: conjunctiva clear, sclera anicteric. Pupils equal round and reactive to light
  - Neck: normal range of motion, no jugular venous distention
  - Cardiac: regular rate and rhythm, normal S1 S2, no murmurs
  - Pulmonary: effort normal. No stridor, wheezing, or respiratory distress
  - Abdomen: *+epigastric tenderness, mild right upper quadrant and left upper quadrant tenderness, voluntary guarding.* Soft. +bowel sounds. No distention. No rebound.
  - Musculoskeletal: normal range of motion, no edema or tenderness
  - Neurologic: oriented to person, place, and time
  - Skin: warm and dry. No rashes or pallor.
  - Psychiatric: normal mood and affect, behavior is normal
- *Stop and Think/Recap*
  - What is the chief complaint?
    - Abdominal pain, nausea
  - What symptoms, past medical history, past surgical history, medications, family history, and social history are relevant to the chief complaint? How do physical exam findings aid in your findings?
    - Nausea, abdominal pain
    - Acute onset of symptoms, constant, severe (9/10), radiates to back (*classic for pancreatitis*)
    - Previous episodes on and off, never this severe
      - This leads to possible gallstone disease—gallstones classically temporarily obstruct the cystic duct, leading to intermittent symptoms of upper abdominal pain.
    - Pregnancy complications
      - Want to keep considering pregnancy complications—especially immediately life-threatening differentials of placental abruption (concealed abruption may not present with vaginal bleeding).
    - Key physical exam findings: epigastric tenderness, right upper quadrant and left upper quadrant tenderness, guarding, and BMI 35
  - List your key differential diagnoses and provide a rationale for each.
    - Gallstone Pancreatitis
      - Epigastric pain radiating to back, history of intermittent on/off symptoms (gallstones previously temporarily blocking cystic duct have now traveled down and are blocking pancreatic duct)
    - Acute Cholecystitis
      - Sudden sharp upper abdominal pain
    - Appendicitis
      - Abdominal pain, and location may be unusual due to gravid uterus
    - Placental Abruption
      - Abdominal pain, pregnancy
    - Peptic Ulcer Disease
      - Upper abdominal, epigastric pain that radiates to the back.
    - Alcoholic Pancreatitis
      - Epigastric pain radiating to the back, but no history of alcohol abuse
    - Hypertriglyceridemia Pancreatitis
      - Epigastric pain radiating to the back, but no history (or family history) of hypertriglyceridemia
  - What lab and imaging studies would you like to order?
    - CBC
    - CMP
    - AST, ALT, lipase, amylase
    - Right upper quadrant ultrasound
      - Evaluate for gallstones.
    - At this point, should also consult an OBGYN service for recommendations

and an ultrasound of the fetus (this is beyond the scope of this case, as the focus is on gallstone pancreatitis and cholecystitis).

- *Labs (reference values in parentheses)*
  - CBC
    - *WBC 13.7 × 10^3 per uL (4–10)*
    - Hgb 12.2 g/dL (12–16)
    - Hct 34.6% (32–52)
    - Neutrophils 89% (50–70)
  - CMP
    - Na 139 mEq/L (135–145)
    - K 3.7 mEq/L (3.5–4.5)
    - Cl 108 mEq/L (95–105)
    - CO_2 20 mEq/L (18–29)
    - BUN 6 mg/dL (8–27)
    - Cr 0.39 mg/dL (0.57–1.00)
    - Ca 8.8 mg/dL (8.8–10.3)
    - Glucose 108 mg/dL (70–115)
    - Tbili 1.2 mg/dL (0.0–1.2)
    - Alk Phos 111 U/L (39–117)
    - *ALT 208 U/L (0–32)*
    - *AST 168 U/L (0–40)*
    - *Amylase > 2400 U/L (60–180)*
    - *Lipase 35,432 U/L (0–160)*
    - LDH 196 U/L (105–333)
- *Imaging*
  - Right upper quadrant ultrasound—radiology report:
    - Pancreas: unremarkable, no peripancreatic fluid
    - Gallbladder: *sludge and mobile gallstone* (0.9 × 0.6 × 0.8 cm), no pericholecystic fluid, *3.5 mm thick* (normal <3 mm)
      - Gallbladder sludge is a collection of cholesterol, calcium, bilirubin, and other compounds that build up in the gallbladder. It is sometimes called biliary sludge because it occurs when bile stays in the gallbladder for too long.
      - Diffuse gallbladder wall thickening (>3 mm by ultrasound) can be seen in such primary gallbladder inflammatory processes as acute, chronic, and acalculous cholecystitis.
    - Biliary: *CBD 4.7 mm* (normal ~4 mm)
      - CBD = common bile duct
- *Diagnosis*
  - Ms. Smith was diagnosed with *gallstone pancreatitis.*
  - What are your recommended next steps for this patient?
    - In patients with gallstone pancreatitis, most stones pass into the duodenum.
    - Next recommended steps: allow resolution of inflammation from pancreatitis (supportive care, nothing by mouth, IV fluids, and monitor labs for decreasing levels of lipase).
    - After resolution of several days, general surgery consultation to evaluate for cholecystectomy so that pancreatitis doesn't recur
    - In patients who have had mild pancreatitis, cholecystectomy can usually be performed safely within seven days after recovery and in the same hospitalization.
- *Surgical Intervention*
  - On Hospital Day 3 she underwent a laparoscopic cholecystectomy and intraoperative ultrasound of the common bile duct.
  - Why was an intraoperative ultrasound of the CBD performed?
    - Looking for stones in the common bile duct which could cause continued symptoms even after the gallbladder is removed (leading to ascending cholangitis or could travel further down and block the pancreatic duct, leading to a second episode of gallstone pancreatitis).
  - The open Hasson technique was used due to the gravid uterus for better visualization during trocar placement.
  - During operative gallbladder dissection:
    - Infundibulum and cystic duct very dilated
    - A very large stone impacted the proximal cystic duct.
  - Intraoperative ultrasound showed no further stones or defects.

  - Normal-appearing gravid uterus
  - No drains were placed, and no intraoperative complications
- *Pathology*
  - Final gallbladder pathology: *chronic cholecystitis with cholelithiasis*
  - How does this pathology relate to our patient's symptoms? How did her pregnancy play a role in her disease course?
    - Chronic cholecystitis—related to her previous intermittent episodes of pain, pathologic evidence that this has been going on for years
      - Symptoms related to gallstones develop when the gallbladder contracts in response to hormonal or neural stimulation, usually due to a fatty meal. Contraction forces stones (or possibly sludge or microlithiasis) against the gallbladder outlet or cystic duct opening, leading to increased intra-gallbladder pressure and pain. The stones often fall back from the cystic duct as the gallbladder relaxes, with amelioration of symptoms.
      - Recent pregnancy likely exacerbated symptoms, leading to this episode of increased gallstone formation and gallstone pancreatitis.
        - Increased levels of reproductive hormones during pregnancy induce a variety of physiologic changes in the biliary system, which promote gallstone formation.
        - A major independent risk factor for gallstones is pre-pregnancy obesity.
- *Postoperative Course*
  - Postoperative Day 1
    - No acute events overnight
    - Afebrile, vital signs within normal limits
    - Pain: improved, mild right upper quadrant pain
    - Diet: advanced from a clear liquid diet and then further advanced to a general diet, with no additional nausea
    - Voiding without difficulty
    - No bowel movement or flatus yet
    - Ambulating without difficulty
    - Antibiotics: Zosyn
      - She was given antibiotics postoperatively to prevent infection.
      - Empiric coverage, directed at Gram-negative enteric organisms
    - Incisions clean, dry, intact
    - Discharged later that day
  - Postoperative Follow-Up in Clinic (POD 7)
    - Minimal pain
    - No fever, chills, vomiting, or diarrhea
    - Low-fat diet, slowly reintroducing foods
    - Lost weight since the onset of symptoms
    - Reports eating better, taking prenatal vitamins
    - Physical exam: incisional scars, no erythema, bleeding, or discharge, minimally tender to palpation
  - 23 weeks later…
    - Delivery of a healthy baby boy
    - No further episodes of biliary colic
- *Social Determinants of Health*
  - Pregnancy, rural healthcare, low income.

End of Case

Answers to Learning Objectives

1. Describe the physiologic changes during pregnancy that contribute to the increased incidence of gallstone formation.

Increased levels of reproductive hormones during pregnancy induce a variety of physiologic changes in the biliary system, which promote gallstone formation:

Estrogen increases cholesterol secretion, and progesterone reduces bile acid secretion, which ultimately causes bile to become supersaturated with cholesterol. A relative overproduction of hydrophobic bile acids, such as chenodeoxycholate, reduces the ability of bile to solubilize cholesterol.

Progesterone slows gallbladder emptying, which further promotes the formation of stones by causing bile stasis.

These changes normalize one to two months following delivery.

Symptoms related to gallstones develop when the gallbladder contracts in response to hormonal or neural stimulation, usually due to a fatty meal. Contraction forces stones (or possibly sludge or microlithiasis) against the gallbladder outlet or cystic duct opening, leading to increased intra-gallbladder pressure and pain. The stones often fall back from the cystic duct as the gallbladder relaxes, with improvement of symptoms.

2. List the incidence and course of gallstone-related disease in pregnancy, and highlight common risk factors for gallstone formation in the general population.

The reported incidence of gallstone-related disease in pregnant women is low, cited in the literature as between 0.05 and 0.33% [1], with reported values depending on patient selection, frequency of assessment, and diagnostic definitions and techniques. In a large prospective serial ultrasound study of over 3200 pregnant women without gallstones at their first ultrasound examination, increased sludge or stones were noted in 7.1% of women on at least one ultrasound by the second trimester, in 7.9% of women by the third trimester, and in 10.2% of women by four to six weeks postpartum. However, among women with sludge or stones, only 1.2% developed symptoms attributable to the gallbladder during pregnancy [2].

In the postpartum period, bile composition and gallbladder function return to normal. Gallbladder sludge is more likely to resolve than gallstones, and smaller stones (less than 10 mm) are more likely to resolve than larger stones [3].

By one year postpartum, most women with sludge during pregnancy have a normal ultrasound examination, but abnormal ultrasound findings can still be seen in patients with stones. This can lead to serious complications such as acute cholecystitis, choledocholithiasis, gangrenous gallbladder, or pancreatitis.

A major independent risk factor for gallstones in pregnant females is pre-pregnancy obesity. Although the prevalence of gallstones has been reported to be higher in multiparous versus nulliparous women, increasing age, obesity, genetic background may account for the persistence and further growth of stones that develop during pregnancy.

The common mnemonic of the 5Fs is a helpful tool to remember the risk factors for the development of cholelithiasis: Female, Forty, Fat (higher BMI), Fertile (multiparous), Fair (blonde, light complexion)

3. *Discuss the differential diagnosis of right upper quadrant and epigastric pain in a pregnant woman.*

In a pregnant woman with right upper quadrant or epigastric pain, both pregnancy-related and nonpregnancy-related clinical diagnoses must be considered, even if gallstones are observed on ultrasound examination, since they may be an incidental finding.

Pregnancy-related conditions Pregnancy-related conditions that may be associated with right upper quadrant or epigastric pain include severe preeclampsia and HELLP syndrome (**H**emolysis, **E**levated **L**iver enzymes, **L**ow **P**latelet count), acute fatty liver, abruptio placentae, uterine rupture, and intra-amniotic infection. These conditions can usually be differentiated from gallstone disease by the clinical setting in which they occur and by obtaining the appropriate diagnostic studies.

Preeclampsia/HELLP Hypertension is the requisite criterion for preeclampsia and is common in HELLP syndrome. Thrombocytopenia is a requisite criterion for HELLP syndrome and is common in preeclampsia. Both disorders occur after 20 weeks of gestation. Gallbladder disease is not associated with hypertension or thrombocytopenia and can occur anytime in pregnancy. Women with severe preeclampsia or HELLP syndrome can have elevated liver enzymes (typically at least twice normal), which can also occur with complicated gallstone disease.

Acute fatty liver Acute fatty liver occurs in the second half of pregnancy, usually in the third trimester. The most frequent initial symptoms are nausea or vomiting, abdominal pain (particularly epigastric), anorexia, and jaundice. Serum aminotransferase elevations are usually higher in fatty liver than in gallbladder disease. Many of these patients have signs of preeclampsia. Hypoglycemia is a feature of severe acute fatty liver but is not present in preeclampsia, HELLP syndrome, or gallbladder disease. Severe acute fatty liver is also characterized by renal failure and disseminated intravascular coagulation, which are not features of gallbladder disease.

Abruption An acute abruption (i.e., decidual hemorrhage leading to the premature separation of the placenta prior to delivery) classically presents with vaginal bleeding, uterine contractions, and abdominal or uterine pain that is typically not limited to the right upper quadrant or epigastrium. In severe cases, the fetal heart rate pattern is abnormal, and disseminated intravascular coagulation occurs. These features distinguish abruption from gallbladder disease.

Uterine rupture Most uterine ruptures occur in laboring women with a prior cesarean delivery or prior transmyometrial surgery. Signs and symptoms of uterine rupture can include an abnormal fetal heart rate tracing or fetal death, uterine tenderness, peritoneal irritation, vaginal bleeding, and shock. Uterine rupture prior to the onset of labor is rare and usually due to sharp or blunt abdominal trauma. This clinical setting is quite different from that in biliary disease.

Intra-amniotic infection Signs and symptoms of intra-amniotic infection include fever, abdominal pain, uterine tenderness, leukocytosis, maternal and fetal tachycardia, and uterine contractions. Intra-amniotic infection is common after premature rupture of the fetal membranes. Women with acute cholecystitis have some of these signs and symptoms, but the location of the pain is different (right upper quadrant or epigastrium versus uterine), and the fetal membranes are typically intact.

Nonpregnancy-related conditions Nonpregnancy-related conditions include non-gallstone-related biliary disease, gastroesophageal reflux, peptic ulcer disease, hepatitis, and right-sided pneumonia. Of note, the location of the appendix migrates cephalad with the enlarging uterus; thus, appendicitis may be more likely to present with right upper quadrant pain in pregnancy.

4. *Describe two possible mechanisms by which gallstone pancreatitis occurs.*

Gallstones are the most common cause of acute pancreatitis; however, only a small minority of patients with gallstones develops pancreatitis. Two factors have been suggested as the possible initiating events in gallstone pancreatitis: reflux of bile into the pancreatic duct due to transient obstruction of the ampulla during passage of gallstones; or obstruction at the ampulla secondary to stones or edema resulting from the passage of a stone. Cholecystectomy and clearing the common bile duct of stones prevent recurrence, confirming the cause-and-effect relationship.

The risk of developing acute pancreatitis in patients with gallstones is greater in men; however, the incidence of gallstone pancreatitis is higher in women due to a higher prevalence of gallstones. Small gallstones are associated with an increased risk of pancreatitis, as these small stones (typically with a diameter of less than 5 mm) are significantly more likely than larger stones to pass through the cystic duct and cause obstruction at the ampulla.

The passage of gallstones through the biliary tract can trigger acute pancreatitis either by obstructing the flow from the pancreatic duct or by obstructing the ampulla, causing bile to reflux back into the pancreatic duct. Patients who present with acute pancreatitis can have elevations in liver enzymes when a gallstone transiently obstructs the ampulla.

5. *Discuss management of gallstone pancreatitis, including timing of cholecystectomy.*

In patients with gallstone pancreatitis, most stones pass into the duodenum. However, in a small proportion of patients, obstructive stones in the biliary tract or ampulla of Vater can cause persistent biliary and pancreatic duct obstruction, leading to acute pancreatitis and cholangitis.

Endoscopic retrograde cholangiopancreatography (ERCP) should be performed early in the course (within 24 hours of admission) for patients with gallstone pancreatitis and cholangitis. Other indications for ERCP include patients with common bile duct obstruction (visible stone on imaging), dilated common bile duct, or increasing liver tests without cholangitis.

In the absence of common bile duct obstruction, ERCP is not indicated for mild or severe gallstone pancreatitis without cholangitis. When in doubt regarding bile duct obstruction in the absence of cholangitis, liver tests can be rechecked within 24 to 48 hours to determine if they improve, or a magnetic resonance cholangiopancreatography (MRCP) or endoscopic ultrasound (EUS) could be performed to determine if there are stones in the common bile duct.

In patients who are found to have stones on EUS or MRCP, ERCP with sphincterotomy and stone extraction is indicated and will prevent future attacks of biliary pancreatitis. However, in the absence of a cholecystectomy, these patients remain at risk for acute cholecystitis, biliary colic, and gallbladder complications of cholelithiasis.

In patients with acute cholangitis and persistent obstruction, urgent ERCP within 24 hours, with papillotomy or surgical intervention to remove bile duct stones, may lessen the severity of gallstone pancreatitis.

In patients with gallstone pancreatitis and persistent obstruction *without* cholangitis, urgent ERCP (within 24 hours) is not indicated. In such patients, therapeutic ERCP can be performed either before the cholecystectomy, if there is a strong suspicion of a stone in the bile duct, or postoperatively if intraoperative cholangiogram demonstrates a stone.

Cholecystectomy should be performed after recovery in all patients with gallstone pancreatitis, including those who have undergone an endoscopic sphincterotomy. In patients who have had mild pancreatitis, cholecystectomy can usually be performed safely within seven days after recovery and in the same hospitalization. In patients who have had severe necrotizing pancreatitis, cholecystectomy should be delayed until active inflammation subsides and fluid collections resolve or stabilize. Supportive care is recommended during the interval period until cholecystectomy.

Failure to perform a cholecystectomy is associated with a risk of recurrent acute pancreatitis, cholecystitis, or cholangitis within 6 to 18 weeks. The risk of recurrent pancreatitis is highest in patients who have not undergone a sphincterotomy.

6. *List the classification of common types of gallstones and their composition.*

Gallstones are composed of a mixture of cholesterol, calcium salts of bilirubinate or palmitate, proteins, and mucin. Based on the predominant constituents, gallstones are broadly classified into the following:

Cholesterol stones Cholesterol stones usually form in individuals with a genetic or environmental predisposition to bile that is supersaturated with cholesterol. Most cholesterol stones have a mixed composition with small amounts of calcium palmitate and bilirubinate salts.

Black pigment stones Black pigment stones result from hemolysis and consist primarily of calcium bilirubinate.

Brown pigment stones Brown pigment stones are associated with a bacterial infection or parasitic infestation of the biliary system. They are also often found in the bile ducts in association with prior biliary manipulation. They may also occur as de novo common bile duct stones following cholecystectomy.

Gallstones in an individual are usually homogeneous in composition.

Exam Questions

1. You are on your third year OBGYN rotation during a clinic day, and your attending has asked you to see the next patient, a 31-year-old female who is 27 weeks pregnant. She brings in a copy of a right upper quadrant ultrasound report from her gastroenterologist, which was obtained after having some intermittent right upper quadrant pain. In the report, she has been diagnosed with gallstones. She has no history of previously diagnosed gallstone formation and asks you if her pregnancy has made her susceptible to forming gallstones. Match the correct answer from the table below, which describes the roles of increased estrogen and progesterone in regards to gallstone formation during pregnancy.

	Estrogen	Progesterone
A	Increases cholesterol secretion	Reduces bile acid secretion
B	Reduces bile acid secretion	Increases cholesterol secretion
C	Slows gallbladder emptying, causing bile stasis	Reduces bile acid secretion
D	No correlation between increased levels of estrogen and gallstone formation during pregnancy	No correlation between increased levels of progesterone and gallstone formation during pregnancy

Answer: A

Learning Objective: Describe the physiologic changes during pregnancy that contribute to the increased incidence of gallstone formation.

Explanation: During pregnancy, elevated estrogen increases cholesterol secretion into bile while progesterone reduces bile acid secretion and gallbladder motility, together promoting gallstone formation. B is incorrect as estrogen (not progesterone) increases cholesterol secretion and progesterone (not estrogen) reduces bile acid secretion. C is incorrect as progesterone (not estrogen) slows gallbladder emptying. D is incorrect as there is indeed a correlation between physiologic changes of pregnancy and increased incidence of gallstone formation.

2. A 37-year-old female who is 16 weeks pregnant presents with a 4 day history of constant epigastric pain that she describes as sharp, severe (9/10 in severity) and radiates to her back. She has some associated nausea and diarrhea. She has had intermittent symptoms over the past several years but never this bad. Admission labs are remarkable for mild leukocytosis with transaminitis, and a lipase of 35,000. RUQ US shows multiple stones, sludge, common bile duct of 4.7 mm. Her findings are consistent with gallstone pancreatitis. The patient is admitted and scheduled for surgery. When is the optimal timing to perform cholecystectomy in this patient?
   A. Immediately
   B. After delivery of the baby
   C. Within a few days of admission, once active inflammation subsides.
   D. Cholecystectomy is not necessary, the patient will recover with supportive care.

Answer: C

Learning Objective: Discuss management of gallstone pancreatitis, including timing of cholecystectomy.

Explanation: In patients who have had mild gallstone pancreatitis, cholecystectomy can usually be performed safely within seven days after recovery (once active inflammation subsides, and lab values such as amylase and lipase decrease), and in the same hospitalization. A is incorrect as it is best to time cholecystectomy within 7 days after recovery (once active inflammation subsides and lab values such as amylase and lipase decrease). For now, the patient should be on an nil per os (NPO) diet and managed with supportive care and fluids. B is incorrect as failure to perform a cholecystectomy is associated with a 25–30% risk of recurrent acute pancreatitis, cholecystitis, or cholangitis within 6–18 weeks. This patient is 24 weeks pregnant and has likely 20–23 more weeks of pregnancy. She is at increased risk of recurrence of her symptoms, which may be much worse the second time. The ideal timing is within 7 days after recovery, once active inflammation subsides, and lab values such as amylase and lipase decrease. D is incorrect as failure to perform a cholecystectomy is associated with a 25–30% risk of recurrent acute pancreatitis, cholecystitis, or cholangitis within 6–18 weeks.

3. You are doing a Capstone rotation in a pathology lab. Today's specimens are from the General Surgery Department, where they performed numerous cholecystectomies the day prior. Your preceptor asks you to correctly identify the type of gallstones and their composition. Which of the following is the correct association with gallstone classification?
   A. Black pigment stones are associated with bacterial infection or parasitic infestation of the biliary system.
   B. Brown pigment stones result from hemolysis and consist primarily of calcium bilirubinate.
   C. Yellow stones are associated with bacterial infection or parasitic infection of the biliary system.
   D. Black pigment stones result from hemolysis and consist primarily of calcium bilirubinate.

Answer: D

Learning Objective: List the classification of common types of gallstones and their composition.

Explanation: Excess calcium bilirubinate from hemolysis crystallizes within the gallbladder, leading to the formation of black pigment gallstones, a specific type of gallstone distinct from cholesterol stones. A is incorrect as brown pigment stones are associated with bacterial or parasitic infections. B is incorrect as black pigment stones result from hemolysis. C is incorrect as brown pigment stones are associated with bacterial or parasitic infections. Yellow stones are typically composed of cholesterol. Cholesterol stones are the most common bile stone formed, comprising up to 80% of gallstones.

References

1. Ellington SR, Flowers L, Legardy-Williams JK, Jamieson DJ, Kourtis AP. Recent trends in hepatic diseases during pregnancy in the United States, 2002-2010. Am J Obstet Gynecol. 2015;212(4):524.e1–7. https://doi.org/10.1016/j.ajog.2014.10.1093.
2. Ko CW, Beresford SA, Schulte SJ, Matsumoto AM, Lee SP. Incidence, natural history, and risk factors for biliary sludge and stones during pregnancy. Hepatology. 2005;41(2):359–65. https://doi.org/10.1002/hep.20534.
3. Maringhini A, Ciambra M, Baccelliere P, et al. Biliary sludge and gallstones in pregnancy: incidence, risk factors, and natural history. Ann Intern Med. 1993;119(2):116–20. https://doi.org/10.7326/0003-4819-119-2-199307150-00004.

17 Persistent Vomiting

Chirag V. Kapadia

Learning Objectives:

1. Understand basic epidemiology and risk factors for HAV, HBV, HCV, HDV, HEV, and HGV.
2. Understand the clinical presentation of viral hepatides as well as the general physical exam (PE) for patients with suspicion of infection.
3. Consider a differential diagnosis and appreciate laboratory evaluation of viral hepatitis.
4. Understand basic treatments for viral hepatitis.

Chief Complaint

A 43-year-old male arrives in your emergency department (ED): "My stomach aches, and I've been throwing up a lot."

Discussion: How broad is abdominal pain? How may the pain be different depending on the location in the abdomen?

Place as many diagnoses as possible into the tablet:

RUQ		*LUQ*
	Periumbilical	
RLQ		*LLQ*

Answer: Pain—in the abdomen—can have many etiologies; one may set up their differential into 9 abdominal quadrants. There can be a multitude of diagnoses in each quadrant, some with overlap as well. Below is a graph that we have created to show a wide variety of diagnoses that may be within your differential. This list does not encompass all diagnoses possible; however, it is a good outline to utilize when thinking about categorizing our diagnoses into a more selective differential (Table 17.1).

C. V. Kapadia (✉)
Department of Hematology / Oncology, Andrew Weil Center for Integrative Medicine, University of Arizona College of Medicine, Tucson, AZ, USA
e-mail: ckapadia1@arizona.edu

C. A. Standley (ed.), *Biomedical Science and Clinical Foundations*,
https://doi.org/10.1007/978-3-031-98353-5_17

Table 17.1 The wide variety of diagnoses that may be within the differential for this patient's pain, based on 9 abdominal quadrants. Cartwright SL, Knudson MP. Evaluation of acute abdominal pain in adults. Am Fam Physician. 2008;77(7):971–8

RUQ	*Epigastric*	*LUQ*
Cholecystitis/cholelithiasis/cholangitis Hepatitis Pneumonia	Esophagitis Gastroesophageal reflux Myocardial infarction Pancreatitis AAA dissection Epigastric hernia	Gastritis Gastric malignancy Pneumonia Myocarditis, pericarditis, MI, ACS (acute coronary syndrome)
	Periumbilical	
Nephrolithiasis Pyelonephritis Vasculitis Perinephric/retroperitoneal abscess Retroperitoneal hematoma	Gastric ulcer Intestinal ulcer Constipation Gastroenteritis Crohn's disease Ulcerative colitis Gaseous distension Ascitic distension	Nephrolithiasis Pyelonephritis
RLQ	*Suprapubic*	*LLQ*
Appendicitis Right diverticulosis/diverticulitis Endometriosis	UTI/cystitis Colorectal malignancy Urinary obstruction/retention Inguinal hernia Pregnancy Epididymitis, testicular torsion	Left diverticulosis/diverticulitis Endometriosis

History of Presenting Illness

A 41-year-old male comes to the ED accompanied by his wife. He complains of right upper quadrant abdominal pain that is dull and constant, rating 5/10 in severity with no radiation. He states that ibuprofen has helped his pain a small amount and did bring down his fever; however, both return shortly thereafter. He has been reporting body aches and having fevers up to 102 degrees for the past 5 days. He states he is nauseous and has vomited 5× with no dark brown, coffee-ground, or red discoloration. His wife states she has noticed some yellow coloring in his eyes worsening over the last few days.

The patient is sitting, itching, and worried about his symptoms. He especially worried because he felt like he did not have an appetite and had been unable to keep anything except broth down over the past two days.

Prompt: What questions might you ask the patient here to probe further?

Answer: One may think to ask a specific review of systems related to this patient's clinical condition (general, head/ears/eye/nose/throat (HEENT), abdominal, integumentary, psychiatric).

- Any significant past medical history?
- Any recent travel or other infectious exposures?
- Any new pets or new food exposures?
- Any recent new drugs utilized or prescribed?

Past Medical History

The patient is healthy and has never experienced this issue before. This is the first time he has come to the ED, other than as a child.

Medications

The patient takes a daily allergy medication, which he believes is cetirizine. He is not sure, but he takes one daily and no other medications.

Allergies

No known drug allergies were reported. The patient does suffer from seasonal allergies around the spring.

Social History

Occupation: He and his wife own a restaurant in the Phoenix Valley; they often find themselves sitting at the bar throughout the day and managing the kitchen flow.

Tobacco: Denies usage and history of tobacco products

Drugs: No known history of recreational, unprescribed, or intravenous drug usage (IVDU) history.

EtOH: He drinks at least two drinks/beers at the bar a day.

Family History

Mother: deceased at age 62, history of colon cancer

Father: hypertension

Children: healthy

Prompt: What would you think is pertinent when obtaining a physical exam in this patient?

Answer:

- Jaundice and other skin changes
- Inspection, auscultation, palpation and percussion of abdomen
- +/− Murphys sign
- McBurney point tenderness
- Splenomegaly, hepatomegaly evaluation
- Costovertebral tenderness evaluation bilaterally
- Obturator sign, Psoas sign, Rovsing Sign
- Presence of rebound tenderness and guarding

Physical exam tips and tricks:

Jaundice – The first areas of your body that often present with yellowing or jaundice include soft tissue membranes such as oral cavity tissue or ocular membranes. Look for scleral icterus as a sign to help clue you into a jaundiced patient.

Murphy's Sign – A sudden cessation of inspiration during inhalation while the examiner pushes against a patient's right upper quadrant [7].

McBurney point – right lower quadrant tenderness implying potential acute appendicitis. When noting tenderness in this region, the following maneuvers may be completed to help further support appendicitis such as:

- *Rovsing Sign* – pain during palpation of left lower quadrant while patient is standing on their right side
- *Psoas Sign* – pain noted when the examiner places their hand above the patient's right knee while asking the patient to simultaneously push up against the examiner's hand
- *Obturator Sign* – increased pain noted when flexing the patient's right thigh at the hip while keeping their knee internally rotated and flexed [23, 24].

PE—Pertinent Findings

Vital Signs

Blood pressure: 125/85

Pulse: 90

Respiration rate: 16

Temperature: 102°

Weight: 210 lb Height: 69 inches

General Appearance: Well-nourished, in slight discomfort, alert and oriented

HEENT: scleral icterus, jaundice of mucosal membrane in mouth

Integumentary: jaundice of skin

Abdominal: No Costovertebral angle (CVA) tenderness. Mild hepatomegaly is appreciated. RUQ abdominal tenderness. Negative Murphy's sign. + Bowel sounds in all 4 quadrants. No splenomegaly was noted.

Prompt: What are you considering higher or lower in your differential diagnosis? What tests might you wish to order and why?

Answer: Complete blood count (CBC)
Basic Metabolic Panel (BMP)
Liver function testing (LFT)
Bilirubin testing and fractionation
Abdominal imaging (Ultrasound, MRI, CT)
Urinalysis and Urine culture

These basic labs may be able to help further elucidate a reason for the patient's abdominal pain and can lead one towards considering further labs which may help narrow the diagnosis.

Lab Review:

CBC shows increased WBC at 11.0.
BMP shows no abnormalities.
Urinalysis within normal limits, UCx pending
Liver enzymes:
AST 4218, ALT 3280, ALK PHOS 300, GGT 150, Bili 23, PT 18 sec, Albumin 25

Prompt: What do the LFT tell us? Why do we get a PT?

Alanine aminotransferase (ALT), aspartate aminotransferase (AST), alkaline phosphatase (ALP), and total bilirubin are all included in the basic LFT, although these tests do not reflect liver function but can rather help reveal a further source for liver injury. For example, elevation of AST and ALT out of proportion to ALP and bilirubin may reveal a hepatocellular disease. However, the elevation of ALP and bilirubin out of proportion to AST and AKT may denote a cholestatic pathology [19].

Prompt: With severely elevated AST and ALT alongside the clinical scenario above what might be a concern at this point?

Stop and Think:
Brainstorm causes of *Hepatitis*

Answer: Hepatotropic viruses: HAV, HBV, HCV, HDV, HEV

Nonhepatotropic viruses: Epstein–Barr Virus (EBV), Cytmegalovirus ((CMV), Herpes Simplex Virus (HSV), coxsackievirus, adenovirus, Dengue virus, Coronavirus-19
Bacteria, fungi and parasites
Toxin related: alcohol, other drugs both recreational and prescribed
Immunologic and inflammatory conditions: autoimmune (AI) hepatitis, primary biliary cholangitis (PBC), primary sclerosing cholangitis (PSC)
Metabolic: hemochromatosis, Wilson's disease, nonalcoholic fatty liver disease / steatohepatitis
Ischemic and vascular: cardiogenic and distributive shock, hypotension, heatstroke, acute Budd-Chiari syndrome
Other causes: malignancy, eclampsia, HELLP syndrome, acute fatty liver of pregnancy [9]

Prompt: What other lab studies would have been IMPORTANT to order?

Answer: An acute hepatitis panel is often ordered in the clinic, screening for antibodies to HAV, HBV, HCV are often the first results obtained. Depending on those, further studies may be completed and are further discussed in detail at the end of this chapter. Other markers may include auto-immune hepatitis markers, EBV antibodies, HSV antibodies, adenovirus antigen testing, HIV testing, serum ceruloplasmin levels, and iron panel with ferritin may also help further narrow the diagnosis.

Results: HAV IgM: +
HAV IgG: –
HAV RNA: +
HBsAg: –
HBeAg: –
Anti-HBc: IgM –
Anti-HBs: +
Anti-HBe: –
HCV RNA: –
HBsAg: –
Anti-HEV IgM: –
HSV: –
Adenovirus: –
HIV: –
EBV: –

AI markers:
antinuclear antibodies: –
anti-smooth muscle antibodies: –
anti-liver/kidney microsomal-1 antibodies: –
anti-soluble liver/liver pancreas: –

Prompt: What is the most likely diagnosis?

Answer: Acute HAV Infection

Prompt: *Would we do a liver biopsy at this time?*

Answer: No this is a procedure that is relatively invasive and can give us more insight into liver damage from things like drug induced liver toxicity for example. In this situation, with viral PCR positive HAV there would be little benefit in liver biopsy while this procedure may in fact harbor increased risk [5].

Prompt: *How do we treat illness?*

Answer: HAV is usually a self-limiting illness and will resolve on its own. Continue supportive care for the patient and observe liver enzyme functions. Return follow-up with hepatology in 4 weeks after discharge [8].

Conclusion:

The patient's AST and ALT return down to below 500, respectively, and he is discharged. He is to follow up with a hepatologist in 4 weeks to observe the status of his disease resolution.

4 Weeks Later:

The patient's AST and ALT have returned to normal limits, and the patient feels much better. He is preparing for the arrival of his son within the month. He feels he has returned to his baseline and is no longer jaundiced.

End of Case

Explanation for Learning Objectives:

1: Understand basic epidemiology and risk factors for HAV, HBV, HCV, HDV, HEV, and HGV.

Viral hepatitis strains (A, B, C, and D) endemic to the United States have been attributed to 90% of acute viral hepatitis cases, with the Hepatitis C virus (HCV) remaining the most common reason attributing to chronic hepatitis. Hepatitis A virus (HAV), an RNA virus, is notably found in the largest concentrations within the stool of infected individuals. Therefore, the largest cause of HAV transmission is related to the fecal-oral route, including contact with food, water, or other items exposed to the fecal matter of an infected individual. Those individuals exposed to infected individuals may also be at risk, with a secondary infection rate reported near 20% in household contacts [8].

Hepatitis B virus (HBV), a DNA virus, is another common cause of viral hepatitis in the United States. HBV remains detectable in bodily fluids such as serum, semen, vaginal mucus, saliva, and tears; however, it has not been noted in urine, stool, or sweat studies. An estimated 2.2 million individuals suffer from chronic HBV infection in the United States. Transmission is notably through parenteral exposure or sexual encounters via contact with mucous membranes. Parenteral exposure, such as needle injuries, blood product transfusions, intravenous drug use (IVDU), or other wounds, accounts for the largest cause of transmission; however, patients with multiple sexual partners, prisoners, and other partners of HBV carriers are other common causes of transmission. HBV may also be transmitted perinatally, with chronic infection being common in those who become infected [28].

HCV, an RNA virus, is most often parenterally transmitted, such as through IVDU and needle sharing. Other common causes of transmission include healthcare exposures, perinatal exposures to HCV, and organ transplantation from HCV-positive patients, among others. A large proportion of patients will develop chronic hepatitis, reportedly 50–80%; however, up to 40% of those cases may resolve spontaneously. Still, there remains a risk of life-threatening complications such as cirrhosis or hepatocellular carcinoma related to HCV infection. Outcomes of HCV infection are often grouped with specific genotypes of various HCV strains [10].

Other hepatitis viruses include the Hepatitis D virus (HDV), which uniquely utilizes Hepatitis B surface antigen (HBsAG) within the formation of its own envelope protein. Therefore, HDV is thought to be only present in those with or resolved hepatitis B infection [20]. Hepatitis E virus (HEV) is most associated with maternal-neonatal transmission [15]. Finally, the Hepatitis G virus (HGV), usually found as a coinfection in those with chronic HBV or HCV, needs more research to determine its mechanism. However, HGV has been associated with acute and chronic liver disease [24].

2: Understand the clinical presentation of viral hepatides as well as general PEs for patients with suspicion of infection.

Viral hepatitis can have various clinical presentations; patients can be asymptomatic or undergoing a multitude of simultaneous symptoms. However, the typical patient with viral hepatitis often has four phases throughout their clinical presentation as detailed below:

Phase 1:

This is often thought to be the incubation phase where viral replications begin to occur. At this phase, patients are most likely asymptomatic; however, studies may become positive for markers of hepatitis.

Phase 2:

Clinical symptoms in this phase may include anorexia, nausea, vomiting, malaise, pruritus, arthralgia, fatigue, and urticaria.

Phase 3:

Also known as the icteric phase, patients here will often present with dark-colored urine and pale-colored stool. Some patients may develop jaundice as well. The liver enzymes will be elevated in this phase.

Phase 4:

The convalescent phase is where patients may start to observe the resolution of symptoms, including lab studies returning to normalized levels as well [11].

When discussing the various viral hepatides, patients can often present with various clinical prodromes. Below, we will discuss common clinical presentations as well as a general PE that may be considered for those patients with concern for viral hepatitis infection.

HAV:

Patients have been reported too often present with symptoms like gastroenteritis or viral respiratory infections. Symptoms may include fever, emesis, fatigue, anorexia, jaundice, among others. Symptoms begin after a 4-week-incubation period and resolve in most patients spontaneously [8].

HBV:

Patients undergo an incubation phase often lasting 12 weeks prior to entering their prodromal phase. At this point, patients often present with common initial symptoms including anorexia, fatigue, and malaise. A few subsets of patients will experience right upper quadrant pain related to inflammation, while others may experience arthralgias and dermatitis. As these patients progress into the icteric phase, they often develop jaundice as well as painful hepatomegaly in addition to dark-colored urine and pale-colored stools. After this phase, some patients may experience swift clinical improvement; however, others may develop a lengthier chronic illness with slow resolution and periodic flare-ups. There remains a small subset of patients who may have prompt progression leading to hepatic failure [11].

HCV:

Patients often undergo an incubation period lasting nearly 8 weeks prior to developing symptoms like those infected with HBV. Once again, common symptoms include malaise, fatigue, and anorexia. It is worth noting that 80% of patients remain asymptomatic [10].

HDV:

Infection with HDV can be considered as a simultaneous infection with HBV or a superinfection in the setting of chronic HBV carriers. Those with simultaneous infections often have a self-limited course; however, those with super infection tend to have a more severe course with a higher risk of developing into chronic HDV infection. When compared to chronic HBV infection, chronic infection with both HBV and HDV carries a greater risk of development of liver failure, severe chronic active hepatitis, and progression to cirrhosis [4].

HEV:

Patients with HEV infection often remain asymptomatic with a disease course like HAV, commonly a self-limited illness. However, the mortality rate increases when pregnant patients are infected with HEV [27].

General Physical Exam:

As we have seen above, physical findings can often vary in individual patients due to the timing of their presentation in relation to when they may have been infected with the virus. It is essential to collect appropriate vital signs of patients, who may show low-grade fevers as well as signs of dehydration, which may be noted with blood pressure recordings.

Dehydration can be further worsened due to emesis episodes and loss of appetite often noted with viral hepatitis. Clinical findings that may be able to help support dehydration may include dry mucous membranes, tachycardia, low blood pressure, and delayed capillary refill.

During the icteric phase, skin and mucous membrane changes may be observable, such as icteric sclerae, jaundiced skin, or even dermatitis. Tender abdominal palpation may also be noted due to hepatic inflammation.

Other findings may show evidence of advanced liver failure in the setting of chronic or acute viral hepatitis. These may include a positive abdominal fluid wave pointing toward abdominal ascites as well as lower extremity or diffuse edema related to malnutrition [3].

3: Consider a differential diagnosis and appreciate laboratory evaluation of viral hepatitis.

As patients may present with a variety of symptoms and a potentially unremarkable PE, one must consider both liver- and non-liver-related disorders. Some of these may include drug-induced hepatitis, AI hepatitis, gastroenteritis, pancreatitis, small-bowel obstruction, cholecystitis, and other biliary issues such as obstruction or cholelithiasis, peptic ulcer disease, and malignancies including pancreatic cancer, hepatocellular carcinoma, and lymphoma, among others.

This differential diagnosis can be further shortened with appropriate lab evaluation. In the case of viral hepatitis, the timing and evaluation of these biomarkers may be able to help hone in on a diagnosis. Initial evaluation when suspecting viral hepatitis includes a hepatic function panel, evaluation of ALP levels, and total bilirubin levels. Further liver function can be tested through prothrombin time (PT) and international normalized ratio, both of which may be prolonged alongside leukopenia and thrombocytopenia. Other lab tests may also include a creatinine level and a serum ammonia level in the setting of altered mental status. However, additional lab tests may be completed that are more specific to the evaluation of viral hepatitis.

HAV:

Testing for diagnosis of acute HAV infection includes evaluation of immunoglobulin M (IgM) antibodies directed to HAV. Although IgM levels decrease some months after acute infection, immunoglobulin G (IgG) antibody levels remain elevated, indicating potential for infection in the past as recently as 2 months ago to several decades. IgG cannot be utilized as a screening test as it does not predict when the infection may have occurred. They may also be positive in the setting of HAV-vaccinated patients [13].

HBV:

Acute HBV Infection:

The first serum marker appearing in HBV-infected patients is the HBsAg, which points to hepatitis B viremia without indicating whether it is an acute or chronic infection. However, the presence of HBsAg likely suggests acute infection; it cannot rule out a flare, chronic infection, or superinfection. HBsAg often lasts about 6 months after acute infection; however, if it persists past that point, then it is considered a chronic HBV infection. Once the infection is cleared, the antibody to HBsAg (anti-HBs) becomes noticeable on lab evaluation.

The first antibody to present itself is the IgM antibody to the hepatitis B core antigen (HBcAg). IgM anti-HBc detectability indicates an acute HBV infection and is required to make a diagnosis. As IgM antibody levels begin to decrease, IgG anti-HBc levels begin to rise.

Another antigen, hepatitis B e-antigen (HBeAg), also presents itself early within the timeline of the infection. HBeAg indicated HBBV replication; once this replication diminishes, the HBeAg becomes undetectable. Afterward, antibodies to HBeAg (anti-HBe) levels become apparent and may persist in the blood indefinitely.

Chronic HBV Infection:

Patients with chronic HBV will have anti-HBc and HBsAg present on labs; whoever the latter may indicate inactive carriers of HBV or active chronic HBV-infected individuals. HBeAg may also be present in those patients with active chronic hepatitis, and if it is present, it would indicate active viral replication. If HBV DNA is detectable at high levels, that may also help indicate active chronic hepatitis. Those with chronic infection would often have an absence of the anti-HBs; however, if present, it may indicate a chronic HBV infection in which the antibody was unable to clear the virus.

Uncommon HBV Infection Scenarios:

Testing for anti-HBc may be positive in the setting of negative HBsAg and anti-HBs. This may indicate a false positive; however, it may also indicate a period where the patient may have cleared the HBsAg without the formation of anti-HBs. Other patients may have cleared their HBV infection and subsequently lost their anti-HBs over some time, which may cause a negative HBsAG and anti-HBs with a positive anti-HBc. Another unusual scenario may be when a patient is positive for anti-HBe and negative for HBeAg, although the virus is active and replicating. This may occur in the setting of a core mutant variant HBV. In this setting, it is generally recommended to complete an HBV DNA PCR assay. Finally, those having received a vaccine for HBV would develop anti-HBs without any other HBV-associated proteins. If patients who receive the vaccine are positive for anti-HBc, then this indicated a previous infection in the setting of vaccinated patients [25].

HCV:

Detection of HCV exposure is done by searching for antibodies to HCV (anti-HCV). Assays for anti-HCV can detect antibodies within 4 to 10 weeks of infection; however, anti-HCV may not become positive for a few months preceding an acute infection. If an assay for anti-HCV does return positive, then a confirmation test needs to be completed, which entails HCV RNA testing. This test can be useful to differentiate between true infections versus false-positive cases, indeterminate cases, as well as rare cases such as perinatal transmission. This test can also illuminate details on viral load as well as HCV genotype.

Once an infection is noted, it becomes important to test for fibrosis. This can be indirectly tested with ALT/AST testing and non-invasively with imaging such as ultrasound-based transient elastography. In certain circumstances, liver biopsy can be considered; however, it remains a largely invasive procedure and is often reserved for cases in which there may be a competing diagnosis [10, 18, 21]. For this reason, often aminotransferase levels may be utilized to help monitor response to treatment; if improving, then likely the infection is resolving; however, in the setting of rising aminotransferase levels after HCV treatment, a relapse may be noted. Still, HCV RNA testing remains the method usually chosen to monitor treatment response [5, 27].

HDV and HEV:

HDV infections are diagnosed through the determination of IgM and IgG antibodies directed to HDV (anti-HDV). When patients test positive, IgM antibody to the HBcAg (anti-HBc) is checked to help elucidate a coinfection versus superinfection. In the case of a coinfection, IgM anti-HBc results are positive; however, in a superinfection, this test would result negative. Another test that is not routinely performed but is available is the HDV RNA test [21].

HEV infections may be determined by evaluating IgM and IgG antibodies to HEV (anti-HEV). HEV RNA may also be evaluated via stool and serum studies [1, 26].

4: Understand basic treatments for viral hepatitis.

In general, most cases of viral hepatitis will be self-limiting, and therefore management is largely supportive in nature. However, patients and providers should be wary of the chances of disease transmission in close contact. Patients should remain cautious of hepatotoxic substances, including medications, alcohol, and others as warranted. However, there remain some more specific treatment options for various viral hepatides.

HAV:

There remains no antiviral therapy available for the treatment of HAV. Often a self-limiting course, most patients will require supportive care. Should patients have considerable symptomatology, they can be admitted under a closer monitored setting [8].

HBV:

Treatment of HBV can be divided into the following two categories:

Acute HBV Infection:

For most cases, treatment remains largely supportive. However, in the setting of more severe infection, medications can be considered. These therapies are often nucleoside or nucleotide analogs. Treatment may be considered include in cases presenting with acute fulminant liver failure, a lengthy course of clinical symptomatology such as greater than four weeks, immunocompromised patients, and those with coinfection of HBV alongside other viruses such as HCV or HDV [12].

Chronic HBV Infection:

The treatment goal is the suppression of HBV DNA and, in turn, the loss of HBeAg. In turn, a reduction of symptoms and prevention of disease progression is the anticipated outcome. In the setting of chronic disease, interferon therapy may be included in the first line. However, in the setting of acute disease, interferon therapy can potentially worsen overall liver inflammation. However, it remains that interferon therapy often causes a wide variety of side effects and is overall not generally well tolerated; therefore, compliance issues have also been reported. Treatment may also be elected with oral nucleoside or nucleotide analog agents [17].

HCV:

Treatment of HCV can be divided into the following two categories:

Acute HCV Infection:

Although acute infections of HCV are not frequently observed, once diagnosed, treatment is recommended. Treatment is like that as below in the chronic HCV section [2].

Chronic HCV Infection:

The foremost goal of treatment for chronic HCV is the eradication of the virus, and a sustained virologic response is defined as the lack of viral detection in the blood 12 weeks after receiving anti-HCV therapy. Those patients who reached this goal have a 99% or greater chance of maintaining a cure [22]. Treatment is further beneficial as curing HCV infection can reverse overall liver inflammation and fibrosis as well as decrease the risk of developing HCC [14, 16]

When selecting a treatment appropriately, a patient's treatment history, degree of fibrosis, cirrhosis history, and decompensation from cirrhosis are all part of the consideration process. Additionally, those with other viral infections (including HIV), pregnant patients, children, and transplant patients may require further additional considerations for treatment. Historically, pegylated interferon alpha and ribavirin were utilized as the mainstays of treatment. However, since the introduction of second-generation direct-acting antiviral agents, the previous mainstay has now become almost obsolete. However, ribavirin can still be used in circumstances on a case-by-case basis [2].

HDV & HEV:

Those with HDV and HBV coinfection often receive pegylated interferon treatment, and oral nucleoside/nucleotide analogs have a limited role in these patients [29].

The treatment for HEV infection is largely supportive. Immunosuppressed patients who may develop chronic HEV infection can have treatment with ribavirin [6].

Exam Questions

1. A 37-year-old male comes to the physician because of a 3-day history of fatigue and yellowish discoloration of his eyes and skin. PE shows mild right upper quadrant abdominal tenderness. The course of different serum parameters over the following 12 months shows the following:
   - IgM anti-HBc peaks at 3 months and then declines to zero at 5 months.
   - HBsAg peaks higher than IgM anti-HBc at 3 months and then declines to zero at 9 months.
   - Anti-HBs begin to rise after 2 months and plateau at 6 months.
   - Total anti-HBc steeply rises after 1 month and stays elevated.
   - Increased ALT at 2 to 4 months

   Which of the following is the most likely explanation for the course of this patient's lab findings?

   A. Chronic hepatitis B infection with high infectivity
   B. Hepatitis B immunity due to vaccination
   C. Acute exacerbation of chronic hepatitis B infection
   D. Resolved acute hepatitis B infection
   E. Chronic hepatitis B infection with low infectivity

   Answer: D

   Learning Objective #3: Consider a differential diagnosis and appreciate laboratory evaluation of viral hepatitis.

   Explanation: The patient's serology results describe the natural history of a resolved or resolving acute hepatitis B infection. Total anti-HBc as well as anti-HBs (both IgGs showing long-term immunity) are formed, and the only by-products of the infection are still left at detection. Furthermore, IgM anti-HBc is declining as the IgGs have begun formation. Additionally, there is no more HBsAg present during detection. A is incorrect as chronic hepatitis B infection with high infectivity would have had no disappearance of the HBsAg. Anti-HBc would become present and would also persist through the infection. Anti-HBc IgM would also be produced but diminish in formation once anti-HBc is formed. HBsAg would not decrease in production. HBsAg allows us to look at infectivity; with low HBsAg, this patient would have a high infectivity profile. B is incorrect as HBV vaccination only involves just the HBsAg. Patients are inoculated with HBsAg and have the chance to form anti-HBs. No other serologies would return positive in this situation. C is incorrect as in an acute exacerbation of chronic hepatitis B, HBsAg would be decreased to a level where the patient would be considered an inactive carrier. However, when HBsAg is once again detectable at a significant level, the patient would be in an acute exacerbation. ALT may increase, as would HBV DNA levels. E is incorrect as chronic hepatitis B infection with low infectivity would have no disappearance of the HBsAg. Anti-HBc would become present and would also persist through the infection. Anti-HBc IgM would also be produced but diminish in formation once anti-HBc is formed. HBsAg would decrease in production, and anti-HBc is formed. HBsAg allows us to look at infectivity; with low HBsAg, this patient would have a low infectivity profile.

2. A 28-year-old woman with a history of intravenous drug use is brought to the E.D. because

of a 1-day history of fatigue, yellow eyes, confusion, and blood in her stools. She appears ill. Her temperature is 38.1 C (100.6 F). PE shows pain in the right upper quadrant, diffuse jaundice with scleral icterus, and bright red blood per rectum. Further evaluation shows virions in her blood, some with a partially double-stranded DNA genome while others have a single-stranded RNA genome. They have the same identical lipoprotein envelope. What is the most likely pathogen infecting this patient?

A. Picornavirus
B. Calicivirus
C. Flavivirus
D. Filovirus
E. Deltavirus
F. Herpesvirus

Answer: E

Learning Objective #1: Discuss the epidemiology and risk factors for HAV, HBV, HCV, HDV, HEV, and HGV.

Explanation: Delta virus consists of both HBV and HDV. These viruses are transmitted sexually, parenterally (for example, with contaminated needles), or perinatally. Although acute HBV infection is often mild or asymptomatic, it can become chronic in approximately 5% of patients. HDV is an interesting virus that is dependent on the HBV surface antigen coat for entry into hepatocytes. Thus, HDV can only cause infection if the patient is also infected with HBV at the same time or if the patient already has a chronic HBV infection. Since there are two viruses present, one may observe the scenario in the question stem where two viral genomes are observed but only one lipoprotein envelope. Without HBV, HDV would be unable to replicate. A is incorrect, as picornavirus is a non-enveloped, positive-strand RNA virus. This virus does not have an envelope. Additionally, it does not have two different RNA types as in the question stem. B is incorrect as calicivirus is a positive-sense, unsegmented, single-stranded RNA virus. It does not have two different RNA types as in this question stem. C is incorrect as flavivirus is a positive-sense, single-stranded, enveloped RNA virus. Although it does have an envelope, it does not have two different strands of RNA as in the question stem. D is incorrect as filovirus is a single-strand, negative-sense RNA virus. It does not have an envelope or two separate forms of RNA as in this question stem. F is incorrect as herpesvirus is a large family of DNA viruses. RNA particles would not be present with this virus.

3. A 31-year-old woman, g2p1 at 24 weeks gestation, is brought to the E.D. by her husband for nausea, vomiting, and lethargy for the past 5 days. She returned from a trip to South Asia 2 weeks prior. Her immunizations are up-to-date, and she has never had a blood transfusion or received any other blood products. Her current temperature is 38.9 C (102 F). She is confused and is unable to answer questions about her name, her location, and the date. On PE jaundice and mild asterixis are both observed. Her PT is 18 seconds (high), serum ALT is 3900 U/L, and serum AST is 3720 U/L. The patient's labs would most likely show an increase in which of the following?

A. Anti-HBV IgM
B. Anti-HDV IgM
C. Anti-HCV IgG
D. Anti-HAV IgM
E. Anti-HEV IgM

Answer: E

Learning Objective: Understand basic epidemiology and risk factors for HAV, HBV, HCV, HDV, HEV, and HGV.

Explanation: Anti-HEV IgM is the most likely correct answer choice. This viral infection, specifically during pregnancy, is associated with a high mortality rate (upward of 10–25%) during the third trimester. This mortality is due to hepatic failure and decompensation as observed in this patient. Moreover, HEV is endemic to southern Asia, to which the patient has a travel history. She has multiple risk factors and is most likely suffering from HEV infection. A is incorrect as HBV is unlikely to cause acute liver failure in most patients. This patient has signs of acute liver failure with decompensation, including encephalopathy. B is incorrect as HDV is unlikely as the patient would have to also be HBV positive. Additionally, she does not have risk factors for HDV infection. C is incorrect as anti-HCV IgG would mean this patient has chronic HCV with an acute exacerbation. HCV is prevalent in West Africa, Eastern Europe, and the Eastern Mediterranean region. The patient does not have this risk factor. Additionally, she does not have social risk factors that would relate back to HCV infection. This is an unlikely answer choice and unlikely to cause hepatic failure in this patient. D is incorrect as anti-HAV IgM is unlikely as HAV is more commonly a self-limiting disease that very rarely causes hepatic failure as in this patient.

References

1. Aggarwal R. Diagnosis of hepatitis E. Nat Rev Gastroenterol Hepatol. 2013;10(1):24–33.
2. Bhattacharya D, et al. Hepatitis C guidance 2023 update: AASLD-IDSA recommendations for testing, managing, and treating hepatitis C virus infection. Clin Infect Dis. 2023;
3. Chin J, et al. Osteopathic physical exam findings in chronic hepatitis C: a case study. Cureus. 2019;11(1):e3939.
4. Farci P, Niro GA. Clinical features of hepatitis D. Semin Liver Dis. 2012;32(3):228–36.
5. Gupta E, et al. Hepatitis C virus: Screening, diagnosis, and interpretation of laboratory assays. Asian J Transfus Sci. 2014;8(1):19–25.
6. Hui W, et al. Treatment of Hepatitis E. Adv Exp Med Biol. 2016;948:211–21.
7. Jeans PL. Murphy's sign. Med J Aust. 2017;206(3):115–6.
8. Koenig KL, et al. Hepatitis A virus: essential knowledge and a novel identify-isolate-inform tool for frontline healthcare providers. West J Emerg Med. 2017;18(6):1000–7.
9. Kwong S, Meyerson C, Zheng W, Kassardjian A, Stanzione N, Zhang K, Wang HL. Acute hepatitis and acute liver failure: Pathologic diagnosis and differential diagnosis. Semin Diagn Pathol. 2019;36(6):404–14. https://doi.org/10.1053/j.semdp.2019.07.005. Epub 2019 Jul 24. PMID: 31405537.
10. Li HC, Lo SY. Hepatitis C virus: Virology, diagnosis and treatment. World J Hepatol. 2015;7(10):1377–89.
11. Liang TJ. Hepatitis B: the virus and disease. Hepatology. 2009;49(5 Suppl):S13–21.
12. Lisotti A, et al. Lamivudine treatment for severe acute HBV hepatitis. Int J Med Sci. 2008;5(6):309–12.
13. Matheny SC, Kingery JE. Hepatitis A. Am Fam Physician. 2012;86(11): 1027–34; quiz 1010–1022.
14. Morgan RL, et al. Eradication of hepatitis C virus infection and the development of hepatocellular carcinoma: a meta-analysis of observational studies. Ann Intern Med. 2013;158(5 Pt 1):329–37.
15. Pérez-Gracia MT, et al. Current knowledge on Hepatitis E. J Clin Transl Hepatol. 2015;3(2):117–26.
16. Poynard T, et al. Impact of pegylated interferon alfa-2b and ribavirin on liver fibrosis in patients with chronic hepatitis C. Gastroenterology. 2002;122(5):1303–13.
17. Rajbhandari R, Chung RT. Treatment of hepatitis B: a concise review. Clin Transl Gastroenterol. 2016;7(9):e190.
18. Regev A, et al. Sampling error and intraobserver variation in liver biopsy in patients with chronic HCV infection. Am J Gastroenterol. 2002;97(10):2614–8.
19. Ribeiro AJS, et al. Liver microphysiological systems for predicting and evaluating drug effects. Clin Pharmacol Ther. 2019;106(1):139–47.
20. Rizzetto M. Hepatitis D virus: introduction and epidemiology. Cold Spring Harb Perspect Med. 2015;5(7):a021576.
21. Safaie P, et al. Hepatitis D diagnostics: utilization and testing in the United States. Virus Res. 2018;250:114–7.
22. Seeff LB, et al. Complication rate of percutaneous liver biopsies among persons with advanced chronic liver disease in the HALT-C trial. Clin Gastroenterol Hepatol. 2010;8(10):877–83.
23. Simmons B, et al. Risk of late relapse or reinfection with hepatitis C virus after achieving a sustained virological response: a systematic review and meta-analysis. Clin Infect Dis. 2016;62(6):683–94.
24. Snyder MJ, et al. Acute appendicitis: efficient diagnosis and management. Am Fam Physician. 2018;98(1):25–33.
25. Soleiman-Meigooni S, et al. Association between hepatitis G and unknown chronic hepatitis. Electron Physician. 2015;7(1):985–9.
26. Song JE, Kim DY. Diagnosis of hepatitis B. Ann Transl Med. 2016;4(18):338.
27. Webb GW, Dalton HR. Hepatitis E: an underestimated emerging threat. Ther Adv Infect Dis. 2019;6:2049936119837162.
28. You CR, et al. Update on hepatitis B virus infection. World J Gastroenterol. 2014;20(37):13293–305.
29. Yurdaydin C. Recent advances in managing hepatitis D. F1000Res. 2017;6:1596.

Worsening Abdominal Pain

18

Alyssa Korenstein

Learning Objectives

1. Explain the pathophysiology of ulcerative colitis and how it compares to that of Crohn's disease, with particular attention to how each disease process affects the histologic layers of gastrointestinal mucosa. Locate where within the gastrointestinal tract each disease process predominates.
2. Define and understand the mechanisms of secretory, osmotic, and inflammatory diarrhea, highlighting common conditions associated with each. Compose a diagnostic algorithm to approach chronic diarrhea in the primary care setting.
3. Understand the electrolyte imbalances that occur with diarrhea and how they impact acid-base status.
4. Review the gastrointestinal and extraintestinal manifestations of ulcerative colitis. Compare and contrast these with the manifestations of Crohn's disease. Recognize common complications associated with each disease.
5. Summarize acute and long-term medical and surgical treatment options for inflammatory bowel disease based on disease staging.
6. Identify the incidence, prevalence, risk factors for, and prognosis of inflammatory bowel disease.
7. Discuss recommendations for appropriate preventive care and screening measures for patients with inflammatory bowel disease.

Chief Complaint: "My stomach hurts!"

Given this information, what body systems or sources might you consider as the cause?

- Systems: gastrointestinal, renal, genitourinary, vascular
- Vascular: abdominal aortic aneurysm, ischemic bowel
- Infection: gastroenteritis, hepatitis, urinary tract infection, pelvic inflammatory disease, pneumonia
- Neoplastic: colorectal cancer or other gastrointestinal malignancy
- Drugs/Toxins: toxic ingestion or overdose
- Inflammatory/Idiopathic: inflammatory bowel disease (IBD), appendicitis, pancreatitis, diverticulitis, cholecystitis, gastritis
- Congenital: volvulus, malrotation, Meckel's diverticulum
- Autoimmune: IBD, celiac disease
- Trauma: gunshot or stab wound, blunt abdominal trauma, abuse
- Endocrine: diabetic gastroparesis, diabetic ketoacidosis, thyroid disease
- Something else: psychosomatic, ulcer, gastroesophageal reflux disease, nephrolithiasis, cholelithiasis, lactose intolerance, ectopic pregnancy, ovarian cyst, testicular torsion, bowel obstruction

A. Korenstein (✉)
Family Physician, One Medical, New York, NY, USA
e-mail: akorenstein@onemedical.com

C. A. Standley (ed.), *Biomedical Science and Clinical Foundations*,
https://doi.org/10.1007/978-3-031-98353-5_18

Essentially, this chief complaint could really be anything! We need more information to narrow this down—gender, age, location of pain, time course, red flags, associated symptoms, and more.

History of Present Illness:

MM is a 27-year-old white male who presents to his primary care physician with a 3-month history of worsening abdominal pain. The pain began gradually as a mild episodic burning and cramping sensation located in his epigastric region after meals. He thought it may have been his acid reflux acting up; however, his pain hasn't remitted with use of over-the-counter reflux medications such as Omeprazole.

Over the last 6 weeks, the pain has become more severe, constant, and diffusely located throughout his abdomen and will now occasionally wake him up at night. He denies any radiation of the pain. Nothing particularly seems to exacerbate the pain, including food. He occasionally has some relief of the pain with defecation. Over the past 6 weeks he has also had increasingly loose stools three to four times per day, and this week he noticed occasional blood in the toilet. He notes that he has also lost about ten pounds unintentionally over the last month. He did travel to Mexico 6 months ago for a vacation with his partner, at which time he developed a brief "stomach flu," which he felt had resolved after a few days. He denies non-steroidal anti-inflammatory drug or recent antibiotic use and has never been tested for Helicobacter pylori.

Here are some additional questions we may want to consider hearing this history:

What red flags are present?

- Unintentional weight loss
- Nighttime awakening with pain
- Blood in stool
  - Dark or tarry stools (melena) would be more likely to represent an upper gastrointestinal source such as a bleeding ulcer, as opposed to bright red blood per rectum, which may be more likely to represent a lower gastrointestinal source.

What is the significance of pain relief with defecation?

How can we further classify this patient's diarrhea to help guide us to a diagnosis?

Let's dive in more to this patient's background.

Past Medical History: Gastroesophageal Reflux Disease (GERD)

Past Surgical History: denies

Medications:

- Famotidine 10–20 mg PO BID
  - Mechanism of Action: reversible H2 receptor blocker which antagonizes H2 receptors in gastric parietal cells, thereby leading to decreased gastric acid secretion.
- Omeprazole 20 mg PO QD before meals
  - Mechanism of Action: Proton Pump Inhibitor (PPI), which irreversibly inhibits gastric parietal cell H^+/K^+/ATPase

Allergies: No known allergies

Family History:

- Father: Deceased at age 62 from colon cancer.
- Mother: Alive, age 65, healthy.
- Brother: Alive, age 33 with psoriatic arthritis.

Social History:

- Works in sales.
- In monogamous relationship with female partner for two years, has no children.
- Never tobacco smoker.
- Alcohol use: two drinks per week.
- Denies illicit drug use.

Review of Systems:

- General: + Ten lbs. unintentional weight loss over the past month, mild fatigue. No fever.

- Head/Ears/Eyes/Nose/Throat (HEENT): + Occasional red itchy eyes. No decreased visual acuity, headache, mouth ulcers, change in hearing, sore throat, or dysphagia.
- Cardiovascular: No chest pain, lower extremity edema, syncope, or palpitations.
- Pulmonary: No shortness of breath, cough, or wheezing.
- Gastrointestinal: + Abdominal pain, loose stool, hematochezia, history of GERD, slightly decreased appetite. No nausea, vomiting, constipation, steatorrhea, melena, abdominal distention, or jaundice.
- Genitourinary: No hematuria, dysuria, or testicular pain or swelling.
- Musculoskeletal: + Occasional back pain and stiffness in mornings for 6 months.
- Endocrine: No polyuria, polydipsia, sensitivity to heat/cold, or sweating.
- Hematologic/Lymphatic: No bruising, bleeding, or lymphadenopathy.
- Neurologic: No numbness, weakness, dizziness, or history of seizures.
- Integumentary/Skin: No rashes, itching, lesions, sores, or changes in hair/nails.
- Psychiatric: No depressed mood, feelings of guilt, loss of interest in activities, difficulty concentrating, suicidal ideation, or hallucinations.

How might these data have modified your differential diagnosis?

- Poorly localized abdominal pain and chronic bloody diarrhea in a young male, associated with back pain/morning stiffness and red eyes, should raise concern for IBD with extraintestinal manifestations. There may also be a possibility of HLA-B27 syndrome with the family history of psoriatic arthritis.
- Recent travel to Mexico raises concern for possible infectious etiology.
- The patient is known for a history of GERD, so a bleeding gastric ulcer or infection with Helicobacter pylori should still be considered.
- The patient's family history of colon cancer is concerning considering him experiencing bloody stool and weight loss, although this patient is young.
- Celiac disease is also still a possibility with bloody diarrhea and can have a variable symptom presentation, although this patient denies any association with food.

Let's move on to his exam.

Exam:

- Vital signs:
  - Blood pressure: 115/76.
  - Pulse: 92 beats per minute.
  - Weight: 120 lbs.
  - Height: 5′ 8″.
  - BMI: 18.2.
  - Temperature. 37 C.
  - Respirations: 12.
  - Oxygen saturation: 98% on room air.
- General Appearance: Alert, conversant, pale-appearing. Mildly uncomfortable/anxious-appearing sitting hunched over on exam table.
- Head/Ears/Eyes/Nose/Throat: Bilateral conjunctival injection. Sclera anicteric. No exophthalmos present. No oral ulcers. No thyromegaly or palpable nodules.
- Heart: Regular rate and rhythm, normal S1, S2, no S3, S4, murmurs, rubs, or gallops.
- Lungs: Clear to auscultation bilaterally, no wheezes, rhonchi, or rales.
- Abdomen: Non-distended. Normal bowel sounds heard throughout. Diffusely tender to light and deep palpation in all quadrants. Mild voluntary guarding. No rebound tenderness. No hepatosplenomegaly.
- Lymph Nodes: No cervical, axillary, or inguinal adenopathy.
- Back: Range of motion is limited in back extension. No costovertebral angle tenderness. No spinous process tenderness to palpation.
- Musculoskeletal: No erythema, swelling, or tenderness in joints.
- Extremities: Two 2–4 cm erythematous nodules on the left anterior tibia, which are mildly

tender to palpation and which the patient attributes possibly to bumping into a coffee table. No rashes. No clubbing, cyanosis, or edema. Dorsalis pedis, posterior tibial, and radial pulses are 2+ symmetrically.
- Rectal: No fissure or hemorrhoids present. Dark brown guaiac positive.

The exam findings of the nodules on the tibia are consistent with erythema nodosum. What diseases are erythema nodosum associated with?

- IBD, sarcoidosis, infections (strep most commonly). Gastrointestinal infections such as salmonella, yersinia, and campylobacter. Fungal infections such as coccidioidomycosis. Tuberculosis), drug reaction (penicillin, sulfa, oral contraceptives), malignancy (lymphoma, other carcinomas), pregnancy. This can also be idiopathic.

What is the significance of the positive non-gastrointestinal exam findings?

- These are likely extraintestinal manifestations of IBD (episcleritis/uveitis, erythema nodosum, ankylosing spondylitis).

How have the exam findings narrowed your differential diagnosis?

- IBD is moving toward the top of the list given exam findings and associated extraintestinal manifestations.
- We would still want to rule out a bleeding ulcer or gastritis, malignancy, celiac, or infectious causes.

What studies should we order next to investigate?

- The following tests should be considered: Complete Blood Count (CBC), Complete Metabolic Panel (CMP), stool culture, stool ova & parasites (O&P), fecal leukocytes and calprotectin, Erythrocyte Sedimentation Rate (ESR), C-reactive Protein (CRP), IgA tissue transglutaminase Antibody (TTG IgA), and Thyroid Stimulating Hormone (TSH), and proceed with a referral to a gastroenterologist to perform upper endoscopy and colonoscopy. Consider also H.pylori testing and HLA-B27 testing.

Lab Results:

CBC:

Lab	Value	Reference range
WBC	10.4 cells × 10^3/mm	4.0–10.9 cells × 10^3/mm
Neutrophils	55%	40–80%
Lymphocytes	30%	12–40%
Monocytes	8%	4–12%
Eosinophils	6%	0–8%
Basophils	1%	0–2%
RBC	4.3 cells × 10^3/mm	4.5–5.9 cells × 10^3/mm
Hemoglobin	10.1 g/dL	13.0–17.0 g/dL
Hematocrit	31%	41–53%
MCV	76 um^3	80–100 um^3
MCHC	30 g/dL	32–36 g/dL
Platelets	500,000 /mm^3	150,000–400,000/mm^3

CMP:

Lab	Value	Reference range
Na	137 mEq/L	135–147 mEq/L
Cl	109 mEq/L	95–105 mEq/L
K	3.2 mEq/L	3.5–5.0 mEq/L
HCO3	18 mEq/L	22–28 mEq/L
Mg	1.3 mg/dL	1.5–2.5 mg/dL
Ca	8.6 mg/dL	8.5–10.3 mg/dL
BUN	25 mg/dL	7–23 mg/dL
Cr	1.0 mg/dL	0.6–1.3 mg/dL
Glucose	90 mg/dL	70–99 mg/dL
AST	20 U/L	10–40 U/L
ALT	23 U/L	7–56 U/L
Alkaline Phos.	47 U/L	44–147 U/L
Total protein	5.8 g/dL	6.1–7.9 g/dL
Albumin	2.7 g/dL	3.5–5.5 g/dL

TSH: 2.0 mIU/L (reference: 0.4–4.0 mIU/L)
Rapid HIV: negative
ESR: 70 mm/hr. (reference: 0–22 mm/hr)
C-reactive protein: 65 mg/L (reference: 0–10 mg/L)

TTG IgA: Negative

Stool microscopy: No cysts or trophozoites visualized

Stool O&P: Negative

Stool culture: No growth

Stool C. difficile toxin: negative

Stool Shiga toxin: negative

Stool E. histolytica antigen: negative

Stool leukocytes: positive (reference: negative)

Fecal calprotectin: positive (reference: negative)

This patient has a microcytic anemia, likely iron deficiency given the gastrointestinal bleeding. Platelet elevation is often seen in inflammatory states. The patient's diarrhea is causing a loss of bicarbonate (HCO_3^-) and potassium (K^+). The loss of HCO_3^- relative to chloride (Cl^-) is contributing to the hyperchloremic metabolic acidosis with a normal anion gap (even when corrected for low albumin). Inflammatory markers (ESR, CRP) are elevated, along with stool inflammatory markers (fecal calprotectin and leukocytes) that are abnormal.

Colonoscopy Report:

Gross appearance: Mucosal surface irregular, friable, and erythematous, with loss of the normal vascular and haustral markings and extensive circumferential ulceration, extending in a continuous segment proximally from the rectum to the splenic flexure. Occasional pseudopolyps noted throughout this area.

Histology: Biopsies obtained from rectum, descending colon, and sigmoid colon are notable for mucosal and submucosal inflammatory infiltrate within crypt lumen (cryptitis). Moderate crypt distortion and atrophy are present. No granulomas present.

Findings from the colonoscopy favor the diagnosis of ulcerative colitis.

Note this is a distinction from the findings of Crohn's disease on colonoscopy, which present in a discontinuous pattern, and histologic biopsy, in which we may more commonly see findings of granuloma.

Questions to consider:

- What is ulcerative colitis, and how does it differ from other forms of IBD?
- What is the long-term prognosis? How is this treated?
- What preventive measures should be taken?
- What complications should we be monitoring for?

Further lab results:

HLA B27: positive

What disease states is this commonly associated with?

- Ankylosing spondylitis, anterior uveitis, ulcerative colitis, reactive arthritis, psoriatic arthritis

Clinical Course:

The patient's presentation being consistent with moderate-to-severe ulcerative colitis, treatment is begun with an anti-tumor necrosis factor (TNF) agent, infliximab, along with an immunomodulator, Azathioprine, and a course of oral glucocorticoids to induce remission of the current flare. Prior to initiating these medications, he receives a negative screening test for tuberculosis and hepatitis. Over the next several days to weeks, his abdominal pain began to subside, and his bowel movements began to return to normal. Under management of a gastroenterologist, he is able to taper off the steroid course after several weeks and is continued on Infliximab therapy for maintenance. His colonoscopy is repeated in 6 months and shows improvement in disease severity, warranting discontinuation of the immunomodulator while continuing Infliximab.

He is referred to an ophthalmologist for evaluation and management of possible uveitis/episcleritis, as well as a rheumatologist for workup of ankylosing spondylitis. He expresses understanding of the importance of maintaining regular follow-up with his primary care doctor and specialists.

One year later

MM is brought to the emergency department by ambulance after his partner returned home from a trip to the grocery store and found him collapsed but somewhat arousable on the floor of the bathroom. He is alert but drowsy in the emergency department and can briefly tell you that he had developed severe, diffuse, disabling abdominal pain over the past day, associated with over ten episodes of diarrhea, which has occasionally been bloody. His partner states MM's ulcerative colitis has otherwise been previously well-controlled on his current medication regimen, and he maintains regular follow-up with his primary care physician, gastroenterologist, and other sub-specialists.

Exam:

- Vital Signs:
  - Temperature: 102.3 F.
  - Pulse: 125 beats per minute.
  - Blood Pressure: 86/52.
  - Respirations: 16.
  - Oxygen saturation: 98% on room air.
- General: Alert but drowsy. Oriented to self and place but not time. Pale and uncomfortable-appearing. Writhing around in bed.
- Head/Ears/Eyes/Nose/Throat: Head normocephalic, atraumatic. Dry oral mucosa.
- Heart: Tachycardic, regular rhythm. No murmurs.
- Lungs: Clear to auscultation bilaterally.
- Abdomen: Tense, mildly distended. Diffuse tenderness to minimal palpation, generally not cooperative with extensive examination of the abdomen.

What might be happening? What should you be most concerned about emergently?

- Consider complications of ulcerative colitis such as bowel perforation or toxic megacolon.

Plain upright abdominal film is obtained and shows distention of the transverse colon associated with mucosal edema. The maximum transverse diameter of the transverse colon is 7.5 cm. No free air under the diaphragm is noted. A CBC is notable for an elevated white blood cell (WBC) count with a left shift and microcytic anemia. A diagnosis of toxic megacolon is made.

A decision is made to proceed with emergent total abdominal colectomy with end ileostomy. He later undergoes a completion proctectomy with reconstruction.

End of Case

Learning Objective 1: Explain the pathophysiology of ulcerative colitis and how it compares to that of Crohn's disease, with particular attention to how each disease process affects the histologic layers of gastrointestinal mucosa. Locate where within the gastrointestinal tract each disease process predominates.

IBD is an idiopathic condition which may be triggered by an overactive immune reaction against the gut microbiome. There are two major classifications of IBD—ulcerative colitis (UC) and Crohn's disease (CD)—each with unique features. Disruptions in inflammatory mediator pathways in genetically susceptible hosts likely influence the development of these conditions. While the exact triggering event is not well understood, this process is thought to be mediated by Helper T cells, type 1 (Th-1) in Crohn's disease, as opposed to Helper T cells, type 2 (Th-2) in UC [10].

Ulcerative colitis, as its name suggests, is limited to affecting the colon and always involves the rectum. Its involvement affects the mucosa in a continuous fashion extending proximally from the rectum. Inflammation of the gastrointestinal tract lining leads to formation of ulcers, bleeding, swelling of the colonic mucosa, and fluid and electrolyte loss. Damage in UC is limited to the mucosal and submucosal layers of the gastrointestinal lining. About a quarter of UC cases remain limited to the rectum, whereas ten percent of individuals may experience 'pancolitis,' meaning the entirety of the colon is diseased [7, 10].

Crohn's disease (CD), contrarily, involves inflammation and stricture formation that may affect any segment of the gastrointestinal tract from the mouth to the anus, occurring in a discontinuous fashion throughout the gastrointestinal tract in a manner referred to as 'skip lesions.' The inflammatory process in Crohn's disease is transmural, in other words, passing through all layers of the gastrointestinal mucosal wall, which is another distinguishing feature from UC. This can lead to the development of clinical manifestations of fissures and fistulae. Although the rectum is often spared from the inflammatory disease process, complications including anorectal fistula and abscess are not uncommon features of Crohn's disease.

Learning Objective 2. Define and understand the mechanisms of secretory, osmotic, and inflammatory diarrhea, highlighting common conditions associated with each. Compose a diagnostic algorithm to approach chronic diarrhea in the primary care setting.

Diarrhea is generally defined as chronic if it lasts for more than 4 weeks in duration. There are multiple ways to categorize diarrhea based on its quality or the underlying pathophysiologic processes at play. Often, overlapping types of diarrhea may coexist in various conditions [1].

Three qualitative categories for diarrhea include watery, fatty (malabsorptive), and inflammatory (containing fecal white blood cells/leukocytes, inflammatory markers such as lactoferrin or calprotectin, or blood). Watery diarrhea may then further be categorized into osmotic, secretory, or functional. In the primary care setting, where the differential diagnosis of diarrhea can be quite broad, using the qualitative categorization of diarrhea first can help narrow down the diagnostic approach and drive a more thoughtful series of testing.

For example, descriptions of diarrhea as 'fatty' may include floating stool (steatorrhea) along with other symptoms suggesting a malabsorptive process, such as bloating. Common conditions that involve fatty diarrhea include lactose intolerance, celiac disease, and infectious processes like giardia, all of which can limit the surface area and capability for fluid absorption by the gastrointestinal tract [1, 2].

Inflammatory diarrhea may manifest as frank blood or pus in the stool. Diarrheal conditions categorized as inflammatory include UC, Crohn's disease, colorectal malignancy, or various types of invasive gastrointestinal infections, including C. difficile secondary to antibiotic use. Further exploration of inflammatory diarrhea should involve obtaining stool inflammatory markers such as a fecal calprotectin level and, pending this result, endoscopic evaluation if the result is abnormal.

Watery diarrhea can be further categorized into osmotic, secretory, or functional on the basis of a fecal osmotic gap.

Osmotic diarrhea, characterized by a high fecal osmotic gap, occurs when nonabsorbable solutes are present in the intestines, drawing more water into the lumen. Lactase deficiency, creating an inability for the body to properly absorb lactose molecules, or use of osmotic laxatives or antacids are common examples of this type of diarrhea. Patients may note improvement of symptoms with fasting.

Secretory diarrhea occurs due to excess fluid secretion by intestinal crypt cells. This excess fluid volume can overwhelm the intestinal absorptive capacity and is characterized by a low fecal osmotic gap and high stool volume. Various infectious pathogens are common culprits, as well as stimulant laxatives, endocrine disorders such as hyperthyroidism, which increases gastrointestinal motility, neuroendocrine tumors, and gastrointestinal surgical procedures. Symptoms related to secretory diarrhea may thereby persist despite fasting.

Functional diarrhea may present with smaller stool volume and a normal fecal osmotic gap. Symptoms are uncommon at night. Irritable bowel syndrome is the most common cause of this type of diarrhea.

Learning Objective 3. Understand the electrolyte imbalances that occur with diarrhea and how they impact acid-base status.

Epithelial cells that line the colon contain sodium channels lining the colonic lumen. These channels are induced by the hormone aldosterone, leading to increased sodium absorption. The basolateral membrane is lined with sodium-potassium-ATPase transporters, which take in the absorbed sodium in exchange for releasing potassium back to the lumen [2].

Normal stool composition is alkaline in pH and contains primarily sodium, potassium, and the major inorganic anion, bicarbonate. Diarrhea causes a decrease in extracellular fluid volume, decrease in intravascular volume, and decreased arterial pressure [4, 5]. The renin–angiotensin II–aldosterone system is activated in attempt to restore blood pressure, but this will be unsuccessful if too much volume is lost and/or too rapidly. In addition to loss of potassium through the gastrointestinal lumen by increased activation of the Na-K-ATPase transport system as mediated by aldosterone, loss of bicarbonate is seen in diarrhea due to high concentration of this in typical gastrointestinal fluids. A loss of bicarbonate relative to chloride causes normal anion gap hyperchloremic metabolic acidosis, along with hypokalemia due to loss of potassium. Renal tubular acidosis follows a similar pattern of hyperchloremic metabolic acidosis, which makes intuitive sense as the cellular mechanisms at the level of the colon are like those of the cells that line the renal tubular cells in the kidney.

Less common electrolyte derangements that may be seen in diarrhea would be metabolic alkalosis in certain congenital forms of diarrhea or in cases of chronic laxative use. Hypernatremia is also an uncommon presentation of diarrhea that may occur in patients with an abnormal thirst response.

Learning Objective 4. Review the gastrointestinal and extraintestinal manifestations of ulcerative colitis. Compare and contrast these with the manifestations of Crohn's disease. Recognize common complications associated with each disease.
The clinical presentations of UC and Crohn's disease can be quite variable in their gastrointestinal and extraintestinal manifestations [7, 9]. There are some shared along with unique distinguishing features of each disease. Although different locations within the gastrointestinal tract may be affected in Crohn's disease as compared to UC, episodic relapsing gastrointestinal symptoms such as diarrhea, fever, abdominal pain, and bloody stool to varying degrees of severity can commonly characterize both disorders. Iron deficiency anemia may develop as a result of blood loss in both, along with electrolyte or other nutrient derangements.

Fibrosing strictures, particularly in the ileum, are seen in Crohn's disease and can lead to complications of bowel obstruction, whereas stricture formation would be rarely seen in UC. Also unique to Crohn's disease, fistulae can develop between bowel loops and may also involve other organs, including the bladder, vagina, and abdominal or perianal skin, predisposing patients to various infections at these sites.

UC is known for producing a greater degree of pseudopolyp formation and more superficial but broad-based mucosal ulcerations as compared to the deeper ulcers seen in Crohn's disease. Non-caseating granuloma formation, thought to be mediated by Th1 cells, is seen on histologic evaluation of the colon in Crohn's disease.

Given the gastrointestinal manifestations in UC are isolated to the colon, colectomy is curative (albeit invasive) as a treatment option, although extraintestinal manifestations would still persist.

Both disease states are associated with a higher risk of development of colon cancer. UC can be associated with the development of the life-threatening gastrointestinal complication of toxic megacolon. The highest risk of this occurring is early in the course of disease, and it presents as a patient with altered sensorium, peritonitis, and signs of high fever, hypotension, tachycardia, leukocytosis, and severe electrolyte disturbance, along with radiographs showing colonic distension. Colon perforation may occur as a result of this, and colectomy is sometimes required if intensive supportive treatment is ineffective.

Extraintestinal manifestations of IBD are common, affecting approximately a third of patients at some point in their disease process. Similar to gastrointestinal manifestations, there are some overlapping and some distinguishing features between UC and Crohn's disease.

- The most common extraintestinal manifestation for both is some form of arthritis—whether migratory polyarthritis or ankylosing spondylitis—as well as other musculoskeletal complications, including osteoporosis.
- Psychiatric conditions such as depression are also common in both in the context of living with a chronic disabling disease.
- Ocular complications of uveitis or episcleritis and skin conditions such as erythema nodosum, pyoderma gangrenosum, and aphthous ulcers are seen in both.
- Nephrolithiasis and cholelithiasis would be more commonly seen associated with Crohn's disease.
- Although iron deficiency may be seen in both conditions due to blood loss, vitamin B12 deficiency may be more commonly identified in Crohn's disease due to the vitamin being absorbed in the small intestine, which Crohn's disease rather than UC affects.
- Cholangitis is a potential complication in both Crohn's disease and UC, but it is more common in the latter.

Learning Objective 5. Summarize acute and long-term medical and surgical treatment options for inflammatory bowel disease based on disease staging.

Several treatment options exist for IBD, including medications or surgical management, and the decision on how to treat varies based on the severity of disease, whether treating Crohn's disease or UC, and if the patient is in a status of treating an active flare to induce remission or maintenance to prevent flares. Often, a "top-down" approach to using biologic or immunomodulator treatment early in the disease process is used in more moderate-to-severe cases [10].

Aminosalicylates, such as 5-aminosalicylic acid, are a common first-line therapy to treat IBD flares and maintain remission and can be administered orally or rectally. Aminosalicylates are more effective in treating UC as compared to Crohn's disease. They are thought to work by modulating the inflammatory response, although the exact mechanism of action is not precisely known.

For IBD flares of moderate severity, corticosteroid tapers are often used to achieve remission; however, they are not useful in long-term maintenance of disease. Antibiotics have not been found helpful in treatment of disease flares and may have undesirable side effects, which can include the risk of development of C. difficile infection. Anti-diarrheal medications should be avoided in times of acute flares, as these can induce the complication of toxic megacolon.

In addition to those with severe disease at onset, other candidates for more advanced medical approaches with anti-TNF monoclonal antibodies and immunomodulator medications may include those who develop frequent flares multiple times per year, flares that require more prolonged steroid use, or in whom flares have become refractory to steroids. Many of these medications can be used to induce and maintain remission in both UC and Crohn's disease. Prior to starting biologic therapy, patients should be screened for hepatitis and tuberculosis.

Surgical treatment is not a common first-line option in IBD. Colectomy would not be curative in Crohn's disease as it may be for UC, given the potential for Crohn's disease to affect all areas of the gastrointestinal tract. However, surgical management may be indicated for patients who develop disease that is refractory to medical management, in the identification of precancerous or cancerous changes, or when other complications of the disease arise, such as colonic perforation, toxic megacolon, or in the treatment of strictures and fistulas.

Learning Objective 6. Identify the incidence, prevalence, risk factors for, and prognosis of inflammatory bowel disease

IBD is common, affecting an estimated 1–2 million individuals in the United States, with an incidence of approximately 70–150 diagnoses made per 100,000 individuals per year [10]. Crohn's disease is equally as common as UC. Males and females are roughly equally affected, with a slightly greater preponderance in females. Morbidity is common, as evidenced by IBD accounting for 100,000 hospitalizations annually. Most cases are diagnosed in young adulthood, between ages of 15 and 40. Tobacco smoking appears to be a risk factor for development of and lack of response to treatment in Crohn's disease, though interestingly there is no correlation between tobacco use and development of UC.

There is a small increase in all-cause mortality in patients with IBD as compared to the general population, mostly driven by the disease itself, although infection risk may also play a role.

Predilection for future flares, disease relapse, and complications of the disease can be variable in both UC and Crohn's disease. Roughly half of patients with UC may have a flare over a 2-year period, though some patients go decades without flares while others exist in a state of persistent disease. Crohn's disease patients may have a lower quality of life than their UC counterparts, perhaps due to the more predictable expectation of a higher rate of disease relapse, which is estimated to be a 90% chance of disease relapse over a decade. The risk of colon cancer is increased in UC patients compared to the general population and for those with Crohn's disease if the colon is affected.

Learning Objective 7. Discuss recommendations for appropriate preventive care and screening measures for patients with inflammatory bowel disease.

IBD patients are at higher risk of developing cancer compared to the general population, specifically colorectal cancer if the colon is affected with prolonged disease in both UC and Crohn's disease, and small bowel malignancy in Crohn's disease patients [6, 10]. Therefore, the current recommendation is to screen patients with IBD for colon cancer with colonoscopy every 1–3 years beginning no later than 8–10 years after the diagnosis is made, ideally when the patient is in disease remission.

Screening for osteoporosis should be considered in patients with prolonged or frequent steroid use and in postmenopausal women.

Patients with IBD may be at risk of malnutrition; therefore, screening for and treating various vitamin deficiencies, such as iron, vitamin B12, and vitamin D, may be necessary [3, 10].

Exam Questions

1. A 27-year-old male presents to clinic with a six-week history of abdominal pain associated with occasional bloody diarrhea. After obtaining a stool sample that is positive for blood, he later undergoes colonoscopy to evaluate the source of bleeding. Colonoscopy reveals circumferential ulceration present in a continuous pattern from the rectum to sigmoid colon. Which of the following is accurate regarding treatment for his likely underlying disease?
   A. Immunomodulators are ineffective.
   B. Anti-diarrheal medications are a useful component of the treatment plan.
   C. Patients may have a moderate response to aminosalicylate therapy.
   D. Colectomy is not curative.
   E. Corticosteroids are effective maintenance therapy.

Answer: C

Learning Objective: 5

Explanation: Aminosalicylates treat ulcerative colitis because they act topically on the colonic mucosa to reduce inflammation by inhibiting prostaglandin and leukotriene synthesis, scavenging free radicals, and modulating cytokine production, thereby decreasing the abnormal immune-driven inflammation characteristic of the disease. A is incorrect: Immunomodulator therapy has shown to be very effective in the treatment of IBD. They are typically administered in advanced disease, however some advocate beginning with a "top down" approach to treatment that utilizes immunomodulator therapy early in the disease course. B is incorrect as anti-diarrheal medications can precipitate toxic megacolon in IBD. D is incorrect as although uncommonly used as a first-line treatment option, colectomy is curative in ulcerative colitis. E is incorrect as corticosteroids are useful for flares only and should not be used long-term as maintenance therapy.

2. After eating a burrito from your favorite take-out venue, you have been suffering from intractable diarrhea for the past two days. What fluid, electrolyte, and acid-base abnormalities would most likely be present?
   A. Hypokalemia, hypovolemia, non-anion gap metabolic acidosis
   B. Hypokalemia, hypovolemia, high anion-gap metabolic acidosis
   C. Hyperkalemia, hypovolemia, non-anion gap metabolic acidosis
   D. Hypochloremia, hypovolemia, metabolic alkalosis
   E. Hyperchloremia, hypovolemia, metabolic alkalosis

Answer: A

Learning Objective: 3

Explanation: Normal function of colon is K+ secretion, so in diarrhea the loss of K+ is exacerbated leading to development of hypokalemia. High flow rate and volume loss causes hypovolemia in addition to hypokalemia. Stool also has high [HCO3−], among other measurable anions, so its loss leads to a non-anion gap metabolic acidosis. More bicarbonate is lost relative to Cl-, so the resulting acidosis is considered hyperchloremic. B is incorrect as while diarrhea is associated with hypokalemia and hypovolemia, anion gap metabolic acidosis is associated with a gain of unmeasurable anions such as lactic acid or ketoacids. C is incorrect as diarrhea is associated with hypokalemia, not hyperkalemia. See above. D is incorrect as this would be the expected response to vomiting, not diarrhea. E is incorrect as diarrhea leads to a metabolic acidosis, not commonly alkalosis.

3. A 27-year-old male presents to clinic with a six-week history of abdominal pain associated with occasional bloody diarrhea. After obtaining a stool sample that is positive for blood, he later undergoes colonoscopy to evaluate the source of bleeding. Colonoscopy reveals circumferential ulceration present in a continuous pattern from the rectum to sigmoid colon. The pathophysiology of this disease involves which of the following?
   A. The pathophysiology involves transmural inflammation.
   B. The pathology is mediated by Th2 cells.
   C. The pathophysiology involves granulomatous inflammation.
   D. The pathology involves any part of the GI tract from mouth to anus.
   E. Reactive Oxygen Species are considered the main underlying mechanism of disease pathology.

Answer: C

Learning Objectives: 1 & 4

Explanation: The main pathophysiologic feature of ulcerative colitis is continuous, superficial mucosal inflammation of the colon starting in the rectum and extending proximally, mediated by an abnormal Th2 cell immune response. A is incorrect as this is a pathophysiologic feature of Crohn's disease, not ulcerative colitis. C is incorrect as this is a feature of the pathophysiology of Crohn's disease, not ulcerative colitis. D is incorrect as this is a pathophysiologic feature of Crohn's disease, not ulcerative colitis. E is incorrect as reactive oxygen species are not a proposed mechanism of disease pathophysiology in either form of IBD.

References

1. Burgers K, Lindberg B, Bevis ZJ. Chronic diarrhea in adults: evaluation and differential diagnosis. Am Fam Physician. 2020;101:472–80.
2. Costanzo L. Costanzo physiology. 5th ed. Elsevier Saunders; 2013.
3. DeLegge MH. Nutrition and dietary management for adults with inflammatory bowel disease. In: UpToDate. 2023. https://www.uptodate.com/contents/nutrition-and-dietary-management-for-adults-with-inflammatory-bowel-disease?search=https%3A%2F%2Fwww-

uptodate-com.ezproxy1.library.arizona.edu%2Fcontents%2Fnutrition-and-dietary-interventions-in-adults-with-inflammatory-bowel-disease%3Fsource%3Dsee_link%23H3594247&source=search_result&selectedTitle=1%7E150&usage_type=default&display_rank=1. Accessed 19 June 2024.
4. Emmett M, Palmer BF. Acid-base and electrolyte abnormalities with diarrhea. In: UpToDate. 2022. https://www.uptodate.com/contents/acid-base-and-electrolyte-abnormalities-with-diarrhea?search=acid+base+electrolyte+abnormalities+diarrhea&source=search_result&selectedTitle=1~150&usage_type=default&display_rank=1. Accessed 19 Jun 2024.
5. Emmett M, Szerlip H. Approach to the adult with metabolic acidosis. In: UpToDate. 2023. https://www.uptodate.com/contents/approach-to-the-adult-with-metabolic-acidosis?search=approach-to-the-adult-with-metabolic-acidosis%3Fsource%3Dsee_link&source=search_result&selectedTitle=1~150&usage_type=default&display_rank=1. Accessed 19 June 2024.
6. Farraye FA, Odze RD, Eaden J, Itzkowitz SH. AGA medical position statement on the diagnosis and management of colorectal neoplasia in inflammatory bowel disease. Gastroenterology. 2010;138:738–45. https://doi.org/10.1053/j.gastro.2009.12.037.
7. Kumar V, Abbas AK, Aster JC, Fausto N. Robbins & Cotran: pathologic basis of disease. 8th ed. Elsevier Saunders; 2009.
8. Lee JM, Lee K-M. Endoscopic diagnosis and differentiation of inflammatory bowel disease. Clin Endosc. 2016;49:370–5. https://doi.org/10.5946/ce.2016.090.
9. Peppercorn MA, Kane SV. Clinical manifestations, diagnosis, and prognosis of ulcerative colitis in adults. In: UpToDate. 2024. https://www.uptodate.com/contents/clinical-manifestations-diagnosis-and-prognosis-of-ulcerative-colitis-in-adults?search=%2Fclinical-manifestations-diagnosis-and-prognosis-of-ulcerative-colitis-in-+adult&source=search_result&selectedTitle=1~150&usage_type=default&display_rank=1. Accessed 19 June 2024.
10. Rowe WA. Inflammatory bowel disease. In: Inflammatory Bowel Disease. 2020. https://emedicine.medscape.com/article/179037-overview?form=login. Accessed 19 June 2024.

Part VII

Endocrine

Elevated Pressures 19

Philip Yue-Cheng Cheung
and Steven Osmond Han

Learning Objectives:

1. Review the normal control and function of the renin-angiotensin-aldosterone system. Explain the mechanism of the hypokalemic metabolic alkalosis observed in this patient.
2. Diagram the synthesis pathways for hormones produced in the adrenal gland, including catecholamines, aldosterone, cortisol, and sex steroids. Distinguish the anatomic zones in which these reactions occur.
3. Differentiate the most common etiologies of hyperaldosteronism. Describe methods to distinguish between these causes.
4. Provide a differential diagnosis for incidentally discovered adrenal masses. Describe an appropriate approach for the workup of adrenal incidentaloma.
5. Discuss the ramifications of our decision to choose a calcium channel blocker (CCB)/angiotensin-converting-enzyme inhibitor (ACEI) combination as first-line therapy for this patient rather than a thiazide diuretic. How might the management of and outcome for this patient have changed?

Chief Complaint: "They said my blood pressure is high. Also, I had the stomach flu."

P. Y.-C. Cheung (✉) · S. O. Han
Department of Radiology, Lewis Katz School of Medicine at Temple University/St. Luke's University Health Network, Bethlehem, PA, USA
e-mail: philip.cheung@sluhn.org; steven.han@sluhn.org

HPI:

JH is a 38-year-old man who presents today to your primary care clinic for high blood pressure. He went to a workplace health screening yesterday after lunch, where he had his blood pressure, blood sugar, and cholesterol checked. He was told that his blood pressure and sugars were high, and that he should follow up with a doctor.

His health screening paperwork shows:

BP 154/90, glucose 215, HDL 48, and LDL 129.

Ask students about the glucose level. They should recognize that JH was screened after lunch (i.e., a non-fasting level), and that this reading cannot be interpreted for the presence or absence of diabetes.

In your office today, vital signs are

BP 158/95, P 88, R 11, T 37.0 °C

Students should immediately notice that the blood pressure remains high.

The low respiratory rate reflects compensation for an acid-base disturbance.

They are *highly* unlikely to notice the slow respiratory rate of 11 (normal is 12–20, though it is almost universally logged as 14–16 because we rarely look for it). If they do not comment on the respiratory rate, consider letting it go and revisiting the missed abnormal vital signs later in the case. If they do notice it, discuss it later in the context of this patient's vomiting.

C. A. Standley (ed.), *Biomedical Science and Clinical Foundations*,
https://doi.org/10.1007/978-3-031-98353-5_19

Stop and Think:

What symptoms will you want to ask JH about?

With a BP this high, students should consider whether this may be hypertensive urgency or emergency. They should consider the symptoms of end-organ damage (primarily in the brain, eyes, lungs, heart, and kidneys).

Reasonable ROS includes headache, confusion, dyspnea, cough, chest pain/discomfort, and changes in urination.

Further History:

He is a generally healthy, athletic man. He recently got the "stomach flu." He experienced 3 days of non-bloody, non-bilious emesis, 4 times per day, which stopped the afternoon before his wellness screening. He is now experiencing some mild diarrhea.

He had not been able to keep much food down for the three days of nausea and vomiting but now has a slight appetite. He is staying hydrated.

He says that he normally would not see a doctor so quickly over his blood pressure, but he wanted to get checked out for the stomach flu, which has made him miserable.

Review of Systems:

General: No fevers, chills, or weight change. Still feels a little sick.

Chest: No dyspnea, cough, or wheezing

CV: No chest discomfort, palpitations

GI: Nausea/emesis improving. Mild diarrhea without hematochezia or melena.

GU: No hematuria

Endo: No heat/cold intolerance, fatigue, polydipsia, or polyuria.

Neuro: No paresthesias

PMH: None

PSH: Appendectomy, age 12

FH:

Father: 68 y/o, hypertension

Mother: 64 y/o, hypertension

Sister: 40 y/o, no medical problems

SH:

Works in the purchasing department of a manufacturing firm; started at a new firm last year. The new firm requires health screenings.

Married, with 3 daughters (ages 8, 4, and 2). They are all in school/daycare.

ETOH: 3 drinks/week

Smoking: None

Drugs: None

Sex: Monogamous with wife. No history of sexually transmitted infections.

Objective

Height 5′10″, weight 160 lb.,

Vital signs: BP 158/95, P 88, R 11, T 37.0 °C

At this point, recognizing the patient's acute GI illness with repeated vomiting, students who have noted the slow respiratory rate should be guided to consider metabolic alkalosis resulting from the loss of stomach acid. If they do not notice this, consider revisiting it much later in the case when hyperaldosteronism is identified.

Physical Exam:

Gen: Well-appearing athletic male, alert, conversant, no acute distress.

Skin: Warm and dry.

HEENT: Normocephalic, atraumatic.

Eyes: Conjunctivae clear, sclerae anicteric. Pupils equal round, reactive to light and accommodation. Fundoscopy shows sharp disc margins and cup-to-disc ratio of <50%. Silver wiring and arteriovenous nicking were noted.

Ask students about the findings of silver wiring and arteriovenous (A/V) nicking, as they are consistent with chronic high blood pressure.

A/V nicking is seen at sites where retinal arteries and retinal veins overlap. Chronically elevated blood pressure in the retinal arterial system is thought to cause compensatory thickening of the vessel wall, thereby compressing the adjacent retinal vein and an engorged "hourglass" appearance of the vein. Students should be very familiar with this appearance and phenomenon.

Silver wiring is another sign of hypertensive retinopathy. Chronic hypertension results in sclerosis (thickening) of the retinal arteriolar walls. Progressive thickening results in increased optical density of the walls. Less advanced sclerosis of the retinal arterioles produces "copper wiring"—the visibly sclerotic walls adjacent to the red blood of the arteriole give a metallic tinge to the vessel, resembling copper wires. As the sclerosis progresses and encircles the vessel, the silvery metallic appearance is all that can be seen, producing silver wiring.

This is a good time to review the appearance of funduscopic findings.

Chest: Clear to auscultation bilaterally. Thoracic expansion is symmetric.

CV: Regular rate and rhythm. No murmurs, gallops, or rubs.

Abd: Soft, nondistended, nontender. No organomegaly or masses. Bowel sounds are hyperactive.

Neuro: Alert and oriented. No focal neurologic findings.

Extremities: Radial, dorsalis pedis, and posterior tibial pulses 2+ bilaterally.

What is JH's problem list today?

1. Gastroenteritis
2. High blood pressure/hypertension

Students should recognize gastroenteritis as the major complaint, given the presence of emesis followed by diarrhea. The patient's children, who are in school and daycare, are likely sources of infection.

The diagnosis of hypertension can be made given two distinct measurements of elevated pressure. Students will likely consider secondary causes of hypertension at this point, recognizing that it is the likely topic of this case. However, they should recognize that primary hypertension (with no known cause) represents 90% of all cases.

Management:

What labs do you want to order today? How would you like to treat JH?

1. Gastroenteritis—conservative management.
2. HTN—his pressures are quite high on two occasions, even with a GI illness that is more likely to decrease pressure than increase it. Additionally, the physical exam is consistent with hypertensive retinopathy. Given that his pressures are more than 20/10 above the goal, first-line combination therapy with a CCB and ACEI is appropriate. We will prescribe amlodipine/lisinopril as a first-line antihypertensive.
3. Labs—Given the high blood pressure, it is appropriate to screen for diabetes. We can also order a CBC/CMP. JH is fasting and does not want to miss more work; he agrees to have blood drawn at your in-clinic lab immediately after the visit.

   It is inappropriate to work up secondary causes of hypertension at this point. While a systolic blood pressure of over 160 or diastolic over 100 may justify screening for aldosteronism, he does not yet meet this threshold.

We will have JH follow up in 10 days to see if he is recovering, review his labs, and monitor his hypertension.

Follow-up visit:

CC: Follow-up

JH has fully recovered from his gastroenteritis and is feeling well with no symptoms. He filled his antihypertensive medication immediately after his visit and has been taking his medication as directed with no missed doses.

VS: **BP 162/94**, P 80, R 11, T 37.4 °C

The labs ordered at his prior visit have resulted, including a CBC, CMP, and hemoglobin A1c (Table 19.1).

Table 19.1 Initial laboratory results

	Patient values	Reference values
WBC	**11.7**	3.6–11.0 K/uL
RBC	5.7	4.5–5.9 M/uL
Hemoglobin	16.4	13.0–18.0 g/dL
Hematocrit	49	40–52%
MCV	92	81–97 fL
MCH	30	26–34 pg
MCHC	33	31–37 g/dL
RDW	14.0	11.5–15%
Platelets	340	150–400 K/uL

CMP:

	Patient values	Reference values
Sodium	141	135–145 mmol/L
Potassium	**3.2**	3.5–4.5 mmol/L
Chloride	**89**	95–110 mmol/L
CO_2	**40**	19–34 mmol/L
Glucose	108	70–110 mg/dL
BUN	18	6–22 mg/dL
Creatinine	1.1	0.6–1.3 mg/dL
Calcium	9.7	8.5–10.9 mg/dL
Protein	6.8	6.3–7.9 g/dL
Albumin	4.1	3.9–5.0 g/dL
Total bilirubin	1.6	0.3–1.9 mg/dL
Direct bilirubin	0.1	0–0.3 mg/dL
Alkaline phosphatase	87	44–147 IU/L
AST	18	8–37 IU/L
ALT	17	0–34 IU/L

Hemoglobin A1C: 5.5 mg/dL < 5.7 mg/dL

Stop and consider these results before proceeding.

CBC:

The mild leukocytosis here reflects an active infection at the point when the labs were drawn.

CMP:

Results are notable for a hypokalemic, hypochloremic metabolic alkalosis.

A somewhat subtle but important distinction should be made here for students. In a BMP/CMP, total CO_2 is measured—because the dominant fraction of CO_2 in the blood exists as bicarbonate, we are effectively measuring bicarbonate. While this measurement is often listed as HCO_3, it is not always. It is intentionally listed here as CO_2, in order to help them recognize this well before ever reaching the wards. This "CO_2" does NOT represent carbon dioxide as a blood gas but instead bicarbonate.

His labs show hypokalemia and hypochloremia. He also has elevated bicarbonate and a subtle finding of decreased respiratory rate, suggesting metabolic alkalosis with respiratory compensation. This all can be consistent with gastric losses given the immediately preceding several-day history of emesis.

Blood gases are not available to confirm metabolic alkalosis, as there would have been little clinical justification for ordering blood gases at the last visit.

His white count is mildly elevated as well, consistent with active infectious disease during his last office visit. Note that he now has normal glucose, as this is a set of fasting labs. The normal A1C excludes diabetes mellitus.

At this point, students have little to go on other than a confirmed diagnosis of hypertension, which is not responding well to a single medication. Students could be guided through a differential diagnosis of primary versus secondary hypertension.

Problem List:

1. Hypertension—Primary versus secondary
   Will increase the dose of amlodipine/lisinopril

Follow up in one month, with follow-up labs including blood gases in the interim.

Follow-up 2:

JH has been taking two antihypertensive drugs now, exactly as directed, with no missed doses. He has been reading about blood pressure and is starting to worry that it is so high. He has been regularly stopping at his neighborhood pharmacy to measure his pressures. He remembers his readings as usually above 160/80.

VS: BP 164/86, P 95, R 16, T 37.0 °C

Labs were obtained as planned prior to this follow-up visit, including repeat CBC, repeat CMP, and an arterial blood gas (ABG) [Table 19.2].

Table 19.2 Follow-up laboratory results

	Patient values	Reference values
WBC	9.7	3.6–11.0 K/uL
RBC	5.7	4.5–5.9 M/uL
Hemoglobin	16.4	13.0–18.0 g/dL
Hematocrit	49	40–52%
MCV	92	81–97 fL
MCH	30	26–34 pg
MCHC	33	31–37 g/dL
RDW	14.0	11.5–15%
Platelets	340	150–400 K/uL
Sodium	136	135–145 mmol/L
Potassium	**3.1**	3.5–4.5 mmol/L
Chloride	104	95–110 mmol/L
CO_2	**38**	19–34 mmol/L
Glucose	108	70–110 mg/dL
BUN	18	6–22 mg/dL
Creatinine	1.1	0.6–1.3 mg/dL
Calcium	9.7	8.5–10.9 mg/dL
Protein	6.8	6.3–7.9 g/dL
Albumin	4.1	3.9–5.0 g/dL
Total bilirubin	1.6	0.3–1.9 mg/dL
Direct bilirubin	0.1	0–0.3 mg/dL
Alkaline phosphatase	87	44–147 IU/L
AST	18	8–37 IU/L
ALT	17	0–34 IU/L

ABG:

	Patient values	Reference values
pH	**7.48**	7.35–7.45
$PaCO_2$	**49**	35–45 mmHg
PaO_2	90	80–95 mmHg
HCO_3	**37**	22–26 mEq/L

Stop and review these new lab results before proceeding.

CBC:

WBC has normalized given the resolution of his infection before these follow-up labs.

CMP: Confirmed hypokalemic metabolic alkalosis

ABG:

Students may need to be walked through the basics of ABG analysis again.

They should first look at the pH. The ABG shows a high pH, indicating alkalosis.

Next, they should qualitatively look at the $PaCO_2$ and HCO_3 to find an explanation for the acid-base disturbance, recognizing that the body does not "overshoot" in correcting a primary disturbance. Here, CO_2 is high, which would decrease pH, while bicarbonate is high, which would increase pH. Qualitatively, the elevated bicarbonate must then be the primary disturbance, indicating a metabolic cause for the alkalosis.

The CO_2 should be interpreted in this context; qualitatively, students will recognize that this likely represents a respiratory compensation for the primary metabolic alkalosis. This would be an appropriate time to call attention to the slow respiratory rate at this and prior visits. Calculating whether or not this is an appropriate level of compensation is probably more effort than needed at this point.

What are you considering now?

Continued hypokalemic metabolic alkalosis in the context of difficult-to-control hypertension should suggest aldosteronism. A screening test should be performed, followed by confirmatory tests if consistent.

Students should be prompted to consider whether our antihypertensive medications could have confounded the lab findings. In this case, a CCB/ACEI combination does not have significant electrolyte side effects, and the persistent hypokalemia is obvious and unexplained. However, thiazides are common and appropriate first-line antihypertensives that can cause hypokalemia.

If this patient had instead been started on a thiazide, and screening labs revealed hypokalemia, we would have explained the finding away as a medication effect. Many patients with aldosteronomas (including the patient who inspired this case) go decades with "difficult-to-treat hypertension" before an appropriate workup makes the diagnosis obvious.

What further tests should be considered?

Plasma aldosterone concentration (PAC) and peripheral plasma renin activity (PRA) are appropriate studies to evaluate for hyperaldosteronism (Table 19.3). Additionally, cortisol and urine metanephrines should be obtained to exclude

Table 19.3 Serum aldosterone and plasma renin activity results

	Patient values	Reference values
PAC	25	<15 ng/dL
PRA	0.4	>1.0 ng/mL/hour
PAC/PRA	62.5	<20

excess production of other hormones in the adrenal glands.

Elevated aldosterone level with reduced renin activity is consistent with pathologic and unstimulated aldosterone secretion, i.e., primary aldosteronism. However, this is only a screening test. The diagnosis should be confirmed by demonstrating inappropriate aldosterone secretion via an oral sodium loading test.

Cortisol and urine metanephrine levels were within normal limits.

Oral sodium loading test:

24-hour aldosterone urinary excretion = 50 nmol (<33)

An oral sodium loading test involves instructing the patient to consume a high-salt diet for three days before measuring 24-hour urinary aldosterone excretion. Alternatively, acute volume expansion with IV saline can be performed. The physiologic response to high salt levels should be to suppress the RAAS system, decreasing aldosterone levels. Non-suppression of aldosterone with an acute sodium load suggests that uncontrolled generation of aldosterone is the primary dysfunctional process.

The majority of cases (~2/3) of primary aldosteronism are a result of bilateral adrenal hyperplasia. In one-third of cases, an aldosterone-secreting adenoma is responsible. Other (rare) causes include unilateral adrenal hyperplasia, ectopic aldosterone-secreting tumors, aldosteronism responsive to glucocorticoids, and functional (hormone-secreting) adrenocortical carcinoma. Distinguishing the etiology of the primary aldosteronism is important, as the management of these conditions differs substantially. Aldosterone-secreting adenomas are managed surgically, whereas bilateral adrenal hyperplasia is necessarily managed medically.

Imaging:

Given laboratory evidence of hyperaldosteronism, a CT abdomen/pelvis was obtained for further imaging evaluation [Figs. 19.1 and 19.2].

The presence of a solitary >1.0 cm solid mass on the adrenal gland, normal contralateral adrenal gland, and the biochemical findings previously presented is consistent with aldosteronoma. As recently as 2005, sources considered this to be diagnostic of the condition and appropriate grounds for referral for surgical management.

However, adrenal vein sampling (to localize the source of biochemical abnormalities) has since returned to prominence as an important diagnostic step. More recent studies that assume adrenal vein sampling as the gold standard have demonstrated that adrenal vein sampling disagrees with cross-sectional imaging (CT or MRI) and changes management in up to 40% of cases.

Students are unlikely to recognize this point in the absence of prior exposure to the topic. It should be emphasized as a learning objective, as it substantially impacts patient management.

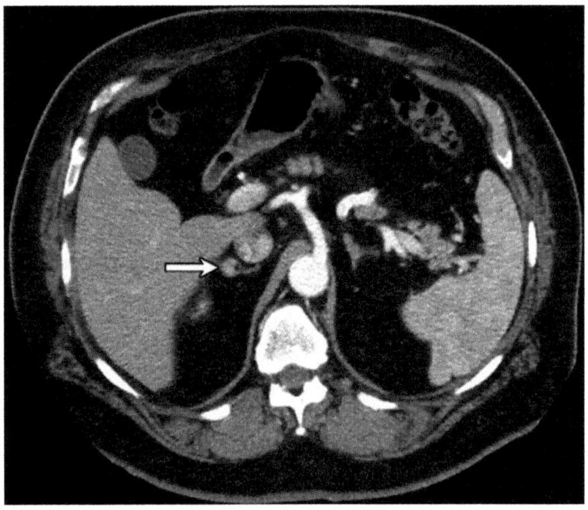

Fig. 19.1 Axial image from a CT abdomen/pelvis with intravascular contrast obtained for evaluation of hyperaldosteronism. A solitary 1.2 cm isodense mass is present on the right adrenal gland (white arrow), which was characterized as an adrenal adenoma on this CT study. The left adrenal gland appears normal. Copyright Dr. Steven Han

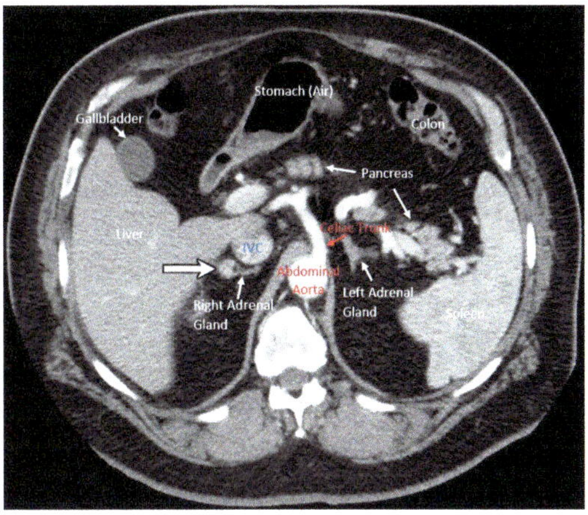

Fig. 19.2 Axial image from a CT abdomen/pelvis with intravascular contrast obtained for evaluation of hyperaldosteronism. A solitary 1.2 cm isodense mass is present on the right adrenal gland (white arrow). The left adrenal gland appears normal. Annotations have been added to identify additional anatomic structures. IV contrast administration can be seen by the bright abdominal aorta and contrast enhancement of the abdominal organs. Neither kidney is visible on this image, as the bilateral adrenal glands are positioned superior to the kidneys. Copyright Dr. Philip Cheung and Dr. Steven Han.

Adrenal Vein Sampling:

The patient is referred to interventional radiology for adrenal vein sampling. During this procedure, femoral venous access is obtained, and catheters are advanced to the right and left adrenal veins. The anatomy of the adrenal glands is demonstrated in Figs. 19.3 and 19.4. After confirming the appropriate catheter position with gentle contrast injections via the catheter (Fig. 19.5), a sample of blood is very gently aspirated from each adrenal vein. Subsequently, ACTH is administered. Most adenomas are sensitive to ACTH and respond to stimulation by increasing hormone secretion. In contrast, normal tissue should not respond to ACTH stimulation due to feedback inhibition by already high levels of circulating aldosterone.

A second sample of blood is aspirated from each of the adrenal veins after stimulation. Samples from the adrenal veins before and after stimulation, along with samples of peripheral

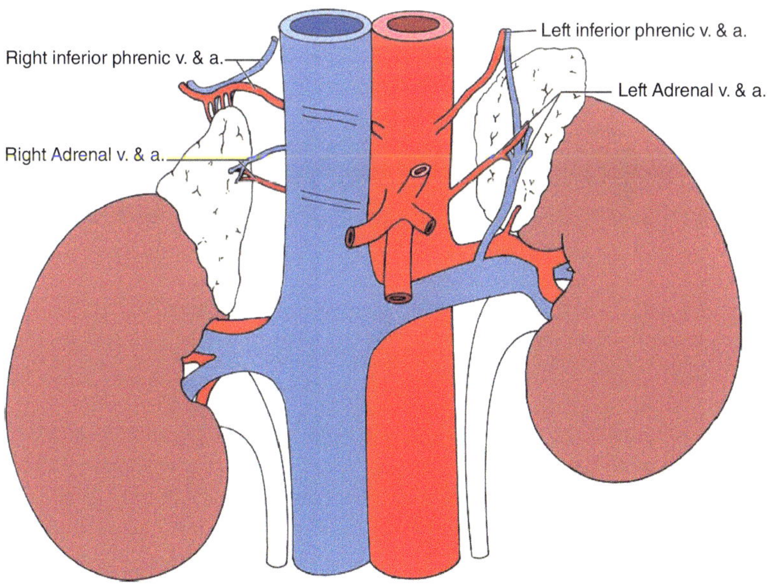

Fig. 19.3 Adrenal gland anatomy. (With permissions from: Kahn SL, Angle JF. Adrenal Vein Sampling. *Tech Vasc Interventional Rad. 2010(13):110–125* [1])

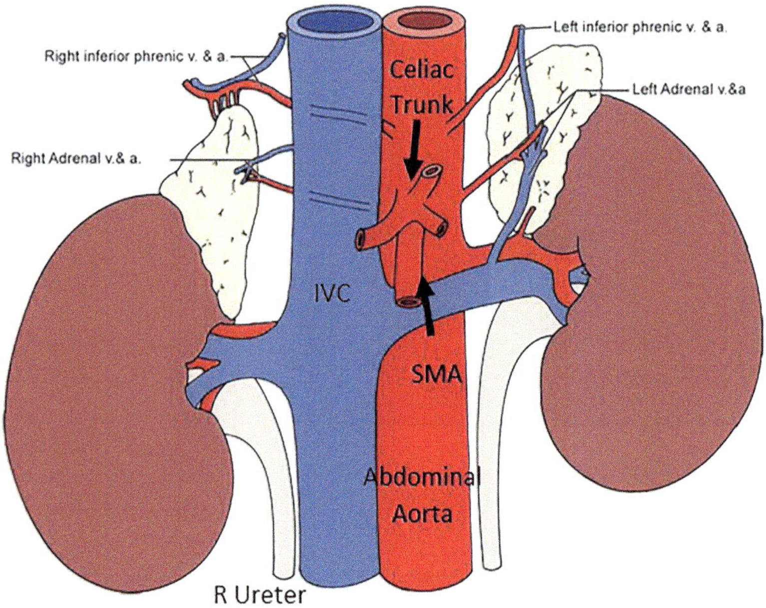

Fig. 19.4 Adrenal gland anatomy and regional vascular anatomy. (Modified from Fig. 19.5 in Kahn SL, Angle JF. Adrenal Vein Sampling. *Tech Vasc Interventional Rad. 2010(13):110–125* [1])

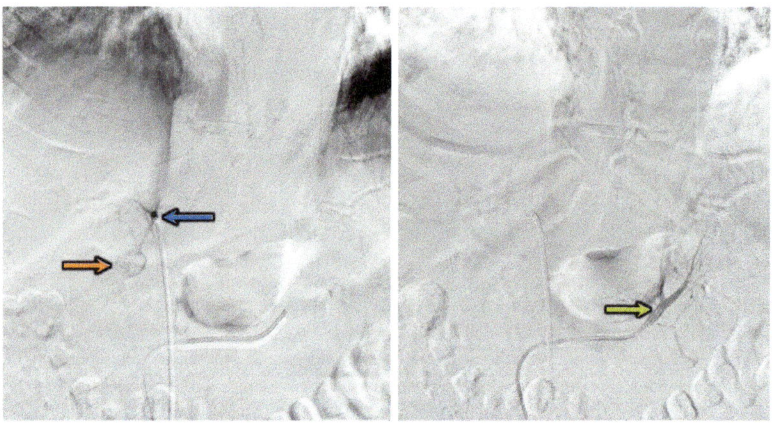

Fig. 19.5 Fluoroscopic images from an adrenal vein sampling procedure. Upon sequential injection of contrast through each catheter, the catheters are confirmed to be appropriately positioned in the R adrenal vein (blue arrow) and L adrenal vein (green arrow). Note the adrenal gland nodule (orange arrow). (Copyright Dr. Steven Han)

blood, are then separately labeled and sent for laboratory analysis.

Students could be asked to identify the anatomical structures in the illustration above, which is reproduced below with labels for major structures they should recognize.

If the students seem particularly comfortable with anatomy, they can be further prompted to identify the three branches of the celiac trunk on this image. The branch directed to the right is the common hepatic artery, the left branch is the splenic artery, and the branch directed superiorly is the left gastric artery.

Students should be shown this fluoroscopic image alongside the anatomical illustration above and should recall or become familiar with the asymmetric drainage of the adrenal veins. The R adrenal vein drains directly into the inferior vena cava; in contrast, the L adrenal vein drains into the L renal vein, which then crosses anterior to the abdominal aorta and inferior to the superior mesenteric artery to drain into the inferior vena cava.

Adrenal vein sampling at baseline confirms normal aldosterone levels at the L adrenal vein, with elevated aldosterone levels measured at the R adrenal vein. After ACTH administration, aldosterone levels remained normal in the L adrenal vein and further increased in the R adrenal vein, consistent with a right-sided aldosterone-secreting adrenal adenoma.

Definitive management:
This patient is referred to an appropriate regional surgical specialist (for example, an endocrine surgeon, urologist, or surgical oncologist) for right adrenalectomy, resulting in complete resolution of his hypokalemia and alkalosis. His hypertension improved significantly and is now well-managed on low-dose, single-agent therapy.

End of Case

Learning Objectives:

1. Review the normal control and function of the renin-angiotensin-aldosterone system. Explain the mechanism of the hypokalemic metabolic alkalosis observed in this patient.

   The renin-angiotensin-aldosterone system is shown in Fig. 19.6. Uncontrolled and excessive aldosterone secretion results in excessive urinary potassium losses (Fig. 19.7).

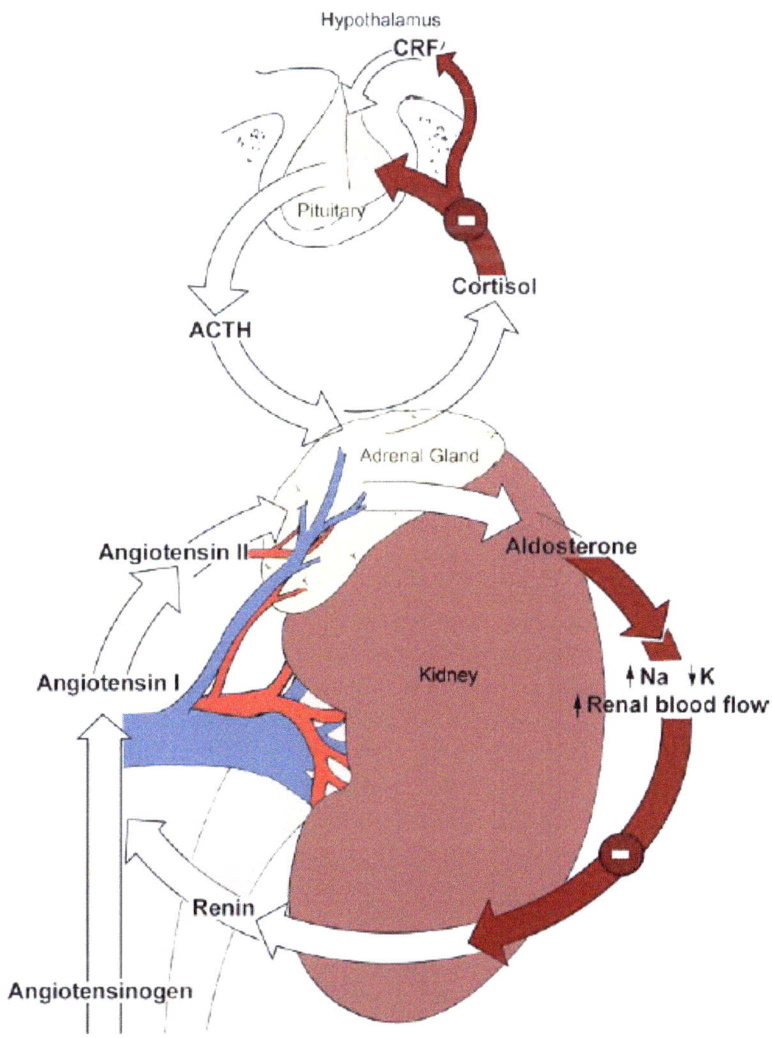

Fig. 19.6 Normal mineralocorticoid pathway. (With permissions from: Kahn SL, Angle JF. Adrenal Vein Sampling. *Tech Vasc Interventional Rad. 2010(13):110–125* [1])

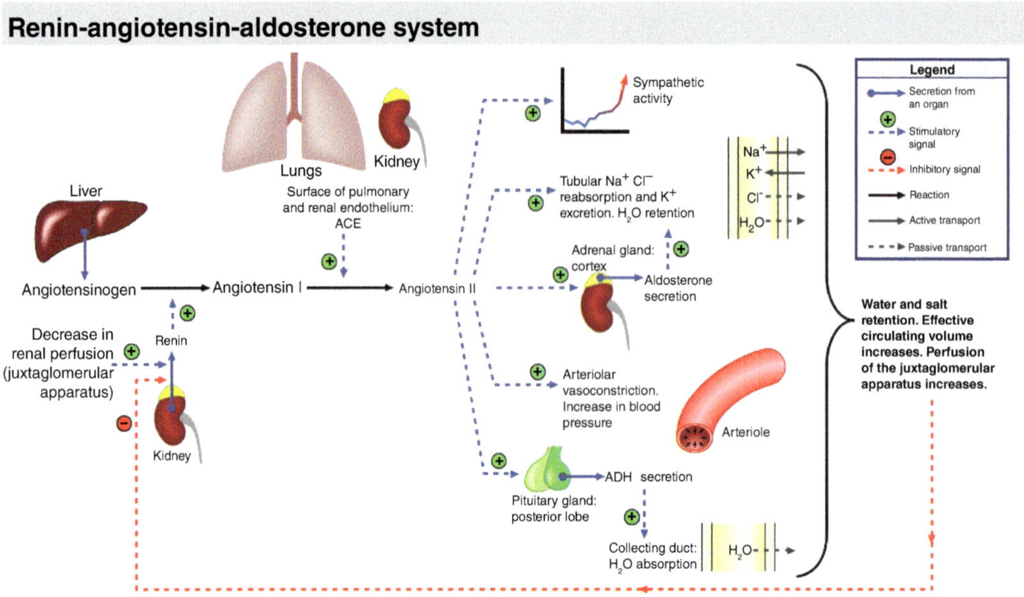

Fig. 19.7 Effects of the renin-angiotensin-aldosterone system. A. Rad, CC BY-SA 3.0 <http://creativecommons.org/licenses/by-sa/3.0/>, via Wikimedia Commons. https://commons.wikimedia.org/wiki/File:Renin-angiotensin-aldosterone_system.png

Aldosterone stimulates basolateral sodium/potassium pumps in the principal cells in the distal tubule and collecting duct in the renal nephron, promoting the resorption of 3 Na + ions in exchange for the excretion of 2 K+ ions into the urine. This is the primary source of hypokalemia.

Aldosterone directly increases the activity of H + -secreting pumps in the apical membrane in alpha-intercalated cells of the distal nephron, resorbing bicarbonate in exchange for chloride ions. This is one factor in the development of metabolic alkalosis.

Hypokalemia further contributes to metabolic alkalosis through two mechanisms:

- It causes potassium to move from cells into the ECF in exchange for sodium and hydrogen ions. This generates extracellular bicarbonate (contributing to alkalosis) and acidifies intracellular fluids. Acidification of intracellular fluid in the kidney stimulates further hydrogen secretion into the urine and bicarbonate reabsorption.
- Hypokalemia stimulates alpha-intercalated cells to attempt to reabsorb and conserve potassium by increasing hydrogen ion secretion into the urine.

2. Diagram the synthesis pathways for hormones produced in the adrenal gland, including catecholamines, aldosterone, cortisol, and sex steroids. Distinguish the anatomic zones in which these reactions occur.

The biochemical pathway for adrenal steroid synthesis is shown in Fig. 19.8.

3. Clinical: Differentiate the most common etiologies of hyperaldosteronism and their respective treatments. Describe methods to distinguish between these causes.

Etiologies of primary aldosteronism include adrenal hyperplasia (unilateral or bilateral), aldosterone-secreting masses (benign adenoma or malignant adrenal cortical carcinoma), or rare genetic diseases (Familial Hyperaldosteronism Types I-IV; Primary Aldosteronism, Seizures, and Neurological Abnormalities (PASNA) syndrome). Of these, bilateral adrenal hyperplasia (60%) and aldosterone-producing adenoma (35%) are most common. Unilateral adrenal hyperplasia is uncommon (2%).

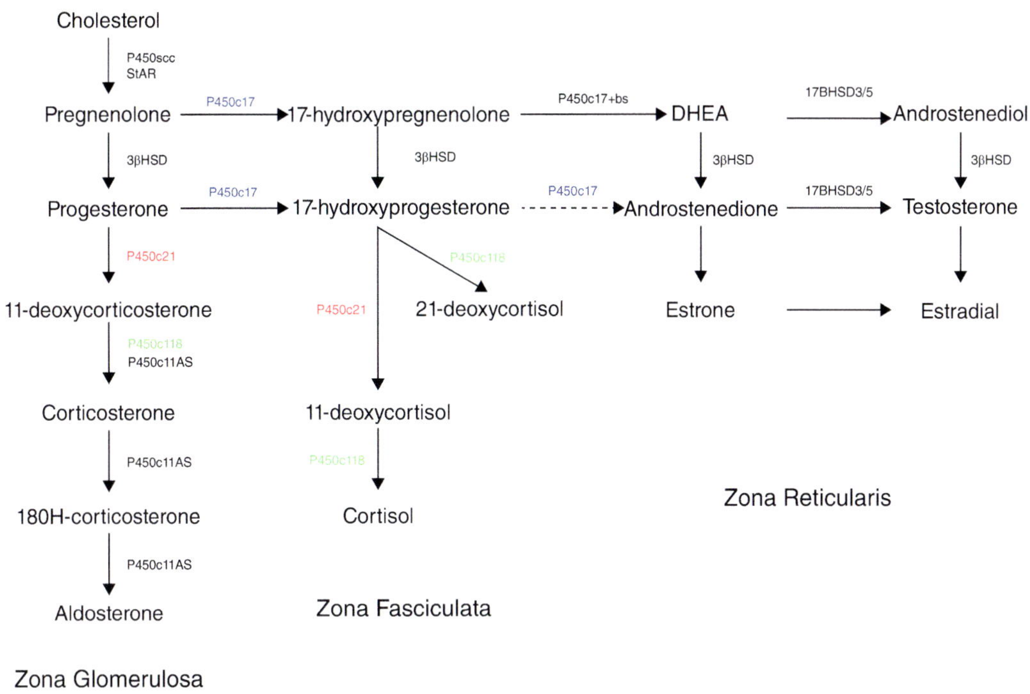

Fig. 19.8 Adrenal steroidogenesis pathway. Biosynthetic pathway of mineralocorticoids (aldosterone), glucocorticoids (cortisol), and sex hormones (testosterone) within the adrenal. Partitioning for the synthesis of key steroids occurring within each of the three zones (zona glomerulosa, zona fasciculata, and zona reticularis) is provided in the shaded areas. Dashed lines with arrowheads, compared to solid lines, denote enzyme steps that have limited affinity for conversion of the substrate to the product. DHEA = dehydroepiandrosterone, 3βHSD = 3β-hydroxysteroid dehydrogenase. With permissions from: Held, Patrice & Bird, Ian & Heather, Natasha. (2020). Newborn Screening for Congenital Adrenal Hyperplasia: Review of Factors Affecting Screening Accuracy. International Journal of Neonatal Screening. 6. 67. 10.3390/ijns6030067.

Adrenal cortical carcinoma rarely presents with pure aldosterone production alone.

Unilateral disease must be distinguished from bilateral disease, as a unilateral source of excess aldosterone production can be treated surgically by adrenalectomy. Students should mainly focus on distinguishing APA/aldosteronoma from bilateral adrenal hyperplasia. Aldosteronoma is surgically managed, often via unilateral laparoscopic adrenalectomy. BAH is managed medically.

It is currently common clinical practice to first confirm the diagnosis of primary aldosteronism biochemically. Cross-sectional imaging, such as CT or MRI, is generally performed second to search for a lesion, followed by adrenal vein sampling to definitively localize the source of the biochemical abnormality. More recently, some authors have advocated instead for AVS followed by imaging, but this is an emerging approach.

Historically, the presence of a unilateral hypodense lesion on CT, > 1.0 cm in size, in the setting of hyperaldosteronism, was considered suggestive of aldosteronoma.

4. Clinical: Provide a differential diagnosis for incidentally discovered adrenal masses. Describe an appropriate approach for the workup of adrenal incidentaloma in the asymptomatic patient.

Adrenal masses are frequently discovered incidentally during imaging studies performed for the workup of unrelated symptoms. The reported prevalence of adrenal incidentalomas on autopsy series ranges from 1.3% to 8.7%, and on abdominal CT from 0.6% to 1.3% [Stifelman]. While the majority of these are nonfunctional, up to 20% of patients with incidentalomas may have subclinical hormonal abnormalities, increasing their risk of metabolic and cardiovascular disease.

Patients with adrenal incidentaloma are generally screened for evidence of hormonal hypersecretion to guide management. A common screening test for hypercortisolism (i.e., Cushing's adenoma) is a 1 mg overnight dexamethasone suppression test. For patients with clinical Cushing's syndrome, the term adrenal incidentaloma is likely inappropriate; workup and management of Cushing's syndrome are beyond the scope of this text. The first-line screening test for excessive catecholamine secretion (i.e., pheochromocytoma) is measurement of plasma-free metanephrines. As discussed in this chapter, the serum aldosterone to plasma renin activity ratio is an important screening test for aldosterone excess.

Adrenal cortical carcinoma is an aggressive malignancy arising from the tissues of the adrenal cortex. These cancers are often functional and can produce any of the adrenal hormones in excess. In addition to the tests above, measurements of serum testosterone, estrogen, dehydroepiandrosterone, and 24-hour urinary 17-ketosteroids can be useful to confirm the diagnosis of hormonal syndromes associated with ACC.

The differential diagnosis for adrenal incidentaloma includes nonfunctional adenoma versus functional adrenal lesions: aldosteronoma, pheochromocytoma, cortisol-secreting adenoma, and adrenal carcinoma. Appropriate testing for these entities is given in Table 19.5.

5. Medical Humanism: Discuss the ramifications of our decision to choose a CCB/ACEI combination as first-line therapy for this patient rather than a thiazide diuretic. How might the management of and outcome for this patient have changed?

Students should recognize that assumptions about medication effects, particularly appropriate and justified assumptions, can and do substantially impact the course of care for patients.

Students should recognize that thiazides, unlike our CCB/ACEI combination, are potassium-wasting diuretics. The known potassium-wasting effect of a thiazide would have masked the hypokalemia in our patient by providing an obvious explanation for the observed electrolyte abnormality. Importantly, we probably would not have ordered a blood gas for this patient at the point we did in this case.

This would have significantly delayed the diagnosis of hyperaldosteronism for this patient. In fact, a substantial proportion of patients with hyperaldosteronism are diagnosed only after decades of "difficult-to-treat hypertension."

Exam Questions

1. A 32-year-old male restrained driver is seen in the emergency department for complaints of abdominal pain after a motor vehicle accident. His vital signs are BP 160/120, P 90, R 14, T 37.0. He has abrasions over his torso from his seat belt that are tender to palpation, but his exam is otherwise unremarkable. A CT of his chest, abdomen, and pelvis is performed, which shows no significant traumatic injury. However, a 1.5 cm nodule is found on his left adrenal gland. What is the appropriate next step in the workup of this nodule?
   A. Blood electrolyte and hormone levels
   B. Low-dose dexamethasone suppression test
   C. Cosyntropin administration test
   D. Fine needle biopsy of the nodule
   E. Referral for consideration of left adrenalectomy

Answer: A

Objective: Biochemical workup of adrenal incidentaloma

Explanation: This patient has an incidentally discovered adrenal mass. Appropriate workup includes screening tests to find evidence of adrenal hormone secretion (i.e., a functional adrenal adenoma). Tests include serum potassium, aldosterone/renin activity ratio, plasma-free metanephrines, and 24-hour urine cortisol. B is incorrect as while a low-dose dexamethasone suppression test is part of the workup for adrenal incidentaloma, it is performed to detect a cortisol-secreting adenoma that is not apparent on the initial urine cortisol screen. It would be the next step following the electrolyte and hormone studies in answer A. C is incorrect as cosyntropin is a synthetic analog of ACTH. It is administered during adrenal vein sampling for confirmation and lateralization of a suspected aldosteronoma. It can stimulate additional pathologic production of aldosterone in aldosteronoma, increasing the diagnostic yield. Adrenal vein sampling is inappropriate in the absence of biochemical evidence that this nodule is producing aldosterone. Electrolyte and hormone studies must come first. D is incorrect as biopsies are performed to obtain a tissue diagnosis in many/most malignancies. Fine needle biopsy is most commonly performed in the context of workup of a thyroid mass. Adrenal incidentalomas are common; the majority are non-functional adenomas with no clinical significance. Appropriate workup involves biochemical studies to determine whether the lesion is functional, which will then dictate further evaluation and management. E is incorrect as adrenalectomy is often the definitive management for a unilateral functional adrenal adenoma. This lesion has not yet been worked up. Appropriate workup involves biochemical studies to determine whether the lesion is functional, which will then dictate further evaluation and management.

2. A 25-year-old woman presents to the emergency department with complaints of an insidiously worsening headache over the last week. Her blood pressure in triage is 185/95. Her blood pressure is controlled with medication, resulting in resolution of symptoms. Her urine pregnancy test is negative, she has no risk factors for intracranial hemorrhage and no history of headache disorders. She believes she is generally healthy and has been feeling well. CBC is within normal limits. Additional labs show a hypokalemic metabolic alkalosis. In this patient, what is the likely mechanism of her hypertension?
   A. Inappropriate retention of electrolytes and water
   B. Increased total peripheral resistance
   C. Direct inotropic effects on cardiac contraction
   D. Increased venoconstriction

Answer: A

Objective: Diagnosis of hyperaldosteronism

Explanation: This vignette involves a young woman presenting with likely hypertensive encephalopathy (insidious headache resulting from very high blood pressure) but no other evidence of hypertensive emergency. Hypokalemic metabolic alkalosis strongly suggests hyperaldosteronism as the etiology. Hyperaldosteronism contributes toward arterial blood pressure through a variety of mechanisms, primarily via the preferential resorption of sodium (with water following the sodium) in exchange for potassium at sites including the distal tubule and collecting duct of the renal nephron. B is incorrect as catecholamines produced by pheochromocytoma and sympathomimetics can increase total peripheral resistance. While pheochromocytoma is a functional adrenal tumor, this vignette does not suggest pheochromocytoma. C is incorrect as catecholamines produced by pheochromocytoma and sympathomimetics exert direct inotropic effects on cardiac muscle. While pheochromocytoma is a functional adrenal tumor, this vignette does not suggest pheochromocytoma. D is incorrect as catecholamines produced by pheochromocytoma and sympathomimetics can produce venoconstriction. While pheochromocytoma is a functional adrenal tumor, this vignette does not suggest pheochromocytoma.

3. A 72-year old-man with a PMH significant for T2DM and HTN presents to your primary care office for follow-up on routine labs. He takes metformin, atorvastatin, atenolol, losartan, and amlodipine. Today, his vital signs are BP 168/93, P 70, R 11, T 36.4 C. He is feeling well, with no headache, dyspnea, chest pain, abdominal discomfort, or urinary changes. He has his usual polyuria and polydipsia without paresthesias. He last saw his optometrist

5 months ago for his annual vision screening, had a colonoscopy 6 years ago that was normal, and all his vaccines are up to date. His lab results are given in Table 19.4.

What is the most appropriate step to take in the care of this patient?

A. Increase metformin to achieve tighter glycemic control
B. Refer for colonoscopy
C. Order CT of the abdomen and pelvis
D. Order plasma aldosterone and peripheral renin activity levels
E. Increase dose of antihypertensive medications to improve BP control

Answer: D

Objective: Workup and management of aldosteronoma

Explanation: This patient has a very high BP of 168/93 despite three antihypertensive medications. Labs demonstrate a hypokalemic metabolic alkalosis that cannot be explained by his medication or current state of health. Any of these findings should raise a suspicion for hyperaldosteronism. Indications for screening for hyperaldosteronism include difficult-to-control hypertension (not well controlled despite three medications), BP > 160/90, hypertension associated with hypokalemic metabolic alkalosis. A is incorrect as while this patient's hemoglobin A1C is elevated, he has a known diagnosis of diabetes. In the elderly, goal A1C levels are between 6.5 and 7.0%, as aggressive control has been shown to be associated with harms including hypoglycemia. His control is appropriate for his age. B is incorrect as this patient has been appropriately screened for colon cancer under USPSTF guidelines. Referring for colonoscopy is not appropriate. C is incorrect as this patient has findings suggestive of hyperaldosteronism. The appropriate next step in workup is to look for biochemical evidence of hyperaldosteronism. While CT of the abdomen and pelvis is appropriate after confirming excess aldosterone secretion to help determine whether or not an aldosteronoma is present (which has implications for management), early CT is inappropriate. A significant proportion of the general population will have clinically irrelevant incidentalomas, which will require unnecessary workup and possible interventions should they be detected on CT. E is incorrect as while his blood pressure is poorly controlled, he is currently on three medications without adequate control. Additionally, the constellation of findings strongly suggest hyperaldosteronism. Continuing to add antihypertensives would be inappropriate; workup for suspected hyperaldosteronism should come next.

Table 19.4 Outpatient labs (hemoglobin A1c, CMP, ABG)

	Patient	Reference
Hemoglobin A1C	6.8	<5.7 %
Sodium	136	135–145 mmol/L
Potassium	3.1	3.5–4.5 mmol/L
Chloride	104	95–110 mmol/L
CO_2	38	19–34 mmol/L
Glucose	145	70–110 mg/dL
BUN	18	6–22 mg/dL
Creatinine	1.1	0.6–1.3 mg/dL
Calcium	9.7	8.5–10.9 mg/dL
Protein	6.8	6.3–7.9 g/dL
Albumin	4.1	3.9–5.0 g/dL
Total bilirubin	1.6	0.3–1.9 mg/dL
Direct bilirubin	0.1	0–0.3 mg/dL
Alkaline phosphatase	87	44–147 IU/L
AST	18	8–37 IU/L
ALT	17	0–34 IU/L
pH	7.48	7.35–7.45
$PaCO_2$	49	35–45 mmHg
PaO_2	90	80–95 mmHg
HCO_3	37	22–26 mEq/L

References

1. Kahn SL, Angle JF. Adrenal Vein Sampling. Tech Vasc Interventional Rad. 2010;13:110–25.
2. Le T, Bhushan V. First aid for the USMLE Step 1 2015. New York: Mcgraw-Hill Education; 2015.
3. Young WF. Primary aldosteronism: renaissance of a syndrome. Clin Endocrinol. 2007;66:607–18.
4. Stifelman MD, Fenig DM. Work-up of the functional adrenal mass. Curr Urol Rep. 2005;6(1):63–71. https://doi.org/10.1007/s11934-005-0069-3. PMID: 15610699.

Part VIII

Reproduction

20 Absence of Periods

Evan Austin

Learning Objectives

1. Differentiate between primary and secondary amenorrhea and identify which one this patient has.
2. Discuss how PCOS interrupts the menstrual cycle and the HPO axis.
3. Describe the Rotterdam Criteria for diagnosis of PCOS and the importance of other testing (TSH, prolactin, 17-OHP, etc.) to exclude other causes of oligomenorrhea.
4. Describe the overall approach to the management of PCOS as well as specific therapeutic mechanisms for the management of its associated menstrual dysfunction, androgen excess, and metabolic abnormalities.
5. Describe the approach to management for women pursuing pregnancy and describe the mechanism of action for ovulation induction therapeutics.
6. Provide an overview of the incidence/prevalence of PCOS as well as its associated risk factors/high risk groups.

Chief Complaint "My periods have stopped"

E. Austin (✉)
Department of Obstetrics and Gynecology, University of Arizona College of Medicine, Phoenix, AZ, USA

STOP AND THINK

- **What diagnoses and/or etiologies should we think about for this chief complaint?**
  - Amenorrhea (absence of periods) is the absence of menses and can be a transient, intermittent, or permanent condition. It often results from dysfunction of neuroendocrine function encompassing the hypothalamus, pituitary, ovaries, uterus, or vagina but can also encompass anatomic or congenital abnormalities in these structures.
  - It is first important to distinguish whether the amenorrhea is primary (absence of menarche by age 15 years) or secondary (absence of menses for more than 3 months in females who previously had regular menstrual cycles, or 6 months in females who had irregular menses).
- **What questions would you want to ask?**
  - Tell me about your periods.
  - What age did they begin?
  - When did your last period begin?
  - Do you have regular periods?
  - What is your usual cycle length?
  - Any possibility you could be pregnant?
  - Are you using any form of birth control/contraception?
  - What other medications do you take?
- **Alarm symptoms/questions to ask:**
  - Any headaches, nipple discharge, or loss of peripheral vision (indicates pituitary

C. A. Standley (ed.), *Biomedical Science and Clinical Foundations*,
https://doi.org/10.1007/978-3-031-98353-5_20

dysfunction).
  - Any significant changes in body weight? (anorexia, polycystic ovary syndrome (PCOS), and thyroid disease).
  - Do you have an impaired sense of smell? (Kallmann syndrome).
  - Have you been having any hot flashes, vaginal dryness, and difficulty sleeping (ovarian insufficiency).

HPI

Ms. Felix is a Hispanic 28-year-old woman presenting to the clinic for evaluation of abnormal menses. She underwent menarche at age 12 and has always had a history of irregular periods. However, over the past 4 years, her periods have become increasingly irregular with several episodes of heavy bleeding. For the past 9 months, her periods have completely stopped.

Because her periods have always been irregular, she never thought much of it or sought evaluation. However, she and her husband have been interested in having a child for some time now, but the home pregnancy tests she takes around once a month are always negative. She also notes a significant amount of weight gain over the past 3 years and has had persistent acne since adolescence. She tearfully confides that her unhappiness with her body image and difficulties in getting pregnant have started to place a strain on her marriage.

She notes she previously saw a dermatologist for her acne when she was 16, but is unaware of any other medical problems. She currently uses over-the-counter face washes to control her acne. She previously tried some diet pills she bought online 2 years ago but stopped them a few months later as they didn't seem to help. She currently takes no medications. She denies headaches, vision changes, cold intolerance, changes in her hair or nails, hot flashes, or changes in libido.

STOP AND THvINK

- **How does this information influence your differential?**
  - Given that she has had periods in the past, we can classify her amenorrhea as secondary amenorrhea. Furthermore, her acne, weight gain, and infertility are most consistent with an endocrinopathy such as PCOS or hypothyroidism. We can consider excluding causes of primary amenorrhea given that she underwent menarche at age 12.
- **What additional information would you like to know?**
  - To exclude other causes of secondary amenorrhea, it is important to obtain a detailed gynecologic history and medication history. It would also be important to look for signs/symptoms of estrogen deficiency (hot flashes/decreased libido), excess prolactin (galactorrhea), or hyperandrogenism (hirsutism and excessive acne).

PMH

History of acne since adolescence
Has not seen a physician since a visit to a dermatologist at 16

Gyn History

Menarche: 12 LMP: 9 months ago
Bleeding lasts 6 days, especially heavy on days 3–6
Has never had a Pap smear

OB History

G0P0

Sexual History

Currently sexually active
3 Lifetime male partners

Has never used any form of contraception/birth control

Never undergone STI testing

No dyspareunia

PSH

None

Medications

None

NKDA

Social History

Ms. Felix lives with her husband of 4 years and two pet dogs.

Feels safe at home. Denies any domestic violence.

Works in a bank, notes her job has been especially stressful lately.

Denies tobacco use.

3–4 alcoholic drinks per week. Tried marijuana in high school but denies other illicit drug use

Has been on and off diet/exercise plans for "as long as I can remember".

Family History

Father alive at 58 with a history of hypertension, diabetes, and nonalcoholic fatty liver disease (NAFLD).

Mother alive at 61 with a history of hypertension and diabetes.

Review of Systems

General: No fevers, chills, diaphoresis, night sweats

Skin: No changes in hair or nails

Hematologic: No lymphadenopathy, abnormal or excessive bleeding

Head: No headaches or head trauma

Eyes: No eye pain, inflammation, discharge, blurring or loss of vision

Ears: No decrease in acuity

Nose: No change in sense of smell or anosmia

Mouth: No change in taste. No bleeding gums

Pharynx: No hoarseness or dysphagia

Respiratory: No cough or sputum, dyspnea, wheezing

Cardiovascular: No chest pain, palpitations

Breast: No pain, mass or discharge

GI: No change in appetite, nausea, emesis

GU: No hematuria or dysuria

Genital: No history of STI or genital lesions

Endocrine: + weight gain × 3 years. No sensitivity to heat or cold

MSK: No pain, tenderness, stiffness, or swelling of muscles/joints

Neurological: No syncope, seizures, or dizziness

Psychiatric: Decreased mood over past 3 months. No memory loss, hallucinations

Stop and Think

- **How does this information inform your differential?**
  - Her weight gain and acne again are consistent with an endocrinopathy such as PCOS or hypothyroidism. However, she is sexually active and has never undergone STI testing, which leaves the possibility of pregnancy or a prior history of pelvic inflammatory disease on the table. Her lack of headache, visual changes, nipple discharge, and no medication use indicate that pituitary pathologies or amenorrhea due to dopamine or GnRH releasing analogues is less likely. The fact that she has never been pregnant or had any uterine intervention also indicates that a process like Asherman's syndrome is less likely.
- **What aspects of the physical exam are most relevant to this patient?**
  - The most important assessment of the physical exam should include BMI and signs of hyperandrogenism (hirsutism, acne, and male-pattern hair loss). A thor-

ough pelvic exam would also be helpful to rule out any structural causes.

Physical Exam:

General: Overweight female, alert and conversant in no acute distress
Skin: Warm and dry. Coarse hair noted on the upper lip and terminal hairs on the chin. Diffuse nodulocystic acne on face
Eyes: Conjunctiva clear, sclera anicteric
Neck: No lymphadenopathy, thyromegaly, or palpable nodules
Breasts: Symmetrical, nontender without masses, nipple discharge, skin changes or retractions. No axillary or supra-clavicular lymphadenopathy
Chest: CTA
Cardiac: RRR, Nl S1, S2 without S3, S4, Murmur, rub
Abdomen: Obese, Bowel sounds active in all four quadrants; nontender, nondistended; Liver span: 10 cm midclavicular line, no hepatosplenomegaly
Extremities: No clubbing, cyanosis, or edema. Capillary refill within 3 s
Pelvic: External genitalia, Bartholin's glands, urethra, and Skeens glands normal. Normal appearing skin and hair distribution. No visible lesions. Vagina pink and moist without discharge or lesions. Pelvic support adequate. Bladder non-tender. Cervix nulliparous/parous, smooth without lesions, discharge, or cervical motion tenderness. Uterus normal size and shape, midline, anteverted, mobile, no masses, nontender. Adnexa nonpalpable.

Stop and Think:

- **What diagnostic testing, imaging, procedures, etc. do you want to order? How will these tests help distinguish your hypotheses?**
  - Given the broad differential for amenorrhea, it is important to order testing that both confirms your suspected diagnosis while also definitely excluding others.
  - For this reason, appropriate diagnostic testing includes:
    - Laboratory evaluation
      - hCG (to rule out pregnancy)
      - TSH (to rule out hypothyroidism)
      - Total testosterone (total testosterone >150 ng/dL requires evaluation for the most serious causes of hyperandrogenism like ovarian and adrenal androgen-secreting tumors) (Testosterone_Threshold)
      - Prolactin (to rule out a pituitary prolactinoma)
      - Serum 17-hydroxyprogesterone (a morning serum 17-hydroxypro gesterone in the early follicular phase helps rule out nonclassical congenital adrenal hyperplasia (NCCAH) due to 21-hydroxylase deficiency. The clinical presentation of NCCAH can be similar if not identical to that of PCOS
      - FSH and estradiol are important as a high FSH in the setting of low estradiol indicates primary ovarian insufficiency (POI). A low/normal FSH and low estradiol indicate hypogonadotropic hypogonadism (functional/hypothalamic amenorrhea or systemic illness) or PCOS if a history of hyperandrogenism
    - Imaging
      - Transvaginal Ultrasound

Ms. Felix's results:

Test	Ms. Felix's result	Reference value
Human chorionic gonadotropin (hCG)	Negative	Negative, not pregnant Positive, pregnant
Prolactin	20 ng/ml	5–25 ng/ml
TSH	3.4 mU/L	0.2–5.4 mU/L
17-Hydroxyprogesterone	1.3 ng/ml	Follicular phase <2 ng/ml
Testosterone:		
Total Free	98 ng/dl 2.2 ng/dl	20–90 ng/dl 0.1–1.3 ng/dl
Follicle stimulating hormone (FSH)	7.0 mU/ml	Follicular: 2.8–11.3 mU/ml Ovulatory surge: 5.8–21 mU/ml Luteal: 1.2–9 mU/ml Postmenopausal: >30 mU/ml
Luteinizing hormone (LH)	20 mU/ml	Follicular: 1.1–11.6 mU/ml Ovulatory surge: 17–77 mU/ml Luteal: 1.2–14.7 mU/ml Postmenopausal: >30 mU/ml
Estradiol	97 pg/ml	Follicular: <20–266 pg/ml Ovulatory surge: 118–335 pg/ml Luteal: 25–165 pg/ml Postmenopausal <20 pg/ml
Transvaginal ultrasound		

Stop and Think

- **How do these results help us refine your diagnosis**
  - The amenorrhea and clinical/biochemical signs of hyperandrogenism (hirsutism, acne, and elevated testosterone) confirm the diagnosis of PCOS as defined by the Rotterdam criteria [21].

What Is Our Final Diagnosis?
Polycystic ovarian syndrome (PCOS).

Stop and Think

- **Are there any additional testing/screenings you would like to perform for Ms. Felix while she is here?**
  - Given the high prevalence of obesity and insulin resistance among women with PCOS, they are at increased risk for type 2 diabetes, dyslipidemia, and coronary heart disease [3]. As a result, patients with PCOS frequently undergo:
    - Fasting lipid profile
    - 2 h oral glucose tolerance test (or fasting glucose with HbA1c)
    - Screen for obstructive sleep apnea and refer to a sleep medicine clinician if necessary
    - Screen for Depression/Anxiety Disorders

So What Happened to Ms. Felix?
She receives counseling for weight loss and is given a referral to a nutritionist. She also receives a pap smear given that she has not had one previously. She plans to start ovulation induction therapy with clomiphene and metformin following weight loss.

Learning Objective Answers

Learning Objective 1 Differentiate between primary and secondary amenorrhea.

Primary amenorrhea is defined as the absence of menses by age 15 in the presence of otherwise normal secondary sexual characteristics or by age 13 if secondary sexual characteristics have not occurred. Secondary amenorrhea is defined as the absence of menses for more than 3 months in a person with previously normal menses or

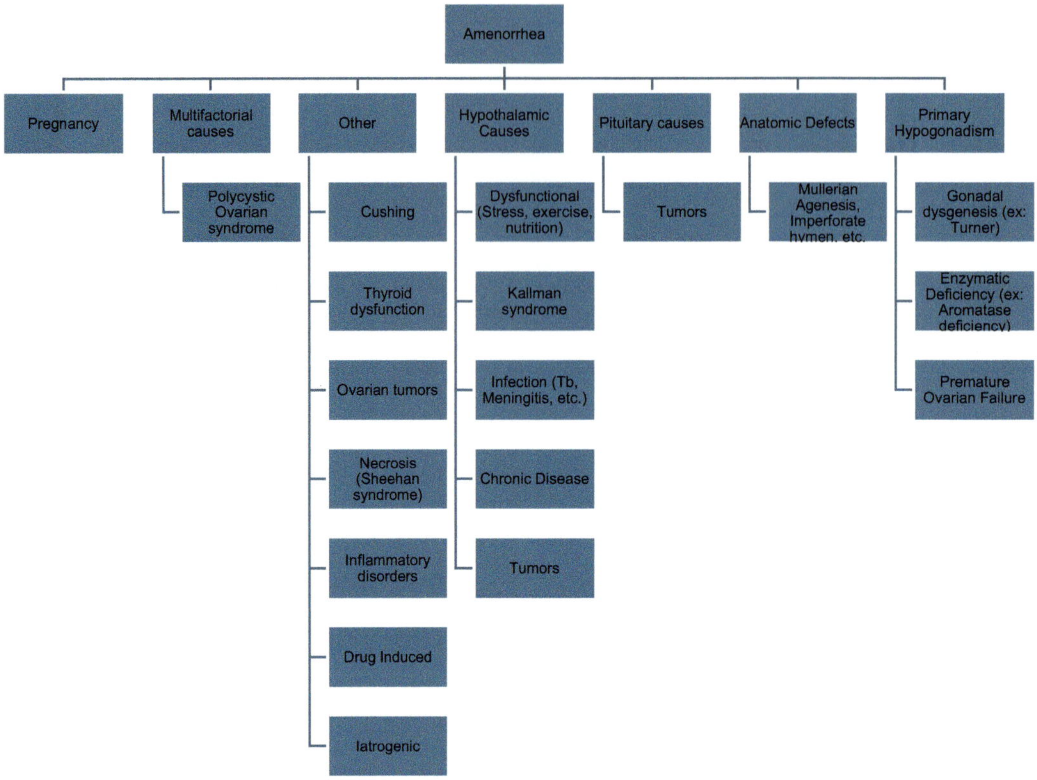

Fig. 20.1 Concept map of causes of amenorrhea

6 months in persons who had irregular cycles. An intermenstrual interval of more than 45 days is also considered abnormal in persons who are greater than or equal to 2 years postmenarche [5].

Out of all the causes of amenorrhea, pregnancy is the most common cause and secondary amenorrhea is more common than primary. Despite the long list of potential causes for amenorrhea (Fig. 20.1), most cases are accounted for by four primary conditions. These conditions include polycystic ovarian syndrome, hypothalamic amenorrhea, hyperprolactinemia, and ovarian failure [13].

Primary amenorrhea is oftentimes the result of a genetic or anatomical abnormality. The most common etiologies include [16]:

- Gonadal dysgenesis (43%)
- Physiologic delay of puberty (15%)
- Mullerian agenesis (14%)
- Polycystic ovarian syndrome (7%)
- Isolated gonadotropin-releasing hormone (GnRH) deficiency (5%)
- Transverse vaginal septum (3%)
- Weight loss/anorexia nervosa (2%)
- Hypopituitarism (2%)

Secondary amenorrhea on the other hand is often due to a neuroendocrine disorder. The most common etiologies for secondary amenorrhea include: [17]

- Ovarian disorders (ex: PCOS and ovarian insufficiency) (40%)
- Hypothalamic disorders (ex: functional hypothalamic amenorrhea)(35%)
- Pituitary disorders (ex: prolactinoma, empty sella, and Sheehan) (17%)
- Uterine disorders (ex: intrauterine adhesions) (7%)

- Other (ex: Congenital adrenal hyperplasia and hypothyroidism) (1%)

As with any chief complaint, it is crucial to obtain an accurate history and physical when working up amenorrhea as this will dictate what steps to implement moving forward. When performing the physical exam, it is prudent to evaluate BMI as an elevated BMI may provide a clue towards PCOS while a very low BMI may provide clues towards functional hypothalamic amenorrhea such as from an eating disorder or very strenuous exercise. Patients should be evaluated for evidence of hyperandrogenism such as hirsutism and acne. Other physical exam findings such as striae, acanthosis nigricans, vitiligo, and breast discharge can also detail as to what is the main etiology. A pelvic exam should be performed universally to identify any potential anatomic causes and to look for any evidence of estrogen deficiency such as vaginal atrophy that could point towards ovarian insufficiency. The physical exam is even more important in cases of primary amenorrhea where the presence or absence of a uterus and/or breasts play a dramatic role in identifying the case for amenorrhea.

Laboratory workup (Fig. 20.2) and imaging can be crucial in helping differentiate causes of amenorrhea as well.

Learning Objective 2 Discuss how PCOS interrupts the menstrual cycle and HPO axis.

The hypothalamic-pituitary-ovarian (HPO) axis is a complex endocrine pathway that is fundamental in regulating the menstrual cycle (Fig. 20.3). To begin, a functioning hypothalamus secretes gonadotropin-releasing hormone (GnRH) in a pulsatile fashion, which causes the anterior pituitary to release follicle-stimulating hormone (FSH) and luteinizing hormone (LH), which then acts on the ovary to release estradiol and progesterone. Specifically, LH acts on theca cells of an ovarian follicle, which helps convert cholesterol to androstenedione via the enzyme, desmolase. FSH acts on the granulosa cell to con-

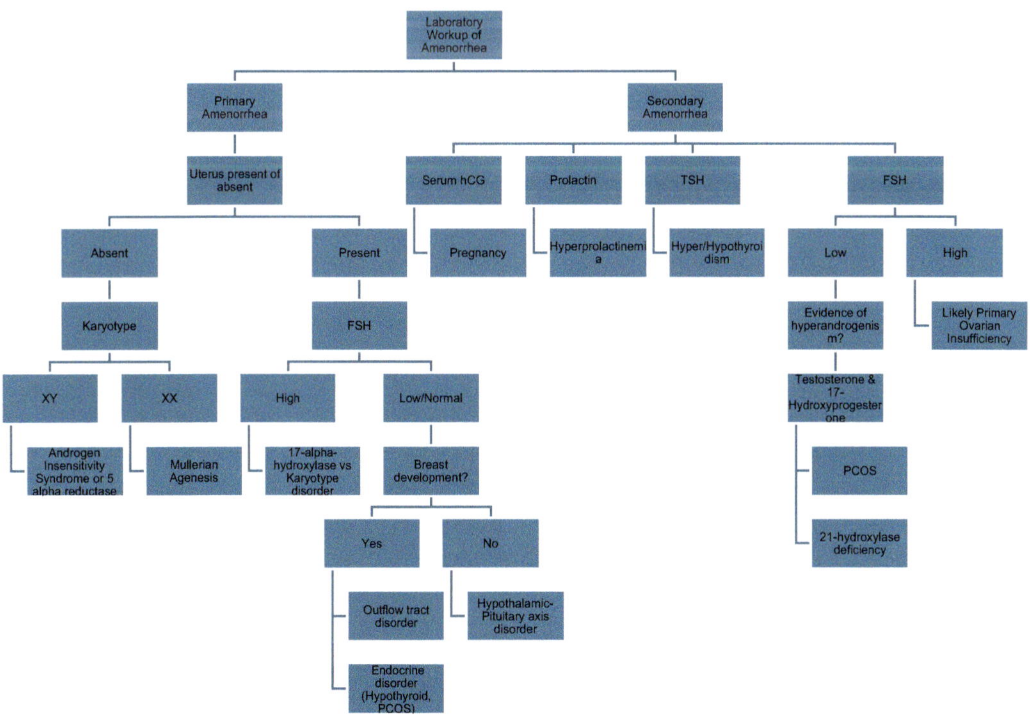

Fig. 20.2 Concept map for the laboratory workup of primary and secondary amenorrhea

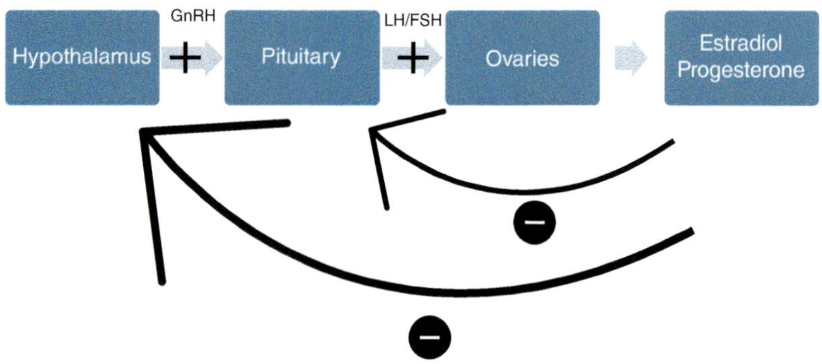

Fig. 20.3 Normal feedback mechanism of the hypothalamic-pituitary-ovarian (HPO) axis

vert androstenedione to estrone (which can then convert to estrogen) via the enzyme, aromatase. Estradiol and progesterone then downregulate the production of GnRH, LH, and FSH via a negative feedback loop.

The menstrual cycle is classically 28 days and is split into two separate phases, the follicular phase (or proliferative phase) and the luteal phase (or secretory phase). In the follicular phase, FSH (as its name implies) works at the level of the ovary to develop a dominant follicle while stimulating endometrial proliferation in the uterus. As estrogen levels increase, a midcycle peak in estrogen triggers an LH surge, which leads to the rupture of the dominant follicle and the release of the oocyte (ovulation). This defines the end of the follicular phase and beginning of the luteal phase. The ruptured follicle is then known as the corpus luteum and releases progesterone, which acts on the endometrium to stimulate proliferation and glandular secretion. In the absence of fertilization, the corpus luteum degenerates to become the corpus albicans, leading to a drop in estrogen/progesterone. This loss of progesterone then leads to endometrial shedding.

While the exact mechanisms for the etiology/pathophysiology are complex and currently up for debate, the overall concept underlying PCOS appears to be related to ovarian hyperandrogenism and hyperinsulinemia, leading to disruptions in the typical HPO axis [19]. Increased LH levels induce excess androgen production from theca cells, which results in hyperandrogenism symptoms like hirsutism, acne, and male pattern baldness. Additionally, androgen is converted to estrone in adipose tissue, and estrone feedback in the HPO axis decreases FSH, which results in the cystic degeneration of follicles. A lack of follicular maturation leads to the failure of a dominant follicle to form and anovulation. This large amount of unopposed estrogen with little progesterone (as a result of no corpus luteum) increases the risk of endometrial cancer.

Learning Objective 3 Describe the Rotterdam Criteria for diagnosis of PCOS and the importance of other testing (TSH, prolactin, 17-OHP, etc.) to exclude other causes of oligomenorrhea.

Given the broad differential for amenorrhea, it is important to order testing that both confirms your suspected diagnosis while also definitely excluding others. PCOS is classically diagnosed via the Rotterdam criteria [7], which states that two out of the following three criteria are required to make the diagnosis:

- Oligo/anovulation
- Clinical/biochemical signs of hyperandrogenism
- Polycystic ovaries by ultrasound

Furthermore, the diagnosis is only confirmed when other conditions that mimic PCOS are excluded (such as thyroid disease, nonclassic congenital adrenal hyperplasia, hyperprolactinemia, and androgen secreting tumors).

For this reason, appropriate diagnostic testing includes:

- hCG (to rule out pregnancy)
- TSH (to rule out hypothyroidism)

- Total testosterone (total testosterone >150 ng/dL requires evaluation for the most serious causes of hyperandrogenism like ovarian and adrenal androgen-secreting tumors)
- Prolactin (to rule out a pituitary prolactinoma)
- Serum 17-hydroxyprogesterone (a morning serum 17-hydroxyprogesterone in the early follicular phase helps rule out nonclassic congenital adrenal hyperplasia (NCCAH) due to 21-hydroxylase deficiency. The clinical presentation of NCCAH can be similar if not identical to that of PCOS
- FSH and estradiol are important as a high FSH in the setting of low estradiol indicates primary ovarian insufficiency (POI). A low/normal FSH and low estradiol indicate hypogonadotropic hypogonadism (functional/hypothalamic amenorrhea or systemic illness) or PCOS if a history of hyperandrogenism
- It was previously common for clinicians to measure LH and FSH in the evaluation of PCOS, and an elevated LH:FSH ratio ≥ 2 was used as evidence to support the diagnosis. However, it is important to note that the LH:FSH ratio was never a criterion for the diagnosis of PCOS and it can be misleading [20] (if there has been recent ovulation, LH will be suppressed and the ratio will be <2:1).

Regarding the typical imaging findings of PCOS:

Ultrasound (US) is typically done in women with hyperandrogenic symptoms but with normal menstrual cycles (thus the US is needed to make it 2/3 for the Rotterdam criteria). There is currently no consensus on optimal ultrasound criteria, but it is important to note that follicle number and size, not cysts, are important in the diagnosis. Classically, the Rotterdam criteria include the presence of 12 or more follicles in either ovary measuring 2–9 mm in diameter and/or increased ovarian volume (>10 mL) [21]. This ovarian volume needs to ensure there are no corpora lutea, cysts or dominant follicles present in the measurement. Only one ovary fitting this definition is sufficient to diagnose. Other morphological features that have been described, but are not a part of the formal diagnostic criteria include hyperchoic central stroma, peripheral location of follicles (string of pearls sign), or follicles of similar size measuring 2–9 mm.

As a result of anovulation in PCOS, the endometrium frequently becomes thickened from the excess estrogen that is not corrected for by the monthly production of progesterone from the ovary that normally follows ovulation. In premenopausal women, the normal endometrial thickness will depend on the stage of the menstrual cycle, but a thickness >15 mm is considered the upper limit of normal in the secretary phase [9]. Above this limit, there is concern for endometrial hyperplasia and progression to endometrial carcinoma, prompting the need for an endometrial biopsy. In this patient, the thickness is 12.06 mm, which is thick but not at the level to warrant a biopsy.

Learning Objective 4 Describe the overall approach to the management of PCOS as well as specific therapeutic mechanisms for the management of its associated menstrual dysfunction, androgen excess, and metabolic abnormalities.

An adequate treatment approach to PCOS requires attending to amenorrhea/oligomenorrhea, hyperandrogenism, anovulatory infertility, and metabolic risk factors. In addition, management should have a focus on reducing metabolic abnormalities contributing to type 2 diabetes and cardiovascular disease, while also preventing endometrial hyperplasia and carcinoma as a result of the unopposed estrogen state from chronic anovulation.

- Lifestyle changes
  - While often overlooked, lifestyle changes like diet and exercise are the most effective treatments for improving insulin resistance and hyperandrogenism [15].
- Oral contraceptives
  - For women not desiring pregnancy, combined estrogen-progestin oral contraceptives are the mainstay of pharmacologic therapy [11].

    - Oral contraceptives decrease the risk of endometrial hyperplasia/carcinoma and reduce hirsutism
  - The chronic anovulation in PCOS increases the risk for endometrial hyperplasia and cancer.
  - Combined oral contraceptives (COCs) increase exposure to progestins, which antagonize endometrial proliferation from estrogen.
  - Alternative treatments for endometrial protection include intermittent progestin therapy or a progestin-containing IUD [4].
    - Contraindications for combined oral contraceptives (in which an alternative treatment would be needed), include age >35 and smoking >15 cigarettes per day, hypertension, history (hx) of venous thromboembolism, hx of thrombogenic mutations, hx of ischemic heart disease, hx of stroke, hx of breast cancer, hx of cirrhosis, hx of migraine with aura, and hx of hepatocellular adenoma.
- Metformin
  - Metformin restores ovulatory menses in 30–50% of women with PCOS and reduces the hyperinsulinemia prevalent in this population [14].
- Spironolactone
  - For women with contraindications to oral contraceptives (such as high VTE risk) or if the hyperandrogenism symptoms persist after 6 months of COC use, spironolactone can be used, although an alternative form of contraception is needed [2].

Learning Objective 5 Describe the approach to management for women pursuing pregnancy and describe the mechanism of action for ovulation induction therapeutics.

Similar to woman not pursuing pregnancy, lifestyle modifications like diet and exercise are the most important factors for PCOS treatment [6]. Pharmacologic interventions to induce ovulation include letrozole, clomiphene citrate, or pulsatile GnRH therapy.

Letrozole is the first-line drug for ovulation induction and is a nonsteroidal competitive inhibitor of the aromatase enzyme system, which is the key enzyme involved in the conversion of androgens to estrogen. [12] This leads to inhibition of the enzyme and a significant reduction in plasma estrogen. For the purposes of ovulation induction, the patient is first subject to a progestin-induced withdrawal bleed. Remember, in anovulation (such as what occurs in PCOS), there is very little progesterone as a result of no corpus luteum. Thus exogenous administration of progesterone mimics this cycle, which is then followed by a "withdrawal bleed" approximately 2–7 days after the progestin is stopped. Then, 2.5 mg of letrozole is given once daily for 5 days, starting on days 3,4, or 5 of menses. This lowers the amount of estrogen present in the follicular phase to restore proper HPO axis function and allow the corresponding development of a primary dominant follicle and LH surge for ovulation.

While previously first line before being surpassed by letrozole, clomiphene is a drug that acts at the level of the hypothalamus. It binds to estrogen receptors for longer durations than estrogen, which effectively inhibits normal estrogenic negative feedback. This lack of feedback results in increased GnRH secretion from the hypothalamus and subsequent pituitary LH and FSH release. Similar to letrozole, clomiphene is typically given following a progestin-induced bleed.

Other options for ovulation induction include direct administration of exogenous GnRH to restore normal HPO axis function [10].

Learning Objective 6 Provide an overview of the incidence/prevalence of PCOS as well as its associated risk factors/high risk groups.

PCOS is the most common cause of infertility and affects 4–20% of reproductive aged women worldwide [18]. Due to the complexity and variance in phenotypes among this metabolic disorder, risk factors are broad and varied. Furthermore, the specific importance of each risk factor towards disorder development is still not fully understood. Given what is known about the syndrome, anything that alters steroidogenesis, ovarian folliculogenesis, neuroendocrine function, metabolism, insulin production, insulin sensitivity, inflammatory factors, and sympathetic nerve function have been theorized to contribute [8]. As such, consumption of large quantities of carbohydrates, hyperinsulinemia, hyperandrogenemia, and persistent low-grade inflammation are postulated to be some of the main contributors to the pathophysiology of PCOS [1]. While certainly not an exhaustive list, some of the risk factors include:

- Oligoovulatory infertility
- Obesity
- Diabetes mellitus
- History of premature adrenarche
- First-degree relative with PCOS
- Ethnicity (Mexican American)
- Antiseizure medication (like Valproate)
- Environmental Toxins
- Genetic Predisposition
- Gut dysbiosis

Exam Questions

1. A 28-year-old female presents to her gynecologist for evaluation of irregular periods for several years. She is interested in becoming pregnant. She states she underwent menarche and has always had irregular periods, but they have become increasingly irregular over the past 1.5 years. On exam, blood pressure is 128/74 mmHg, pulse is 88 BPM, temperature is 37 C, and BMI is 29. She has coarse hair on her upper lip/chin, and acne on her face/back. Pelvic exam reveals a normal-sized uterus and ovaries are not palpable. Serum testosterone is 101 ng/dl (ref 20–90 ng/dl). She is diagnosed with PCOS and is started on the first-line medication to induce ovulation. Which of the following is a mechanism of action of this medication?
   (a) Competitive inhibitor of enzymes in granulosa cells
   (b) Competitive inhibitor of enzymes in theca cells
   (c) Increases levels of plasma estrogens
   (d) Contains combination of estrogen and progestin

   Answer: A.

   Learning Objective #4.

   Explanation: The first line treatment for ovulation in patients with PCOS is letrozole, a nonsteroidal competitive inhibitor of the aromatase enzyme system, which catalyzes the conversion of androgens to estrogens. At the ovarian follicle, aromatase is present in granulosa cells, which would make A the correct answer. B is incorrect because aromatase is not present in the theca cell. Instead, the theca cell functions to convert cholesterol to androstenedione via the enzyme, desmolase. C is incorrect because letrozole would decrease plasma estrogen levels as a result of aromatase inhibition. Combined oral contraceptives (choice D) are frequently used for the treatment of PCOS, but not in the context of ovulation induction.
2. A 24-year-old female presents to her primary care physician for worsening acne. She has had acne since adolescence but notes it has been worse in the past year or so. She has also noticed more hair growth on her chin, has started to gain weight despite a consistent exercise regimen, and her periods have been irregular for the past year. She is started on a combined oral contraceptive and her symptoms improve. In addition to improving her symptoms, which of the following is also true about her medication?
   (a) Decreases risk for developing a venous thromboembolism
   (b) Decreases risk of endometrial carcinoma
   (c) Can also be used for migraine prophylaxis
   (d) Decreases risk of stroke

   Answer: B.

   Learning Objective #4.

   Explanation: Combined oral contraceptives (COCs) have a number of medical uses. In this case, they are an effective treatment for PCOS, which is what this patient most likely has. Despite their wide use, COCs do have several contraindications. Notably, they increase, rather than decrease, the risk for venous thromboembolism (choice A). They are also contraindicated in those with a history of migraine with aura (choice c) and those with a history of stroke (choice D). The increased exposure to the progestins present in COCs antagonize endometrial proliferation, therefore decreases the risk of endometrial hyperplasia and carcinoma (choice B).

3. You are on your OB/GYN rotation when you see a 29-year-old woman in the clinic with a concern for infertility. After taking a thorough history/physical and reviewing her labs, you suspect the cause of her infertility is due to PCOS. Which of the following criteria could you use to justify your diagnosis?
   (a) History of anovulation and LH:FSH ratio > 2:1
   (b) Clinical signs of hyperandrogenism and polycystic ovaries on ultrasound
   (c) LH:FSH ratio > 2:1 is all that is needed to confirm the diagnosis
   (d) Polycystic ovaries on ultrasound is all that is needed to confirm the diagnosis

   Answer: B.

   Learning Objective #3.

   Explanation: PCOS is most commonly diagnosed by the Rotterdam criteria [21], which states that two of the three following criteria are required to make the diagnosis:

- Oligo- and/or anovulation
- Clinical and/or biochemical signs of hyperandrogenism
- Polycystic ovaries (by ultrasound)

While it was previously common to use an LH:FSH ratio $\geq$ 2 as evidence to support the diagnosis of PCOS, this ratio has never been a formal criterion for the diagnosis and can be misleading, as the LH will be suppressed if there has been recent ovulation. Thus, choices A and C are both incorrect. Choice D is incorrect as one other component of the Rotterdam criteria beyond the polycystic ovaries is needed to confirm the diagnosis. Choice B meets two criteria for diagnosis and therefore could appropriately be used to justify the diagnosis.

References

1. Barrea L, M. P. Source and amount of carbohydrate in the diet and inflammation in women with polycystic ovary syndrome. Nutr Res Rev. 2018;31:291.
2. Barrionuevo P, N. M. Treatment options for hirsutism: A systematic review and network meta-analysis. J Clin Endocrinol Metab. 2018;103:1258.
3. Committee AA. American Association of Clinical Endocrinologists Position Statement on metabolic and cardiovascular consequences of polycystic ovary syndrome. Endocr Pract. 2005:126–34.
4. Dumesic DA, L. R. Cancer risk and PCOS. Steroids. 2013;78:782.
5. Efthimios Deligeoroglou 1, N. A. Evaluation and management of adolescent amenorrhea. Annals of the New York Academy of Science; 2010.
6. Escobar-Morreale HF, B.-C. J.-B. The polycystic ovary syndrome associated with morbid obesity may resolve after weight loss induced by bariatric surgery. J Clin Endocrinol Metab. 2005;90:6364.
7. Group, R. E.-S. Revised 2003 consensus on diagnostic criteria and long-term health risks related to polycystic ovary syndrome. Fertility Sterility; 2004.
8. Ibáñez LOS. An International Consortium Update: Pathophysiology, Diagnosis, and Treatment of Polycystic Ovarian Syndrome in Adolescence. Horm Res Paediatr. 2017;88:371.
9. Isabela Corrêa Barboza, 1. D. Analysis of endometrial thickness measured by transvaginal ultrasonography in obese patients. In: Einstein. Sao Paulo; 2014. p. 164.
10. Kelly AC, J. R. Alternate regimens for ovulation induction in polycystic ovarian disease. Fertility and Sterility; 1990.
11. Legro RS, A. S. Diagnosis and treatment of polycystic ovary syndrome: an Endocrine Society clinical practice guideline. J Clin Endocrinol Metab. 2013;98:4565.
12. Legro RS, B. R. Letrozole versus clomiphene for infertility in the polycystic ovary syndrome. N Engl J Med. 2014;371:119.
13. Medicine PC. Current evaluation of amenorrhea. Fertil Steril. 2006;
14. Moghetti P, C. R. Metformin effects on clinical features, endocrine and metabolic profiles, and insulin sensitivity in polycystic ovary syndrome: a randomized, double-blind, placebo-controlled 6-month trial, followed by open, long-term clinical evaluation. J Clin Endocrinol Metab. 2000;
15. Moran LJ, H. S. Lifestyle changes in women with polycystic ovary syndrome. Cochrane Database Syst Rev. 2011;

16. Reindollar RH, B. J. Delayed sexual development: a study of 252 patients. Am J Obstet Gynecol. 1981;140:371.
17. Reindollar RH, N. M. Adult-onset amenorrhea: a study of 262 patients. Am J Obstet Gynecol. 1986;155:531.
18. Ritu Deswal VN. The prevalence of polycystic ovary syndrome: A brief systematic review. J Human Reprod Sci. 2020;
19. Rosenfield RL, E. D. The pathogenesis of polycystic ovary syndrome (PCOS): the hypothesis of PCOS as functional ovarian Hyperandrogenism revisited. Endocr Rev. 2016;37:467.
20. Saadia Z. Follicle stimulating hormone (LH: FSH) ratio in polycystic ovary syndrome (PCOS)—obese vs, vol. 74. Medical Archives: Non-Obese Women; 2020. p. 289.
21. Teede HJ, M. M. Recommendations from the international evidence-based guideline for the assessment and management of polycystic ovary syndrome. Fertility Sterility; 2018.

21 Short Stature

Cynthia A. Standley

Learning Objectives

1. Compare and contrast hypogonadotropic vs. hypergonadotropic hypogonadism and describe the initial workup for primary amenorrhea.
2. Describe the pathways and hormones responsible for pubertal development and how these changes correlate with the Sexual Maturity Rating and clinical changes that occur during puberty in girls and boys.
3. Define mosaicism and discuss methods of genetic testing in patients with suspected Turner syndrome. Review the different genotypes of Turner syndrome.
4. Describe the clinical features and common abnormalities associated with Turner syndrome.
5. Discuss the role of growth hormone and estrogen therapy in the treatment of Turner syndrome.
6. Describe other X-chromosome abnormalities that can cause infertility.
7. Consider the psychological, social, and emotional issues a young girl with delayed puberty may experience. Explain this patient's future fertility and discuss the options for her to have children in the future.

C. A. Standley (✉)
Department of Bioethics and Medical Humanism, University of Arizona College of Medicine-Phoenix, Phoenix, AZ, USA
e-mail: cstand@arizona.edu

Chief Complaint

A mother brings her 15-year-old daughter to the clinic with the concern that "she hasn't developed like other girls in her school."

Prompt: *Given only this information, what systems are you considering?*

Possible differentials for this chief complaint include:

- constitutional growth delay (late bloomer)
- genetic /chromosomal/congenital
- pituitary dysfunction
- CNS mass/tumor
- chronic systemic disease
- hypothyroidism

History of Present Illness

Amy H. is a 15-year-old female who is brought in by her mom for concerns that she has not developed in ways that other girls her age have. Amy has not noticed any breast development but does have pubic hair growth that began at age 13. She is noticeably shorter than other children, and she does not think she ever had a growth spurt. She notes that she feels well and performs well in school.

C. A. Standley (ed.), *Biomedical Science and Clinical Foundations*,
https://doi.org/10.1007/978-3-031-98353-5_21

Prompt: Define primary vs secondary amenorrhea.

Primary amenorrhea: the failure of menses to occur by age 16 years, in the presence of normal growth and secondary sexual characteristics. If by age 13 menses has not occurred and the onset of puberty, such as breast development, is absent, a workup for primary amenorrhea should start.

Secondary amenorrhea: When at least one menstrual period has occurred, but menstruation has subsequently ceased for six months or longer.

Past Medical History
Recurrent otitis media.

Past Surgical History
Tonsillectomy at age 10.

Medications
Daily multivitamin

Allergies
No known drug allergies

Family History
No history of growth delay or pubertal health issues in the family

Mom had menarche at age 12

Dad is 6′3 and Mom is 5′5″

Prompt: *Why is absence of delayed puberty in the family a pertinent negative?*

There is less likely to be a constitutional growth delay in this patient.

Social History

Mom is asked to leave the room for a HEEADSSS assessment.

- **H (Home/Environment)**—Lives at home with Mom, Dad, and 3 brothers; feels safe at home and has a good relationship with family
- **E (Education/Employment)**—ninth grade, gets mostly A's, does not have a job but does chores around the house
- **E (Eating)**—Eats junk food "sometimes"
- **A (Activities)**—Plays guitar and plays volleyball
- **D (Drugs)**—Denies drug use
- **S (Sexuality)**—Denies history of sexual activity; not dating
- **S (Suicide/Depression)**—feels "down" from time to time regarding height; admits to beginning to struggle with self-image but denies anxiety/depression/suicidal ideations
- **S (Safety)**—no guns in the home, no violence in home

Review of Systems

Gen: + occasional fatigue. No fevers
HEENT: No headaches, visual problems, or URI symptoms
CV: No chest pain or palpitations
Resp: No cough or shortness of breath
GI: + occasional constipation. No abdominal pain, nausea, or vomiting
GU: No dysuria, polyuria
Endo: No polydipsia, no sensitivity to heat or cold
Neuro: No dizziness, tremors, or numbness
MS: + Occasional joint pain. No limitations to movement

Prompt: What will you be looking for on a physical exam?

When suspecting primary amenorrhea in a patient, a physical exam would primarily focus on assessing the development of secondary sexual characteristics like breast development, pubic hair (Tanner staging), and genital anatomy through a pelvic exam, Also a good idea to check for signs of underlying conditions like Turner syndrome through physical features like a webbed neck or low hairline.

Physical Exam

Temperature: 36.7 °C
BP: 118/78 mmHg
Pulse: 85 bpm

Resp rate: 12 breaths per minute
Height: 135 cm
Weight: 23 kg

The patient's data is plotted on a growth curve and compared to her previous growth metrics as detailed in her medical chart. Her growth curve demonstrates a normal growth velocity early on but eventually results in a poor growth velocity. There is a distinct absence of an increasing growth velocity around puberty.

Prompt: Is her growth curve a concern?
Yes! The best test to differentiate pathologic causes of short stature such as growth hormone deficiency and serious underlying illness from constitutional delay of growth and puberty is the growth velocity.

Prompt: Calculate this patient's estimated adult height using her parents' heights.
Mid-parental (MP) target height is calculated as (Paternal height in inches + maternal height in inches)/2 + 2.5 inches for boys and minus 2.5 inches for girls. This gives the mean predicted height with SD of 2 inches. Patient's MP target height is 67.5inches (50%) suggesting her current growth is abnormal for her genetic potential.

Physical Exam (Continued)

General: Alert and interactive, overweight female, in no acute distress
HEENT: Normal cephalic/atraumatic; extraocular muscles intact; pupils equal, round, and reactive to light and accommodation. Oropharynx clear, mucous membranes moist, no pharyngeal edema
Chest: Chest clear to auscultation bilaterally. Good aeration
CV: Regular rate and rhythm with normal S1 and S2, without murmurs/rubs/gallops
GI: Soft, nontender/nondistended. + bowel sounds (BS), no hepatosplenomegaly
Skin: No rashes or lesions noted
Extremities: Warm, well-perfused. Capillary refill <2 sec
Genitourinary: Normal external genitalia. Breast growth sexual maturity rate 1/5, pubic hair growth sexual maturity rating 5/5

Prompt: *What is on your problem list for this patient?*

- Delayed puberty (no breast development and no menses).
- Short stature.
- Adrenarche appropriate.

Prompt: *Has your preliminary diagnosis changed based on the physical exam?*
Some diagnoses to consider for this patient can be divided into those originating centrally, those related to a peripheral cause, and those having been acquired.

Central
Constitutional delay of growth and puberty
Pituitary dysfunction from mass, genetic abnormality
CNS space occupying lesion with resulting pituitary dysfunction
Chronic systemic illness (diabetes, malignancy)
Hyperprolactinemia
Hypothyroidism
Malnutrition with resulting leptin deficiency
Excessive exercise/energy expenditure (female athletic triad of amenorrhea, dietary dysfunction, osteoporosis)

Peripheral
Chromosomal, genetic, and congenital
Gonadal dysgenesis (45 XO, 45X/46XY, 46XX/46XY, 47XXY)
LH/FSH receptor mutations
Androgen or partial androgen insensitivity syndromes
Testicular regression or anorchia
Galactosemia and other metabolic conditions

Acquired
Autoimmune gonadal dysfunction

Chemotherapy
Infection/Infiltrative gonadal disorders
Torsion
Trauma
Irradiation
Surgical

Prompt: What tests are you considering at this point and how do they help determine the diagnosis?

- CMP to evaluate kidney function, liver function, electrolytes.
- CBC to evaluate for anemia, leukemia, or marrow suppression from chronic disease.
- Karyotype to determine if XX, XY or XO.
- FSH/LH levels: to discriminate central vs peripheral causes of delayed puberty.
- Bone Age: for height prediction, determine growth potential.
- Testosterone level: to help determine if central or peripheral.
- TSH: to determine if hypothyroidism is cause of pubertal delay, (by unknown mechanism).
- IGF-1:mediator for the growth promoting actions of growth hormone (GH), reflects GH concentration, GH varies during day but IGF more stable.
- Prolactin level: to determine if hypothalamic or pituitary disorder/CNS lesion is leading to loss of hypothalamic inhibition of prolactin secretion, if HIGH, need CNS imaging!

Abnormalities in puberty are classified as central (gonadotropin dependent) or peripheral (gonadotropin independent). These are discriminated by FSH/LH levels. For delayed puberty low or normal FSH/LH levels indicate a central process (hypogonadotropic hypogonadism) that can be benign (constitutional delay) or pathologic (CNS abnormality resulting in decreased pituitary gonadotroph function). A peripheral cause (gonad dysfunction or peripheral androgen resistance) would be associated with high FSH/LH levels because of failed feedback. The testosterone level will be low in central or peripheral causes and is only marginally helpful in discrimination between benign and pathologic causes in borderline cases. Bone age does not discriminate between pathologic or benign causes of delayed puberty but can be helpful with height prediction. All height predictions suppose a NORMAL growth velocity and therefore are not applicable in conditions with abnormal growth velocities such as GH deficiency, hypothyroidism, or underlying systemic illness.

Laboratory Findings

CMP and CBC are normal

Test	Patient result	Normal range
FSH	17.6 mIU/mL	1.1–7.4 mIU/mL
LH	12.2 mIU/mL	0.3–5.6 mIU/L
Total testosterone	546 ng/dL	185–886 ng/dL
Prolactin	10 ng/mL	4–23 ng/mL
IGF-1	205 ng/mL	109–485 ng/mL
TSH	8.4 ∫U/mL	0.5–5 ∫U/mL
Free T4	0.3 ∫U/mL	0.7–1.8 ∫U/mL

Prompt: What are the next steps for diagnosis/treatment?

Since FSH/LH high, indicates a peripheral process. A normal prolactin rules out a prolactinoma. High TSH with a low free T4 indicates hypothyroidism, a common comorbidity with Turner syndrome. Patient also had fatigue, constipation, joint pain. Next step: karyotype analysis.

Karyotype Analysis

Karyotyping reveals a 45,X/46,XX mosaicism.

Prompt: What is the diagnosis?

The diagnosis is Turner syndrome, mosaic form.

Patient Follow-up

The patient and her mom are told about the diagnosis of Turner syndrome. They are told that Amy will need to start estrogen therapy to address her delayed puberty and begin taking growth hormone to improve her height. She is also noted to have hypothyroidism and is started on a trial of levothyroxine.

10 Years Later

Amy returns to your clinic with her husband and expresses frustration that they have been unable to conceive. You refer her to your OB/GYN colleague for further evaluation.

End of Case

Answers to Learning Objectives

1. **Compare and contrast hypogonadotropic vs. hypergonadotropic hypogonadism, and describe the initial workup for primary amenorrhea.**

Table 21.1 shows a comparison of hypogonadotropic and hypergonadotropic hypogonadism according to various features. A key difference is that hypogonadotropic hypogonadism stems from a central issue (hypothalamus or pituitary), whereas hypergonadotropic hypogonadism originates from a peripheral issue (gonadal failure) [1]. A key similarity is that both result in low sex steroid levels, leading to delayed puberty, infertility, and other signs of hypogonadism.

When working a patient up for primary hypogonadism, it is important to follow a systematic approach to determine the underlying cause [2]. The initial assessment starts with obtaining a clinical history and physical examination. Look for pubertal milestones, signs of virilization, presence of chronic illness or stress, past abdominal or pelvic surgeries that might indicate genital tract abnormalities, and plot the growth chart. Evaluate sexual maturity staging for breast and pubic hair development and examine the external genitalia.

Laboratory investigations helpful to include in an investigation of the cause of amenorrhea include:

- Pregnancy test to rule out pregnancy
- FSH and LH levels to help determine cause of hypogonadism
- TSH and prolactin to assess for presence of hypothyroidism or hyperprolactinemia
- Estradiol levels to evaluate ovarian function
- Androgen levels to evaluate for androgen-secreting tumors or polycystic ovarian syndrome
- 17-hydroxyprogesterone level to rule out congenital adrenal hyperplasia
- Karyotype analysis

Finally, imaging studies can be conducted, such as a pelvic ultrasound to assess the uterus and ovaries and identify any structural abnormalities. A brain MRI can be considered if a central

Table 21.1 A comparison between hypogonadotropic hypogonadism and hypergonadotropic hypogonadism

Feature	Hypogonadotropic hypogonadism	Hypergonadotropic hypogonadism
Definition	Low gonadal function due to insufficient stimulation from the hypothalamus to the pituitary	Low gonadal function due to primary gonadal failure
Cause	Dysfunction in the hypothalamus or pituitary	Dysfunction of the gonads (ovaries/testes)
Gonadotropin levels (LH/FSH)	Low	Elevated
Sex steroid levels (estrogen/testosterone)	Low	Low
Feedback mechanism	Defective gonadotropin-releasing hormone secretion or signaling leads to low LH/FSH and downstream hypogonadism	Gonadal failure leads to low sex steroids, which remove negative feedback causing high LH/FSH

cause of amenorrhea is suspected. Lastly, a bone age X-ray can help to evaluate delayed puberty.

2. **Describe the pathways and hormones responsible for pubertal development and how these changes correlate with the Sexual Maturity Rating and clinical changes that occur during puberty in girls and boys.**

Puberty culminates in sexual maturity. Onset is between the ages of 8 and 13 in girls and 9 and 14 in boys. During this time, maturation of the hypothalamic-pituitary-gonadal axis occurs, including the initiation of pulsatile gonadotropin hormone release, the appearance of secondary sex characteristics, an acceleration of growth, and the capacity for fertilization [3].

In girls, the start of puberty is marked by thelarche, the development of breast tissue. The mean age is 10.9 years. Following is pubarche, the development of pubic hair, occurring at a mean age of 11.2 years. Menarche, the first menstrual period, occurs 2.25 years after the onset of puberty and usually by the 13th year. Peak growing time for girls occurs 1.3 years before menarche, with an average growth during this growth period of 9 inches. Pubertal maturation is complete in about 2 years, when adult height is achieved, mature breasts have formed, broader hips have developed due to adipose tissue deposition, and an inverted triangle of pubic hair is seen.

In boys, the first clinical sign of puberty is enlargement of the testes, along with development of pubic hair and penile enlargement. Facial and body hair increase, muscle bulk increases, and the voice deepens as the larynx enlarges. Sperm production and ejaculatory capability are present by 13.5–13.7 years of age. Adult testicular volume and penile size are achieved by 16 years of age, and final adult height is achieved at 18 years of age.

Other changes of puberty include a growth spurt under the influence of growth hormone and IGF-1. In girls, the growth spurt begins early in puberty, with a peak velocity of growth attained at menarche. In boys, the growth spurt begins near the end of puberty, almost 2 years later than in girls, and they gain an average of 11 inches in height. Acne begins to appear due to an increase in sebaceous gland activity related to the effects of testosterone and adrenal androgens. This is also the age when gingivitis begins to appear due to the effects of sex steroids. Elevated hormone levels cause an exaggerated response to dental plaque on teeth and gums.

Both genetic and environmental factors are involved in the timing of puberty. While puberty begins when the hypothalamus increases secretion of gonadotropin-releasing hormone (GnRH), what triggers this is not completely understood. What has received the most attention is the hormone leptin from adipose tissue. Having enough body fat seems to be a crucial indicator that the body is ready to become sexually mature. Leptin from adipocytes appears to function as a permissive factor in the onset of human puberty. Leptin released by the high-fat content of adipose tissue acts in the brain to suppress feeding and stimulate metabolism (by inhibiting neuropeptide Y). Neuropeptide Y is a neuromodulator implicated in the control of energy balance at the level of the hypothalamus. Additionally, leptin stimulates norepinephrin (NE) release, which then triggers increased pulsatility of GnRH neurons. Overall, the interplay between genetics, hormones, and environmental factors shapes the timing of puberty, with the hypothalamic-pituitary-gonadal axis acting as the central control system.

Once triggered, the increasing secretion of gonadotropin-releasing hormone (GnRH) leads to the release of luteinizing hormone (LH) and follicle-stimulating hormone (FSH) from the pituitary gland. These hormones stimulate the gonads to produce sex steroids (estrogen and testosterone), initiating the physical changes associated with puberty.

Sexual Maturity Rating (SMR), also known as Tanner Staging, is a system used to assess physical development during puberty [4]. It categorizes the progression of secondary sexual characteristics into five distinct stages, ranging from Stage 1 (prepubertal) to Stage 5 (full maturity). In clinical practice, SMR helps healthcare providers track pubertal development. For girls, it primarily evaluates breast development and pubic hair growth to determine their progression through puberty. In boys, SMR focuses on testicular enlargement, genital growth, and pubic hair as key indicators of maturity. This rating system is crucial for identifying normal growth patterns, diagnosing early or delayed puberty, and guiding appropriate medical interventions when needed.

3. **Define mosaicism and discuss methods of genetic testing in patients with suspected Turner syndrome. Review the different genotypes of Turner syndrome.**

Mosaicism refers to the presence of two or more populations of cells with different genotypes within a single individual, originating from a single fertilized egg. This genetic variation arises due to mutations occurring after fertilization, leading to distinct cell lines that can affect various tissues, including blood, skin, and reproductive cells.

Mosaicism is a common occurrence in Turner syndrome (TS). TS is a chromosomal disorder affecting females, characterized by the partial or complete absence of one X-chromosome. Mosaic TS means that some cells have the typical two sex chromosomes (XX), while others have only one X-chromosome (45,X) or other variations. More than half of all patients with TS have a mosaic chromosomal complement. This cell line mosaicism results from sex chromosome nondisjunction occurring during post-zygotic cell division. Absence of mosaicism in a karyotype from a peripheral blood sample does not universally preclude mosaicism in other tissues.

Genotypes of TS:

- Classic Turner syndrome (45,X)
- Mosaic Turner syndrome (45,X/46,XX or other variants)
- Turner syndrome with Y variant (45,X/46,XY or other Y variants)
- TS with isochromosome X (46,X,i(Xq)): Instead of a normal second X-chromosome, there is an abnormal X with duplicated long arms (isochromosome X).

TS is occasionally diagnosed incidentally during prenatal testing. More commonly, it is suspected based upon characteristic clinical features that show themselves from infancy through adolescence. The diagnosis is confirmed by karyotype analysis. A karyotype analysis for TS should be performed in any female with suspect characteristic features [5]. Prenatally, cases of TS are discovered incidentally during testing that was performed for unrelated reasons, such as advanced maternal age. TS may also be suspected because of certain congenital anomalies noted on fetal ultrasonography, including cardiac defects, nuchal thickening, or short femur. TS may be apparent at birth, presenting with congenital lymphedema of the hands and feet, webbed neck, nail dysplasia, narrow and high-arched palate, and short fourth metacarpal. In infants and children, TS should be suspected in any female with unexplained growth failure, defined as a growth velocity less than the tenth percentile for age or stature that is substantially less than predicted from parental heights. It should also be suspected in patients with other characteristic features, including webbed neck, left-sided cardiac defects (e.g., aortic coarctation or hypoplastic left heart syndrome), high-arched palate, and short fourth metacarpal. Finally, TS should be suspected in adolescent girls who fail to start or complete breast development or those with amenorrhea, especially if short stature and/or other features suspicious of TS are present. Prompt diagnosis is important to permit management of comorbidities, including effective treatment of short stature.

4. **Describe the clinical features and common abnormalities associated with Turner syndrome.**

TS is one of the most common chromosome anomalies in humans and represents an important cause of short stature and ovarian insufficiency in females [6]. The most consistent characteristic of girls and women with TS is short stature. Nearly all individuals with TS exhibit a shorter than average height, often noticeable by age 5. Due to underdeveloped ovaries, most affected females experience premature ovarian failure, leading to delayed or absent puberty and infertility. Common physical characteristics include a webbed neck, low-set ears, low hairline at the back of the neck, broad chest with widely spaced nipples, and swelling of hands and feet, especially at birth. The broad chest and short stature can sometimes give a disproportionately stocky appearance.

Common abnormalities in individuals with TS affect the heart, kidneys, skeleton, hearing, and metabolism. Girls may have congenital heart defects such as coarctation of the aorta or bicuspid aortic valve. Structural kidney anomalies are more prevalent, potentially leading to hypertension or urinary tract infections. Conditions such as scoliosis, osteoporosis, and other orthopedic issues are more common. An increased incidence of ear infections and progressive hearing loss is observed in those with TS. Metabolically, there is a heightened risk for obesity, hypertension, and liver abnormalities, including steatosis and steatohepatitis.

5. **Discuss the role of growth hormone and estrogen therapy in the treatment of Turner syndrome.**

As short stature is the most common clinical feature of TS, recombinant human growth hormone therapy starting in early childhood is recommended to maximize adult height [7]. Therapy should begin as soon as the height of a girl with TS falls below the fifth percentile for age, which usually occurs between two and five years of age, rather than starting this therapy later in childhood. Treatment of children involves daily injections of growth hormone, usually for as long as the child is growing. Lifelong continuation may be recommended for those most severely deficient as adults. Girls can return to adult height with growth hormone therapy. Note that growth hormone secretion testing is not indicated because patients with TS do not have growth hormone deficiency despite their short stature. Nonetheless, growth hormone therapy in pharmacologic doses improves growth.

Almost all girls with TS will need treatment with exogenous estrogen for inducing and maintaining the development of secondary sex characteristics and promoting optimal bone health [8]. Later, cyclic progestins are added to induce cyclic uterine bleeding and prevent endometrial hyperplasia. The timing and dosing of estrogen therapy should be selected to reflect normal puberty. Beginning treatment with low-dose estradiol around 11 to 12 years of age permits a normal timing and pace of puberty without compromising adult height. Growth hormone and estrogen may be given together until epiphyseal fusion occurs, following which the growth hormone is stopped.

6. **Describe other X-chromosome abnormalities that can cause infertility.**

Two other X-chromosome abnormalities that can cause infertility are Klinefelter syndrome and Fragile X syndrome. Klinefelter syndrome (KS) is the most common congenital abnormality causing primary hypogonadism, occurring in approximately 1 in 1000 live male births [9]. The most common genotype is 47,XXY, but greater and lesser numbers of X chromosomes have also been reported, resulting in mosaicism. The 47,XXY genotype results from non-disjunction of the sex chromosomes of either parent during meiotic division, while mosaicism likely results from non-disjunction during mitotic division after conception. The greater the number of extra X chromosomes, the greater the phenotypic consequences, both gonadal and extragonadal.

A hallmark of KS is small, firm testes and reduced testosterone production, leading to underdeveloped secondary sexual characteristics. Individuals may have sparse facial and body hair due to decreased androgen levels. Approximately one-third of adolescents with KS develop enlarged breast tissue, which may persist into adulthood. Individuals with KS often exhibit taller than average height, with disproportionately long legs and arms. Most males with KS experience azoospermia (absence of sperm), leading to challenges with natural conception. Early diagnosis and tailored interventions, including testosterone replacement therapy and educational support, can significantly improve quality of life and mitigate some of the associated challenges of KS.

Fragile X syndrome (FXS) is a genetic disorder resulting from a loss-of-function mutation in the fragile X mental retardation 1 (*FMR1*) gene on the X-chromosome and is the most common inherited cause of intellectual disability [10]. Both males and females can be affected. Fragile X is caused by an unstable expansion of a CGG trinucleotide repeat at the 5′ untranslated region.

This condition leads to a spectrum of phenotypic manifestations encompassing cognitive, behavioral, and physical features depending upon the mutation state, degree of methylation, sex, mosaicism, and degree of the fragile X mental retardation protein (FMRP) deficit. Individuals with FXS often experience learning disabilities and cognitive impairments such as autism spectrum disorder, attention deficit/hyperactivity disorder, anxiety, and mood disorders, with males typically more severely affected than females. Common physical traits include a long, narrow face, prominent ears, and a prominent forehead [11]. Post-pubertal males often present with enlarged testicles. Early diagnosis and tailored interventions, including educational support and behavioral therapies, are crucial in managing the diverse manifestations of FXS and enhancing the quality of life for affected individuals.

7. **Consider the psychological, social, and emotional issues a young girl with delayed puberty may experience. Explain this patient's future fertility and discuss the options for her to have children in the future.**

Adolescence is a difficult phase of life and may be more difficult for those experiencing an abnormal puberty. A young girl with pubertal maturation problems may feel like an outcast and begin to isolate herself. She might be made fun of or bullied at school. She may start to exhibit signs of anxiety or depression. As a healthcare practitioner, it is important to counsel the family to monitor for significant changes in behavior, such as retraction from social interactions, team sports, or other group activities. Reassure the family that puberty is variable and can occur later in some children. Provide the patient and family with goals and expectations when it comes to pubertal changes, and if these goals are not being met, assure them that further testing will be done to find out why. Offer the family psychological and family counseling in addition to support groups. Follow-up often to assess for psychological changes.

While TS results in primary ovarian failure, patients with TS CAN become pregnant using methods such as in vitro fertilization with oocyte donation [12]. However, pregnancy in women with TS carries significant health risks, including a heightened likelihood of cardiovascular complications. Therefore, before attempting to become pregnant, women with TS should undergo a complete medical evaluation, with particular attention to cardiovascular and renal function. Given the increased health risks associated with pregnancy in TS, some individuals opt for gestational surrogacy. Another alternative to build a family without the medical risks associated with pregnancy is adoption. Many individuals with TS find this to be a fulfilling path to parenthood. Collaborating with a multidisciplinary medical team ensures personalized care and informed decision-making tailored to each individual's health status and reproductive goals.

Acknowledgement The case scenario was provided by Gregory Norris, MD.

Exam Questions

1. A 14-year-old female is brought in by her mother due to amenorrhea. The patient reports she has never had a period in the past and became concerned when her friends talked about "changes." She has Sexual Maturity Stage 1 breast development. What is the best next step in evaluation?
   A. Reassurance
   B. Karyotype analysis
   C. Ultrasound
   D. Urine β-HCG
   E. FSH
   F. LH

Answer: D
Learning Objective: Compare and contrast hypogonadotropic vs. hypergonadotropic

hypogonadism and describe the initial workup for primary amenorrhea

Explanation: First test is always human chorionic gonadotropin (HCG) in a female of reproductive age with amenorrhea. Urine HCG is a quick, non-invasive test that has high sensitivity and specificity for detecting a common cause of amenorrhea. While seen more uncommonly in a younger female, pregnancy should always be high on the differential when a patient presents with amenorrhea at any premenopausal age. A is incorrect, as reassurance is inappropriate—primary amenorrhea needs to be ruled out. While an ultrasound (option C), karyotype analysis (option B), FSH (option E), and LH (option F) would be helpful tests, they are considered only after a urine HCG.

2. An 11-year-old female presents to the clinic for developmental changes. Her mom is concerned that she "looks different" from the other kids in class. On physical exam, she exhibits SMR Stage 2 breast development and SMR Stage 3 pubic hair growth. Her pubarche is caused primarily by activity of which of the following?
   A. Hypothalamic ACTH
   B. Ovarian estrone
   C. Ovarian estradiol
   D. Adrenal zona reticularis
   E. Adrenal zona glomerulosa
   F. Adrenal zona fasciculata

Answer: D

Learning Objective: Describe the pathways and hormones responsible for pubertal development and how these changes correlate with the SMR and clinical changes that occur during puberty in girls and boys.

Explanation: Pubarche, the development of pubic hair, is due to the actions of androgens, particularly from the adrenal gland in females. The adrenal zona reticularis is responsible for secreting androgens in response to pituitary ACTH. ACTH is not produced by the hypothalamus (option A). Ovarian estrone (option B) and ovarian estradiol (option C) are related to secondary sex characteristics in the developing female, not pubarche. The adrenal zona glomerulosa (option E) does not produce androgens (it produces mineralocorticoids). While some androgens are produced by the adrenal fasciculata (option F), the majority are produced in the deeper zona reticularis.

3. A 13-year-old female presents to the family practice clinic with amenorrhea. Her mom reports that she has never had a period and "isn't developing like the other girls." On physical exam, she is noted to be short in stature, has a shield-shaped chest, and has SMR 1 breast development. A karyotype analysis is done and shows 45,X/46,XY. Which of the following is the most likely mechanism of her mosaicism?
   A. Germline chromosomal non-disjunction during cell division
   B. Somatic chromosomal non-disjunction during cell division
   C. Y-linked disorder
   D. Spontaneous mutation

Answer: A

Learning Objective: Define mosaicism and discuss methods of genetic testing in patients with suspected TS. Review the different genotypes of TS.

Explanation: The karyotype of this patient suggests this is a case of TS. Mosaicism is most commonly a result of a germline chromosomal non-disjunction during cell division. While some diseases are caused by somatic non-disjunction (option B), TS is defined by anomalies of the X-chromosome. While a small percentage of patients can have a structurally abnormal Y chromosome, TS is defined by anomalies of the X-chromosome and is not caused by spontaneous mutation (option D).

References

1. Melmed S, Polonsky KS, Larsen PR, Kronenberg HM, editors. Williams textbook of endocrinology. 14th ed. Philadelphia: Elsevier; 2020. Section: Disorders of the Hypothalamus and Pituitary & Gonadal Disorders

2. Laufer MR, Grady AE. Evaluation and management of primary amenorrhea. UpToDate; 2023. Retrieved from www.uptodate.com
3. Plant TM. Neuroendocrine control of the onset of puberty. Front Neuroendocrinol. 2015;22(38):73–88.
4. Claude JA, Sapra A. Physiology. StatPearls: Sexual maturity rating; 2022. Retrieved from https://www.ncbi.nlm.nih.gov/books/NBK551691
5. Welt CK. Clinical manifestations and diagnosis of primary ovarian insufficiency (premature ovarian failure). UpToDate; 2025. Retrieved from www.uptodate.com
6. Kikkeri NS, Nagalli S. Turner syndrome. StatPearls; 2023. Retrieved from https://www.ncbi.nlm.nih.gov/books/NBK554621
7. Irzyniec T, Jez W, Lepska K, Maciejewska-Paszek I, Frelich J. Childhood growth hormone treatment in women with turner syndrome—benefits and adverse effects. Sci Rep. 2019;9:15951.
8. Klein KO, Rosenfield RL, Santen RJ, Gawlik AM, Backeljauw PF, Gravholt CH, Sas TCJ, Mauras N. Estrogen replacement in turner syndrome: literature review and practical considerations. J Clin Endocrinol Metab. 2018;103(5):1790–803.
9. Los E, Leslie SW, Ford GA. Klinefelter syndrome. StatPearls; 2023. Retrieved from https://www.ncbi.nlm.nih.gov/books/NBK482314
10. Garber KB, Visootsak J, Warren ST. Fragile X syndrome. Eur J Hum Genet. 2008 Jun;16(6):666–72.
11. Van Esch H. Fragile X syndrome: clinical features and diagnosis in children and adolescents. UpToDate; 2024. Retrieved from www.uptodate.com
12. Folsom LJ, Fuqua JS. Reproductive issues in women with turner syndrome. Endocrinol Metab Clin N Am. 2015 Dec;44(4):723–37.

Part IX

Psyche

22 Lingering Tiredness

Jasper Puracan

Learning Objectives

1. Explain the mechanism of action for SSRI & SNRI medications and side effects related to these classes of medications .
2. Describe the mechanism of action for cyclic antidepressants and monoamine oxidase inhibitors, identify atypical antidepressants, and discuss related side effects.
3. Identify the potential causes of serotonin syndrome, outcomes of elevated serotonergic transmission, and describe the mechanism of action for the antidote to serotonin syndrome should standard resuscitation efforts fail.
4. Differentiate between the DSM-V clinical criteria for generalized anxiety disorder and major depressive disorder. Examine the clinical questionnaires (GAD-7, PHQ-2, and PHQ-9) utilized in assessing patients who may have these conditions.
5. Identify key nonpharmacological treatment modalities for anxiety and/or depression, spanning interpersonal therapies to possible procedures.
6. Describe the epidemiology and risk factors associated with the development of generalized anxiety disorder and major depressive disorder.
7. Identify potential roadblocks to treatment within the context of cultural norms and perceptions towards mental health and how clinicians can treat patients with better cultural awareness.

J. Puracan (✉)
Department of Psychiatry, Banner University Medical Center, Phoenix, AZ, USA

REBLS CBI

Chief Complaint: You're reviewing the chart of your next outpatient clinic patient. Mr. Adam Villanueva, a 24-year-old Filipino American male, is coming in today with a chief complaint of weight changes as well as fatigue (lingering tiredness).

What Is Your Differential Diagnosis?

V—vascular—anemia, lymphedema
I—infectious—pneumonia, COVID-19, infectious diarrhea
N—neoplastic—Hodgkin's lymphoma, testicular cancer, pancreatic cancer
D—drug reaction—SSRI/SNRI use
I—idiopathic/iatrogenic—supplement/OTC medication use, bariatric surgery
C—congenital/ cardiac—heart failure
A—autoimmune/allergic—cystic fibrosis, Addison disease, IBD
T—traumatic—s/p abdominal injury, trauma surgery

C. A. Standley (ed.), *Biomedical Science and Clinical Foundations*,
https://doi.org/10.1007/978-3-031-98353-5_22

E—endocrine/metabolic—diabetes, malnutrition, hypo/hyperthyroidism
R—Renal/Respiratory—Sleep apnea, acute renal failure
p**S**ychiatric—anxiety, depression, substance use disorders, eating disorders

History

Adam is a calm 24-year-old male who reports that over the past 4 months, he has felt consistently fatigued and has noticed his weight has been dropping in that time period. He estimates that he has lost roughly 15 pounds. Additionally, during this time he describes a feeling of being "on edge," and that he can't shake the sensation. When this happens, he feels like his heart is "jumping around in his chest." He says he worries most about COVID-19 as well as the stresses of "application season." He reports occasional headaches and muscle aches as well. Some nights, he is unable to sleep due to the restlessness. He reports trying to use melatonin to sleep at night and energy drinks during the day to deal with insomnia and fatigue, respectively, but neither of them alleviates his symptoms. He is concerned that this will impact his work as an assistant in a research laboratory.

How does this expanded HPI change your current differential?

Students should be able to narrow differential diagnosis; given specific history elements of stressors, along with constellation of restlessness, insomnia, fatigue refractory to stimulants and worries. Psychiatric concerns should predominate and take precedence over other differential diagnoses, though causes of cardiac origin may play a role in this presentation.

V—vascular—anemia, lymphedema
I—infectious—pneumonia, COVID-19, infectious diarrhea
N—neoplastic—Hodgkins lymphoma, testicular cancer, pancreatic cancer
D—drug reaction—SSRI/SNRI use
I—idiopathic/iatrogenic—supplement/OTC medication use, bariatric surgery
C—congenital/ cardiac—heart failure, arrhythmias
A—autoimmune/allergic—cystic fibrosis, Addison disease, IBD
T—traumatic—s/p abdominal injury, trauma surgery
E—endocrine/metabolic—diabetes, malnutrition, hypo/hyperthyroidism
R—Renal/Respiratory—Sleep apnea, acute renal failure
p**S**ychiatric—**anxiety, depression, substance use disorders, eating disorders**

PMH Adam denies having any prior surgeries, hospitalizations, or accidents. He reports that he has seasonal allergies, but no other health conditions. Adam was born in America and is up to date with his immunizations. He reports no sick contacts at his workplace or apartment complex.

Medications
10 mg Melatonin nightly
10 mg cetirizine (Zyrtec) nightly
500 mg acetaminophen (Tylenol) as needed
Multivitamin one tablet daily

Allergies No known drug allergies

Family History Parents are immigrants from the Philippines. Mother has HTN (hypertension), diabetes, and hypercholesterolemia. Father has mild HTN, GERD, and is on a DASH diet per his PCP. Has one older sibling who lives in New York, says he is healthy. Adam also provides information on his extended family, stating "I've heard that almost all of my aunts and uncles are 'crazy' in some way or another, and a lot are alcoholics. Guess my parents didn't want me ending up like that." He says that he is not aware of any mental health concerns in his immediate family.

Social History Lives alone in Tempe, AZ. Currently working in a research lab at ASU. Graduated from NAU *summa* cum *laude* in

May 2020 with a biology degree, a second degree in political science, and a minor in French. He states that he completed his applications for medical school 2 months ago, and is now awaiting offers to interview with different medical schools across the country. Says that "unless I have to go to work or get gas, I stay at home. I don't have contact with anyone I don't need to be in contact with because of COVID."

High Risk Behaviors When you begin asking Adam about HRBs, you notice he becomes somewhat shy with his answers, but responds to your questions. He says that he doesn't use tobacco in any form. He reports that he normally doesn't drink but that "when I feel super on edge, I usually take a shot of tequila or a beer or two and that usually calms me down." When you ask him how often that happens, he reports that its once every 1 to 2 weeks. He denies the use of any drugs, stating "I don't want to even risk trying them because I'm applying to medical school." He says that he usually has three to four energy drinks a day to stay awake and alert while at work. He reports having had three prior female partners, but is presently single, not sexually active, and has no hx of STIs.

ROS

General: No fevers, chills, diaphoresis, night sweats.

Hematopoietic: No enlarged or tender lymph nodes, abnormal or excessive bleeding or bruising.

HEENT: No present headache, vision or hearing changes, nasal discharge, sore throat.

Lungs: No cough, wheezing or shortness of breath.

Heart: Reports palpitations, no chest pain, lightheadedness.

Urinary: No dysuria, frequency, urgency.

Endocrine: 15 lb. weight loss over last four months, fatigue, occasional insomnia, no hot or cold intolerance or increased thirst.

Musculoskeletal: Occasional muscle pain as per HPI. No pain, tenderness, or stiffness of joints.

Neurological: No weakness, numbness.

Psychiatric: When asked about his mood, he appears guarded as he states "I'm feeling fine, but I'm not sure why I'm tired all the time."

Stop and Think

What symptoms, past medical history, medications, family, and social history are relevant to a chief complaint?

This is intended to help guide students to Learning Objective 4. Students will likely identify the weight loss, fatigue, insomnia, and the noticeable "guarding" with questioning on HRBs as relevant to the chief complaint, along with the isolated palpitations. Due to the limited opportunities that the patient has to interact with others during pandemic times, the likelihood of an infectious cause is low. Students may also take note of the extended family history and the comments that the patient makes about them and his parents. It is vital for students to understand that with psychiatric issues, listening to what the patient says is oftentimes as valuable as the facts contained within their statements. The lack of knowledge of any mental health conditions within the immediate family may be factual, or could be due to a cultural drive to not admit mental health concerns on the part of the parents and brother. Attention must also be paid to the discussion on the patient's HRB (High Risk Behaviors) responses—while he does respond to the questions about sexual activity and tobacco/alcohol/drug use, it is important to note that in some cases the patient may be holding back information. In this case, the combination of the patient appearing reluctant to share information as well as the use of alcohol as a compensatory mechanism for anxiety symptoms may cause students to wonder if the patient is telling the truth. Hypothetically, if there was a weight gain along with fatigue and compensatory eating for emotional distress, as opposed to this case presentation, students may also include the family history of HTN, DM, and hypercholesterolemia as an aggravating factor. However, these details do not align with the reported weight loss and fatigue originally stated in the chief complaint. Students may also catch onto this patient's distinguished academic achievements so far, along with the desire to become a physician, and may describe academic pressures as part of the concerns this patient presents with. This is intended to tie into the cultural aspects of "the model minority" that many Asian Americans are confronted with in present society. This will be touched on later.

Physical Examination

Vitals:

T = 36.2 °C (97.8 °F)	Normal
P = 122	Tachycardic
BP = 136/80	Within normal limits
RR = 19	Within normal limits
Resting O_2 sat = 99%	Normal

General: Adam is a neatly dressed Asian male with a slightly overweight body habitus. Appears anxious.
Skin: Warm and dry
HEENT: Unremarkable
Neck: Unremarkable
Chest/Lungs: Breath sounds equal bilaterally; no crackles or wheezing
Cardiovascular: Tachycardia, regular rate, normal S1 and S2, no murmurs
Abdomen: Bowel sounds present, soft, nontender; no hepatosplenomegaly
Extremities: No edema, DP/PT 2+ bilaterally
Neurological: CNII-XII intact, strength and sensation intact in all extremities

Stop and Think

1. How does this information help you to prioritize your differential diagnosis?

This is overall a very benign physical exam. This should continue to lead students to consider more psychiatric concerns are in motion here. The subjective palpitations are corroborated by an objective tachycardia, observation of a slightly anxious affect, and an almost elevated respiration rate. It is important to emphasize that when assessing a patient in real time, it will appear much different compared to this scenario. Observation of an anxious affect in person can take many forms—shifting eyes, body language, mannerisms and speech. Conversely, observation of a depressed affect can be represented more by a constellation of downcast eyes, distractibility, low energy, poor eye contact, and even slower than expected motion in the absence of an injury or neurological deficits. These are all observations that a physician can make regardless of specialty or training, and may help identify potential other stressors that they may be able to help address for patients.

2. How can you better refine your differential diagnosis? What further form of assessment can you perform in this type of situation?

This is intended to guide students to the MSE. In the absence of a physical exam, and oftentimes in both outpatient and inpatient settings, the core of the psychiatrist's workup is the mental status exam. It provides a framework to assess a patient's thought process, mood, affect, and other potential psychological factors at play that helps to determine their present state as well as helping to narrow down a potentially broad psychiatric differential. It is important to note, again, that much of this requires observation during interactions with patients, something that cannot be replicated perfectly in a CBI setting. As such, inferences will be made based upon the patient's upcoming conversation. However, students may already be aware of some of the terms listed in the next section, relating to the mental status exam and will likely be practicing elements of the MSE during their Doctoring course. Of note, it is still vital that for a general workup, obtaining basic labs such as a CBC, CMP, and thyroid levels would be indicated here as well, in order to investigate more physiological causes of some of this patient's symptoms.

Mental Status Exam

Mental Status Exam

Client Name					Date
OBSERVATIONS					
Appearance	◻ Neat	◻ Disheveled	◻ Inappropriate	◻ Bizarre	◻ Other
Speech	◻ Normal	◻ Tangential	◻ Pressured	◻ Impoverished	◻ Other
Eye Contact	◻ Normal	◻ Intense	◻ Avoidant	◻ Other	
Motor Activity	◻ Normal	◻ Restless	◻ Tics	◻ Slowed	◻ Other
Affect	◻ Full	◻ Constricted	◻ Flat	◻ Labile	◻ Other
Comments:					
MOOD					
◻ Euthymic ◻ Anxious	◻ Angry	◻ Depressed	◻ Euphoric	◻ Irritable	◻ Other
Comments:					
COGNITION					
Orientation Impairment	◻ None	◻ Place	◻ Object	◻ Person	◻ Time
Memory Impairment	◻ None	◻ Short-Term	◻ Long-Term	◻ Other	
Attention	◻ Normal	◻ Distracted	◻ Other		
Comments:					
PERCEPTION					
Hallucinations	◻ None	◻ Auditory	◻ Visual	◻ Other	
Other	◻ None	◻ Derealization	◻ Depersonalization		
Comments:					
THOUGHTS					
Suicidality	◻ None	◻ Ideation	◻ Plan	◻ Intent	◻ Self-Harm
Homicidality	◻ None	◻ Aggressive	◻ Intent	◻ Plan	
Delusions	◻ None	◻ Grandiose	◻ Paranoid	◻ Religious	◻ Other
Comments:					
BEHAVIOR					
◻ Cooperative	◻ Guarded	◻ Hyperactive	◻ Agitated	◻ Paranoid	
◻ Stereotyped	◻ Aggressive	◻ Bizarre	◻ Withdrawn	◻ Other	
Comments:					
INSIGHT	◻ Good	◻ Fair	◻ Poor	Comments:	
JUDGMENT	◻ Good	◻ Fair	◻ Poor	Comments:	

This is done in addition to the physical exam if a clinician suspects that there may be an active psychiatric concern for one of their patients. It relies heavily on observation and conversation with patients in order to get a better understanding of how their current mental state is influencing their lived experience.

Next Steps

With a concern that there is some type of mental health issue at play, and the relative lack of physical exam findings that might point to a physiological cause of Adam's symptoms, you decide to spend more time talking with him. You look at your clinic schedule as you document your physical exam and see that your next patient canceled last minute, giving you another half hour before you need to wrap things up with Adam.

"Adam, so far I don't see a physical cause for what you've been feeling the last few months. Overall your physical exam tells me you're in decent shape. I want to spend more time talking with you, especially since it seems that the last few months have been particularly stressful for you. How have you been holding up?"

1. The key point here is to show that starting to investigate psychiatric concerns with patients necessitates that the physician starts with an

open ended question. This is to allow the patient to feel that they have a space to share their true thoughts and to build trust. Echoing the sentiment that the patient appears and reports being stressed works to help the patient feel heard, and may compel them to open up more. Much of this is emphasized in the students' Doctoring course in the NEURS (Name, Explore, Understand, Respect, Support) emotional validation framework.

Adam starts to open up to you, and starts to take on a more sullen appearance as he starts to look at the floor more. He says "Well, honestly it's been going on longer than the last few months. I've felt like this for close to a year now. I'm always so worried about whether or not I'll actually be able to go to medical school. This is my second time applying, and I thought I would've gotten in the first time and could avoid doing a gap year. During all of my senior year, I was really on edge. Every month went by without an interview offer until the season ended. I really thought I had a good application, good enough test scores. People were expecting me to get a lot of interviews, and probably even make it into an Ivy League program. But as the year went on, I felt worse and worse. More and more restless, unable to sleep. Started drinking more to try to relax, as long as I was off the next day. What few friends I had in college said I got more irritated too. Over time, I started to hate myself too, for not being good enough. Now that it's another application season, it feels like all these thoughts and feelings are coming back again. I'm not hungry anymore, I barely sleep and I'm always tired. Barely can concentrate at work. I'm always worried about what people think of me not being in medical school because they think I'm really smart. You want to know the worst part about all of this is? My parents didn't believe me when I told them about all of this four months ago. They got real angry when I told them I was drinking, and said that 'it's all in your head'. They already think I'm a screwup for not getting into medical school. They said that if I don't get in this year, they're cutting me off from the family completely. My friends have also been wondering why I haven't gotten into medical school yet. I feel like trash and I don't think I'll ever do enough or be enough to make people happy. Every shortcoming makes me feel even more anxious and sad. And honestly, you're the only person I've tried to tell besides my parents."

Prompt:

2. With this conversation, how would you report this patient's MSE in regards to your observations, mood, and cognition?

There is a lot of information to unpack and process from the patient. He has provided additional, key information to the students that will help them guide the discussion on how to best describe these aspects of the MSE. In regards to observations, we can assume his appearance is neat (from the general section of the physical exam), speech is normal, eye contact is avoidant, motor activity can be assumed to be normal, and affect is full (given the ability to shift from calm to sullen in this case so far). Regarding mood, he can be described as both anxious and depressed. Cognition can be inferred as intact—he remembers details about college, recent memories about earlier parts of the clinic visit, and does not appear to be distractible or disoriented.

To complete your MSE, you say to Adam "I hear you, and I am incredibly glad that you chose to speak with me today about all of what's been going on the past several months. There's some additional questions I need to ask you to make sure you're safe and so that I can develop a good treatment plan. Is it alright if we talk some more?," to which Adam agrees.

You ask if he hears or sees things that are not really there, which he denies.

(Auditory/Visual Hallucinations)

You ask if he has any thoughts or hurting or killing himself. He denies that, but also says "when I feel my worst, I feel like I wouldn't mind getting hit by a bus. It's not that I want to die or would jump in front of one, but the thought of that happening to me doesn't bother me when I feel really low."

(Suicidality, he reports passive ideation but no active ideation, plan, or intent)

You then ask if he has any thoughts of hurting or killing anyone else, which he denies.

(Homicidality)

Based on the conversation, there does not appear to be any active delusions. After he has opened up to you, he appears more cooperative rather than shy or guarded.

3. How would you rate a patient's insight and judgement? Given that Adam is not in an altered state of consciousness, what would you rate his insight and judgement as?

Insight and judgement are two key aspects of the MSE: for psychiatric patients and to assess a patient's capacity to make medical decisions for themselves. In the context of the MSE, assessing insight refers to how well a patient is aware of themselves and their psychiatric condition, whereas judgement is an assessment of whether the patient has an ability to avoid behavior that might be hazardous to themselves. There are more marked derangements of both insight and judgement in more severe psychiatric cases, including florid mania, untreated schizophrenia, or extreme substance use disorder. In this patient's case, he appears to have fair insight into his anxiety and depression. He can identify what is causing him to feel restless and down, but does not have enough knowledge about himself to connect these sources of stress to why they cause him to psychologically respond in the ways that he does, or to connect the symptoms themselves to one another in a constellation that he can recognize. In line with this, the patient has fair judgement. He can identify some ways to try and deal with the symptoms he is experiencing (melatonin, caffeine), but does not meet "good." This is due to the fact that he indulges in compensatory alcohol use when feeling severe symptoms of anxiety. While he avoids use if it may impair his work the next day, it is not an ideal coping mechanism. Now conversely, his judgement would be poor if at any presence of anxiety symptoms, he drank profusely regardless of any responsibilities he may have the next day. There are formal and informal ways to assess insight and judgement, and in this case we interpret his present state based on the conversation as an indirect way.

Stop and Think

With all of this information now available, and having talked with Adam through a very difficult conversation, what is your updated diagnosis? Are there other tools that clinicians might be able to use to help with diagnosis?

The mixture of the symptoms he's had for some time now should signal students to conclude that he has a mixture of both anxiety and depression. Students are likely familiar with key clinical symptoms that, when in relation to each other, would indicate that a patient likely has anxiety or depression. Given that there is a high prevalence of co-presenting anxiety and depression, this case is intended to highlight the more organic application of their psychiatric knowledge, and to show the all too common fact that there are considerable overlaps and comorbidities of psychiatric conditions both in their psychological etiology and in their presentation. The board exams and block tests will much more likely test students on these diagnoses and their related components in isolation of one another.

In regards to tools, students will likely mention the GAD-7 and the PHQ, whether it is the 2 item or the 9 item variant. These questionnaires have been studied and shown to have had a utility in helping clinicians diagnose generalized anxiety disorder and major depressive disorder. Oftentimes outpatient clinics will integrate these as additional forms for patients to fill out after arriving for their scheduled appointment, or for their initial intake and visit at the facility.

With no physical health conditions that are causing Adam any issues, there is no indication of any lab testing. You then talk to him about treatment. Since there is no active suicidal or homicidal ideation, and he doesn't represent a threat to anyone, you feel that you can manage him in an outpatient setting.

What are possible pharmacological treatments for mixed anxiety and depression? What would you turn to first?

SSRI/SNRIs
TCAs
MAOIs
Atypicals

Generally, SSRIs are the first choice and most often prescribed of these medications. However, the choice of what to use depends greatly on other factors including other medications, patient preference of what side effects they'd like to avoid, and response to different antidepressant classes, amongst other drivers. As such, the choice of which medication to use first becomes more complicated. There was an effort by Banner Health to investigate use of genetic sequencing in service to targeted pharmacogenetics for mental health diagnoses such as depression, identifying which patients may be responsive or resistant to certain antidepressants.. This represents another example of an emerging field where pharmacogenetics is intended to become a powerful asset for physicians as they try to optimize treatment for their patients in order to achieve the greatest health benefits.

In terms of non-pharmacological treatments, what are options for patients on an outpatient treatment plan?

Cognitive behavioral therapy, interpersonal psychotherapy, behavioral activation, and psychodynamic psychotherapy, amongst others, form the bedrock of non-pharmacological treatment. Cognitive behavioral therapy is the most often utilized, due to a greater dearth of research on its utilization for various mental health conditions.

Transcranial Magnetic Stimulation and Electroconvulsive Therapy are used for more resistant forms of depression, and would not be the first line treatment. Valleywise utilizes TMS for outpatient treatment for patients, and actually still also conducts ECT for patients with the most severe and resistant conditions, such as marked catatonia and severe major depression.

You recommend to Adam that he start on escitalopram as a daily medication, emphasizing that he do not take more than the dose recommended. You also refer Adam to a clinical psychologist, explaining that he may benefit from some cognitive behavioral therapy as an adjunct to pharmacological treatment. He inquires about what to do with sudden spikes of anxiety, and you discuss the use of hydroxyzine on an as-needed basis, to which he agrees to try as well.

Why is it vital that patients avoid overdosing on medications such as SSRIs? What kind of unique reaction could take place in the event of an overdose?

Serotonin syndrome is a characteristic, and board-tested, concept that is important for clinicians starting patients on SSRI medication regimens to monitor and be aware of. In a setting where there is increased serotonergic neurostimulation, the risk of serotonin toxicity is present, which can manifest as a classic triad of mental status changes, autonomic hyperactivity, and neuromuscular abnormalities. This can potentially be lethal, and requires monitoring and prompt treatment.

Adam seems to agree it would help, but he expresses some concerns.

"Is this all confidential? Would I be able to keep word of these treatments from getting out? I don't want people to think I'm insane. It feels like besides my parents, a lot of other people expect a lot out of me, and I don't think I can let them know about anything I've told you."

Prompt: How might the idea of "the model minority" and similar concepts influence the care that patients might accept and receive?

This, along with the next prompt, are intended to guide students towards Learning Objective 7. In essence, the model minority myth is that Asian Americans are not out to cause trouble or make noise, and are incredibly successful in America. This overlooks variable SES between different Asian populations in America, and places extremely high and oftentimes unfair expectations upon Asian Americans within American culture, that can both drive and influence responses to mental health conditions such as MDD and GAD.

Prompt: What are some ways that clinicians can integrate cultural nuances and socioeconomic determinants of mental health (SDOMH) into their practice?

Clinicians can engage with cultural awareness organizations to provide educational resources to their colleagues, in efforts to broaden the understanding of the background of an ever changing patient population in the US. Seeking out opportunities to share knowledge and hold conversations with colleagues from other cultural backgrounds would be beneficial as well. There is also some research that state that utilization of culturally sensitive and complementary treatment modalities into mental health treatment, dependent on the cultural identity of the patient, may provide greater health outcomes compared to standard practice. This necessitates an integration of knowledge of different cultural norms and drivers into a clinician's practice.

You reassure Adam, stating that HIPAA laws restrict access to medical health records and that the psychologist you have referred him to is experienced in navigating the interaction between Asian cultural norms and mental health concerns. You ask him to follow up in 1 month to assess how the treatment plan is progressing.

One month later, Adam returns to the clinic. He seems more calm and at ease as you go in to speak with him. He reports that the escitalopram has seemed to make him feel less on edge and down gradually over the last month, and that the psychologist you referred him to has helped him start working on mindfulness and understanding his emotions better. On top of that, he's ecstatic to tell you that he's also received four invitations to interview with medical schools. He can't thank you enough for being someone he could trust with his anxiety and depression.

End of Case

Learning Objective 1 Explain the mechanism of action for SSRI & SNRI medications and side effects related to these medication classes.

Key Points:

1. SSRIs operate primarily by preventing the reuptake of serotonin neurotransmitters at the pre-synaptic surface, elevating the levels of serotonin within the synaptic cleft.
2. SNRIs operate similarly, and also inhibit the reuptake of norepinephrine at the pre-synaptic surface.
3. SSRI and SNRI side effects span weight gain, sexual dysfunction, drowsiness, insomnia, anxiety, and many others at varying incidences.

Standard transmission of serotonergic signals starts with the release of serotonin neurotransmitters from the pre-synaptic membrane into the synaptic cleft. These then interact with 5-HT receptors on the post-synaptic membrane to propagate signals forward. Attenuation of serotonergic signal transmission is driven by the 5-HT monoamine transporter on the pre-synaptic membrane (called SERT). The serotonin that returns to the pre-synaptic membrane can then be degraded by monoamine oxidase A and B. The mechanism is similar for norepinephrine.

SSRIs and SNRIs work by inhibiting the reuptake of solely serotonin, or both serotonin and norepinephrine [1, 2]. This then leads to an increasing amount of affected neurotransmitters in the synaptic cleft. As a result, with higher amounts of neurotransmitter present in the cleft, there is continued interaction with their respective receptors on the post-synaptic cleft, thereby increasing serotonin and norepinephrine activity.

Both of these medication classes have important side effects to keep track of. The three most common side effects for SSRIs include sexual dysfunction (17%), drowsiness (17%), and weight gain (12%), whereas SNRIs have had reported common side effects of nausea, dizziness, and diaphoresis. Important to note for both of these medication classes is that there are differing risks of suicidality based on age. Consulting patients on the use of these antidepressants should include a conversation about suicide risk, as in those aged 18–24, they may raise the risk of suicidal ideation and completion, whereas there is no change for those aged 24–30, and a decrease in risk for those aged 31 and older.

Learning Objective 2 Describe the mechanism of action for cyclic antidepressants and monoamine oxidase inhibitors, identify atypical antidepressants, and discuss related side effects.

Key Points:

1. Tricyclic and tetracyclic antidepressants inhibit the reuptake of serotonin and norepinephrine from the synaptic cleft as well.

2. Tricyclics are in one of two categories—tertiary amines have two methyl groups at the end of its side chain, whereas secondary amines have only one methyl group.
3. MAOi medications interfere with the function of monoamine oxidase A, a key enzyme that normally degrades serotonin and norepinephrine in the presynaptic membrane.
   (a) Tranylcypromine, phenelzine, and selegline have varying functions in relation to MAOa and MAOb.
4. Atypical antidepressants that are used include bupropion and mirtazapine.
5. Side effects for these medications are very similar to that of SSRI/SNRI medications.

TCAs operate along the same principles as SSRIs and SNRIs. These, along with MAOIs emerged as the first utilized antidepressants, finding use in the late 50 s and 60 s. The caveat with the tricyclics in particular is the differentiation between tertiary amines and secondary amines in the side chain of different tricyclic antidepressants. Tertiary amines (amitriptyline, clomipramine, doxepin, imipramine, and trimipramine) have two methyl groups on the side chain and have been found to have greater potency in inhibiting the reuptake of serotonin compared to norepinephrine. In comparison, TCAs that are secondary amines, with only one methyl side chain group (desipramine, nortriptyline, and protriptyline) and have greater efficacy in blocking the reuptake of norepinephrine compared to serotonin. Tertiary amines tend to have more severe side effects than secondary amines due in part to causing more anticholinergic adverse effects, and TCAs in general cause more side effects compared to SSRIs/SNRIs. As such, clinicians won't resort to these unless necessary.

MAOIs such as tranylcypromine, selegiline, and phenelzine work by directly inhibiting the monoamine oxidase enzymes, namely A and B [3]. Overall, the mechanism of action leads to the inactivation of these enzymes, halting the breakdown of serotonin and norepinephrine in the presynaptic membrane thereby increasing the amount of these neurotransmitters that can be repackaged into synaptic vesicles for continued transmission. Tranylcypromine is an irreversible inhibitor of MAOa primarily, and also appears to have some similar effect on MAOb, and also blocks serotonin reuptake. Phenelzine irreversibly inhibits both MAOa and MAOb. Selegiline has a dose-dependent function, where at lower doses selectively inhibits MAOb and increases dopaminergic neurotransmission, whereas at higher doses inhibits both MAO enzymes while increasing serotonergic, noradrenergic, and dopaminergic activity. All of these, in addition to the risks of causing serotonin syndrome, can also cause hypertensive crisis if used with sympathomimetic agents or foods containing tyramine.

Two commonly used (relatively speaking) atypical antidepressants in the United States are bupropion and mirtazapine [4]. These drugs have been tested on in board examinations and are included in this CBI debrief for completion's sake. Bupropion is a monocyclic aminoketone that has utility in depression as well as treating obesity and tobacco dependence, with common side effects of dry mouth, nausea, and insomnia. Of note, this is contraindicated for anyone with bulimia nervosa or anorexia nervosa. Mirtazapine has a similar structure to tetracyclines, but works to increase 5-HT1 neurotransmission indirectly by inhibiting postsynaptic 5-HT2 and 5-HT3 receptors and presynaptic a2 adrenergic receptors. Common side effects include dry mouth, drowsiness, and sedation.

A table of side effects for all classes of antidepressants from UpToDate is included below for reference.

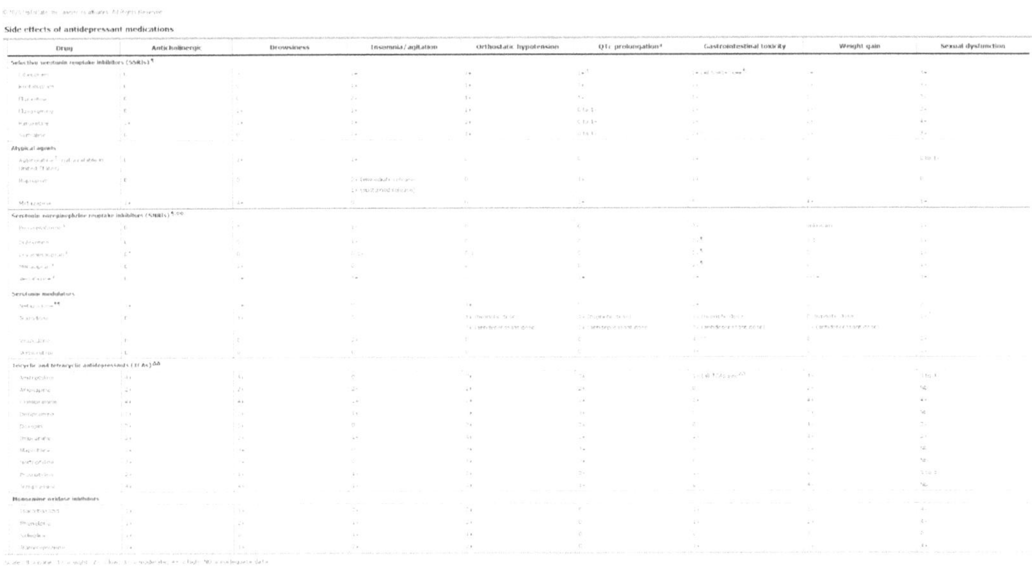

Side effects of antidepressant medications

Drug	Anticholinergic	Drowsiness	Insomnia / agitation	Orthostatic hypotension	QTc prolongation	Gastrointestinal toxicity	Weight gain	Sexual dysfunction
Selective serotonin reuptake inhibitors (SSRIs)								
Atypical agents								
Serotonin norepinephrine reuptake inhibitors (SNRIs)								

Learning Objective 3 Identify the potential causes of serotonin syndrome, predict outcomes of elevated serotonergic activity, and describe the mechanism of action for the antidote to serotonin syndrome should standard resuscitation efforts fail.

Key Points:

1. Associated with stimulation of postsynaptic 5-HT1A and 5-HT2A receptors and can be precipitated by any number of ways that elevate serotonergic activity.
2. Elevated serotonergic activity has consequences throughout the body, including autonomic symptoms, mental state changes, and neuromuscular hyperactivity.
3. Normal course of care to treat serotonin syndrome is to utilize benzodiazepines and supportive care. Should that fail, the use of cyproheptadine is recommended as an antidote, as it is an antagonist for both 5-HT1A and 5-HT2A receptors.

Serotonin syndrome is a key concern for physicians and patients as they begin and continue medical therapies for various psychiatric concerns [5]. Of the other side effects, outside of tyramine-induced hypertensive crisis, this represents a severe complication of antidepressant pharmacology. Serotonin syndrome can take place in a variety of situations, all revolving around continued stimulation of 5-HT1A and 5-HT2A receptors. The different etiologic categories for serotonin syndrome are listed below, along with examples of common causative agents.

(a) Impairment of serotonin reuptake (SSRIs/SNRIs, cocaine, MDMA)
(b) Increased release of serotonin (amphetamines, cocaine, MDMA)
(c) Increased serotonin formation (tryptophan)
(d) Monoamine oxidase inhibition (MAOIs)
(e) Direct serotonin receptor agonist activity (buspirone, triptans, ergots, LSD)

The consequences of elevated serotonergic activity are expressed through new autonomic symptoms, mental state changes, and neuromuscular hyperactivity. Autonomic nervous system consequences include diaphoresis, tachycardia, hyperthermia, elevated blood pressure, emesis, and diarrhea. Shifts in mental state encompass delirium, agitation, anxiety, restless, and disorientation. Also, tremors, muscle rigidity, myoclonus, and hyperreflexia can appear. Normally, after workup is complete and serotonin syndrome is the leading diagnosis, standard of care is to stop all potential serotonergic agents, attempt to normalize vital signs, and achieve sedation with benzodiazepines. Importantly, if these measures do not work to help stabilize the patient, clinicians must then turn to the use of cyproheptadine as an antidote. It is a histamine-1 receptor antagonist, and also a 5-HT1A and 5-HT2A antagonist, working to reverse the increased serotonergic transmission and its associated symptoms.

Examples of agents that can precipitate serotonin syndrome

Mechanism	Agent involved
[illegible]	[illegible]
[illegible]	[illegible]
[illegible]	[illegible]
[illegible]	[illegible]
[illegible]	[illegible]
[illegible]	[illegible]

Learning Objective 4 Differentiate between the DSM-V clinical criteria for generalized anxiety disorder and major depressive disorder. Examine the clinical questionnaires (GAD-7, PHQ-2, and PHQ-9) utilized in assessing patients who may have these conditions.

Key Points:

1. Clinical criteria for generalized anxiety disorder include excessive worry/anxiety for at least 6 months, inability to control the worry, the anxiety causes significant distress, not due to a substance or another mental disorder, and at least three of the symptoms in the GAD-7.
2. Clinical criteria for major depressive disorder involves a history of one or more depressive episodes without a history of mania or hypomania, involving five of the nine symptoms listed on the PHQ-9 for at least 2 weeks, nearly every day.
3. GAD-7 and the PHQ-9 are validated tools used by clinicians that convert the clinical stigmata of both GAD and MDD into forms that patients and physicians can use.

Clinical criteria for both GAD and MDD are outlined by the DSM-5. For GAD, clinical criteria focus on the worries or anxiety itself, the length of time it has been occurring, and whether it is able to be controlled or not. Regarding MDD, in the absence of factors that may lead to a diagnosis of cyclothymic disorder, bipolar I or bipolar II disorder, clinical diagnosis focuses on elements that characterize the patient's depressive episode(s) as well as a minimum length of 2 weeks for the symptoms to have been occurring. The clinical criteria for both were utilized in designing the GAD-7 and the PHQ-9, shown below [6]. These aid clinical decision-making and diagnosis, and often times are integrated into the intake paperwork for patients in outpatient settings. Validated in prior studies, these instruments allow the clinician to determine both the presence and severity of any GAD or MDD. Of note, there has also been use of the PHQ-2, a quicker version of the PHQ-9 that only utilizes the first two questions of the PHQ-9 which were also converted from a numeric scale to a simple yes/no response. Any positive response would compel the clinician to utilize the PHQ-9 to better characterize the patient's symptoms.

GAD-7

Over the last 2 weeks, how often have you been bothered by the following problems?	Not at all	Several days	More than half the days	Nearly every day
1. Feeling nervous, anxious or on edge	0	1	2	3
2. Not being able to stop or control worrying	0	1	2	3
3. Worrying too much about different things	0	1	2	3
4. Trouble relaxing	0	1	2	3
5. Being so restless that it is hard to sit still	0	1	2	3
6. Becoming easily annoyed or irritable	0	1	2	3
7. Feeling afraid as if something awful might happen	0	1	2	3

Total Score ___ = Add Columns ___ + ___ + ___

If you checked off any problems, how difficult have these problems made it for you to do your work, take care of things at home, or get along with other people?

Not difficult at all	Somewhat difficult	Very difficult	Extremely difficult
☐	☐	☐	☐

PHQ-9 depression questionnaire

Name:	**Date:**			
Over the last 2 weeks, how often have you been bothered by any of the following problems?	**Not at all**	**Several days**	**More than half the days**	**Nearly every day**
Little interest or pleasure in doing things	0	1	2	3
Feeling down, depressed, or hopeless	0	1	2	3
Trouble falling or staying asleep, or sleeping too much	0	1	2	3
Feeling tired or having little energy	0	1	2	3
Poor appetite or overeating	0	1	2	3
Feeling bad about yourself, or that you are a failure, or that you have let yourself or your family down	0	1	2	3
Trouble concentrating on things, such as reading the newspaper or watching television	0	1	2	3
Moving or speaking so slowly that other people could have noticed? Or the opposite, being so fidgety or restless that you have been moving around a lot more than usual	0	1	2	3
Thoughts that you would be better off dead, or of hurting yourself in some way	0	1	2	3
Total ___ =	___	+ ___	+ ___	+ ___
PHQ-9 score ≥10: Likely major depression				
Depression score ranges:				
5 to 9: mild				
10 to 14: moderate				
15 to 19: moderately severe				
≥20: severe				
If you checked off any problems, how difficult have these problems made it for you to do your work, take care of things at home, or get along with other people?	Not difficult at all	Somewhat difficult	Very difficult	Extremely difficult

Learning Objective 5 Identify key non-pharmacological treatment modalities for anxiety and/or depression, spanning interpersonal therapies to possible procedures.

Key Points:

1. CBT is most common and most researched, but dependent on the context of the patient's situation with their mental health, other modalities may be more optimal.
2. Transcranial magnetic stimulation and electroconvulsive therapy are still in use as well, indicated for more resistant forms of depression and other more severe mental health conditions.

Nonpharmacological modalities typically include cognitive behavioral therapy, psychodynamic psychotherapy, interpersonal psychotherapy, behavioral activation, problem-solving therapy, and supportive psychotherapy [7, 8]. Cognitive behavioral therapy is the most often utilized and most researched talk therapy modality presently, focused on shifting perceptions of cognitive distortions and encouraging better insight into one's own mental and emotional state, in preparation for present and future challenges. However, dependent upon the patient's comfort level and preferences, as well as any potential comorbid mental health conditions and engagement with the therapeutic course, these other modalities may be more beneficial and appropriate. As an example, for a patient that may have both depression as well as borderline personality disorder, dialectical behavioral therapy may be a more effective therapy modality than the others.

Transcranial magnetic stimulation and electroconvulsive therapy are two interventions focused primarily on treating more resistant forms of depression, which do not respond as well to the standard pharmacotherapy & talk therapy combination. ECT is reserved for the most severe and resistant forms of depression, including marked catatonia, depression with psychotic features, or a persistent suicidal intent. Both of these are more invasive options, and TMS can be done on an outpatient basis. ECT requires a procedure room and anesthesia, thus requiring visits to the hospital. Notably, Valleywise (Maricopa) has continued to provide both services for patients.

Learning Objective 6 Describe the epidemiology and risk factors associated with the development of generalized anxiety disorder and major depressive disorder.

Key Points:

1. MDD
   (a) Prevalence has been rising over the last few years
   (b) Estimated lifetime prevalence in the United States is 17%
   (c) Two times greater in females than males
   (d) Prevalence of depression declines with increasing age overall
2. GAD
   (a) Lifetime prevalence in the United States is between 5.1% and 11.9%
   (b) Twice as common in women compared to men
   (c) Most common anxiety disorder amongst elderly
   (d) 66% of those with GAD had a comorbid diagnosis
3. MDD/GAD Risk Factors—mixture of genetic, external, and behavioral sources can lead to the development of these mental health diagnoses

Both MDD and GAD have been found to be present in a fairly large contingent of the American population [9, 10]. Likely due to a greater awareness and slightly decreased stigma surrounding mental health, the prevalence of MDD has been rising, more than doubling between 1991 and 2001 within the United States alone. Estimated lifetime prevalence of MDD in the US is 17%, and a 12-month prevalence between 2 and 6%. It is far more prevalent in women relative to men, however this may be also due to differences in both the etiology and symptomatology of depression between genders. Interestingly, age has been found to have a negative correlation with prevalence, with findings that there is a lower prevalence in those 65 years and older compared to those younger. This must be considered with the additional fact that these elderly adults also tended to be in good health, without chronic conditions that would negatively impact their emotional state.

GAD has a lifetime prevalence between 5.1% and 11.9% within the United States and is one of the most common mental health diagnoses encountered in primary care settings. Like MDD, it is twice as common in women as it is in men yet this may also be driven, again, by differences in behaviors and help-seeking between genders. Of note, 66% of those with GAD have at least one comorbid mental health diagnosis in their lifetime, including social phobia (34.4%), specific phobia (35.1%), and panic disorder (23.5%). Clinicians must be vigilant for any indication that a patient either has or is beginning to develop an additional mental health concern to address in tandem with their existing GAD.

Risk factors for both GAD and MDD encompass biological, psychological, and external drivers. These encompass trauma/stressful life events, loss of loved ones, genetics, history, neuroticism, low SES, low education, unstable family structure, and other prior mental health diagnoses. This is to illustrate the multifactorial nature of many mental health conditions including GAD and MDD, such that an integrative and multidisciplinary therapeutic approach that embodies the biopsychosocial model of care is vital to patients' clinical improvement.

Learning Objective 7 Identify potential roadblocks to mental health treatment within the context of cultural norms and perceptions and how clinicians can treat patients with better cultural awareness.

Key Points:

1. How mental health is viewed is greatly influenced by culture
   (a) The "model minority" myth greatly influences Asian Americans
   (b) Higher levels of stigma
   (c) Collectivistic values may pressure patients away from seeking help, seen as individualistic
2. Adaptations of care to cultural nuances are important
   (a) Provision of culturally sensitive care
   (b) Education on different cultures
   (c) Entering into conversations and encounters with no judgment

Filipino culture, as well as several other Asian cultures, emphasizes the importance of educational attainment. Couched in the context of the immigration of highly successful persons from India, China, Japan, Korea, and the Philippines, there has been a persistent belief in the "model minority" here in America. This concept essentially revolves around the notion that the Asian immigrant population represents the successes of the United States in giving minority segments of the populace the opportunity to attain success and stature without complaint or becoming obtrusive in American society. This concept disregards the markedly more complex picture within the Asian cultural "monolith" in America, where less advantaged populations such as the Hmong and Cambodians do not enjoy the same opportunities for success as the other previously mentioned groups. On top of creating division within and between ethnocultural groups in the United States, this "model minority" myth represents a considerably negative pressure on patients who may not live up to these expectations, or those who suffer from mental health issues such as the patient in this case. There is also a considerable cultural undercurrent wherein many Asian populations are greatly reluctant to speak about any mental health issues, if at all. This cultural norm can negatively influence patients' readiness to begin mental health treatment, seek it out in the first place, and even develop a support group of trusted individuals. Each of these factors can amplify issues relating to an already tenuous mental state and must be addressed effectively in order to provide effective and compassionate care.

Understanding the interactions between culture and a patient's present mental health is an important tool for clinicians. While treatment courses can be recommended to patients once enough diagnostic criteria are met, much of the clinical improvement that may be achieved is highly reliant on the patient's comfort, willingness, and ability to be an active participant in their care. Cultural norms and perceptions can influence that ability. As an example, within Asian communities, there is a considerable stigma against talking about mental health, to the point where it may go unaddressed by the community at large and would earn a patient scorn from others from the same background for discussing their issues. Furthermore, American-born children of immigrants face a generational conflict between what their parents' culture and what American culture dictate for behavior and norms. Comparatively, Asian cultures are more collectivistic and deferential to elders in nature, whereas American culture is centered around individualism and independence. This cultural conflict can manifest as and be the driver of mental health issues for first-generation Asian Americans, resembling a hesitance to talk about mental health concerns as seen in this CBI case.

For patients facing cultural pressures alongside their mental health concerns, it is important for physicians to be informed about how perceptions and norms interact with mental health, and how to best approach a patient with a different cultural background than the clinicians. This encompasses educating oneself on other cultures, meeting with patients, and avoiding judgmental comments, and integrating cultural awareness into treatment plans and clinical practice. These all help to establish rapport and trust between the patient and the physician, which are vital to adherence to treatment plans and ultimately improved clinical outcomes.

Exam Questions

1. A 32-year-old female patient who you recently started on a treatment regimen for comorbid generalized anxiety disorder and major depressive disorder is presenting to the ED with complaints of muscle stiffness, diarrhea, tachycardia, and agitation. Collateral information from her boyfriend reveals that she took a bottle of pills, but that he wasn't sure of the name of the medication. You need to give an antidote for her condition. Which of the following molecular receptors will the antidote bind to?
   A. Benzodiazepine
   B. μ-opioid
   C. Acetylcholine
   D. 5-HT1A and 5-HT2A

Answer: D

Learning Objective: Identify the potential causes of serotonin syndrome, outcomes of elevated serotonergic transmission, and describe the mechanism of action for the antidote to serotonin syndrome should standard resuscitation efforts fail.

Explanation: Serotonin receptor types 5-HT1A and 5-HT2A describe the target receptors for cyproheptadine, the definitive antidote used to treat the serotonin syndrome that this patient has developed from the antidepressant overdose. The symptoms listed in the vignette represent continued serotonergic transmission by way of these two post-synaptic receptors, and with the history of MDD, it is likely that this patient was started on an SSRI treatment regimen but was not fully assessed for suicide risk, contributing to this scenario. A is incorrect this receptor is for benzodiazepines, and the associated antidote for a benzodiazepine overdose that targets this receptor is flumazenil. In an isolated benzodiazepine overdose, the patient would present with CNS depression and normal vital signs. Given the complaints of agitation and tachycardia, the patient likely wouldn't have overdosed with a BZD, regardless of their GAD, nor would they have the symptoms listed here. B is incorrect as this receptor is implicated in cases of opioid overdoses, which are characterized by respiratory depression, depressed mental status, and absence of bowel sounds. The antidote is naloxone, which directly competes with opioids at these receptors and inhibits signal transmission. These symptoms do not match up with the symptoms of serotonin syndrome listed in the vignette. C is incorrect as acetylcholine receptors are implicated in cholinergic toxicity cases, which are reversed by the use of atropine, competitively inhibiting the action of acetylcholine at muscarinic receptor sites. Patients with signs of cholinergic toxicity will present with bradycardia, lacrimation, miosis, diarrhea, and diaphoresis. While this patient does have diarrhea, the history points away from a potential organophosphate poisoning, making serotonin syndrome secondary to an SSRI the more likely cause.

2. In your outpatient clinic, you are speaking with a 48 y/o male who you've just diagnosed with major depressive disorder, and are now discussing treatment possibilities. He denies the use of tobacco, drugs, or alcohol, has no other ongoing health concerns, and has not been treated for MDD before. In tandem with sertraline, what additional treatment would be most appropriate for this patient?
   A. Olanzapine
   B. Cognitive behavioral therapy
   C. Alprazolam
   D. Amitriptyline
   E. Transcranial magnetic stimulation

Answer: B

Learning Objective: Identify key non-pharmacological treatment modalities for anxiety and/or depression, spanning interpersonal therapies to possible procedures.

Explanation: Cognitive behavioral therapy is the most often utilized non-pharmacological treatment modality for MDD, and is frequently employed in conjunction with SSRIs/SNRIs to treat patients diagnosed with MDD. A is incorrect as Olanzapine is a second-generation antipsychotic indicated for treating patients with schizophrenia and treatment-resistant major depressive disorder. While this may become part of this patient's future treatment regimen, this patient has not been treated for MDD before and should be treated with first-line modalities before escalating to an antipsychotic. C is incorrect as Alprazolam is a benzodiazepine indicated for generalized anxiety disorder and anxiety associated with depression. Given that this patient has MDD in isolation from other health conditions, this medication would not be utilized in this case. D is incorrect as Amitriptyline is a tertiary amine tricyclic antidepressant, and it has been utilized as an initial medication for MDD in the past. However, the side effect profile, along with the emergence of more tolerable medications (SSRIs/SNRIs), make this less likely to be used for a treatment-naïve patient. E is incorrect as transcranial magnetic stimulation is a procedure utilized for patients who are suffering from a treatment-resistant form of MDD. While this patient may use this modality later on in his treatment, this would not be indicated for use with SSRIs in a case of newly diagnosed MDD.

3. A 57 year-old male comes into the emergency department complaining of nausea and vomiting after attending a cocktail party 2 hours ago. He reports not drinking due to being a designated driver, but that he had several hors d'oeuvres consisting of cured meats and cheeses. He reports that he is being treated for depression and recently switched to a new medication, but has no history of hypertension. On exam, he appears uncomfortable, and his blood pressure is 192/97. Which of the following is the most likely new medication he is taking and is responsible for his present condition?
   A. Phenelzine
   B. Amitriptylin.
   C. Citalopram
   D. Mirtazapine

Answer: A

Learning Objective: Describe the mechanism of action for cyclic antidepressants and monoamine oxidase inhibitors, identify atypical antidepressants, and discuss related side effects.

Explanation: This patient is presenting with hypertensive crisis as a result of consuming tyramine containing foods at the cocktail party. As a result of the mechanism of MAOIs such as phenelzine, tyramine (a sympathomimetic) is not broken down in the GI tract and as a result enters systemic circulation, causing a hypertensive crisis, leading to the nausea and vomiting as a secondary effect due to elevated intracranial pressure from the elevated blood pressure. B is incorrect as Amitriptyline is a tertiary amine cyclic antidepressant that can cause serotonin syndrome as a major side effect, characterized by vomiting and elevated blood pressure, amongst other symptoms. However, given the recent change in the patient's medication and a precipitating event involving tyramine-containing foods, serotonin syndrome, and by extension use of a TCA, is less likely. C is incorrect as Citalopram is an SSRI that can cause serotonin syndrome as a major side effect, characterized by vomiting and elevated blood pressure, amongst other symptoms. However, given the recent change in the patient's medication and a precipitating event involving tyramine-containing foods, serotonin syndrome, the use of an SSRI is less likely. D is incorrect as Mirtazapine is an atypical antidepressant and has a similar structure to tetracyclic antidepressants. It works to increase 5-HT1 neurotransmission indirectly by inhibiting postsynaptic 5-HT2 and 5-HT3 receptors and presynaptic a2 adrenergic receptors. Common side effects include dry mouth, drowsiness, and sedation, which are not consistent with the symptoms presented in this clinical vignette.

References

1. Hirsch M, Birnbaum RJ. In: Solomon D, editor. Selective serotonin reuptake inhibitors: pharmacology, administration, and side effects. UpToDate; 2023. https://www.uptodate.com/contents/selective-serotonin-reuptake-inhibitors-pharmacology-administration-and-side-effects.
2. Nelson C. In: Solomon D, editor. Serotonin-norepinephrine reuptake inhibitors: pharmacology, administration, and side effects. UpToDate; 2023. https://www.uptodate.com/contents/serotonin-norepinephrine-reuptake-inhibitors-pharmacology-administration-and-side-effects.
3. Hirsch M, Birnbaum RJ. In: Solomon D, editor. Monoamine oxidase inhibitors (MAOIs): pharmacology, administration, safety, and side effects. UpToDate; 2023. https://www.uptodate.com/contents/monoamine-oxidase-inhibitors-maois-pharmacology-administration-safety-and-side-effects.
4. Hirsch M, Birnbaum RJ. In: Solomon D, editor. Atypical antidepressants: pharmacology, administration, and side effects. UpToDate; 2023. https://www.uptodate.com/contents/atypical-antidepressants-pharmacology-administration-and-side-effects.
5. Boyer EW. In: Ganetsky M, editor. Serotonin syndrome (serotonin toxicity). UpToDate; 2024. https://www.uptodate.com/contents/serotonin-syndrome-serotonin-toxicity.
6. Williams J, Nieuwsma J. In: Swenson S, editor. Screening for depression in adults. UpToDate; 2025. https://sso.uptodate.com/contents/screening-for-depression-in-adults.
7. Craske M. In: Friedman M, editor. Generalized anxiety disorder in adults: cognitive-behavioral therapy and other psychotherapies. UpToDate; 2024. https://www.uptodate.com/contents/generalized-anxiety-disorder-in-adults-cognitive-behavioral-therapy-and-other-psychotherapies.
8. Rush AJ. Major depressive disorder in adults: approach to initial management. In: Swenson S, Solomon D, editors. . UpToDate; 2025. https://www.uptodate.com/contents/major-depressive-disorder-in-adults-approach-to-initial-management.
9. Baldwin D. In: Friedman M, editor. Generalized anxiety disorder in adults: Epidemiology, pathogenesis, clinical manifestations, course, assessment, and diagnosis. UpToDate; 2025. https://www.uptodate.com/contents/generalized-anxiety-disorder-in-adults-epidemiology-pathogenesis-clinical-manifestations-course-assessment-and-diagnosis.
10. Krishnan KRR. In: Swenson S, Solomon D, editors. Major depression in adults: epidemiology. UpToDate; 2024. https://www.uptodate.com/contents/major-depression-in-adults-epidemiology.

23 Strange Behavior

Robert Yang

Learning Objectives

1. Compare and contrast the clinical presentation of delirium, dementia, and depression.
2. Identify the risk and protective factors for delirium.
3. Identify the methods of diagnosing delirium and list tools that can be utilized to assist with diagnosing patients.
4. List the treatment plan and medical management for delirium. Also include management of agitation, pharmacologic, and non-pharmacologic.
5. Describe the prognosis and potential complications and consequences of delirium on patient function after discharge.
6. Analyze the incidence and prevalence of delirium. Are there any groups that are particularly susceptible? How often does the diagnosis get missed? Are there any studies that examine better ways to assess for delirium?

Chief Complaint "My husband is not acting like himself"

Differential Diagnosis

- Intoxication
- Psychosis—schizophrenia, schizoaffective, etc.
- Dementia
- Delirium
- Mood disorder—depression, anxiety, mania
- Sundowning
- Non-convulsive seizures
- Encephalopathy
- Stroke
- Meningitis
- Hyper/hypothyroid
- Hypo/hyperglycemia

R. Yang (✉)
Department of Psychiatry, University of Arizona College of Medicine Phoenix, Phoenix, AZ, USA
e-mail: Robert.yang@bannerhealth.com

History of Presenting Illness

You are asked to consult on Jim, an 82-year-old male post-op day 4 from a laparoscopic cholecystectomy whose wife is complaining that he is acting differently than he has the past few days. She states that he sometimes does not make any sense with some of his sentences. Also, he has been forgetting some of the recent conversations he has had with her at the hospital. Patient has been stable since his operation and his Foley catheter was removed last night. Patient is able to report that he is currently not in any pain but other history is difficult to obtain from him as he is lethargic. Per staff, mentation has been fluctuant and on assessment today he is A x O 2 to person and place.

Prompt: What is important to ask patient's family right now? How does his mental state right now compare with his baseline at home?

C. A. Standley (ed.), *Biomedical Science and Clinical Foundations*,
https://doi.org/10.1007/978-3-031-98353-5_23

Prior to the hospital stay, patient has been having some difficulty with memory because he misplaces things more often over the past 5 years. She states that he is still sharp and solves a daily sudoku puzzle otherwise. His gets around 5 hours of sleep a night and she thinks that his mood is "ok."

PMH
HTN
High cholesterol
COPD
Chronic back pain

Medications
Lisinopril 10 mg QD PO
Atorvastatin 40 mg QD PO
Oxycodone-Acetaminophen 1 tablet Q6h PRN could be contributing to altered status

Allergies
NKDA

Social History
Patient was previously diagnosed with alcohol use disorder.
Wife reports that he has been sober for the past 5 years.
He smokes 1 pack of cigarettes a day for the past 30 years.
No other drug use.

Note: Some patients may be able to hide things from the spouse, so just because wife says that he has been sober, we cannot rule out completely.

FH:
Father was diagnosed with bipolar I disorder.
Mom was diagnosed with depression and Alzheimer's.
Older sister diagnosed with epilepsy.
HTN runs in the family.

Stop and Think
- What is the chief complaint?
  - Altered mental status
- What symptoms, PMH, medications, FH, social hx are relevant to the chief complaint?
  - difficulties with memory
  - lethargy
  - hx of substance abuse
  - oxycodone-acetaminophen
  - FH of psychiatric and neurological disorders
- What is our differential?
  - Delirium secondary to either an infection post-op or from medications.
  - Dementia—less likely due to the acute nature. Patient's baseline is showing that he is just having normal cognitive decline from age. This acute episode goes beyond his baseline.
  - Depression
  - Substance intoxication/withdrawal
  - Seizure/Neurological etiology—less likely due to no personal history of having seizures and he is now in his 80 s.
- What physical exam findings and ancillary studies (labs, imaging) can be used to narrow down the differential?
  - Comprehensive physical exam will be difficult so focus on vital signs, hydration status, skin condition, and infectious loci. Patient's appearance can help indicate if there are any signs of intoxication or underlying organ failure. Vital signs can also help examine for signs of infection or any signs of withdrawal/intoxication.
  - Neurological exam can be difficult depending on patient status, emphasizing on consciousness, attention, cranial nerves, and motor deficits. If indicated, can also perform LP or EEG.
  - Mental status exam—MMSE, BCAM.
  - CBC, CMP—to assess for infection and electrolyte abnormalities; UA for possible UTI; UDS—for intoxication, ethanol level—intoxication.
  - Possible imaging would be CT head but would be done last if all other tests come up negative to look for any neurological etiologies.
  - If positive abdominal exam, could CT abdomen to see if there are any post-op complications occurring.

Physical Examination:
Vitals: Pulse 80 bpm, RR 16, T 98.6; normal temperature does not rule out all possible eti-

ologies of infection in this patient (UTI), SpO2 99% RA, BP 134/86

Gen: lethargic thin male, somnolent

Skin: warm, pink, and dry

HEENT: NC/AT, PERRLA, EOMI, nasal passages clear, oropharynx without exudate or erythema

Neck: supple with full ROM, no JVD, no carotid bruits, no thyromegaly or masses

Lungs: CTAB

CV: RRR, nl s1, s2, no s3, s4, murmurs, rubs, PMI fifth ICS MCL

Abdomen: incision sites w/ mild erythema, no drainage, healing well. Non-tender, non-distended, no HSM

Extremities: No clubbing, cyanosis, edema

Pulses: radial, femoral, DP, PT 2+ bilat sym

Neuro: CN could not be properly assessed due to limited cooperation by the patient; motor and sensory unable to assess; patellar and Achilles reflex 2+ symmetrical; normal tone; toes down-going; gait unable to be assessed

Mental Status Exam:

Appearance: male appears as stated age

Behavior: no eye contact, somnolent

Speech: slowed, soft

Affect: flat

Mood: depressed

Thought process: tangential

Psychomotor: decreased movement

Attention: poor

Memory: short-term

Insight: lacking

Prompt: How do we perform the mental status exam?

A mental status exam is an important part of a comprehensive assessment. It involves a structured assessment of the patient's psychological and cognitive functioning through observation of components such as appearance, general behavior, speech, language, mood, affect, thought process and perception.

BCAM (Brief Cognitive Assessment Test)

Positive

Prompt What is the BCAM useful for diagnosing?

The Brief Cognitive Assessment Test is useful for diagnosing delirium. It includes 4 features: Feature 1 = acute onset or fluctuating course, Feature 2 = inattention, Feature 3 = disorganized thinking, and Feature 4 = altered level of consciousness. The diagnosis of delirium by this method requires the presence of features 1 and 2 and either 3 or 4 [1].

CBC

Component	Patient
RBC	4.00 × 10^12/L
MCV	90 fL
RDW-CV	12%
Platelets	300 × 10^9/L
WBC	9.8 × 10^9/L

Note: CBC is normal. Patients with UTI may not show any signs of infection on their CBC

CMP

Component	Patient
Na	143
K	4.2
Cl	107
CO2	27
Glucose	100
BUN	52
Creatinine	2.73
Ca	9.6
Albumin	4.1
Bilirubin	0.5
Protein	7.6
Albumin	4.1
ALT	40
AST	32
Alk Phos	83

What do the CBC and CMP suggest? What other studies do we still need?

The CBC is normal. Patients with UTI may not show any signs of infection on their

CBC. Creatinine is elevated suggesting some decreased kidney function. UA should be acquired to analyze urine in some more detail.

UA

Component	Patient
pH	6.0
Protein	+1
Glucose	Negative
Ketones	Negative
Bilirubin	Negative
Urobilinogen	0.3
Blood	Trace
Leukocytes	+3
Nitrite	Positive
WBC	>100/hpf
RBC	10–15/hpf

Having nitrites and leukocytes indicates that this patient has a UTI.

Urine drug screen: negative

Negative ethanol

Do we need to perform any imaging at the moment?

Probably not at the moment.

How do these test results help rule out and define your hypothesis?

Based on history and physical exam, it seems that patient's symptoms are acutely different than baseline but physical exam shows mostly just mentation deficits. Through lab results, we know that patient does not have any drugs on board and is showing signs of UTI. Because of the combination of being post op, being an elderly patient, previous catheter, and diagnosis of UTI, patient has a lot of risk factors for delirium [2].

Stop and Think

- *What is the diagnosis and what were we able to rule out?*
  - Patient has delirium due to a UTI.
  - Symptoms are acute, less likely to be dementia or a mood disorder. Given baseline report from wife, patient has normal mood and no hx of seizure disorder so less likely. Lab results show no sepsis, drug use, or ethanol in his system.
  - Patient had Foley catheter and is post -op, likely UTI is causing the delirium.
- *How does this relate to the patient's initial chief complaint?*
  - Patient had acute change in mental status.
  - Risk factors are old age, UTI, post-op day 3, opioid use, hx of alcohol use disorder.
- *What is the next step in management?*
  - Treat the underlying condition.
  - Delirium is managed by treating the mental status as well as the underlying condition. In this patient's case, we would treat the patient's UTI with antibiotics.

Next Steps

Patient was treated empirically with ceftriaxone 1 g IV and urine cultures were sent off.

The next night

You get paged by the night nurse saying that patient has been agitated and screaming at the nurses. There was an event where he began threatening them and swinging his arms around.

What do we do next?

Options include:

Low-dose haloperidol (0.5 to 1 mg) PRN most commonly used to manage patient behaviors.

Consider using Olanzapine—it is sedating, does not need to be adjusted renally or hepatically, and can come in a dissolvable tablet. It can be provided 2.5 mg–5 mg PRN with a max dose of 20 mg within a day. Also it comes in IM formulations.

Ziprasodone—sedating, no renal or hepatic adjustments; it comes in PO and IM. It can provide 10 mg BID PRN; max of 160 mg.

Patient was able to rest and was continued to be treated with antibiotics. His mental status has gone down to baseline, and he was able to be discharged home.

End of Case

Learning Objective Answers

1. Compare and contrast the clinical presentation of delirium, dementia, and depression.

Table 23.1 provides a quick comparison of depression, delirium, and dementia.

Delirium

A disturbance of consciousness and altered cognition are essential components of delirium and associated confused states. This condition can develop over a short period of time and can fluctuate throughout the day. An early sign of delirium is a change in awareness and ability to focus, sustain, or shift attention. This can be subtle, but family members are essential to relay how behaviors have changed from baseline. Another change is that patients can be more distractible during conversation. Patients also can appear drowsy, lethargic, or even semi-comatose. The opposite is more likely to occur in cases with alcohol or sedative drug withdrawal and is less common in older adults.

Changes in cognition can occur as well. Patients may have perceptual disturbances where they misidentify people in the room or believe that certain objects represent people. These hallucinations can range from being visual, auditory, or somatosensory, and the patient generally does not have insight on these hallucinations. Alongside these hallucinations, delusions of harm may appear.

Delirium develops over hours to days and can persist for days to months. Symptoms generally become more severe at night, and patients can be relatively lucid during morning rounds. Additionally, patients can complain of fatigue, sleep disturbance, depression, anxiety, restlessness, irritability, and hypersensitivity to light or sound. In older patients, the most common presentation is a relatively quiet, withdrawn state that frequently is mistaken for depression.

Dementia and Mild Cognitive Impairment

Most patients do not present with self-complaint of dementia symptoms. Most often, a caretaker or spouse will bring patient in describing increasing memory issues. Dementia, like delirium, has to be represented by a change in cognition from baseline [4]. However, unlike delirium, the change is gradual. Usually the patient will have difficulty with normal activities of daily living such as driving or managing finances. Forgetfulness is usually the chief complaint for dementia syndromes. They will have difficulty with retaining new info, handling complex tasks, reasoning, spatial ability, language, and behavior. Specific dementia syndromes such as Alzheimer's and vascular dementia have specific presentations that are diagnosed presumptively.

There are also different causes for cognitive impairment so the entire clinical picture must be considered. Conditions that include parkinsonism along with dementia include Lewy body dementia, progressive supranuclear palsy, multiple system atrophy, and corticobasal degeneration.

Table 23.1 Characteristics of depression, delirium, and dementia

	Depression	Delirium	Dementia
Onset	Weeks to months	Hours to days	Months to years
Mood	Low/apathetic	Fluctuates	Fluctuates
Course	Chronic; responds to treatment	Acute; responds to treatment	Chronic, with deterioration over time
Self-awareness	Likely to be concerned about memory impairment	May be aware of changes in cognition; fluctuates	Likely to hide or be unaware of cognitive deficits
Activities of daily living (ADLs)	May neglect basic self-care	May be intact or impaired	May be intact early, impaired as disease progresses
Instrumental activities of daily living (IADLs)	May be intact or impaired	May be intact or impaired	May be intact early, impaired before ADLs as disease progresses

Source: Ref. [3]

Normal cognitive decline associated with aging is distinguished from dementia because they are not very progressive and typically do not affect daily function. Delayed recall or forgetting remained relatively stable. Mild cognitive impairment is an intermediate between normal aging and dementia. Patients categorized with mild cognitive impairment (MCI) do not meet criteria for dementia but have some increased severity of cognitive change. They are at a higher risk for developing dementia but also may remain stable.

Depression in the Elderly

Patients with depression are often more likely to complain about memory loss than those with dementia. Depressed patients often present on their own instead of having a family member or caretaker bring them in. These patients often have more psychomotor retardation and have poor effort on testing for symptoms. They often say phrases such as "I just can't do this." This is distinguished from dementia because dementia patients often put the effort in, but their responses are incorrect. These patients will also describe the typical depression symptoms such as loss of interest, change in appetite, sleep disturbance, fatigue, impaired concentration, suicidal ideation (SI), and guilt. Patients who respond to affection from family/caregivers, retain humor, look forward to visits, and accept assistance and care are less likely to be suffering from depression.

2. Identify the risk and protective factors for delirium.

Predisposing risk factors:

- Dementia
- Cognitive impairment
- History of delirium
- Functional impairment
- Vision impairment
- Hearing impairment
- Severity of illness
- Depression
- Stroke
- Alcohol abuse
- Older age

Precipitating Factors:

- Medications
- Psychoactive medications
- Sedatives-hypnotics
- Use of physical restraints
- Use of bladder catheter
- Abnormal electrolytes
- Infection
- Surgery

Prevention:

Orientation protocols—Provision of clocks, calendars, windows, verbal reorienting, familiar faces.

Cognitive stimulation—Regular visits from family and friends, avoiding overstimulation at night especially.

Facilitation of physiologic sleep—Nursing and medical procedures should be avoided during sleeping hours if possible. Reduce night-time noise.

Early mobilization and minimized use of physical restraints.

Visual and hearing aids for patients with impairments.

Ensuring adequate intake and output.

Addressing infection if it is suspected.

Review medication regimen and try to optimize it.

Managing pain—Use of non-opioid medications should be used where possible. Must balance the benefits of opioid use to treat pain vs potential for opioid related delirium.

3. Identify the methods of diagnosing delirium and list tools that can be utilized to assist with diagnosing patients.

Two important parts of delirium are to recognize that it is occurring and uncover the underlying cause. Clinicians often fail to recognize delirium; in some reports, this happens in more than 70 percent of cases. Behavioral problems or cognitive impairment may be readily apparent but wrongly attributed to the patient's age, to dementia, or to other mental disorders.

Next, the DSM-5 can help form a framework for assessing delirium. A change in the level of consciousness is often the first observable clue. Clinicians must not "normalize" lethargy or somnolence by assuming that illness, sleep loss, fatigue, or anxiety are causing the changes. In cases where the patient appears awake, the ability to focus, sustain, or shift attention can be assessed during attempts to obtain a history; a global assessment of the patient's "accessibility" during conversation or the performance of a mental status examination is a sensitive indicator of delirium. Conversation with the patient may elicit memory difficulties, disorientation, or speech that is tangential, disorganized, or incoherent. The clinician should be aware of superficially appropriate conversation that follows social norms but is poor in content. When in doubt, formal mental status testing should be performed, such as the Mini-Mental State Examination or brief bedside tests of attention. Serial-sevens and spelling a word such as "farm" or "world" backward are other simple tests of attention.

History—clues to etiology can be obtained from family, e.g., Hx of recent illness, organ failure, med list, hx of abuse, etc.

General exam—often difficult and impossible to obtain due to state of patient. It should assess for vital signs, hydration status, skin condition, and potential infectious foci. General appearance may be suggestive. Signs can show potential drug use (track marks), CO poisoning, or ketones. A bitten tongue or posterior shoulder fracture-dislocation could suggest a convulsive seizure as well as other head injuries. It must be kept in mind that there are false-positive findings as well.

Neurologic exam—It can be confounded by inattention and altered consciousness. It should emphasize level of consciousness, degree of attention, visual fields, and unambiguous cranial nerve and motor deficits. It can help distinguish any focal neurologic disease. If there is no obvious cause for delirium, it can use neuroimaging, LP, and EEG. It can also look for signs of metabolic or toxic causes such as having asterixis, nystagmus, or other encephalopathic signs.

Review medications to determine if patient is toxic or taking any medications that can contribute to an overmedicated state. Other medical processes should be evaluated for such as fluid balance and electrolytes.

Confusion Assessment Method (CAM) is a tool that is used in the hospital setting to quickly assess a patient for possible delirium. It has a sensitivity of 94 to 100% and a specificity of 90 to 95%. This can be incorporated for routine bedside assessment by nurses for patients that are at risk for delirium. Evidence shows that the CAM is the best test that can be used to identify delirium. There are variations that have been developed for the ICU to allow mechanically ventilated patients the ability to respond to similar questions to assess for delirium.

4. List the treatment plan and medical management for delirium. Also include management of agitation, pharmacologic and non-pharmacologic.

While patient is being worked up for the underlying cause of delirium, supportive care should be initiated for the patient. Depending on what they're in the hospital for, patient should be adequately hydrated and have adequate pain control. Once the underlying condition is identified, therapy should target that etiology to help relieve the delirium. Prevention factors mentioned above should be initiated. Patient should be encouraged to have good nutrition and mobility. Family and other caregivers should discuss how to approach treatment as well as it can be extremely taxing to take care of delirious patients and resources must carefully be assessed.

Managing Agitation

Hyperactive delirium is less common in older patients but cause many barriers to patient care. The patient has increased risk of falls, wandering off, removing tubes, and cause harm to themselves. In these cases, symptomatic control is necessary. In these instances, nonpharmacological resources can be utilized first as psychotropic medications have had mixed responses.

Non-pharmacological interventions include noise control, adequate lighting, and frequent reassurance, touch, and verbal orientation. Having these things adjusted by family or familiar people is preferred. If the patient begins to develop hallucinations and delusions, they should not be endorsed nor challenged. Physical restraints can be used but only as a last resort as they can increase agitation and create additional problems.

Antipsychotics can be used to treat agitation in delirium when symptoms are going to cause harm to the patient and there are not any effective alternatives. As mentioned earlier, there are options of using haloperidol, olanzapine, or ziprasidone as the common choices for medication. Of the antipsychotic medications, low-dose haloperidol is one of the more commonly used medications to help with agitation as it has been around longer and there is limited evidence in regards to the newer antipsychotics.

Benzodiazepines should not be used to treat agitation unless the case is related to drug or alcohol withdrawal or when antipsychotic medications are contraindicated. Some studies show that benzos have increased the risk of delirium so they should be avoided when possible.

In hypoactive delirium, symptomatic treatment is not usually necessary as patients will not usually be at risk for self-harm.

5. Describe the prognosis and potential complications and consequences of delirium on patient function after discharge.

Patients with delirium experience prolonged hospitalizations, functional and cognitive decline, higher mortality, and higher risk for institutionalization even after adjusting for baseline differences in age, comorbid illness, or dementia.

Mortality associated with delirium is high. Several studies have estimated that the one and 6 month mortality to be 14 and 22 percent, respectively. This comes out to approximately twice that of patients without delirium. Some studies have also found a relationship between duration of delirium and mortality. Protracted delirium was associated with increased 1 year mortality compared with those whose symptoms had resolved more quickly, regardless of underlying dementia.

Signs of delirium may persist for 12 months or longer, especially if patients had underlying dementia. One long-term follow-up study showed that after 2 years only 1/3 of patients who experienced delirium still lived independently in the community. Other studies have shown that post-op patients were more likely to have a persistent drop in MMSE scores over baseline at 6 months compared to those who did not suffer delirium. Though delirium is considered a diagnosis that can be treated and reversed, it still seems to cause some impairments that may be prolonged or permanent.

6. Analyze the incidence and prevalence of delirium. Are there any groups that are particularly susceptible? How often does the diagnosis get missed? Are there any studies that examine better ways to assess for delirium?

Nearly 30% of older medical patients experience delirium at some time during hospitalization. Depending on the setting and medical conditions, delirium rates can fluctuate between 18%–64% of patients.

High rates of delirium have been demonstrated in ICUs, EDs, hospice units, nursing homes, and post-acute care settings. Typically, patients who have multiple different medications, especially those that can alter consciousness and cognition, are older, and have poor nutritional status and mobility issues are more likely to be susceptible to get delirium.

Exam Questions

1. A 81-year-old female presents to the ED with altered mental status for the past 2 days as reported by her son. He states that the patient keeps talking to other people occasionally but no one is in the room and she cannot focus on conversations compared to normal. She has a past medical history of ESRD, HTN, high cholesterol, T2DM, anxiety, COPD, and CHF for which she is taking medication for all of these. She does not use any alcohol, drugs, or tobacco. Her physical exam is unremarkable, and vitals are currently stable. A CBC and CMP have been

sent off for work-up. What is the next step of work-up for this patient?
(a) Administer haloperidol 0.5 mg
(b) Head CT
(c) Medication reconciliation
(d) Administer lorazepam 2 mg
(e) Teach the son how to redirect the patient

Answer: C
Objective: #4
Explanation: Patient has multiple comorbidities and is elderly. She is most likely taking a large amount of medications which may be causing her delirium. It should also be noted whether or not she is taking any medications that could potentially be exacerbating this condition. A is incorrect: Patient is not currently agitated, so it is unnecessary for any measurements that require sedation. B is incorrect: Patient does not indicate that there is any trauma at this moment in time. She has been having hallucinations and distractibility. There are other things that can be done first that are more likely causes of delirium. D is incorrect: Patient is not currently agitated and does not require sedation. Benzodiazepines could also exacerbate this current condition. E is incorrect: While important for long-term management, not appropriate at this time because it does not help us assess what is occurring in the patient right now.

2. Surgery calls to ask you to consult on their 78-year-old male patient who is post op day 4 from a hernia repair because patient's wife says he has been more forgetful than normal. Patient has lived a healthy life and has only been diagnosed with HTN that he manages with lifestyle changes. Physical exam is benign, and his vitals are stable. Labs are sent off to assess for fluid status, electrolyte balance, UDS, and to assess for potential sites of infection. Which of the following is not something that can be done to help decrease the risk of further decline in cognition?
   (a) Adequate pain control
   (b) White noise at night
   (c) Frequent family visits
   (d) Good lighting
   (e) Verbal reorientation

Answer: B
Objective: #2
Explanation: Noise should be limited for patients at risk for delirium. They should also have maintained sleep-wake cycles. If patients are overstimulated, and not sleeping well, then they have a higher risk for developing delirium. White noise at night may potentially be too much stimulation and disrupt the patient's sleep. A is incorrect: Though opioids can contribute to delirium, adequate pain control can help patients. Clinicians must weigh the benefits against the cons to determine the amount of medication patients receive. C is incorrect: Having familiar people around patients is helpful for patient comfort, and family can help reorient the patient. D is incorrect: Creates an environment that may help the patient stay oriented. E is incorrect: If staff or family could redirect the patient when distracted or forgetful, it can help the patient not have worse delirium.

3. A 76-year-old male presents to your clinic with his wife as she states that he has become more forgetful over the past few years. She states that because of the forgetfulness, he cannot drive or go shop for groceries anymore. She also states that he seems to lack motivation and just sits on the couch and watches TV for most of the day. He has a PMH of HTN and DM with no pertinent family history or substance use history. His vitals and physical exam are normal. When conducting the mental status exam, patient is able to respond but does not successfully perform the tasks requested. What is his most likely diagnosis?
   (a) Delirium
   (b) Dementia
   (c) Depression
   (d) Absence seizure
   (e) Catatonia

Answer: B
Objective: #1
Explanation: Patient's condition has been declining for a few years and has gotten to a point where he cannot perform ADLs anymore. There are no other influences at this time other than cognitive decline. He does not have any other external factors that could be affecting his mentation. A is incorrect: Patient seems to be going

through a chronic process. Delirium is more acute and related to prolonged hospital stays, metabolic/toxic influences, etc. Patient is relatively healthy and has been having some decline to the point where he is unable to perform ADL. C is incorrect: Though patient seems to have lost motivation, he is willing to participate in the mental status exam. Usually depressed patients would respond that they could not do the activity. If patient was depressed, he most likely would have self reported the symptoms instead having his wife bring him into the hospital. D is incorrect: Usually diagnosed in children. Patient also does not have a PMH or FH of any seizure disorders so unlikely to be any type of seizure at this age. E is incorrect: Patient is still responsive and able to communicate with the clinician. He was able to participate in the mental status exam so unlikely to be in a catatonic state.

References

1. Delirium: prevention, diagnosis and management in hospital and long-term care. London: National Institute for Health and Care Excellence (NICE); 2023 Jan 18. (NICE Clinical Guidelines, No. 103.) Available from: https://www.ncbi.nlm.nih.gov/books/NBK553009/
2. Inouye SK, Westendorp RG, Saczynski JS. Delirium in elderly people. Lancet. 2014 Mar 8;383(9920):911–22. doi: 10.1016/S0140-6736(13)60688-1. Epub 2013 Aug 28. PMID: 23992774; PMCID: PMC4120864.
3. Gagliardi JP. Differentiating among depression, delirium, and dementia in elderly patients. Virtual Mentor. 2008;10(6):383–8. https://doi.org/10.1001/virtualmentor.2008.10.6.cprl1-0806. PMID: 23212038
4. Gogia B, Fang X. Differentiating Delirium Versus Dementia in the Elderly. [Updated 2023 Feb 20]. In: StatPearls [Internet]. Treasure Island (FL): StatPearls Publishing; 2024 Jan-. Available from: https://www.ncbi.nlm.nih.gov/books/NBK570594/

Part X

Hematology

24 Acute Confusion

Joshua I. Gordon

Learning Objectives:

1. Discuss some therapies for CLL and their mechanisms of action: purine analogs, alkylating agents, monoclonal antibodies, and small molecule inhibitors.
2. Analyze the pathophysiology of TLS and understand how the various electrolyte abnormalities develop.
3. Compare and contrast the Rai and Binet staging systems for CLL and how these play into the treatment decisions.
4. Correlate the sequelae of TLS and the objective findings that patients may demonstrate.
5. Outline the preventative and treatment measures for TLS.
6. Role-play to practice what a conversation would be like with a patient that had failed multiple treatments and is now facing an end-of-life decision.

J. I. Gordon (✉)
Department of Internal Medicine, Division of Pulmonary, Critical Care and Sleep Medicine, Wexner Medicine Center, The Ohio State University, Columbus, OH, USA

Center for the Advancement of Team Science, Analytics, and Systems Thinking in Health Services and Implementation Science Research (CATALYST), The Ohio State University, Columbus, OH, USA
e-mail: Joshua.Gordon@osumc.edu

Chief Complaint

You are on night float as a third-year medical student covering another team's service when you are paged by the night nurse saying, "Mr. Miller is acting a little funky." She insists that someone come see the patient, but the intern is swamped with 3 new admissions, so off you go!

Prompt: *Does this warrant immediate evaluation?*

This is a common occurrence for night-float residents to encounter. Often, they are seeing a patient with an acute problem for the first time and are forced to read up quickly on the hospital stay and the ongoing issues. While this holds little value for Step 1 preparation, the role of effective communications is a theme that can be discussed, as it will be of the utmost importance during the later years of medical school and residency.

The point is that when you are called about a patient that has had an acute change in consciousness or has decompensated in some way, this warrants immediate evaluation by the physician. Sending the medical student to go see a patient that is being called on would be less ideal. This is especially true during night shifts; personnel are limited from a nursing and physician standpoint.

Prompt: *Develop an initial diagnostic list. What are you concerned about with this patient? What other information would you like to have?*

C. A. Standley (ed.), *Biomedical Science and Clinical Foundations*,
https://doi.org/10.1007/978-3-031-98353-5_24

Review the causes of recent onset altered mental status, focusing on those that may be seen in hospitalized patients. The following are some suggestions, organized according to organ system [1]:

- Cardiac
  - Global hypoxia or ischemia
  - Congestive heart failure
  - Hypertensive encephalopathy
- Pulmonary
  - Decreased PaO_2
  - Hypercapnia
- Gastrointestinal
  - Hepatic failure/encephalopathy
  - Wilson's disease
- Renal
  - Uremia
  - Hypo/hypernatremia
- Endocrine
  - Hypoglycemia
  - Diabetic ketoacidosis
  - Hypercalcemia
  - Addisonian crisis
- Neuro
  - Cerebrovascular accident
  - Intracerebral hemorrhage
  - Seizures
  - Neurodegenerative disorder
- Infectious Disease
  - Pneumonia
  - Urinary tract infection
  - Sepsis of unknown origin
- Medication overdose/reaction
- Alcohol/Intoxication
  - Opioids, other illicit drug(s)

Infection should be a major concern given that the patient is hospitalized with a hematologic malignancy and may not mount aneffective immune response.

History of Present Illness

This patient is an 80-year-old male who was admitted to the hospital earlier that day for initiation of cancer treatment. He received his first dose today and was doing well this afternoon. His wife noticed he was having more trouble moving around as the day went on, and this evening, he had some trouble answering questions for the nurse when she checked on him after dinner.

Prompt: *What might be some common malignancies in an 80-year-old male?*

Some possible malignancies that the patient could be treated for include colon cancer, prostate cancer, lung cancer, skin cancer, or a hematologic malignancy such as leukemia and lymphoma [2]. These should all be considered when initially evaluating older male patients. Students should note that a new treatment was started today.

Past Medical History
Chronic lymphocytic leukemia (CLL) diagnosed 9 years ago, refractory to multiple treatments
Hypertension for the past 17 years
Hyperlipidemia for the past 17 years

Past Surgical History
Appendectomy at 10 years old
Inguinal hernia repair at 50 years old

Medications
Home Meds
Lisinopril 20 mg po qd
Atorvastatin 40 mg po qHS
Hospital Meds
Pantoprazole 40 mg po qd
Heparin 5000 U SQ TID
Oxycodone 5 mg po q4h prn
Ondansetron 4 mg IV q4h prn
Allopurinol 300 mg po qd
Acetaminophen 650 mg po q4h prn

Allergies
Sulfa rash

Family History
Mom died of breast cancer in her 70 s
Dad died of heart attack in 80 s
No siblings

Social History
Born and raised in Texas
Mechanical engineer until he retired at 67

Former smoker, started at 20 and quit at 40; smoked 0.5 pack per day
Minimal ethanol
No drugs
Married to his wife of 15 years, she is a former teacher

Prompt: *Summarize the key information from this history.*

Of note, aside from his lymphoma, the patient has a relatively unremarkable past medical history. He has a remote smoking history, but no other high-risk behaviors.

His hospital medications are standard for an inpatient setting. Students may discuss the utility of a proton pump inhibitor (i.e. Pantoprazole) and anticoagulation (i.e. Heparin) when he does not have any identifiable problems, like gastroesophageal reflux disease or history of venous thromboembolism. However, patients receive anticoagulant prophylaxis as an inpatient and often receive GI ulcer prophylaxis [3, 4]. His ondansetron would be for any nausea he has with his new treatment, and oxycodone would be for any cancer-related pain he has been having. Allopurinol is used to prevent increased uric acid levels in patients receiving cancer chemotherapy. These patients can have increased uric acid levels due to release of uric acid from dying cancer cells.

Oncologic History

Diagnosed 9 years ago with Rai stage III CLL.

Treated initially with obinutuzumab + acalabrutinib with complete response achieved.

Progression of disease with new splenomegaly and retroperitoneal lymphadenopathy; admitted for initiation of venetoclax + rituximab. He has received the first doses of each of these.

Prompt: *What does "stage III" indicate?*

Students will cover the Rai staging as a learning objective. In general, cancer staging is a way to measure the extent of cancer in the body [5]. When a cancer is staged, factors such as tumor size and growth, location, and whether the cancer has spread beyond its original site are considered. As with all other cancers, a higher stage means a more extensive disease burden and should therefore require treatment. Stage III suggests the tumor has grown deeper into surrounding tissues and spread to nearby lymph nodes.

Students will cover some of the treatments that can be used for CLL, but something to note are the different strategies to treat cancer. Specifically, obinutuzumab is a monoclonal antibody, which the students should recognize given the –umab suffix.

Review of Systems

The patient is unable to provide a full review of systems secondary to his altered mental status.

Prompt: *What questions would you want to ask his wife if she is at bedside?*

Some considerations for this would be to gauge a timeline of how long the patient has been acting unusually. Inquire as to any recent medication changes, including new medications that may have been started or discontinued. Ask about ethanol history.

Review of Systems (cont.)

His wife at his bedside tells you that he started "acting funny" right before dinner. She says he has not thrown up but has been coughing a bit. She thinks he looks uncomfortable and keeps wiggling in bed and mumbling incoherently.

Physical Exam

General: frail elderly man, unable to provide coherent answers to questions, in minimal acute distress. Not alert or oriented, not responding appropriately to questions

Vital signs: T 36.8 °F, BP 110/68 mmHg, HR 116 bpm, RR 26 breaths/min, O_2 94% on room air

HEENT: Conjunctiva clear, sclera anicteric, pupils equal and round, reactive to light and accommodation

Cardiovascular: Tachycardic, regular rhythm, normal heart sounds, no murmurs

Pulmonary: Diminished breath sounds bilaterally, increased respiratory effort, tachypnea

Abdominal: + splenomegaly, soft, nontender, nondistended, + bowel sounds x4

Extremities: Trace pitting edema R > L, distal pulses palpable and symmetric

Skin: No skin lesions, sporadic chronic ecchymoses noted

Neuro: No gross motor or sensory deficits; difficult to gauge due to inattention and inability to follow commands during assessment, negative Babinski

Prompt: *What are the key findings in the physical exam?*

The vitals are relatively unremarkable. While the students may not recognize this at the time, the splenomegaly and skin findings may be representative of progressive CLL. Additionally, he is tachycardic and tachypneic, and is altered without acute focal neuorlogic deficits. The splenomegaly and skin findings reflect his progressed CLL, while the respiratory and neurologic findings are more reflective of a concurrent acute process.

Prompt: *What are the next steps you want to take in evaluating this patient?*

Investigation to rule out infection should begin with blood cultures, chest X-ray, and complete blood count (CBC). Other laboratories should include a comprehensive metabolic panel (CMP), uric acid, calcium, phosphorus, and urinalysis, and an arterial blood gas (ABG).

Table 24.1 Complete blood count

Component (units)	Patient	Reference range
WBC (x10^9/L)	42	4–10.5
RBC (x10^{12}/L)	3.8	4.1–5.6
Hemoglobin (g/dL)	10.2	12.5–17.0
Hematocrit (%)	30.0	36.0–50.0
MCV ($\int$m^3)	86	80–98
MCH (pg/cell)	29.6	27.0–34.0
MCHC (g/dL)	34.3	32.0–36.0
RDW (%)	14.0	11.7–15.0
Platelets (x10^9/L)	64	140–415
Neutrophils (%)	70	40–74
Lymphocytes (%)	21	14–46
Eosinophils (%)	5	4–13
Basophils (%)	2	0–7
Monocytes (%)	2	0–3
ANC (x10^9/L)	2.5	1.8–7.8

WBC White blood count, *RBC* Red blood count, *MCV* Mean corpuscular volume, *MCH* Mean corpuscular hemoglobin, *MCHC* Mean corpuscular hemoglobin concentration, *RDW* Red cell distribution width, *ANC* Absolute neutrophil count

Table 24.2 Comprehensive metabolic panel

Component (units)	Patient	Reference range
Na (mEq/L)	132	136–144
K (mEq/L)	6.5	3.7–5.2
Cl (mEq/L)	102	96–106
CO_2 (mEq/L)	19	20–29
BUN (mg/dL)	42	7–20
Cr (mg/dL)	1.8	0.7–1.3
Glu (mg/dL)	106	70–100
Ca (mg/dL)	8.2	8.5–10.9
Albumin (g/dL)	4.0	3.9–5.0
Total protein (g/dL)	7.0	6.3–7.9
ALP (units/L)	52	44–147
AST (IU/L)	30	8–37
ALT (IU/L)	32	10–34
Bilirubin (mg/dL)	1.0	0.2–1.9

ALP Alkaline phosphatase, *AST* Aspartate aminotransferase, *ALT* Alanine aminotransferase

Table 24.3 Urinalysis

Component (units)	Patient	Ref
Color	Yellow	–
Clarity	Slightly turbid	–
pH	5.0	4.5–8
Specific gravity	1.020	1.005–1.025
Glucose (mg/dL)	0	< 20
Ketones (mg/dL)	0	< 3
Nitrites (mg/dL)	0	0–1
Leukocyte esterase	Neg	Neg
Bilirubin (mg/dL)	0	<1.8
Urobilinogen (mg/dL)	0.2 mg/dL	< 1.6
Protein (mg/dL)	Trace	<20
RBC (cell/hpf)	1	<3
WBC (cell/hpf)	0	< 2
Casts (#/lpf)	0	0–2
Crystals	Occasional needle-shaped crystals	–

RBC Red blood cell, *WBC* White blood cell

Next Steps

You decide to order a CBC (Table 24.1), CMP (Table 24.2), and urinalysis (Table 24.3). In addition, an EKG, ABG, chest X-ray, and blood cultures are ordered.

Further Testing

Uric Acid: 10.2 (mg/dL) (Ref 3.4–7.0)
Phosphorus: 4.9 (mg/dL) (Ref 2.5–4.5)
ABG: pH 7.32, pCO2 20, pO2 82, HCO3 18
Blood Cultures—pending

Prompt: *Summarize the key laboratory findings.*

The laboratory findings for our patient reflect multiple simultaneous disease processes. The anemia, thrombocytopenia, and leukocytosis that are seen in his CBC are evidence of his progressive CLL. As the malignant process becomes more prominent, RBC and platelet precursors are pushed out of the marrow, causing a lack of maturation for those blood components and subsequent anemia/thrombocytopenia.

As far as the chemistries go, the patient is hyperkalemic, hypocalcemic (even when corrected for albumin), hyperuricemic, and hyperphosphatemic. There is also evidence of acute kidney injury with an elevated creatinine and BUN. Additionally, he has a metabolic acidosis (non anion gap), and a blood gas with a mild metabolic acidosis with incomplete respiratory compensation. The urinalysis shows needle-shaped crystals, evidence of uric acid deposition.

EKG

EKG shows peaked T-waves consistent with hyperkalemia without QRS widening. Rate and rhythm are regular.

Prompt: Are you concerned about the EKG results?

The EKG for our patient shows increased T wave amplitude, which is a classic sign for hyperkalemia. However, there is no significant QRS widening that would suggest impending rhythm issues. The findings here are enough to treat the hyperkalemia aggressively so as to avoid any of the potential arrhythmias, like V-tach or V-fib.

Imaging

Chest X-ray shows no acute abnormality. Lung volumes are low, but there are no infiltrates or alveolar filling opacities.

Diagnosis

Based on the findings of hyperkalemia, hyperuricemia, hypocalcemia, and hyperphosphatemia in a CLL patient that started a new treatment, the patient is diagnosed with tumor lysis syndrome.

You attribute his altered mental status to uric acid nephropathy leading to acute kidney injury.

Treatment

Aggressive IV hydration is begun. Diuretics are added, the dose of allopurinol is increased, and electrolyte abnormalities are addressed.

Blood cultures are returned as no growth to date after day 4.

Electrolytes are corrected and remain within normal limits during the rest of his inpatient stay.

The patient achieves therapeutic dosing of his venetoclax and is discharged with close outpatient follow-up by his primary hematologist.

The Case Continues

- The patient continues venetoclax treatment and follows up with his hematologist several weeks later.
- Unfortunately, his CBC has continued to worsen; he has developed acute pain due to his splenomegaly and progressive lymphadenopathy, which is only partially relieved by oxycodone.
- The hematologist discusses with him the pros and cons of continuing treatment.

Prompt: *What types of things would you discuss and how would you handle this conversation?*

This is explored in the answer to learning objective #7.

End of Case

Learning Objective Answers

1. **Discuss some therapies for CLL and their mechanisms of action: purine analogs, alkylating agents, monoclonal antibodies, small molecule inhibitors.**

CLL is managed using various therapeutic agents, each with distinct mechanisms of action [6].

- **Purine analogs**
  Purine analogs, such as cytarabine, fludarabine, and pentostatin, are antimetabolites that interfere with DNA synthesis. They prevent correct replication of DNA, thereby destroying the genetic material of many cells, but most importantly those that divide quickly (i.e., tumor cells).
- **Alkylating agents**
  Alkylating agents, including chlorambucil and bendamustine, work by adding alkyl groups to DNA bases, causing cross-linking and strand breaks. This disrupts DNA replication and triggers cell death. Bendamustine uniquely combines properties of both alkylating agents and purine analogs, offering efficacy with reduced hematological toxicity.
- **Monoclonal antibodies**
  Monoclonal antibodies target specific antigens on CLL cells. Anti-CD20 autoantibodies (found on B-cell neoplasms) such as rituximab and obinutuzumab bind to the CD20 antigen on B-cells, inducing antibody-mediated cellular cytotoxicity and complement-dependent cytotoxicity; they can also induce apoptosis of B-cells. Anti-CD52 antibodies such as alemtuzumab target the CD52 antigen, leading to direct cytotoxic effects on both normal and malignant lymphocytes.
- **Small molecule inhibitors**
  Small molecule inhibitors disrupt specific signaling pathways essential for CLL cell survival. Bruton Tyrosine Kinase (BTK) Inhibitors, such as ibrutinib, permanently bind to and inhibit BTK; they can drive the cell toward apoptosis and inhibit cellular migration. BCL-2 inhibitors such as venetoclax target the BCL-2 protein, a key survival protein in CLL, restoring apoptotic processes in CLL cells.

These therapies, either as monotherapies or in combination, have significantly improved CLL management by targeting specific aspects of the underlying cell biology of the disease.

2. **Analyze the pathophysiology of TLS and understand how the various electrolyte abnormalities develop.**

Tumor lysis syndrome (TLS) is a life-threatening medical emergency that occurs when large numbers of cancer cells rapidly die and release their contents into the bloodstream. This sudden influx can overwhelm the body's homeostatic mechanisms, causing significant metabolic disturbances [7]. It is seen most commonly in hematologic malignancies but can be seen in some solid tumors. Spontaneous TLS can be seen with **hyperuricemia**. The degradation of nucleic acids from lysed tumor cells leads to increased production of uric acid. Elevated uric acid levels can result in the formation of urate crystals, which may precipitate in the renal tubules, causing acute kidney injury.

Massive tumor cell lysis releases large amounts of potassium into the bloodstream, leading to elevated serum potassium levels (**hyperkalemia**). This can result in cardiac arrhythmias and neuromuscular dysfunction.

The breakdown of cancer cells releases intracellular phosphate into the circulation. The kidneys may struggle to excrete the excess phosphate, leading to **hyperphosphatemia**.

Elevated phosphate levels can precipitate with calcium and reduce serum calcium concentrations, leading to the formation of calcium phosphate crystals. These may deposit in renal tissues and contribute to acute kidney injury. Additionally, **hypocalcemia** can manifest as neuromuscular irritability, including tetany, seizures, and cardiac arrhythmias.

These metabolic abnormalities can lead to severe clinical consequences, including renal failure, cardiac arrhythmias, seizures, and, if not promptly managed, death.

3. **Compare and contrast the Rai and Binet staging systems for CLL and how this plays into the treatment decisions.**

CLL is staged primarily using two systems: the **Rai** and **Binet** staging systems. Both aim to assess disease progression and guide treatment decisions, though they differ in methodology and regional preference. The Rai staging system for CLL classifies the disease into five stages (0-IV) based on lymphocyte count and the presence or absence of enlarged lymph nodes, spleen, or liver, and anemia or thrombocytopenia, with stages 0, I, and II considered low to intermediate risk and stages III and IV as high risk [8]. The Binet system has three stages of CLL and is used in the United Kingdom for classifying CLL based on clinical and laboratory parameters [9]. It helps determine the extent of the disease and guide treatment decisions. The Rai system is more common in America.

Rai Staging System emphasizes blood counts and the presence of anemia or thrombocytopenia: [8].

- Stage 0 (low risk): Lymphocytosis in blood and bone marrow without other symptoms
- Stage I (intermediate risk): Lymphocytosis with enlarged lymph nodes
- Stage II (intermediate risk): Lymphocytosis with hepatomegaly and/or splenomegaly, with or without lymphadenopathy
- Stage III (high risk): Lymphocytosis with anemia, with or without organ enlargement
- Stage IV (high risk): Lymphocytosis with thrombocytopenia, with or without anemia or organ enlargement

Binet Staging System focuses on the number of affected lymphoid tissue areas and blood counts [9].

- Stage A: Fewer than three areas of lymphoid tissue enlargement without anemia or thrombocytopenia
- Stage B: Three or more areas of lymphoid tissue enlargement without anemia or thrombocytopenia
- Stage C: Presence of anemia and/or thrombocytopenia, irrespective of the number of lymphoid tissue enlargements

Both staging systems assist in prognostication and treatment planning. For early-stage CLL (Rai 0, Binet A), immediate treatment may not be necessary. Instead, a "watch and see" approach is often adopted. For intermediate-stage CLL (Rai I-II, Binet B), treatment decisions are based on disease symptoms, progression rate, and patient factors. For advanced-stage CLL (Rai III-IV, Binet C), active treatment is recommended due to significant cytopenias or symptomatic disease.

4. **Correlate the sequelae of TLS and the objective findings that patients may demonstrate.**

TLS is an oncologic emergency arising from the rapid destruction of malignant cells, leading to the release of intracellular contents into the bloodstream. This process results in several metabolic disturbances, and most sequelae are secondary to the electrolyte abnormalities that develop [10].

As potassium is primarily an intracellular ion, when cells are damaged, as in TLS, large quantities of potassium are released, elevating potassium levels and leading to hyperkalemia. Clinical manifestations of hyperkalemia are evident as muscle weakness or paralysis and palpitations. Cardiac conduction abnormalities and arrhythmias (seen on an EKG as peaked T-waves and QRS widening) can also occur and are potentially fatal if not recognized and treated early.

The release of intracellular phosphate during TLS leads to elevated phosphate levels known as hyperphosphatemia. The excess phosphate binds to calcium, forming insoluble calcium phosphate complexes (that appear as crystals in a urinalysis), thereby reducing serum calcium levels, leading to secondary hypocalcemia. Clinical manifestations of this scenario include muscle cramps, twitching, paresthesias such as numbness or tingling, and tetany.

The breakdown of nucleic acids from lysed tumor cells increases uric acid levels, causing hyperuricemia. Elevated uric acid can precipitate in the renal tubules, leading to acute kidney injury. Clinical manifestations of this include nausea, vomiting, lethargy, altered mental status, decreased urine output, and edema.

Recognizing these clinical manifestations is crucial for the timely diagnosis and management of TLS, aiming to prevent severe complications and improve patient outcomes.

5. **Outline the preventative and treatment measures for TLS.**

As TLS is a life-threatening oncologic emergency, effective prevention and management strategies are essential to mitigate the associated metabolic disturbances. To prevent and treat TLS, the focus is on aggressive hydration, uric acid lowering therapies (allopurinol), and close monitoring of electrolytes and kidney function [11]. For prevention, aggressive intravenous hydration with isotonic saline should be initiated at 2–3 liters/m^2/day to enhance renal perfusion and promote urinary excretion of uric acid and electrolytes. A xanthine oxidase inhibitor, such as allopurinol, can be started 1–2 days before chemotherapy and continued for up to a week to reduce the formation of uric acid. Phosphate binders may be used to reduce phosphate levels. Serum electrolytes, renal function, and urine output should be frequently monitored to detect early signs of TLS.

Despite appropriate prevention, 3–5% of patients undergoing chemotherapy will develop TLS [12]. If TLS is diagnosed, aggressive hydration should be initiated or continued to ensure high urine output [10, 11]. Hyperkalemia poses a significant risk; thus, dietary potassium intake can be restricted, and should hyperkalemia occur, potassium-lowering agents can be used. Additionally, dietary phosphate intake can be restricted, and phosphate binders used to reduce absorption. Calcium gluconate can be administered parenterally to manage hypocalcemia, to stabilize cardiac membrane, and to avoid risk for arrhythmia [10]. However, often correcting the elevated phosphate will correct the calcium without direct intervention.

Diuretics can be used to ensure adequate urine output. In cases of acute kidney injury or refractory electrolyte imbalances, hemodialysis can be initiated. Early identification of at-risk patients and prompt implementation of these strategies are crucial in preventing and managing TLS effectively.

6. **Role-play to practice what a conversation would be like with a patient that had failed multiple treatments and is now facing an end-of-life decision.**

A conversation with a patient facing an end-of-life decision after failed treatments should be a compassionate, open, and patient-centered dialogue, focusing on understanding their wishes, fears, and goals for the remaining time, while offering support and resources for palliative care [13].

Establish a safe and empathetic space. Acknowledge the difficult situation and validate their emotions. Always ask who they want present during this conversation. Some patients may want to be alone with the doctor; some may want to have a large support system with them during these difficult conversations.

A main concept to recognize in this objective is that the physician should attempt to shield the patient from the physician's inherent biases. Let the patient express their desires and wishes regarding future treatments. Allow them to express their concerns and questions without judgement.

Use simple language, avoiding medical jargon, and speak in a clear, straightforward manner, ensuring that the patient understands the information. Completely inform them about what each choice would mean, what further steps could be taken on each path, and gauge their interests. Allow time for patients to come to their own decision; don't pressure them into deciding right away. Offer your input and advice when solicited.

Discuss end-of-life care options. Explain the benefits of palliative care, which focuses on alleviating suffering and improving quality of life. Discuss hospice care as an option for those with a limited prognosis, emphasizing comfort and dignity at the end of life. Encourage the patient to discuss their wishes with their family and create an advance directive or living will.

Support the patient and family by providing information about support groups, counseling services, and other resources that can help the patient and their family cope with the situation. Offer ongoing support and reiterate that the patient and their family can ask questions at any time.

Exam Questions

1. You are called to evaluate an 86-year-old male with non-Hodgkin's lymphoma who recently started treatment. He complains of lethargy and reports that he nearly fell during his walk around the ward this morning during physical therapy. On exam, he demonstrates 4/5 strength in his lower extremities and 3/5 strength in his upper extremities. His vitals are within normal limits. What is the most urgent test to order at this time?
   A. Urinalysis
   B. Electrocardiogram
   C. Chest radiograph
   D. Complete blood count
   E. Abdominal computed tomography

Answer: B

Learning Objective: #2 Analyze the pathophysiology of TLS and understand how the various electrolyte abnormalities develop.

Explanation: This patient is potentially hyperkalemic secondary to tumor lysis syndrome. It is essential to evaluate their cardiac status and determine whether they need urgent correction of their hyperkalemia, which would be indicated by EKG changes, such as widening of the QRS and peaking of the T-waves. While the other choices may yield notable abnormalities, the EKG is the most pertinent because of the need to rapidly correct the potassium.

2. In the clinic, you see a familiar patient who has progressive diffuse large B-cell lymphoma. Despite treatment, her cancer has continued to progress. She is here to discuss the next best steps. You feel it is correct to inquire as to whether she wants to continue treatment of her cancer. What do you say first during this conversation with her and her husband, who is at the appointment with you today?
   A. I'd like to talk about the need for hospice care in the future.
   B. Are you sure you want to continue with another aggressive treatment?
   C. I'd like to discuss the future of your care with you alone. Would your husband mind stepping out for a moment?
   D. I think it might be wise to address what our goals of care are at this time. Would you be ok with having this conversation?
   E. I have a new treatment I want you to try. It may work, so we should give it a fighting chance.

Answer: D

Learning Objective: #6 Role-play to practice what a conversation would be like with a patient that had failed multiple treatments and is now facing an end-of-life decision.

Explanation: This question aims for students to recognize that the treatment choices should ultimately belong to the patient. All choices except D are physician-centered and don't allow the patient to drive the tenor of the conversation.

3. A 58-year-old male presents to the clinic with the complaint of early satiety and weight loss. He has unintentionally lost about 15 lbs. in the last 2 months. He also has noticed some new bruising on his arms over the last several months. Physical exam reveals splenomegaly, and CBC shows a WBC of 42 with a 50% lymphocytosis. The platelet count is 62. A bone marrow biopsy is done and reveals chronic lymphocytic leukemia. Based on these results, which of the following do you conclude?
   A. The patient has stage III disease and should be treated with combination therapy.
   B. The patient has a low-risk form of cancer and can be managed conservatively with watchful waiting.
   C. The patient should follow up in 6 weeks to trend his blood counts.
   D. The patient has a high-risk form of cancer and should receive workup to begin treatment.
   E. The patient needs to be rushed to the emergency room and start treatment this evening.

Answer: D

Learning Objective: #3 Compare and contrast the Rai and Binet staging systems for CLL and how these play into the treatment decisions.

Explanation: Based on the Rai staging, the patient has high-risk CLL (stage IV) due to thrombocytopenia, splenomegaly, and systemic symptoms. He should receive further workup to guide treatment initiation, making option D the best answer. A is incorrect, as this patient is in stage IV rather than stage III, and targeted therapy (e.g., BTK inhibitors like ibrutinib) is often preferred over traditional chemo-immunotherapy. B is incorrect, as while watchful waiting is appropriate for low-risk CLL, this patient has significant symptoms which are high-risk features; thus, he requires treatment rather than observation. C is incorrect, as while blood count monitoring is used in some cases of CLL, this patient already has high-risk features, and simply waiting and trending his counts would delay necessary treatment. E is incorrect. CLL even in advanced stages, is not a medical emergency. This patient needs treatment soon, but he does not require immediate hospitalization or emergency care.

References

1. Veauthier B, Hornecker JR, Thrasher T. Recent-onset altered mental status: evaluation and management. Am Fam Physician. 2021;104(5):461–70.

2. Cinar D, Tas D. Cancer in the elderly. North Clin Istanb. 2015;2(1):73–80.
3. Badireddy M, Mudipalli VR. Deep Venous Thrombosis Prophylaxis. [Updated 2023 May 7]. In: StatPearls [Internet]. Treasure Island (FL): StatPearls Publishing; 2025 Jan-. Available from: https://www.ncbi.nlm.nih.gov/books/NBK534865/
4. Clarke K, et al. Indications for the use of proton pump inhibitors for stress ulcer prophylaxis and peptic ulcer bleeding in hospitalized patients. Am J Med. 2022;135(3):313–7.
5. Brierley J, Gospodarowicz M, O'Sullivan B. The principles of cancer staging. Ecancermedicalscience. 2016;10:ed61.
6. Sánchez Suárez MDM, Martín Roldán A, Alarcón-Payer C, Rodríguez-Gil MÁ, Poquet-Jornet JE, Puerta Puerta JM, Jiménez Morales A. Treatment of chronic lymphocytic leukemia in the personalized medicine era. Pharmaceutics. 2024;16(1):55.
7. Howard SC, Jones DP, Pui CH. The tumor lysis syndrome. N Engl J Med. 2011;364(19):1844–54.
8. Rai KR, Sawitsky A, Cronkite EP, et al. Clinical staging of chronic lymphocytic leukemia. Blood. 1975;46:219–34.
9. Binet JL, Auquier A, Dighiero G, et al. A new prognostic classification of chronic lymphocytic leukemia derived from a multivariate survival analysis. Cancer. 1981;48:198–206.
10. Adeyinka A, Kaur A, Bashir K. Tumor Lysis Syndrome. [Updated 2024 Oct 5]. In: StatPearls [Internet]. Treasure Island (FL): StatPearls Publishing; 2025 Jan-. Available from: https://www.ncbi.nlm.nih.gov/books/NBK518985/
11. Coiffier B, Altman A, Pui C-H, et al. Guidelines for the management of pediatric and adult tumor lysis syndrome: an evidence-based review. J Clinical Oncol. 2008;26(16):2767–78.
12. Puri I, Sharma D, Gunturu KS, Ahmed AA. Diagnosis and management of tumor lysis syndrome. J Community Hosp Intern Med Perspect. 2020;10(3):269–72.
13. Balaban RB. A physician's guide to talking about end-of-life care. J Gen Intern Med. 2000;15(3):195–200.

25 Bloody Urine

Ashley Lukefahr

Learning Objective Answers

1. Identify the normal stages of red blood cell (RBC) maturation and the normal morphological characteristics of RBCs.
2. Describe iron metabolism and how this relates to the laboratory parameters found in iron studies (ferritin, total iron-binding capacity (TIBC), etc.). What changes in these laboratory parameters are expected during states of iron deficiency anemia?
3. Discuss the components of blood measured in a complete blood count, including mean corpuscular volume (MCV), red cell distribution width (RDW), mean corpuscular hemoglobin (MCH), and mean corpuscular hemoglobin concentration (MCHC). Explain how and why these components change during states of iron deficiency anemia.
4. Describe the signs and symptoms consistent with the clinical presentation of iron deficiency anemia. What explains this patient's red urine?
5. Review the available treatments for iron deficiency anemia. When should we expect to see changes in Mrs. Armstrong's symptoms, and when should we expect to see changes in Mrs. Armstrong's hematologic parameters?
6. Describe the etiologies of iron deficiency and the prevalence among populations stratified by age and gender.

A. Lukefahr (✉)
Department of Pathology, The University of Arizona College of Medicine – Phoenix, Phoenix, AZ, USA
e-mail: lukefahr@arizona.edu

Chief Complaint (CC) "There's blood in my urine!"

History of Present Illness (HPI)

Mrs. Armstrong is a 34-year-old female who presents to your health clinic because she states that she saw blood in her urine this morning. She states that her urine was bright red throughout urination. She is concerned because she has never had this symptom before.

She denies dysuria (pain with urination), trauma to her flank or abdomen, weight loss, change in appetite, subjective fevers, recent sore throat, nausea, vomiting, or rash.

She is 24 weeks pregnant with her third child in 3 years. She has seen an obstetrician only once during this current pregnancy and is not taking any prenatal vitamins. Mrs. Armstrong also states that she has been feeling very tired for the past few months. Although she denies a change in appetite, she states that she has become more "picky" about what she eats during her pregnancy; she consumes large amounts of vegetables, including bell peppers and beets. Lately, she has developed a taste for eating ice. She has no other complaint.

C. A. Standley (ed.), *Biomedical Science and Clinical Foundations*,
https://doi.org/10.1007/978-3-031-98353-5_25

Past Medical History (PMH)
Gravida 3 Para 2.

24 weeks pregnant by last menstrual period and ultrasound at 16 weeks.

Medications (Meds)
None.

No known drug allergies (NKDA).

Social History (SH)
Mrs. Armstrong lives with her husband and 2 children. She is a librarian at a local elementary school. She smoked half a pack of cigarettes per day for 3 years in college but has not smoked since. She does not drink alcohol or use illicit drugs. She does prenatal yoga three times a week for exercise.

Family History (FH)
Her father is 65 years old and has hypertension. Her mother is 62 years old and has a history of breast cancer. She is an only child. She denies a family history of renal disease.

Review of Systems (ROS)
General: No fevers, chills, or change in weight.
Hematopoietic: No problems with easy bruising, history of anemia, or excessive bleeding.
Urinary: Hematuria (see HPI). No dysuria, frequency, urgency, tenderness in back or flank, or history of UTIs.
Genital: G3P2. No history of problems with irregular menses, no history of sexually transmitted infections (STIs).
Endocrine: Easy fatigue. No history of thyroid problems.
Other systems: Negative.

1. What is the chief complaint?

Red urine/Blood in the urine.

2. What symptoms, past medical history, medications, family, and social history are relevant to the chief complaint?

Gross (macroscopic) hematuria is visible to the naked eye and appears pink, bright red, or brown. The patient is describing red urine throughout urination, which is concerning for a renal or ureteral source. The color is not indicative of the concentration of red blood cells (RBCs) present in the urine, because as little as 1 mL of whole blood per liter of urine can produce a visible color change. Bleeding at the onset of urination occurs when the bleeding source is the urethra. Bleeding at the end of urination suggests the bladder trigone as the possible source. Bleeding throughout urination may suggest the source is the bladder, ureter, or kidney.

The acute onset of her symptoms during pregnancy is concerning, as it is important to rule out any vaginal bleeding, urinary tract infection, cystitis, etc. that may be a threat to mother and fetus.

She has no alarm symptoms, such as increased age (older than 40–50 years), constitutional symptoms (weight loss, appetite loss, chronic fatigue), back or flank pain, recent sore throat, or a family history of renal disease, that would be concerning for malignancy, chronic infection, or acute glomerulonephritis.

She is not using any medications, such as aspirin, antibiotics, or non-steroidal anti-inflammatory drugs (NSAIDs) that would raise concern for interstitial nephritis.

She does not have risk factors, such as advanced age or a substantial history of cigarette smoking, which would raise concern for bladder cancer.

3. Review your key hypotheses.
   (a) Urinary Tract Infection: The most common etiology for hematuria in pregnant women is infection, followed by stones, underlying renal disease, medications, trauma, tumors, and obstruction.
   (b) An etiology specific to pregnancy: such as placenta percreta (placental invasion of the bladder).
   (c) Benign cause: There are many causes of red urine, and it should not automatically be assumed that urine is red because of blood. Vegetable dyes, drugs such as phenazopyridine (Pyridium), and excessive ingestion of beets can also cause urine to appear red.

(d) Idiopathic: In 8–10% of cases, no cause for hematuria is identified in the initial evaluation.

4. What physical examination findings and ancillary studies (laboratory tests, imaging studies, etc.) can be used to distinguish the hypotheses given in question 3 above?

Pelvic examination
Complete blood count (CBC)
Comprehensive metabolic panel (CMP)
Urinalysis/Urine dipstick test for hemoglobin

Physical Examination

General appearance: Well-developed, well-nourished female, alert and conversant, in no acute distress.

Vital signs: blood pressure: 119/79 mm Hg; heart rate 89 beats per minute; temperature: 98 degrees Fahrenheit; respiratory rate 16 breaths per minute; O_2 saturation, 98%.

Height 165 cm; **Weight** 65 kg [BMI = 23.9 kg/m^2].

Skin: Pale.

HEENT: Normocephalic atraumatic (NCAT); pupils are equal, round, and reactive to light and accommodation (PERRLA); extraocular muscles intact (EOMI). Pale conjunctiva. Hearing intact bilaterally; nasal passages clear; oropharynx without exudate or erythema; dentition intact. Tongue appears smooth.

Neck/Thyroid: Supple with full range of motion (ROM). No jugular vein distention. No carotid bruits. No thyromegaly or masses.

Chest/Lungs: Clear to auscultation (CTA); breath sounds equal bilaterally. No crackles, rhonchi, or wheezing.

Heart: Regular rate. Normal S1, S2, without S3, S4. II/VI systolic murmur at left lower sternal border.

Abdomen: Non-tender. No flank/costovertebral angle (CVA) tenderness. No suprapubic tenderness.

Genital: Normally developed genitalia with no external lesions. Vagina and cervix show no lesions, inflammation, discharge, or tenderness.

Stool guaiac: Negative for occult blood.

Extremities: No clubbing, cyanosis, or edema. Mild spooning of nails.

Laboratory Findings

Laboratory value	Patient	Normal
Sodium	140 mEq/L	135–147 mEq/L
Potassium	4.2 mEq/L	3.5–5.0 mEq/L
Bicarbonate (HCO_3)	25 mEq/L	24–28 mEq/L
Chloride	102 mEq/L	95–105 mEq/L
Hemoglobin	7.1 g/dL	Male: 13.6–16.9 g/dL, Female: 11.9–14.8 g/dL
Hematocrit	23%	Male: 40–50%, Female: 35–43%
MCV	74 fL	82.5–98 fL
RDW	17.1%	11.4–13.5%
MCH	21 pg	27.6–33.3 pg
MCHC	28 g/dL	32.5–35.2 g/dL
White blood count	5.5 × 10^9/L	3.8–10.4 × 10^9/L
Platelet count	220 × 10^9/L	Male: 152–324 × 10^9/L, Female: 153–361 × 10^9/L
Blood Urea Nitrogen (BUN)	10 mg/dL	8–18 mg/dL

Urinalysis

Laboratory Value	Patient	Normal
Color	Pale yellow	Yellow
Clarity/turbidity	Clear	Clear
pH	5.2	4.5–8
Specific gravity	1.010	1.005–1.025
Glucose	115 mg/d	≤ 130 mg/d
Ketones	None	None
Nitrites	Negative	Negative
Leukocyte esterase	Negative	Negative
Bilirubin	Negative	Negative
Urobilinogen	0.6 mg/dL	Small amount (0.5–1 mg/dL)
Protein	110 mg/d	≤ 150 mg/d
RBCs	0 RBCs/hpf	≤ 0–2 RBCs/hpf
WBCs	1 WBCs/hpf	≤ 0–2 WBCs/hpf
Squamous epithelial cells	10 squamous epithelial cells/hpf	≤ 15–20 squamous epithelial cells/hpf
Casts	0 hyaline casts/lpf	0–5 hyaline casts/lpf
Crystals	None	Occasionally
Bacteria	None	None
Yeast	None	None

Stop and Think

1. How do these test results help you to refine your hypothesis (i.e., what do they confirm or rule out?)

The normal urinalysis puts hematuria (gross and microscopic), infection, or renal causes of hematuria low on the list of diagnoses.

The low hemoglobin and hematocrit are consistent with Mrs. Armstrong's complaints of fatigue and are concerning enough to be worked up. The low MCV and high RDW point to a possible hematologic cause of Mrs. Armstrong's symptoms.

The symptoms of craving for ice (see HPI) and the physical exam findings of pale conjunctiva, spooning of the nails, and the heart murmur are also concerning for another etiology of her symptoms.

The benign and/or idiopathic causes of red urine are now more likely.

2. What other tests would you now consider ordering? Defend your rationale for ordering these additional tests.

Peripheral smear.

Iron studies.

Bone marrow biopsy with Prussian Blue staining (gold standard).

The patient's red urine symptoms are best explained by a benign and/or idiopathic cause. Her stated over-ingestion of beets is concerning for beeturia. Given the changes in her hematologic parameters and the abundance of other symptoms that are present, a more thorough work-up of her hematologic status is warranted.

Iron Studies

Laboratory value	Patient	Normal
Serum iron	10 mcg/dL	Male: 65–175 mcg/dL, Female: 50–170 mcg/dL
Total iron-binding capacity (TIBC)/ transferrin	470 mcg/dL	250–460 mcg/dL
Transferrin saturation	2.5%	Male: 20–50%, Female: 15–50%
Serum ferritin	10 mcg/L	18–300 mcg/L

Peripheral blood smear: Microcytic, hypochromic red cells. Poikilocytes.

Bone marrow aspirate: Microscopic examination of a Prussian Blue reaction on a bone marrow aspirate shows iron stores are absent (normal: abundant Prussian Blue positivity indicates iron as hemosiderin in reticuloendothelial system/macrophages).

Stop and Think

1. What is your diagnosis?
   Iron deficiency anemia
2. How does this relate to Mrs. Armstrong's initial chief complaint?
   To be answered by the learning objectives.

End of Case

Learning Objective Answers

1. Identify the normal stages of RBC maturation and the normal morphological characteristics of RBCs.
   - In adults, hematopoiesis primarily takes place in the bone marrow. RBCs are derived from pluripotent hematopoietic stem cells [1].
   - In the bone marrow, the earliest identifiable cell committed to the RBC lineage is the proerythroblast. The stages of maturation into a mature red cell are as follows: proerythroblast - > basophilic erythroblast - > polychromatic erythroblast - > pyknotic erythroblast - > reticulocyte - > mature RBC [2].
   - The proerythroblast is a relatively large cell with basophilic cytoplasm and dispersed nuclear chromatin [2].
   - The more differentiated erythroblasts become progressively smaller and contain increasing amounts of hemoglobin, with the cytoplasm taking on a more polychromatic (multicolored) appearance and the nuclear chromatin becoming more condensed [2].
   - Erythroblasts mature in close proximity to macrophages in an "erythroid nest." This may facilitate access to iron in the macrophages, allowing the iron to be incorporated into heme [2].

- The nucleus is enucleated to form a relatively spherical reticulocyte, which is released from the bone marrow. At this point, the reticulocyte contains messenger ribonucleic acid (mRNA) that synthesizes hemoglobin. This mRNA will stain basophilic with supravital stains (such as new methylene blue, which bind nucleic acids). Within a week, the mRNA is lost [2].
- Mature RBCs are nonnucleated, flexible, biconcave disks with a mean diameter of 7–8 um, similar in size to the nucleus of a small lymphocyte. On a peripheral blood smear stained with a Romanowsky stain (such as a Wright's stain), they appear round with eosinophilic cytoplasm. On a peripheral blood smear, the biconcave shape of the RBC produces a central area of pallor, approximately 1/3 the diameter of the cell. Minimal variations in size (anisocytosis) and shape (poikilocytosis) can be observed [2].

2. Describe iron metabolism and how this relates to the laboratory parameters found in iron studies (ferritin, total iron-binding capacity (TIBC), etc.). What changes in laboratory parameters do we expect during stages of iron deficiency anemia?
   - The normal total body iron content is approximately 50 mg/kg body weight in adult males and approximately 35 mg/kg body weight in adult females [1].
   - All cells of the body contain iron in the form of iron-containing compounds. Most iron is found within the heme moiety of a heme protein (hemoglobin, myoglobin, cytochromes, catalases, peroxidase). Iron may also be stored in the form of ferritin or hemosiderin. Some iron circulates in the plasma bound to transferrin [1].
   - Most storage iron is stored in the form of ferritin. Ferritin is made from a protein shell that encloses an iron core. Iron stored in ferritin may be mobilized when the body needs to restore hemoglobin levels, such as following bleeding [1].
   - Transferrin is the main protein that transports iron in the plasma. Approximately 0.1% of the total body iron content is found circulating in the plasma, bound to transferrin [1].
   - Iron is derived from RBC destruction, iron stores, and gastrointestinal absorption [1].
   - Iron cycles between the reticuloendothelial system (RES) and bone marrow. Macrophages of the reticuloendothelial system detect senescent RBCs and internalize them for degradation. Every day, approximately 20 mL of RBCs undergo destruction by the RES, with subsequent liberation of iron. Macrophages can transport iron to the plasma, where it binds transferrin. Dietary iron is also transported through plasma while bound to transferrin. RBC precursors in the bone marrow have transferrin receptors that allow them to bind transferrin, internalize the iron, and then incorporate the iron into hemoglobin [1, 2].
   - Only 10% of dietary iron is absorbed via the gastrointestinal system (primarily the duodenum). Heme iron is more readily absorbed than nonheme iron, which requires ferric (Fe^{3+}) iron to be reduced to ferrous (Fe^{2+}) before it can be absorbed [1].
   - Iron cannot be excreted. Instead, iron is lost from the body when cells (such as epithelial cells of the gastrointestinal tract) are lost [1].
   - Regarding iron studies, decreased serum ferritin and absence of iron in the bone marrow are the earliest changes seen with iron deficiency anemia, followed by decreases in serum iron, decreases in transferrin saturation, and increases in TIBC; see Table 25.1 [3, 4].
   - Serum ferritin, a marker of total body storage iron, will decrease with iron deficiency and depletion. Ferritin may be falsely elevated to normal levels during periods of inflammation, as ferritin is an "acute-phase reactant" [1]. Ferritin levels of less than 30 ng/mL are 92% sensitive and 98% specific for iron deficiency [3, 4].

- Serum iron will decrease, with the depletion of storage iron [1].
- Serum transferrin, also reported as the TIBC, is increased in iron deficiency, as iron-binding proteins are upregulated when iron stores are low. Transferrin saturation refers to the percentage of iron-binding proteins that are saturated with iron and is decreased during iron deficiency. This parameter is calculated from serum iron and TIBC [3, 4].
- Soluble transferrin receptor testing measures proteins cleaved from the transferrin receptors on erythroid precursor cells in the bone marrow. The concentration of soluble transferrin receptors is directly proportional to the rate of erythropoiesis and inversely proportional to iron availability. In individuals with iron deficiency, the soluble transferrin receptor will be increased; see Table 25.1 [3, 4].
- RBC protoporphyrin or RBC zinc protoporphyrin are elevated during iron deficiency, because intestinal zinc absorption increases, and zinc becomes incorporated into developing RBCs; see Table 25.1 [3, 4].
- The absolute reticulocyte count and the reticulocyte hemoglobin content are decreased with iron deficiency; see Table 25.1 [3, 4].
- Although not routinely used in the clinical setting (due to expense and invasiveness of the procedure), staining of the bone marrow for storage iron is the gold standard test for iron deficiency anemia. Intracellular iron staining in macrophages and erythroid precursors (sideroblasts) by a Prussian blue stain will be absent due to iron depletion from the bone marrow [3, 4].

Table 25.1 Iron study abnormalities in iron deficiency anemia [3, 4]

Laboratory study	Abnormality in iron deficiency anemia
Serum ferritin	Decreased
Transferrin or Total iron-binding capacity (TIBC)	Increased
Transferrin saturation (serum iron/TIBC × 100)	Decreased
Soluble transferrin receptor	Increased
Free erythrocyte porphyrin (FEP) or erythrocyte zinc protoporphyrin	Increased
Reticulocyte hemoglobin concentration	Decreased

3. Define the components of blood measured in a CBC, including MCV, RDW, MCH, and MCHC. Explain how and why these parameters change during states of iron deficiency anemia.
   - The components of blood that are measured in a CBC are RBC count, hemoglobin, MCV, reticulocyte count, platelet count, and white blood cell count. The parameters that are calculated are the RDW, MCH, and MCHC. Hematocrit may be measured or calculated. See Table 25.2 for CBC parameters in adults [6].
   - The RBC count is the number of RBCs per microliter of blood. Iron deficiency is associated with a decrease in the number of RBCs [6].
   - Hemoglobin refers to the concentration of hemoglobin in whole blood. Iron deficiency anemia is associated with a decreased hemoglobin [6].
   - Hematocrit is the packed spun volume of blood comprised of RBCs. Iron deficiency anemia is associated with a decreased hematocrit [6].
   - MCV refers to the average volume/size of the RBCs. Iron deficiency anemia is associated with a decreased MCV [6].
   - The RDW measures variation in MCV. Iron deficiency anemia is associated with an increased RDW, consistent with a large variation in the size of RBCs [6].
   - MCH is the average hemoglobin content in the RBCs. Iron deficiency anemia is associated with a decreased MCH [6].
   - MCHC is the average hemoglobin concentration per RBC. Iron deficiency anemia is associated with a decreased MCHC [6].
   - Automated counting can provide an absolute reticulocyte count. Iron deficiency anemia is associated with a decreased reticulocyte count [6].

Table 25.2 Complete blood count (CBC) parameters in adults [5]

Parameter	Calculation	Normal range	Abnormality in iron deficiency anemia
Red blood cell number (RBC)		Male: 4.2–5.7 × 10^6/microL Female: 3.8–5.0 × 10^6/microL	Decreased
Hemoglobin (Hgb)		Male: 13.6–16.9 g/dL Female: 11.9–14.8 g/dL	Decreased
Hematocrit (Hct)	RBC × MCV/10; roughly equivalent to Hgb × 3	Male: 40–50% Female: 35–43%	Decreased
Mean corpuscular volume (MCV)	MCV = Hct/RBC	82.5–98 fL	Decreased
Mean corpuscular hemoglobin (MCH)	MCH = Hgb/RBC	27.6–33.3 pg	Decreased
Mean corpuscular hemoglobin concentration (MCHC)	MCHC = Hgb/Hct	32.5–35.2 g/dL	Decreased
Red cell distribution width (RDW)	RDW = (standard deviation of MCV/MCV) × 100	11.4–13.5%	Increased
Reticulocyte count		Male: 16–130 × 10^3/microL Female: 16–98 × 10^3/microL	Decreased
Platelet count		Male: 152–324 × 10^3/microL Female: 153–361 × 10^3/microL	May be increased
White blood cell count		3.8–10.4 × 10^3/microL	No change

- The platelet count is the number of platelets per microliter of blood. Iron deficiency anemia may be associated with thrombocytosis, or an elevated platelet count [6].
- The white blood cell count is the number of white blood cells per microliter of blood. No changes in the white blood cell count are expected with iron deficiency anemia [6].
- Anemia is defined as a reduction in hemoglobin, hematocrit, or the RBC count [5].
- Changes in CBC parameters are usually detectable after changes in iron studies [3, 4].
- As iron stores become depleted, there is no longer enough iron to sustain RBC production [1].
- The first detectable CBC abnormality in iron deficiency anemia is an increase in RDW, followed by a decrease in the MCV [1].
- The peripheral blood smear shows hypochromic (with an increased area of central pallor), microcytic (smaller than normal) RBCs with some anisocytosis and poikilocytosis. These abnormalities are the result of the production of RBCs with reduced hemoglobin content. As more microcytic cells appear in the blood, and mix with the normocytic RBCs that are already present, the RDW will become elevated. Smaller cells will result in a decreased MCV [1].
- As fewer newly formed RBCs are produced and released, the reticulocyte count may decrease [2].
- Thrombocytosis may be present, especially if blood loss is occurring [1].

4. Describe the signs and symptoms consistent with the clinical presentation of iron deficiency anemia. What explains this patient's red urine?
   - Symptoms of anemia include the following: fatigue, weakness, decreased exercise

tolerance, dyspnea on exertion, palpitations, pica (the dietary intake of substances with no nutritional value, such as ice (pagophagia), starch (amylophagia), clay (geophagia), and paper), hair loss, headache, hearing loss/tinnitus, mood changes/irritability, and restless legs syndrome [3, 4].
   - Beeturia, a red appearance of the urine associated with ingestion of beets, is found with increased frequency in those with iron deficiency. A reddish pigment in beets (betalaine) shows increased intestinal absorption in the iron deficient state and is a redox indicator that becomes decolorized by ferric ions [3, 4].
   - Physical examination findings include the following: pallor, dry/roughened skin, angular cheilitis (cracking of the edges of the lips), koilonychia (spooning of the nails), tachycardia, systolic flow murmurs, atrophic glossitis (loss of tongue papillae, beginning at the tip and lateral borders of the tongue and moving posteriorly and centrally), and dysphagia with esophageal webs/strictures (due to a web of mucosa forming at the junction of the hypopharynx and esophagus) [3, 4].
   - Other signs/symptoms may be present and related to the underlying cause of iron deficiency (e.g., abdominal pain from a duodenal ulcer) [3, 4].
5. Review the available treatments for iron deficiency anemia. When should we expect to see changes in Mrs. Armstrong's symptoms, and when should we expect to see changes in Mrs. Armstrong's hematologic parameters?
   - If an etiology is identified, correction and management of the underlying cause of the anemia is warranted [1].
   - Duodenal absorption of iron is enhanced in those with iron deficiency, making oral iron replacement a preferred treatment modality. Many oral iron formulations are available. It is estimated that the maximum amount of daily elemental iron that can be absorbed with an oral preparation is 25 mg. As an example, a 325 mg tablet of ferrous sulfate contains 65 mg of elemental iron. Once daily dosing or dosing every other day are both acceptable dosing schedules, dependent on side effects and patient preference. Enteric-coated and sustained-release capsules are not recommended, as they are less efficient for oral absorption. The recommended duration of therapy depends on the severity of iron deficiency and may extend up to 6 months ([1, 3, 4], Treatment).
   - Oral iron is associated with nausea, constipation, and dark/tarry stools [1].
   - Vitamin C may enhance oral iron absorption, as iron is best absorbed in the ferrous ($Fe2+$) state in a mildly acidic solution. Certain foods (e.g., tea, grains, eggs, dairy products) and drugs/supplements (e.g., calcium supplements, proton pump inhibitors) impair oral iron absorption ([1, 3, 4], Treatment).
   - Parenteral iron is recommended for those patients with an intolerance to oral therapy, non-compliance with therapy, ongoing blood loss, or a malabsorption state ([1, 3, 4], Treatment).
   - Transfusion of blood products should be used in patients with clinical signs and symptoms of cardiovascular compromise. A unit of packed RBCs is expected to raise the hemoglobin by 1 g/dL [1].
   - Pica/pagophagia often ends upon initiation of therapy, before any hematologic changes occur, with feelings of well-being reported within the first few days of treatment ([3, 4], Treatment).
   - Glossitis will resolve within weeks to months of iron repletion therapy ([3, 4], Treatment).
   - Following the initiation of iron repletion, hemoglobin levels should rise by approximately 1 g/dL each week. Peripheral blood smears will show an increase in reticulocytes, beginning 7–10 days after the initiation of iron repletion therapy [1].
   - Hemoglobin levels are expected to normalize by 6–8 weeks after the initiation of iron repletion therapy ([3, 4], Treatment).

6. Describe the etiologies of iron deficiency and the prevalence among populations stratified by age and gender.
   - The etiologies of iron deficiency include the following: traumatic hemorrhage, gastrointestinal bleed, menstruation, pregnancy (increased demand for iron), lactation, neoplasms, epistaxis, hematemesis, hemoptysis, hematuria, medications, dietary inadequacy, malabsorption (e.g., surgical gastrectomy/gastric bypass, celiac disease), high-intensity athletics, and inherited/genetic disorders [1, 3, 4].
   - Healthy infants born at full-term usually have adequate iron for the first 4–6 months of life. Risk factors for the development of iron deficiency in the infant include the following: maternal iron deficiency (resulting in inadequate iron stores at birth), prematurity (as most of the iron stores are deposited during the last trimester of fetal development), fetal-maternal hemorrhage, perinatal hemorrhagic events, and twin-twin transfusion syndrome. Infants that are solely breastfed require iron supplementation, with breastmilk providing adequate iron until approximately 4 months of age. Unfortified cow's milk increases intestinal blood loss and introduction before 12 months of age is a risk factor for iron deficiency anemia [7].
   - In 2010, the global prevalence of anemia was estimated to be 32.9% [2].
   - In the United States, iron deficiency anemia is most commonly seen in women during their reproductive years. Data from the third National Health and Nutrition Examination Survey (NHANES III) indicates the prevalence of iron deficiency anemia in the United States is 9–16% among females aged 12–49 years, 7% among toddlers aged 1–2 years, 6% among females aged 70 years or more, 3% among males aged 70 years or more, and 2–5% among males aged 12–69 years [8].

Exam Questions

1. An 18-year-old female is seen for a general medical examination. Review of systems is remarkable for generalized weakness, lethargy, and inability to perform routine work for the previous few months. On further questioning, she reveals that she has had excessive bleeding during menstruation for the previous 6 months. On physical examination, she has tachycardia, pale gums, and a swollen tongue. The physician suspects that the patient is anemic and orders laboratory tests. On the peripheral smear, the lab reports microcytosis, hypochromia, mild anisocytosis, and polychromasia. There is no basophilic stippling. A certain population of cells is noted to be 0.4% of the total peripheral cell population (normal: 0.5–1.5%). These cells contain messenger ribonucleic acid, lack a nucleus, and are found in both the bone marrow and peripheral blood of normal individuals. Which of the following is the name for this type of cell?
   A. Basophilic erythroblast
   B. Polychromatic erythroblast
   C. Proerythroblast
   D. Pyknotic erythroblast
   E. Reticulocyte
   Answver: E.
   Learning Objective #1.
   Explanation: Reticulocytes contain messenger ribonucleic acid (mRNA), and they are present in both the bone marrow and peripheral blood. The other cell types (Options A, B, C, and D) are only seen in the bone marrow of normal, healthy adults. Therefore, option E is the most correct answer.
2. A 28-year-old female visits her primary care physician for her yearly physical examination. During her review of systems, she states that she has been feeling fatigued. She denies weight loss, diarrhea, and menorrhagia. Physical examination shows pallor. Blood studies show the following: hematocrit 32%

(normal: 35–43%), hemoglobin 11.1 g/dL (normal: 11.9–14.8 g/dL), and platelets 300 × 10^9/L (normal: 153–361 × 10^9/L). Further iron studies are ordered. Which of the following variables in an iron study is most likely to be lower than normal in this patient?
   A. Red cell distribution width (RDW)
   B. Serum ferritin
   C. Total iron-binding capacity (TIBC)
   D. Transferrin saturation
   Answer: D.
   Learning Objective #3.
   In iron deficiency, the following variables are increased: RDW, TIBC, FEP, and transferrin receptor. The following variables are decreased: hemoglobin, MCV, RBC, serum ferritin, transferrin saturation, and reticulocyte hemoglobin concentration. Therefore, option D is the most correct answer.
3. A 36-year-old female presents with a feeling of weakness, listlessness, and easy fatigability. Physical examination shows conjunctival pallor. Hemoglobin is 10.0 g/dL (normal: 11.9–14.8 g/dL). Additional laboratory studies are most likely to reveal which of the following in this patient?
   A. Low MCV, High RDW
   B. Low MCV, Normal RDW
   C. High MCV, High RDW
   D. High MCV, Normal RDW
   E. Normal MCV, High RDW
   Answer: A.
   Learning Objective #3 and 4.
   Explanation: Iron deficiency anemia causes microcytosis (low MCV) from impaired hemoglobin synthesis and anisocytosis (high RDW) due to the presence of both small and normal-sized red blood cells. Option B is incorrect; this characterizes thalassemia trait. Option C is incorrect; this characterizes B12 deficiency, folate deficiency, immune hemolysis, liver disease, and myelodysplasia. Option D is incorrect; this characterizes aplastic anemia, liver disease, and certain medications. Option E is incorrect; this characterizes early iron deficiency, early folate deficiency, early B12 deficiency, sickle cell anemia, and SC disease. As this patient's signs and symptoms reflect advanced iron deficiency, these values would not be expected.
4. A 37-year-old woman is admitted to the hospital with a one-week history of dyspnea on exertion, fatigue, and dizziness. Her laboratory data revealed iron deficiency anemia with a hemoglobin of 5.7 g/dL (normal: 11.9–14.8 g/dL). Which other symptom is most likely to be present in this patient?
   A. Aversion to eating ice
   B. Enhanced convexity of the nails
   C. Cracking of the edges of the lips
   D. Increased papillation of the tongue
   E. Tonic-clonic seizures
   Answer: C.
   Learning Objective #4.
   Explanation: Inflammation and cracking at the corners of the mouth is a condition known as angular cheilitis and is a symptom of iron deficiency anemia. Option A is incorrect: pagophagia, or affinity for eating ice, is associated with iron deficiency anemia. Option B is incorrect: spooning of the nails (koilonychia) is seen in iron deficiency anemia, and with this symptom, nails are concave instead of convex. Option D is incorrect: glossitis is a symptom of iron deficiency anemia and is characterized by a smooth, waxy-appearing, red tongue with atrophy of papillae. Option E is not associated with iron deficiency anemia.
5. A 40-year-old male presents to your clinic with a chief complaint of fatigue. The patient's history is remarkable for gastric bypass surgery a year ago. Postoperative nutritional surveillance and nutrient supplementation have not been adopted. The patient has trouble digesting food due to his inability to maintain an acidic environment in his stomach. Physical examination is remarkable for a pale appearance. Lab results are as follows: WBC 7.0 × 10^9/L (normal: 3.8–10.4 × 10^9/L), hemoglobin 6.2 g/dL (normal: 13.6—16.9 g/dL), hematocrit 19.8% (normal: 40–50%), platelets 278 × 10^9/L (normal: 152–324 × 10^9/L),

MCV 60 fL (normal: 82.5–98 fL), RDW 20% (normal: 11.4–13.5%). Which of the following is the best treatment option for this patient?

A. Ferrous sulfate 325 mg PO daily for 6 months
B. Ferrous sulfate 325 mg PO daily until symptoms improve
C. Ferrous sulfate 325 mg PO daily with calcium supplements
D. A single infusion of 1000 mg of IV iron
E. Patient should receive a blood transfusion

Answer: D.

Learning Objective #5.

Explanation: This patient has a decreased acidity of the stomach, which means that there is not enough acid to keep iron from being converted to insoluble ferric hydroxide. This makes IV iron (choice D) a better therapeutic choice than oral iron (choices A, B, and C). Blood transfusions (choice E) are reserved for hemodynamically unstable patients or those with evidence of end-organ ischemia. Calcium supplements (choice C) can impair iron absorption.

6. A 22-month-old boy presents to a health care clinic with a chief complaint of pallor. A visiting relative who has not seen the child for 4 months told his mother that the boy appears pale. On review of systems, you find that he is an active toddler, with no recent fatigue or change in sleeping habits. He consumes 36–48 ounces of breast milk per day. His birth was remarkable for a postmature delivery at 42 weeks 2 days gestational age (normal: 38–42 weeks). His mother consumed iron supplements during pregnancy. The mother states that the house they live in was built before 1950. Physical examination is remarkable for a pale appearance. Lab results are as follows: WBC 6.1 × 10^9/L (normal: 3.2–9.8 × 10^9/L), hemoglobin 6.2 g/dL (normal: 11–13.7 g/dL), hematocrit 19.8% (normal: 34–44%), platelets 389 × 10^9/L (normal: 130–400 × 10^9/L), MCV 54 fL (normal: 75–86 fL), RDW 21% (normal: 12–14.6%). On the peripheral blood smear, the laboratory reports microcytosis, hypochromia, mild anisocytosis, and polychromasia. There is no basophilic stippling. Which of the following is the most likely explanation for the infant's physical examination and laboratory findings?

A. Infant's mother consumed iron supplements during pregnancy
B. Infant is fed with breast milk alone
C. Lead poisoning
D. This is a normal stage of development
E. Postmature delivery

Answer: B.

Learning Objective #4 and 6.

Explanation: The infant's physical examination and laboratory findings are most consistent with iron deficiency anemia. The amount of iron necessary for a growing child cannot be provided in breast milk alone. Option A is incorrect, as iron supplements would ensure that the mother had adequate iron stores during pregnancy. Iron deficiency in the mother during pregnancy would result in inadequate iron stores at birth. Option C is incorrect; although living in a house built before 1950 is a risk factor for having lead paint in the home, the lack of basophilic stippling points away from lead poisoning. Option D is incorrect, as the clinical presentation, physical examination, and laboratory findings are not normal for an infant. Option E is incorrect, as prematurity is a risk factor for iron deficiency, as half of the infant's iron stores are deposited in the last month of fetal life.

References

1. Lazarus HM, Schmaier AH. Concise guide to hematology. 2nd ed. Cham: Spring International Publishing AG; 2019.
2. Hoffbrand V, Vyas P, Campo E, Haferlach T, Gomez K. Color atlas of clinical hematology: molecular and cellular basis of disease. 5th ed. Newark: Wiley, Incorporated; 2019.
3. Auerbach M, DeLoughery TG. Causes and diagnosis of iron deficiency and iron deficiency anemia in adults.

In: Connor RF, editor. UpToDate. Wolters Kluwer; 2024a. Accessed 27 June 2024.
4. Auerbach M, DeLoughery TG. Treatment of iron deficiency anemia in adults. In: Connor RF, editor. UpToDate. Wolters Kluwer; 2024b. Accessed 27 June 2024.
5. Means RT Jr, Brodsky RA. Diagnostic approach to anemia in adults. In: Connor RF, editor. UpToDate. Wolters Kluwer; 2024. Accessed 27 June 2024.
6. George TI. Automated complete blood count (CBC). In: Connor RF, editor. UpToDate. Wolters Kluwer; 2024. Accessed 27 June 2024.
7. Powers JM. Iron deficiency in infants and children <12 years: Screening, prevention, clinical manifestations, and diagnosis. In: Connor RF, editor. UpToDate. Wolters Kluwer; 2024. Accessed 27 June 2024.
8. Centers for Disease Control and Prevention (CDC). Iron deficiency—United States, 1999–2000. MMWR Morb Mortal Wkly Rep. 2002;51(40):897–9.

Part XI

Emergency Medicine

Subjective Fever 26

George Nguyen

Learning Objectives

1. Explain the HIV replication cycle and how HIV infects host T-cells and other immune cells. Describe the mechanism in which HIV leads to severe T-cell immunodeficiency/AIDS. Comment on the HIV genome and which viral proteins are produced.
2. Compare how viral RNA, p24 antigen, anti-p24 antibodies, anti-gp120 antibodies, and CD4+ lymphocytes levels relatively change from initial HIV infection over time.
3. List the major pathogens that lead to opportunistic infections associated with AIDS. Comment on the relative CD4 T-cell counts in relation to these opportunistic pathogens. Evaluate malignancies closely associated with AIDS.
4. Identify the clinical presentation and risk factors of acute HIV infection (acute retroviral syndrome) and compare this with the symptomatology of AIDS-induced Pneumocystis jiroveci pneumonia.
5. Describe the diagnostic tests used for HIV (focus on fourth generation) and its utilization for disease progression, response to therapy, and immune status.
6. Describe the pharmacologic treatment available to treat HIV and list their mechanism of actions and associated toxicities. Comment on the treatment of Pneumocystis jiroveci pneumonia.
7. Explain the role physicians play in HIV prevention when patients are newly diagnosed HIV-positive in the constraints of existing state laws in the American Medical Association Code of Medical Ethics guidelines.

Setting: Emergency Medicine

Scenario: You are the physician team seeing a patient who called into his family medicine clinic for symptoms of shortness of breath and coughing but was promptly told to go to the emergency room due to his current conditions. You diligently try to know more about your patient and find a note in the EMR from 6 years ago.

EMR Will Display the Following Note from 6 Years Ago

Chief Complaint: Fevers and Malaise.

HPI: Geoffrey Danlin is a 21-year-old Caucasian male with no significant PMH who presents into clinic with a 2-day history of headache, fevers, sore throat, and myalgia.

Geoffrey recently returned from a trip to Rocky Point for his fall break with his former classmates where he was in good health initially. Geoffrey could not recount any event that led to

G. Nguyen (✉)
Department of Internal Medicine, University of Arizona College of Medicine Phoenix – Banner University Medical Center, Phoenix, AZ, USA
e-mail: George.Nguyen@bannerhealth.com

C. A. Standley (ed.), *Biomedical Science and Clinical Foundations*,
https://doi.org/10.1007/978-3-031-98353-5_26

him feeling this way but began feeling malaise and a subjective fever 2 days prior to coming into the clinic. He also returned from Mexico on that same day. The fever has been constant, and he gets some chills. Geoffrey has not taken any medication for the fever and feels the same as he did the first day of illness. He has begun to feel a sore throat but does not have any coughs or sputum production. He ultimately was told to see the clinic due to his mother worrying. He notes no other symptoms.

PMH

- Asthma diagnosed at age 8
- Eczema diagnosed at age 8
- No prior surgical procedures

Medications

- Albuterol inhaler before exercise only
- Hydrocortisone cream for eczema during flares

Allergies

- Allergic to Sulfa drugs (may come into play with Bactrim)
- Causes anaphylaxis

Family History

- Mother: Cervical cancer and breast cancer; proud survivor
- Father: HTN, HF
- No other cancers in the family

Social History/High-Risk Behavior

- Living: He lives in the off-campus housing down the street from where he recently dropped out of college. He has had no sick contacts
- Occupation: Currently unemployed
- Travel: He came from Rocky Point for fall break last week
- Pets: He does not have any pets at home or contact with pets
- Immunizations: Up to date on immunizations for school, but he did not receive influenza vaccination this year
- Alcohol: "On the weekends when there are get-togethers, but I left my binge drinking days behind me"
- Smoking: "Have tried marijuana once or twice, but no tobacco"
- Illicit Drug Use: Denies
- Sexual History: Sexually active, lifetime partners of 2

Review of Systems

- General: + Fevers, chills, diaphoresis; no night sweats, or weight change.
- Skin: + Rash; no lesions, pruritus, sores, or change in hair or nails.
- Hematologic: + Cervical tender lymphadenopathy, no abnormal or excessive bleeding, ecchymosis, or history of anemia.
- Head: +Headaches; no head trauma.
- Eyes: No glasses/contacts, no eye pain, inflammation, discharge, infection, injury, blurring, or loss of vision.
- Ears: No tinnitus, pain, infection, discharge, or vertigo.
- Nose: No discharge, sinus pain, or epistaxis.
- Mouth: No change in taste or pain in mouth/tongue. No lesions on the mouth, gums, lips, or tongue.
- Pharynx/larynx: +Pharyngitis; no hoarseness, or dysphagia.
- Respiratory: No cough, sputum, hemoptysis, dyspnea, wheezing, or pleuritic chest pain.
- Cardiovascular: No chest pain, palpitations, light-headedness, syncope, or edema. No h/o heart murmurs, DVTs, DOE, or change in exercise tolerance.
- GI: +Nausea, no change in appetite, dyspepsia, reflux/GERD or abdominal pain. No emesis, hematemesis, or coffee-ground emesis. No hernia, jaundice/icterus, pain with BM, recent changes in frequency/consistency/color of BM, melena, diarrhea, constipation, hemorrhoids, or hematochezia.
- GU: No dysuria, frequency, urgency, polyuria, nocturia, incontinence, hematuria, flank/CVA tenderness.

- Genital: No h/o of STIs, genital lesions, rashes, pain, or discharge.
- Endocrine: No weight changes, easy fatigue, change in sleep pattern.
- MSK: +Pain in extremities. No stiffness or swelling of the joints or muscles. No limitation of movement of the neck, trunk, or extremities. No h/o deformity or injury of the bones or joints.
- Neurological: No syncope, seizures, dizziness, weakness, or paresthesia, or abnormal clumsiness/difficulty with balance. No difficulty with bowel or bladder control.
- Psychiatric: No change in moods, prolonged crying. No previous treatment of a psychiatric illness.

Physical Exam

- Vital Signs: Temp: 39C (102.2F), BP: 105/55 mmHg, Pulse: 98 bpm, R: 20 breaths/min
- Gen: Normal weight male, alert, and conversant in NAD
- Skin: Maculopapular rash seen on collar region, warm, hair normal texture/distribution.
- HEENT:
- Head: Normocephalic and atraumatic
- Eyes: Conjunctiva clear, sclera anicteric, visual acuity 20/20 OU, Pupils 5 mm, PERRLA, EOMI
- Ears: Canals c cerumen, TMs pearl grey with nl light reflex. Hearing grossly intact.
- Nose: Septum midline, turbinates non-edematous
- Throat: Erythematous without exudates
- Neck: Tender cervical lymphadenopathy; no thyromegaly or nodules, carotid nl upstroke s bruit.
- Chest: Excursion or expansion is symmetric; CTA&P bilaterally
- Cardiac: RRR, nl S1, S2 s S3, S4, M, R. PMI 5ICS MCL
- Abdomen: Non-distended, non-tender; +bowel sounds all four quadrants, without hepatosplenomegaly. No rebound/rigidity
- Extremities: s CCE. Tenderness to palpation for UE and LE, but full ROM for UE and LE
- Pulses: radial, bronchial, femoral, DP, PT are 2+ symmetric,
- Lymph node survey: no axillary lymphadenopathy

Labs: CBC (Table 26.1)/BMP (Table 26.2)

Specific test for EBV - > Heterophile antibody test pending

Specific test for CMV - > CMV serology pending

Specific for HIV - > HIV serology pending

Hepatitis panel pending

Imaging: None

Assessment and Plan

- Acute fever, malaise, and lymphadenopathy 2/2 to possible influenza, EBV, HIV or other viral illness vs bacterial infection
  - Did CBC/BMP in clinic
  - Will get HIV, EBV, and CMV testing
  - Will get hepatitis panel
  - Symptomatic treatment
  - RTC in a week for follow-up and progression of symptoms

Prompt Are there other causes for vague symptoms as these?

Syphilis, disseminated gonococcal infection, viral hepatitis, new-onset systemic lupus erythematous (Students should note possible infectious/viral etiology).

Addendum: Patient never returned back to clinic for follow-up and never did continual lab studies of EBV, CMV, or HIV testing.

End of Chart Review and Beginning of Case

Chief Complaint: "I…can't…breathe…too much coughing…".

HPI: Geoffrey Danlin is a 27-year-old male with a history of asthma presents to the emergency department urgently with coughing and shortness of breath.

Table 26.1 Complete Blood Count (CBC)

Component	Patient	Reference
Hemoglobin	14	12–15 g/dL
Hematocrit	41	33–43%
White blood count	4500	3200–9800/mm^3
Differential	64% neutrophils, 5% bands, 28% lymphocytes, 2% monocytes, 1% eosinophils, 1% basophils	60–70% neutrophils, 2–6% bands, 25–40% lymphocytes, 2–8% monocytes, 1–4% eosinophils, 0–1% basophils
Platelet count	130	130–400 × 10^3/mm^3

Table 26.2 Basic Metabolic Panel (BMP)

Component	Patient	Reference
Sodium	139	135–147 mEq/L
Potassium	4.1	3.5–5.0 mEq/L
Bicarbonate	25	24–28 mEq/L
Chloride	99	95–105 mEq/L
BUN	16	8–18 mg/dL
Creatinine	0.8	0.6–1.2 mg/dL
Glucose	95	70–100 mg/dL

Prompt What is your differential diagnosis?

V—vascular (e.g., heart failure, myocardial infarction, PE)
I—infectious (pneumonia, bronchitis, viral illness, immunodeficient)
N—neoplastic (e.g., lung cancer, etc.)
D—drug reaction (ACE inhibitors, etc.)
I—idiopathic (psychogenic cough or tic)/primary inflammatory (post-viral syndrome)
C—congenital/cardiac (chest deformity, CF, congenital heart disease, valvular disease)
A—autoimmune/allergic (e.g., allergic/asthmatic cough; anaphylactic reaction)
T—traumatic/toxins (foreign body, pneumothorax, hemothorax, ingestion)
E—endocrine/metabolic (e.g., gastrointestinal reflux, malnutrition, Mallory-Weiss, Borhaave's)
R—Renal/respiratory
pSychiatric

PMH

- Asthma diagnosed at age 8
- Eczema diagnosed at age 8
- No prior surgical procedures

Medications

- Albuterol inhaler before exercise only
- Hydrocortisone cream for eczema during flares

Allergies

- Allergic to sulfa drugs (may come into play with bactrim)
- Causes anaphylaxis

Family History

- Mother: Cervical cancer and breast cancer; proud survivor
- Father: HTN, HF
- No other cancers in the family

Social History/High-Risk Behavior

- Living situation: In and out of the streets; recently moved back in with mother
- Occupation: Currently unemployed; college dropout
- Travel: none
- Sick contacts: Recalls some who were sick with similar cough when he was at homeless shelter
- Pets: None
- Immunizations: No influenza virus, but up to date on immunizations
- Tobacco: Weekly marijuana use with no tobacco use
- Alcohol: None; no withdrawal symptoms
- Illicit Drug Use: IV drug user for last 3 years. Last use was 6 months ago with heroin
- Sexual History: Sexually active with men; lifetime partners of 10+; does not use condoms

Prompt What parts of this patient's history are concerning? Are there risk factors? How does this relate to the patient's presentation from 6 years ago?

Patient has been on the streets and in homeless shelters, which raises concern for cocci, TB, and other infections. IV drug use and men who have sex with men are increased risks for HIV. Endocarditis could also be on the differential at this point due to IV drug use.

From the CDC, the following are risk factors for HIV: anal sex, vaginal sex, oral sex, injection drug use, HIV risk and prevention estimates, pre-exposure prophylaxis (PrEP), post-exposure prophylaxis (PEP), HIV treatment as prevention, condoms, and male circumcision (see Learning Objective #4).

Students should be able to recognize and begin to be prompted that the patient has risk factors for HIV and, given the initial EHR note, could possibly have a chronic HIV at this point of time since the initial note may have described an acute HIV infection.

Review of Systems

- General: + Fevers, chills, diaphoresis, night sweats, decrease in weight (lost 10 lbs. in last year).
- Skin: No rash, lesions, pruritus, sores, or change in hair or nails.
- Hematologic: No, lymphadenopathy, abnormal or excessive bleeding, ecchymosis, or history of anemia.
- Head: No headaches; no head trauma.
- Eyes: No glasses/contacts. No eye pain, inflammation, discharge, infection, injury, blurring, or loss of vision.
- Ears: No tinnitus, pain, infection, discharge, or vertigo.
- Nose: No discharge, sinus pain, or epistaxis.
- Mouth: No change in taste or pain in mouth/tongue. No lesions on the mouth, gums, lips, or tongue.
- Pharynx/larynx: +Pharyngitis; no hoarseness, or dysphagia.
- Respiratory: + cough, + sputum, + dyspnea; no, hemoptysis, wheezing, or pleuritic chest pain.
- Cardiovascular: + Chest Pain; no palpitations, light-headedness, syncope, or edema. No h/o heart murmurs, DVTs, DOE, or change in exercise tolerance.
- GI: +Nausea and decreased appetite; no dyspepsia, reflux/GERD or abdominal pain. No emesis, hematemesis, or coffee-ground emesis. No hernia, jaundice/icterus, pain with BM, recent changes in frequency/consistency/color of BM, melena, diarrhea, constipation, hemorrhoids or hematochezia.
- GU: No dysuria, frequency, urgency, polyuria, nocturia, incontinence, hematuria, flank/CVA tenderness.
- Genital: No h/o of STIs, genital lesions, rashes, pain, or discharge.
- Endocrine: No weight changes, easy fatigue, change in sleep pattern.
- MSK: No stiffness, tenderness, or swelling of the joints or muscles. No limitation of movement of the neck, trunk, or extremities. No h/o deformity or injury of the bones or joints.
- Neurological: No syncope, seizures, dizziness, weakness, or paresthesia, or abnormal clumsiness/difficulty with balance. No difficulty with bowel or bladder control.
- Psychiatric: No change in moods, prolonged crying. No previous treatment of a psychiatric illness.

Prompt What could be possible causes to the patient's positive ROS findings? How does this change your differential?

Sources of infection could be pulmonary, GI, or skin flora and less likely to be from a UTI, or meningitis. Weight loss and night sweats have concern for malignancy, TB, or cocci. Chest pain includes many possibilities, but should explore myocardial infarction, pulmonary embolism, and pneumonia as lethal causes.

Physical Exam

- VS: Temp: 38.1C (100.6 F), BP: 98/58 mmHg; pulse: 101 bpm, R: 26 breaths/min, O2 sat: 90% RA
- Gen: Cachectic appearing male, alert and conversant, but with increased work of breathing

- Skin: Warm. There are purple lesions on the inner thigh. No itching or painful lesions noted
  (Kaposi Sarcoma)
- HEENT:
- Head: Normocephalic and atraumatic
- Eyes: Conjunctiva clear, sclera anicteric, visual acuity 20/20 OU, pupils 5 mm, PERRLA, EOMI
- Ears: Canals c cerumen, TMs pearl grey with nl light reflex. Hearing grossly intact
- Nose: septum midline, turbinates non-edematous

Prompt What is the significance of the patient's vital signs?

The patient's vital signs are positive for multiple factors in the Systemic Inflammatory Response Syndrome (SIRS) which put the patient in the sepsis category that is compensated due to no hypotension. Other labs will be needed to confirm multi-organ dysfunction for possible upgrade to septic shock.

From Up To Date:

Sepsis is a systemic inflammatory response to a confirmed or suspected infection. Clinically, the Systemic Inflammatory Response Syndrome (SIRS) is the occurrence of at least two of the following criteria: fever >38.0 °C or hypothermia <36.0 °C, tachycardia >90 beats/min, tachypnea >20 breaths/min, leukocytosis >12*109/l or leucopoenia <4*109/l.

The development from sepsis to septic shock represents a continuum with increasing mortality. The in-hospital/28-day mortality in severe sepsis is 10–40% and in septic shock it is 30–60% [1]. Early treatment with antibiotic and fluid resuscitation has been found to be strongly related to increased survival, which makes severe sepsis a condition which is important to identify and treat as early as possible. (https://www.ncbi.nlm.nih.gov/pmc/articles/PMC2806258/)

Prompt What skin lesion does he likely have?

The cutaneous lesion is Kaposi sarcoma and appears most often on the lower extremities, face, oral mucosa, and genitalia. The lesions are often elliptical and may be arranged in a linear fashion along skin tension lines; they may be symmetrically distributed. The lesions are not painful or pruritic and usually do not produce necrosis of overlying skin or underlying structures.

The assortment of colors associated with these lesions is due to their vascularity and includes many hues of pink, red, purple, and brown. Early lesions can easily be mistaken as purpura, hematomas, angiomas, dermatofibromas, or nevi. More commonly, however, Kaposi sarcoma lesions are papular, ranging in size from several millimeters to several centimeters in diameter.

Lymphedema, particularly in the face, genitalia, and lower extremities may be out of proportion to the extent of the disease and may be related to both vascular obstruction by lymphadenopathy and the cytokines involved in the pathogenesis of Kaposi sarcoma.

- Throat: white collection on tongue that is scrapable, with minor erythema of posterior pharynx; no exudates
  (Oral Thrush)
- Neck: Cervical lymphadenopathy bilaterally; no thyromegaly or nodules, carotid nl upstroke s bruit.
- Chest: Crackles heard bilaterally, intercostal retractions seen
- Cardiac: Tachycardia, nl S1, S2 s S3, S4, M, R. PMI 5ICS MCL
- Abdomen: Non-distended, non-tender; +Bowel sounds all four quadrants, without hepatosplenomegaly. No rebound/rigidity
- Extremities: s CCE
- Pulses: radial, DP, PT are 1+ symmetric
- Lymph node survey: generalized bilateral axillary lymphadenopathy

Prompt What parts of the patient's subjective history are important and what parts of the patient's physical exam are noteworthy? How does this change your differential?

Noteworthy physical exam findings:

Oral Thrush—Students should be able to differentiate that the white discoloration that is scrapeable is related to oral thrush or oral candidiasis compared to leukoplakia which is associated with squamous cell carcinoma and HPV infections, in which these white oral lesions are non-scrapeable. Up to 90% of persons with advanced untreated HIV infection develop oropharyngeal candidiasis, with 60% having at least 1 episode per year with frequent recurrences (50–60%). Esophageal candidiasis occurs less frequently (10–20%) but is the leading cause of esophageal disease.

Crackles, Intercostal retractions: Patient's pulmonary condition is worsening and shows signs of pneumonia. Because the crackles are heard throughout the lungs and not focused on the bases, the diagnosis of pulmonary edema is less likely.

Generalized lymphadenopathy with cervical lymphadenopathy—correlation with disseminated gonococcal infections, syphilis, HIV, and systemic infections. Chronic HIV should now be priority due to the addition of oral thrush and generalized lymphadenopathy.

Prompt What further lab work should be ordered?

Students can be prompted to look-up diagnostic tests necessary for HIV, which will be shown below.

CBC (Table 26.3) and CMP (Table 26.4)—Looking for differentials and possible lymphocytopenia for HIV; white count for sepsis.

Lactate dehydrogenase to see how badly septic patient is appearing.

Blood cultures

Infections: Hep A, B, C, RPR (syphilis), gonorrhea, and chlamydia (G/C).

Arterial blood gas

1–3-beta-D-glucan levels—specific to Pneumocystis jiroveci pneumonia

EKG, Echo, troponins due to patient's chest pain to rule out MI, endocarditis

Chest X-ray and CT—Thorax

HIV-Related Tests: CD4 Count, HIV viral load, HIV-1/HIV-2 antigen/antibody immunoassay, HIV genotyping/phenotyping

Hep A, B, C—Negative

RPR (Syphilis)—Negative

Gonorrhea and Chlamydia (G/C) —Negative

Lactate Dehydrogenase Levels: 362 IU (140 IU–280 IU)

1–3-beta-D-glucan levels: 90 pg/mL (normal average is 17 pg/mL)

(https://academic.oup.com/labmed/article/42/11/679/2657644)

Prompt What is the significance of these lab findings?

CBC shows a decreased in the white blood cell count and more specifically an increase in bands (acute infection) with lymphocytopenia on the differential. This should signal to students that the patient is most likely immunocompromised from HIV/AIDS with a coexisting pulmonary infection. AIDS is the most common infectious disease causing lymphocytopenia, which arises from destruction of CD4+ T cells infected with HIV. Thrombocytopenia is a result of chronic HIV infections.

> During the end of the physical exam, Geoffrey started becoming increasingly tachypneic and having worsening respiratory distress. He was given nasal cannula oxygen and immediately admitted to the inpatient units for further work-up.

Lactate dehydrogenase levels are elevated signaling a septic outlook for the patient. Results of a study of 62 patients (54 with advanced HIV disease) showed that only 7% of those with documented PJP had normal serum LDH levels; the mean LDH level in patients with PCP was 362 IU. The mean initial level in surviving patients was 340 IU, vs 447 IU for non-survivors.

1–3-beta-D-glucan levels are elevated. From Up To Date: Elevated plasma levels of 1–3-beta-D-glucan, a component of the cell wall of P. jirovecii, have been found in HIV-infected patients with PJP. Elevated levels can also be observed in

Table 26.3 Complete Blood Count (CBC)

Component	Patient	Reference
Hemoglobin	12	12–15 g/dL
Hematocrit	33	33–43%
White blood count	2800	3200–9800/mm^3
Differential	60% neutrophils, 7% bands, 15% lymphocytes, 8% monocytes, 4% eosinophils, 1% basophils	60–70% neutrophils, 2–6% bands, 25–40% lymphocytes, 2–8% monocytes, 1–4% eosinophils, 0–1% basophils
Platelet count	100	130–400 × 10^3/mm^3

Table 26.4 Complete Metabolic Profile (CMP)

Component	Patient	Reference
Sodium	142	135–147 mEq/L
Potassium	4.2	3.5–5.0 mEq/L
Bicarbonate	20	24–28 mEq/L
Chloride	100	95–105 mEq/L
BUN	16	8–18 mg/dL
Creatinine	1.1	0.6–1.2 mg/dL
Glucose	108	70–100 mg/dL
ALT (SGPT)	17	5–35 U/L
AST (SGOT)	15	0–30 U/L
Alkaline phosphatase	50	44–147 U/L
Bilirubin, total	0.3	0.1–1.2 mg/dL
Total protein	6.2	6.3–7.9 g/dL
Albumin	3.8	3.9–5.0 g/dL

patients infected with other fungi (in particular histoplasmosis), and false positives can be seen as a result of other clinical variables. Therefore, potential confounding factors must be considered when interpreting the results of this test and should be supported by imaging.

The patient's decrease in total protein and albumin levels is a sign of malnourishment since this patient has lost 10 lbs over the last few months and has had decreased oral intake recently.

Bicarb being down to 20 mEq/L should signal to students of an acid-balance issue and a sign that an ABG should be done, which follows.

ABG: pH: 7.1 (7.38–7.42) / PaCO2: 30 mmHg (38–42 mmHg) / PaO2: 80 mmHg (80–100 mmHg)

CMP: Na: 142 mEq/L / Cl: 100 mEq/L

Bicarb from CMP: 20 mEq/L

Prompt What acid–base state in this patient in? What is the differential diagnosis of anion-gap metabolic acidosis?

pH value is less than 7.4, which means the patient is in an acidotic state.

PaCO2 being low suggests a respiratory alkalosis (hyperventilation, in which this patient has tachypnea).

Anion Gap = Na—(Cl + Bicarb) = 142–100—20 = 22, which is greater than 12 suggesting an anion gap metabolic acidosis.

CO2 respiratory compensation evaluation is done by Winter's formula = Expected CO2 = (Bicarb x 1.5) + 8 +/− 2; Expected CO2 = (20 x 1.5) + 8 +/− 2 = 36–40.

Because the patient's PaCO2 is 30, which is less than the expected CO2; the patient has a concurrent respiratory alkalosis.

Ultimately, this patient is diagnosed with an *anion gap metabolic acidosis and respiratory alkalosis.*

Differential for anion gap metabolic acidosis includes:

M—Methanol (formic acid)
U—Uremia
D—Diabetic ketoacidosis
P—Propylene glycol
I—Iron tablets or isoniazid
L—Lactic acidosis (such as by metformin toxicity)
E—Ethylene glycol
S—Salicylates (late)

EKG

The patient's EKG is shown in Fig. 26.1.
Troponins: Negative
Transthoracic Echo: Negative with preserved ejection fraction.

Prompt What is the significance of the EKG and troponin levels? And the echo?

Students can be asked to read EKG in terms of rate, rhythm, axis, and special features.

It should be noted that the EKG shows sinus tachycardia, a sign for a severe infection brewing in the patient that requires an increased heart rate to maintain perfusion in the patient's body. Tachycardia is one of the criteria for SIRS and shows the patient may be in sepsis. Because the patient complained of chest pain as well, the ideas of a myocardial infarction and pulmonary embolism remain lower on the differential now with no STEMI or NSTEMI seen. A pulmonary embolism will require a CT-angio to be confirmed. Endocarditis is unlikely with normal echo.

CD4+ Count: 180 cells/mm^3 (500–1400 cells/mm^3)
HIV viral load: 80,000 copies/mL
HIV-1/HIV-2 Antigen/Antibody Immunoassay: Pending
HIV Genotyping/Phenotyping: Pending
Blood Culture: Pending

Prompt What is the importance of CD4+ count in quantifying the extent of the patient's HIV infection?

As HIV infection progresses, the number of CD4+ cells declines. When the CD4 count drops below 200, a person is diagnosed with AIDS and becomes prone to opportunistic infections. A normal range for CD4 cells is about 500–1500. Specific opportunistic infections based on CD4+ counts is a learning objective for patients and should be hinted at here.

In early infection w/ viremia the viral load range is > 100,000 copies/mL while chronic HIV infection is 10,000–30,000 copies/mL. This patient stands to be in a chronic HIV infection range that is uncontrolled which stands to be the reason he has PJP.

The HIV-1/HIV-2 Antigen/Antibody Immunoassay allows for quicker response than Western Blot in diagnosing HIV infection and specifies which strand of HIV it is; HIV screens are generally done using an ELISA and confirmed with a Western Blot, but this patient's index of suspicion is high, allowing for one to confirm with the immunoassay.

HIV genotyping/phenotyping is used to see degree of resistance in HIV strand to antiretroviral medication.

Prompt What is the patient diagnosed with at this point in time before imaging is done?

Chronic HIV progressing to acquired immunodeficiency syndrome (AIDS).

Imaging

A chest X-ray is obtained. The trachea is midline with no signs of a tension pneumothorax. There are no rib fractures, scapula fractures, and the humerus is placed well in the glenoid fossa. There is no cardiomegaly, but pulmonary arteries/veins are difficult to assess with patchy infiltrates. The diaphragm is not unequally elevated on one side nor is there signs of pulmonary edema since diaphragmatic angles are clearly shown and appropriate. In the AP view, bilateral interstitial infiltrates are seen; predominantly perihilar in distribution; no pleural effusions. In the lateral view: interstitial infiltrates seen anterior and posteriorly.

CT-Thorax

Findings: Diffuse patchy bilateral upper and lower lobe ground-glass opacities. Differential considerations include PJP and CMV pneumonia as well as other opportunistic infection.

Bronchoalveolar Lavage (BAL) Specimen:
Methenamine Silver Stain Positive
Acid Fast Bacilli Stain Negative
Cocci—Negative
Fungal KOH Negative
Gram Stain: gram positive diplococci in chains
Culture: pending

Prompt What is your impression of the BAL?

Students should be able to note that methenamine silver stain is definitive diagnosis for Pneumocystis jiroveci pneumonia (PJP) and that PJP is often coexisting with a community-acquired pneumonia, in which this case streptococcus pneumoniae is the most likely culprit from the gram stain [2].

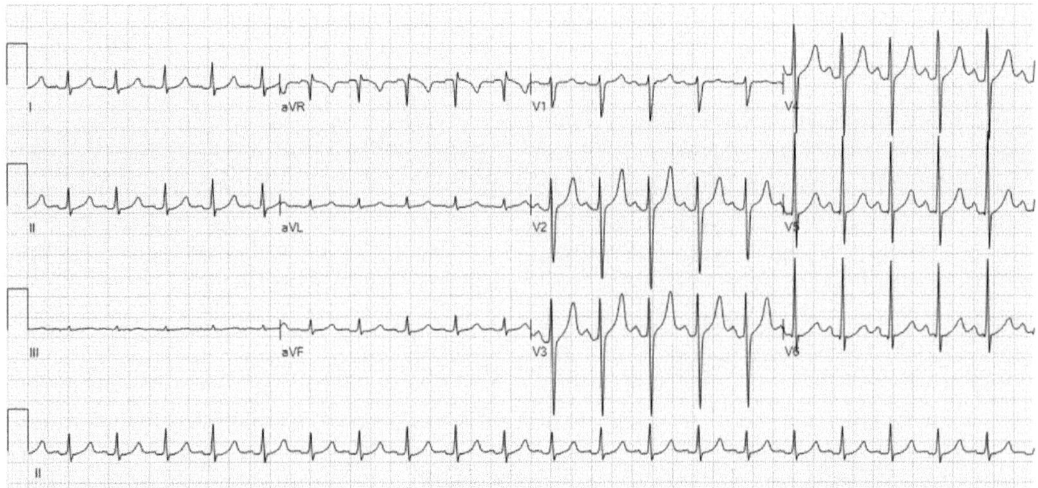

Fig. 26.1 EKG. Ewingdo, CC BY-SA 4.0 https://creativecommons.org/licenses/by-sa/4.0, via Wikimedia Commons. (https://commons.wikimedia.org/wiki/File:ECG_Sinus_Tachycardia_125_bpm.jpg)

Prompt What is the treatment for Pneumocystis jiroveci pneumonia (PJP)? Is there anything in the patient's history that complicates treatment regimens?

Atovaquone and dapsone are used for minor/moderate PJP; trimethroprim-sulfamethoxazole is first-line therapy [3].

Geoffrey Danlin was admitted to the inpatient units and was placed on IV ceftriaxone and azithromycin for his CAP and pentamidine and prednisone for his severe PJP due to his allergy to sulfa-containing drugs.

Further Results

HIV-1/HIV-2 Antigen/Antibody Immunoassay: HIV-1 Positive; HIV-2 Negative.

HIV Genotyping/Phenotyping: Susceptible to protease inhibitors, nucleoside RT inhibitors, non-nucleoside RT inhibitors.

Geoffrey Danlin was then placed on 2 nucleoside reverse transcriptase inhibitors (tenofovir alafenamide and emtricitabine) and 1 integrase inhibitor (raltegravir) for antiretroviral therapy.

Sample of Drug Resistance Mutations based off of genotyping and phenotyping can be found here: https://hivdb.stanford.edu/pages/genotype-phenotype.html

Students normally are not tested on the USMLE on specific gene mutations towards resistance to medication, but should understand the use of genotyping and phenotyping in the susceptibilities of HIV drug medications.

Prompt How would you approach telling the patient about his HIV diagnosis and the chronicity and progression of it? What social issues does he have in terms of follow-up appointments?

Delivering an HIV diagnosis requires a compassionate, clear, and supportive approach. Ensure the conversation happens in a private, quiet setting with ample time for discussion. State the diagnosis clearly and compassionately. Anticipate emotional reactions and be ready to offer immediate resources and next steps. Explain how HIV is now a chronic, manageable disease with antiretroviral therapy. With consistent treatment, HIV can be suppressed to undetectable levels, preventing illness and transmission [4]. Reinforce this with hope and control.

In terms of follow-up appointments, HIV care requires ongoing medical visits. Social factors that might create barriers to care include stigma and disclosure—fear of judgement may lead to hesitation to disclose their status even to close contacts. Medication and appointments can be costly. Some patients may lack reliable transportation to clinics. Long wait tiles or difficulty scheduling appointments may deter follow up.

Prompt Should the patient be placed on prophylactic treatment to prevent PJP from reoccurring?

Trimethroprim-sulfamethoxazole would be initiated as prophylaxis in a normal patient, but because this patient is allergic to sulfa-containing drugs, he would be placed on dapsone and pyrimethamine due to his CD4+ count being < 200 cells/mm^3.

Geoffrey Danlin was told of his diagnosis after initiation of treatments, but while he was still inpatient. He was told that his HIV diagnosis has progressed to AIDS, which is the reason why he had the worsening pneumonia symptoms and that he will be prone to infections in the future due to this diagnosis. The providers on the case showed sincerity and were sorry that they could not be there for the patient when he first came to the clinic to stress the importance of follow-up at the time of his initial presentation of acute HIV, but will be with the patient for the remainder of his journey.

Promt As Geoffrey Danlin's primary physician, what responsibility do you have as a physician for his previous partners? What responsibilities does he have to his previous partners?

Students can provide initial thoughts on contacting previous partners of Geoffrey's HIV diagnosis.

End of Case

Learning Objective Answers

Learning Objective 1: Explain the HIV replication cycle and how HIV infects host T-cells and other immune cells. Describe the mechanism in which HIV leads to severe T-cell immunodeficiency/AIDS. Comment on the HIV genome and which viral proteins are produced.

The genome of HIV consists of 9 genes encoding for a total of 15 proteins. The three most important gene codes on the HIV genome include the *pol* gene, *gag* gene, and the *env* gene. The *pol* gene codes for the polyproteins needed for the creation of protease, reverse transcriptase, and integrase, which all have roles described further below. The *gag* gene codes for the gag protein (produces p24 and p17) which is necessary for the creation of matrix proteins, nucleocapsids, and capsid proteins necessary for the budding process. The *env* gene codes for surface glycoproteins gp160, which cleaves to form gp120, which is necessary for HVI to attach to CD4+ T-lymphocytes and gp41, which allows for the fusion an entry into the immune cells.

The key points of the HIV replication cycle can be summarized in the below steps (Fig. 26.2):

1. Entry—HIV enters the body through mucosal lesions or through infected immune cells and attaches to CD4+ receptors of target cells with gp120 glycoprotein (binding). CD4+ receptor cells include T-lymphocytes, macrophages, monocytes, and dendritic cells.
2. Fusion—The HIV viral envelope interacts with the CD4 receptor and coreceptor of the immune cell, which would be CCR5 in macrophages and CCR5 or CXCR4 in T-cells. These components allow for the viral envelope to fuse with the immune cell and releasing the virion's RNA into the cell. Of note, individuals who do not possess a CCR5 receptor are resistant to HIV.
3. Reverse Transcription—Using the *pol* gene, the virion is able to use the enzyme reverse transcriptase to convert the virion's RNA into DNA, where the DNA product migrates into the nucleus of the cell.
4. Integration—Using the *pol* gene, the virion uses the enzyme integrase to insert the viral DNA into the DNA of the host CD4+ cell. Upon integration, the CD4+ cell is considered infected for the remainder of its life.
5. Replication—Using the host CD4 cells, transcription and translation are preferentially done to create new viral RNA, which are fur-

ther translated into polyprotein chains for viral budding and maturation.

6. Assembly—Viral proteins and enzymes from the translation of viral RNA move to the cell's outer membrane and assemble into an immature, non-infectious HIV particle or bud, which is released from the host CD4+ cell.
7. Post-budding and Maturation—The viral enzyme protease from the *pol* gene cuts the long HIV polyprotein chain into smaller, but still functional HIV proteins creating mature, infectious viral particles. Upon the completion of budding, the host CD4+ cell undergoes apoptosis or cell death.

Currently, the exact mechanism of HIV causing AIDS is unknown. Most scientists think that HIV causes AIDS by directly inducing the death of CD4+ T cells or interfering with their normal function, and by triggering other events that weaken a person's immune function. Over a period of years, the high viral load eventually accumulates in lymphoid tissues, which causes an increased production of cytokines such as TNF-alpha and IL-6, which recruits more immune cells in the lymphoid tissue, making these uninfected cells at risk of being easily infected. These cells undergo the HIV replication cycle and ultimately, cell death leading to the lower CD4+ counts with chronic HIV infections. In addition, T cells infected with HIV lose the capacity to produce IL-2, which enhances the growth of other T cells to fight invading organisms, further causing immunodeficiency.

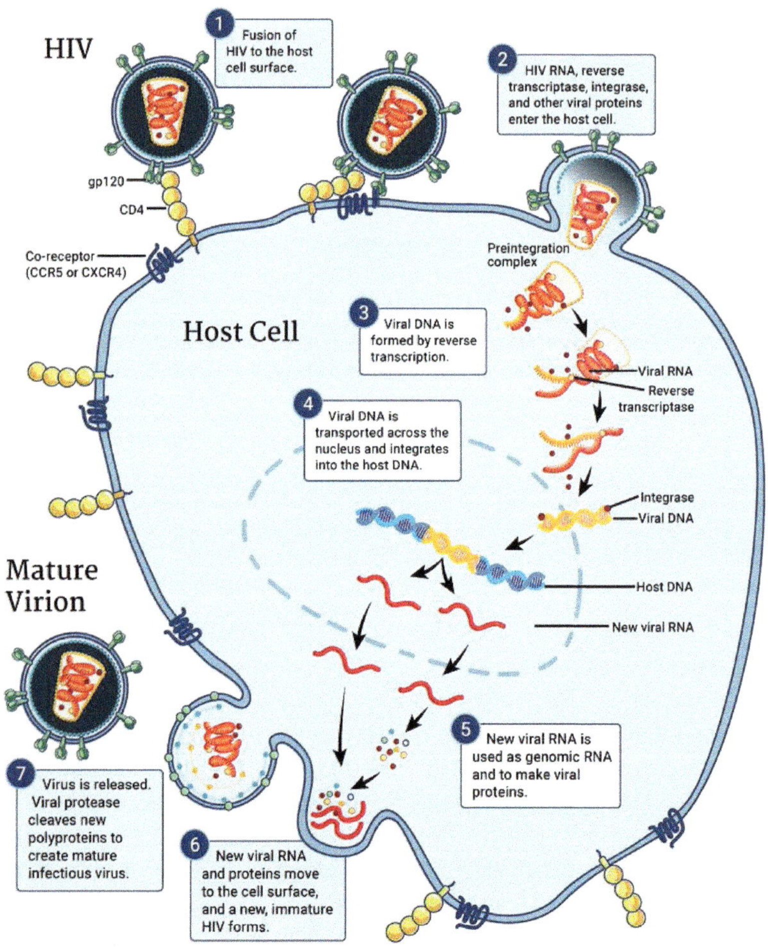

Fig. 26.2 Demonstration of HVI Replication Cycle. Image Credit: NIAID CC BY 2.0. (https://www.flickr.com/photos/niaid/5057022555)

Learning Objective 2: Compare how viral RNA, p24 antigen, anti-p24 antibodies, anti-gp120 antibodies, and CD4+ lymphocytes levels relatively change from initial HIV infection over time.

The viral RNA levels, p24 antigen, anti-p24 antibodies, anti-gp120 antibodies, and CD4+ lymphocytes levels change drastically over the time course of HIV infection.

When evaluating the HIV RNA levels, one should note that the body enters a period called the "Eclipse Phase," in which 10–12 days after initial HIV infection in which no diagnostic test is capable of detecting HIV. The RNA levels will continue to increase and reach nadir at approximately 20–25 days, in which viral loads are typically >100,000 copies/mL of plasma. This is typically the point where individuals will feel the symptoms of acute HIV infection or acute retroviral syndrome. CD4+ cell counts may also see a dip during the peak levels of HIV viral loads and can be seen as dropping to levels as low as 500 cells/mm^3, but still within normal range. The CD4+ cells will rebound upwards weeks after the peak viral loads and will remain stable until approximately 6 years on average if no antiretroviral treatment is given, in which patients will reach AIDS with CD4+ <200 cells/mm^3.

HIV p24 antigen will begin to accumulate approximately 5 days after initial HIV infection and will peak at the 25-day mark. Antibodies to both p24 antigen and gp120 antigens will be produced after 14 weeks post-initial infection and will remain stably elevated during the asymptomatic chronic phase that happens 2–10 years from initial infection. Levels will begin to drop as the patient enters AIDS and begins losing CD4+ cells and is unable to communicate with B-cells to form further antibodies against these antigens. A summary of the time frame can be found in Fig. 26.3 below.

Learning Objective 3: List the major pathogens that lead to opportunistic infections associated with AIDS. Comment on the relative CD4 T-cell counts in relation to these opportunistic pathogens. Evaluate malignancies closely associated with AIDS.

The leading major source of morbidity and mortality in HIV-infected patients include the acquisition of opportunistic infections from bacteria, viruses, fungi, and protozoa due to the increased risk these patients possess. Opportunistic infections are defined as more frequent or more severe infections as a result of immunosuppression. Due to the progressive reduction in cell-mediated immunity, HIV and eventual AIDS will lower the CD4+ count of patients. Opportunistic infections still occur in the modern day and mostly comprise of patients who are not receiving antiretroviral therapy.

For board examinations, students are expected to know the opportunistic infections and specific CD4+ counts related to HIV and eventual AIDS (when the CD4+ count is <200) (Table 26.5).

The primary prevention and treatment of opportunistic infections include the use of antimicrobial prophylaxis and initiation of antiretroviral therapy [4]. The use of antiviral therapy alone have reduced the rate of opportunistic infections from 140 per every 1000 person-years to less than 20 per 1000 person-years in studies.

Due to the HIV's mechanism of action of causing immunosuppression, cancers with a viral association have been shown to have a higher incidence within HIV patients [5, 6]. A general list is shown next:

- Human herpesvirus 8 (HHV-8) causes Kaposi sarcoma and some subtypes of lymphoma.
- Epstein–Barr Virus (EBV) leads to subtypes of non-Hodgkin lymphoma and Hodgkin lymphoma, nasopharyngeal carcinoma, and oral hairy leukoplakia.
- Human papillomavirus (HPV) leads to cervical cancer, anal cancer, oropharyngeal cancer, penile cancer, vaginal cancer, and vulvar cancer.
- Hepatitis B and Hepatitis C virus both lead to hepatocellular carcinoma.

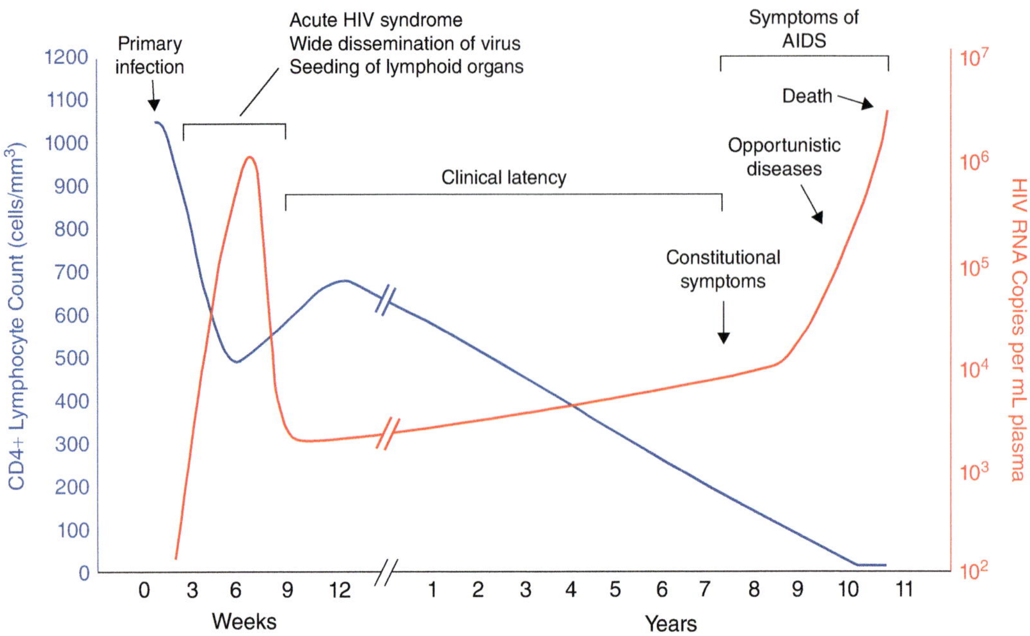

Fig. 26.3 Laboratory profile of HIV infection over time. Sigve, CC0, via Wikimedia Commons https://commons.wikimedia.org/wiki/File:Hiv-timecourse_copy.svg, https://creativecommons.org/publicdomain/zero/1.0/

Several studies have shown that the introduction of antiretroviral therapy has lowered the incidence of certain cancers in HIV-infected patients, namely Kaposi sarcoma and non-Hodgkin lymphoma. The reasoning suggested includes the lowering amounts of HIV RNA circulating in the blood, which restores the immune system to fend off these viruses listed above. It is important to note that individuals with HIV infection follow their own protocol in terms of cancer screenings. For example, pap smears are done on HIV-infected women upon the diagnosis of HIV with a follow-up pap test in 6 months to a year if normal rather than the every 3 years protocol in normal women. Some experts have also suggested anal paps be done as well.

Learning Objective 4: Identify the clinical presentation and risk factors of acute HIV infection (acute retroviral syndrome) and compare this with the symptomatology of AIDS-induced Pneumocystis jiroveci pneumonia.

Risk factors for HIV infection include: injection drug use, sexual contact (anal, vaginal, or oral), blood products, vertical transmission from mother to child, or organ transplants. The rate and risk index is shown in Table 26.6.

The clinical presentation of acute HIV infection presents as a constellation of non-specific symptoms that is similar to that of a mononucleosis type of syndrome [7, 8] (Table 26.7). If there is no high degree of suspicion of HIV, the diagnosis is often missed. Although an estimate of 10–60% of individuals with early HIV infection are asymptomatic depending on the study, the usual time for development of symptoms is 2–4 weeks after HIV exposure. Studies have shown that this correlates with the peak viremia that appears at the two-week mark. The most common findings include fever, generalized lymphadenopathy, sore throat, rash, myalgia/arthralgia, diarrhea, weight loss, and headaches. Other symptoms that are specific to acute HIV infection include the prolonged duration of symptoms and presence of sharply demarcated,

Table 26.5 CD4+ count and related opportunistic infections

CD4+ count	Opportunistic Infection	Associated findings	Prophylactic treatment
<500 mm^3	Candida Albicans	Oral thrush that is scrapable; pseudohyphae under microscope	–
	Epstein–Barr virus	Oral hairy leukoplakia	–
	HHV-8	Kaposi sarcoma	–
	HPV	Squamous cell carcinoma of anus or cervix	–
	Reactivated TB	Fevers, hemoptysis, night sweats, weight loss	
<200 mm^3	Histoplasma capsulatum	Fevers, night sweats, chills, weight loss macrophages contain oval yeast cells on microscope	–
	JC virus reactivation	Progressive multifocal leukoencephalopathy	–
	Pneumocystis jiroveci	Ground-glass opacity on chest CT; pneumonia	Trimethoprim-sulfamethoxazole
	Cryptosporidium parvum	Watery diarrhea; Acid-fast oocytes in stool	Nitazoxanide
<100 mm^3	Aspergillus fumigatus	Hemoptysis, pleuritic chest pain, cavity in upper lung lobe	–
	Bartonella henselae	Bacillary angiomatosis	–
	Candida albicans	White plaque esophagitis	–
	Cytomegalovirus	Retinitis, esophagitis, encephalitis intranuclear inclusion bodies (owl eyes) on microscope	–
	Epstein–Barr virus	B-cell lymphoma	–
	Toxoplasma gondii	Ring-enhancing brain abscesses	Trimethoprim-sulfamethoxazole
	Mycobacterium avium-intracellulare	Fever, night sweats, weight loss	Azithromycin

Table 26.6 Risk index of HIV by exposure route

Exposure route	Estimated risk per 10,000 exposures
Blood transfusion	9250
Needle-sharing injection drug use	63
Receptive anal intercourse	138
Insertive anal intercourse	11
Receptive penile-vaginal intercourse	8
Insertive penile-vaginal intercourse	4
Receptive oral sec (with ejaculation)	Low, but not precisely quantified
Insertive oral sex	Very low
Needlestick injury (healthcare setting)	23
Mother-to-child transmission (without treatment)	2000–4000 per 10,000

Ref: Centers for Disease Control and Prevention (CDC). HIV Risk Behaviors. Available at: https://www.cdc.gov/hiv/

painful mucocutaneous ulcers. Fevers often range from 38 °C to 40 °C, and lymphadenopathy is primarily non-tender and involved the axillary, cervical, and occipital nodes. The rash typically erupts 48–72 h after the onset of fevers and will include the upper thorax, collar region, and face most often. Laboratory features will often include high viral RNA levels that are >100,000 copies/mL with normal CBC (although a transient CD4 cell count drop occurs early in infection, the numbers often rebound quickly at the time of symptoms). Table 26.7 shows the likelihood of symptoms to occur with acute HIV infections.

Often, chronic HIV infection will go unnoticed and asymptomatic until the patient progresses to a CD4+ count <200mm^3, in which the patient becomes classified with AIDS and is at risk of opportunistic infections, which can be seen in Learning Objective #3. This case explores the most common opportunistic infection seen in

Table 26.7 Symptoms of acute HIV infection in terms of frequency

Symptom	Estimated frequency (%)
Fever	80–90%
Fatigue	70–90%
Rash	40–80%
Headache	50–70%
Sore throat	50–70%
Swollen lymph nodes	40–70%
Muscle and joint pain	50–70%
Night sweats	50–60%
Nausea, vomiting, or diarrhea	30–60%
Weight loss	30–50%
Mouth ulcers	10–20%
Genital ulcers	10–20%

Ref: Centers for Disease Control and Prevention (CDC). *HIV Symptoms and Stages*. Available at: https://www.cdc.gov/hiv/

HIV-infected patients in industrialized countries, Pneumocystis jiroveci pneumonia (PJP).

PJP's clinical manifestation begins with a gradual onset of symptoms that include a fever, cough, and dyspnea that usually progresses over days to weeks. Patients on average begin to have pulmonary symptoms at 3 weeks and will often note fatigue with exertional activities (i.e., climbing stairs, shaving, etc.). Less occurring symptoms include chills, chest pain, and weight loss. About 5–10% of patients will exhibit no symptoms. Physical exam findings will show crackles and rhonchi on auscultation 50% of the time while normal chest examinations will occur in the other 50% of cases. Patients will often have oral thrush on oropharyngeal examination. Laboratory findings will include CD4+ counts decreased below 200 cells/microL, hypoxia, elevated lactate dehydrogenase levels (average 362 IU), lowered diffusion capacity, and elevated 1, 3-beta-D-glucan levels. Chest x-ray will demonstrate diffuse, bilateral, interstitial or alveolar infiltrates. Associated chest x-ray findings of PJP could also show a pneumothorax. High-resolution computed tomography offers a high sensitivity and specificity for diagnosis of possible PJP with the presence of patchy/nodular ground-glass attenuation. Definitive diagnosis of PJP is ultimately done with the appearance of cystic or trophic forms of the organism from either a sputum sample, bronchoalveolar lavage, or tissue biopsy.

Learning Objective 5: Describe the diagnostic tests used for HIV (focus on fourth generation) and its utilization for disease progression, response to therapy, and immune status.

There are multiple different diagnostic tests available to confirm if a patient is infected with HIV, but the CDC has created an algorithm for testing for diagnosis/screening upon high suspicion for HIV infection [9, 10]. Routine screening is recommended at least one time in patients aged 13–75 who do not have risk factors. Individuals who are injection drug users, men who have sex with men, sex-traffic workers, sex partners to HIV-infected individuals, bisexual individuals, or IV drug users; or patients who have sex with HIV unknown people should be screened at least annually for HIV. The purpose and importance to screening is that early course diagnosis of HIV with successful treatment of antivirals can lead to patients having life expectancies similar to that of the general population, but a late diagnosis can lead to a 33% chance of developing AIDS within 1 year of initial HIV diagnosis [11].

The available tests that diagnose HIV can be separated into categories of screening and confirmatory tests. ELISAs that detect HIV antibodies are used as the initial screening test and are referred to as third-generation antibody tests that detect IgM and IgG antibodies to HIV-1 and HIV-2 as early as 3 weeks after virus exposure, but cannot discern between the two. There are various ELISA tests available with some that are laboratory-based that require greater than 3 h of time while some are rapid and can be done in less than 20 min. The longer the test, the higher the sensitivity and specificity, which approach 100% for chronic HIV infections, but are less sensitive than the combination antigen/antibody test (fourth-generation). The combination antigen/antibody test (fourth generation) defers from its predecessor in that it is able to detect both HIV antibody and HIV p24 antigen as well as group

M and O infections. The sensitivity and specificity of fourth-generation tests approach 100% and are said to identify acute HIV infection in 80% of patients whose HIV diagnosis was missed by the third generation test. Examples of fourth-generation combination tests include the ARCHITECT HIV Ag/Ab combo test and the determine HIV 1/2 Ag/AB combo which produce rapid results within 30 min.

The preferred confirmatory test is with the HIV-1/HIV-2 differentiation immunoassay, which generally takes <20 min to confirm the fourth-generation screening test and distinguish between a HIV-1 or HIV-2 infection. The available differentiation immunoassays on the market include Bio-Rad Geenius HIV1/2 confirmation assay or the Bio-Rad Multispot HIV-1/HIV-2 (99.3–100% sensitivity for both). Before the immunoassay, Western blots would be done after an initial positive ELISA, but the disadvantage to such a test is the long turnaround, which required several days to 2 weeks to return with a result.

An alternative approach includes the viral detection, which can be done with a viral load test and can be used to establish an HIV diagnosis. The use of viral detection over diagnostic assay is indicated for neonatal HIV infection, patients with indeterminate serologic testing, a patient in the "window period" of HIV seroconversion, or screening blood donors. Plasma HIV RNA can be done qualitatively or quantitatively, with the quantitative measurements being used clinically to monitor the management of HIV-1 infected individuals on antiretrovirals. The plasma HIV-1 RNA viral load is often the first indicator to see if a patient is responding or resistant to initial antiretrovirals used. Disease progression and immune status are done with a CD4+ count, which indicates the need for prophylactic medication and the urgency to initiate antivirals (more in Learning Objective #3). Typical CD4+ counts range from 500 to 1500 cells/mm^3 with AIDS being diagnosed with a CD4+ count below 200 cells/mm^3. In patients who remain untreated for whatever reason, CD4 counts should be monitored every 3–6 months to assess the urgency of antiretroviral initiation and the need for opportunistic infection prophylaxis.

Learning Objective 6: Describe the pharmacologic treatment available to treat HIV and list their mechanism of actions and associated toxicities. Comment on the treatment of Pneumocystis jiroveci pneumonia.

As described in Learning Objective #1, HIV infection has multiple steps that can be targeted by antiretroviral medications. A schematic description of the mechanism of the four classes of currently available antiviral drugs against HIV is shown in Fig. 26.4. Most often an HIV-infected naïve treatment patient will begin a drug regimen that includes 2 nucleoside reverse transcriptase inhibitors and an integrase inhibitor or three nucleoside reverse transcriptase inhibitors. A summary of the available treatment from 6 major classes is given below with the most common side effects. All newly diagnosed HIV-infected individuals should undergo drug resistance testing through genotyping to further narrow down options for antiretrovirals. In certain studies, individuals with a newly diagnosed early HIV infection, 15–20% of them harbored viral isolates that were resistance to at least one drug. Genotyping is preferred over phenotyping due to the associated costs and time comparisons.

Class: Nucleoside reverse transcriptase inhibitors

Example drugs: Zidovudine, Lamivudine, Emtricitabine, Abacavir, Satvudine, Didanosine

Mechanism of Action: Acts as a nucleoside analog that competitively inhibits reverse transcription of RNA to DNA by preventing the formation of 3′ to 5′ phosphodiester linkages.

Toxicities: Bone marrow suppression, myopathy, neuropathy, HIV-associated lipodystrophy (abnormal distribution of fat)

Class: Non-nucleoside reverse transcriptase inhibitors

Example drugs: Nevirapine, Efavirenz

Mechanism of Action: non-competitive inhibitors of viral reverse transcriptase

Toxicities: Hepatotoxicity, CNS toxicity, associated with Stevens-Johnson syndrome

Class: Nucleotide analogs

Example drugs: Tenofovir

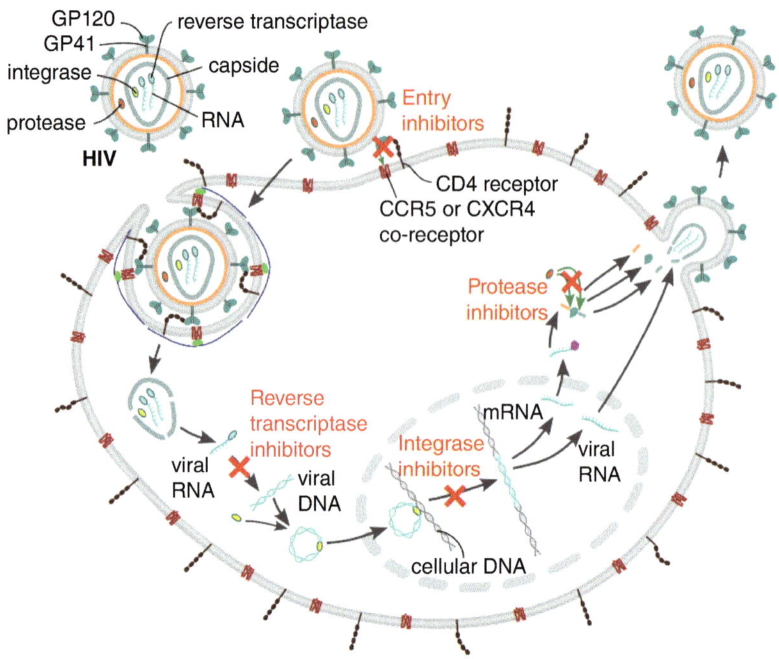

Fig. 26.4 Antiretrovirals and their mechanism of action. Fusion inhibitors (interfere with the binding, fusion or entry of an HIV virion0, reverse-transcriptase inhibitors (interfere with the translation of viral RNA to DNA), integrase inhibitors (block the viral enzyme integrase, that inserts the viral genome into the DNA of the host cell), and protease inhibitors (block proteolytic cleavage of protein precursors that are necessary for the production of infections viral particles). Thomas Splettstoesser (www.scistyle.com), CC BY 3.0 https://creativecommons.org/licenses/by/3.0, via Wikimedia Commons (https://upload.wikimedia.org/wikipedia/commons/d/d5/HIV-drug-classes.svg)

Mechanism of Action: Acts as a nucleotide analog that competitively inhibits reverse transcription of RNA to DNA

Toxicities: Nephrotoxicity

Class: Integrase inhibitors

Example drugs: Raltegravir, Dolutegravir

Mechanism of Action: Inhibits viral integrase

Toxicities: Hepatotoxicity, hypersensitivity reactions

Class: Fusion inhibitor

Example drugs: Enfuviritide

Mechanism of Action: Competitively binds to the viral protein gp41 and prevents fusion of HIV virus into the cell

Toxicities: Skin hypersensitivity reactions

Class: Protease inhibitors

Example drugs: Indinavir, Ritonavir, Nelfinavir, Lopinavir

Mechanism of Action: Inhibits viral protease causing the virus to be unable to cleave viral polypeptides leading to only immature/non-infectious virions to be produced

Toxicities: Lipodystrophy, nephrolithiasis, hyperglycemia, and insulin resistance

Class: CCR5-antagonist

Example drugs: Maraviroc

Mechanism of Action: blocks the CCR5 coreceptor needed for certain HIV genotypes for HIV infection into cells

Toxicities: GI intolerance

For PJP, the preferred treatment regimen includes trimethoprim-sulfamethoxazole (Bactrim) for 21 days with a standard dose of 15–20 mg/kg/day orally or intravenously three to four times a day [3]. Bactrim is also used for prophylaxis of PJP when CD4+ counts are <200 cells/mm^3. Alternatives to patients who hold contraindications to bactrim may use trimethoprim-dapsone, clindamycin-primaquine, atovaquone, or pentamidine. Corticosteroid treatment with oral prednisone has shown reduced risks for respiratory failure.

Learning Objective 7: Explain the role physicians play in HIV prevention when patients are newly diagnosed HIV-positive in the constraints of existing state laws and in the American Medical Association Code of Medical Ethics guidelines.

Physicians initially have a clinical approach to HIV prevention that includes biomedical interventions and behavioral interventions. The HIV epidemic is a multifaceted issue with a large magnitude that must be tackled in multiple interventions that are patient-specific.

Biomedical interventions include the initiation and maintenance of antiretroviral therapy, pre-and post-exposure prophylaxis, and voluntary medical circumcision for uninfected heterosexual males. Antiretroviral therapy suppresses the viral load in plasma, which ultimately minimizes the risk of transmission sexually and perinatally. In the United States, antiretroviral therapy is recommended for all patients infected with HIV regardless of CD4+ count due to the benefit of lowered morbidity and mortality from AIDS and non-AIDS associated conditions. Thus, treatment success can be done with improved adherence to medication, which can be done by lowering pill burden, flexible dosing frequencies, and frequent counseling and encouragement by providers.

Behavioral interventions include counseling on condom use and routine risk reduction assessments for injection drug users and screens for sexually transmitted infections (STIs). Condom use has been shown to reduce the risk of sexual transmission, but has shown to be no longer essential if patients have the virus completely repressed with the use of antiretrovirals. Injection drug users should be given addiction treatment (i.e., buprenorphine-naltrexone for opioid users) to decrease the use of injection needles [12]. Ongoing sexual partners should be placed on pre-exposure prophylaxis for the uninfected partner to prevent transmission.

According to the American Medical Association Code of Medical Ethics, the recommended guidelines are posted below:

To protect the welfare and interests of individual patients and fulfill their public health obligations in the context of HIV, physicians should:

(a) Support routine, universal screening of adult patients for HIV with opt-out provisions.
(b) Make efforts to persuade reluctant patients to be screened, including explaining potential benefits to the patient and to the patient's close contacts.
(c) Continue to uphold respect for autonomy by respecting a patient's informed decision to opt out.
(d) Test patients without prior consent only in limited cases in which the harms to individual autonomy are offset by significant benefits to known third parties, such as testing to protect occupationally exposed health-care professionals or patients.
(e) Work to ensure that patients who are identified as HIV-positive receive appropriate follow-up care and counseling.
(f) Attempt to persuade patients who are identified as HIV-positive to cease endangering others.
(g) Be aware of and adhere to state and local guidelines regarding public health reporting and disclosure of HIV status when a patient who is identified as HIV-positive poses significant risk of infecting an identifiable third party [13]. The doctor may, if permitted, notify the endangered third party without revealing the identity of the source person.
(h) Safeguard the confidentiality of patient information to the greatest extent possible when required to report HIV status.

Exam Questions

1. A 27-year-old man presents to the emergency department with progressive dyspnea on exertion, dry cough, fatigue, intermittent fevers, and chills for the past 4 weeks. The patient does not use tobacco or illicit drugs, but occasionally drinks alcohol. He is allergic to

sulfur-containing drugs. His sexual history includes a monogamous relationship with a male partner for the past 2 years, but he has previously had multiple partners. Temperature is 38.2 C (100.8 F), blood pressure is 138/82 mmHg, pulse is 93/min, and respirations are 28/min with a pulse oximetry of 89% on room air. Oropharyngeal exam is significant for scattered white plaques and lung auscultation reveals bilateral diffuse crackles. Chest CT-Thorax shows ground glass opacities. Which of the following treatment regimens will be most effective for this patient's pulmonary condition?

A. Ceftriaxone and Azithromycin
B. Rifampin, Isoniazid, Pyrazinamide, and Ethambutol
C. Amphotericin B
D. Trimethoprim-sulfamethoxazole and Prednisone
E. Pentamidine.

Answer: E

Key Learning Objectives: LO#4 and LO#6

Explanation: The correct answer choice is E. Pentamidine, which is the second line treatment for Pneumocystis jiroveci pneumonia (PJP) in individuals who have a sulfa-allergy or other contraindication to sulfur-containing drugs.

A is not the correct answer choice as it is the normal treatment for community-acquired pneumonia, but the question stem includes key features of a most-likely chronic HIV (i.e., men who have sex with men, oral thrush) as well as a confirmed diagnosis of PJP with ground-glass opacities seen bilaterally on CT-Thorax.

B is the treatment choice of primary and active tuberculosis, in which is less likely without symptoms of hemoptysis, night sweats, weight loss, and history of recent travel into endemic regions.

C is the treatment for coccidiomycosis, which is less likely due to the explanation seen in A.

D is the first-line treatment of PJP, but the question stem notes that the patient has an allergy to sulfur-containing drugs, which would not be the most effective treatment compared to answer E, Pentamidine.

2. A 40-year-old pet shop employee with a past medical history significant for cervical cancer presents to emergency room with onset of fever, focal seizures without post-ictal states, and visual changes. Temperature is 38.3 C (101 F), blood pressure is 127/73 mmHg, pulse is 97/min, and respirations are 18/min with a pulse oximetry of 97% on room air. Head CT shows a single ring-enhancing lesion. Patient receives the appropriate initial medical treatment for the neuropathology consistent with his CT and clinical presentation. Which of the following prophylactic medication should also be initiated for this patient?

A. Trimethoprim-sulfamethoxazole only
B. Azithromycin and Clindamycin
C. Trimethoprim-sulfamethoxazole and Clindamycin
D. Trimethoprim-sulfamethoxazole and Azithromycin
E. Trimethoprim-sulfamethoxazole, Azithromycin, and Nitazoxanide

Answer: E

Learning Objective: LO#3 and LO#5

Explanation: The correct answer choice is E. Trimethoprim-sulfamethoxazole, Azithromycin, and Nitazoxanide. The patient is presented with a single-ring enhancing lesion on Head CT, which is consistent with Toxoplasma gondii rather than CMV, which appears as a double-ring enhancing lesion on Head CT. Because the ptatient has Toxoplasma gondii, their CD4+ count can be assumed to be <100 mm^3 since Toxoplasma gondii presents clinically in a majority of cases below this threshold. With CD4 + counts below <100 mm^3 patients will need prophylactic treatment for the following opportunistic infections: Pneumocystis jiroveci and Toxoplasma gondii (Trimethoprim-sulfamethoxazole), Mycobacterium avium-intracellulare (Azithromycin), and Cryptosporidium parvum (Nitazoxanide).

3. Which of the following matches of the genes responsible for HIV infection, viral protein, and treatment medications are correct?

Answer Choice	Specific Gene	Viral Protein	Treatment
A	Gap	Gp41	Enfurviritide
B	Pol	Gp120	Maraviroc
C	Env	Integrase	Raltegravir
D	Pol	Protease	Saquinavir
E	Env	Reverse transcriptase	Tenofovir

Answer: D

Learning Objective: LO#1 and LO#6

Explanation: Of the answers choices, only answer choice D is correct.

The env gene produces gp120 and gp41, which are responsible for the attachment and fusion of HIV into immune cells, which are targeted by fusion/entry inhibitors (i.e., enfuvirtide or maraviroc).

The gag gene leads to the production of p24 and p17 used in the viral capsid and viral matrix formation of HIV, which are not targeted by FDA approved HIV medication.

The pol gene produces the proteins reverse transcriptase, protease, and integrase which are targeted by nucleoside reverse transcriptase inhibitors (i.e., zidovudine, tenofovir, etc.), protease inhibitors (i.e., saquinavir, indinavir, etc.), and integrase inhibitors (i.e., raltegravir), respectively.

References

1. Kales CP, et al. Early predictors of in-hospital mortality for Pneumocystis carinii pneumonia in the acquired immunodeficiency syndrome. Arch Intern Med. 1987;147(8):1413–7.
2. Wilkin A, Feinberg J. Pneumocystis carinii pneumonia: a clinical review. Am Fam Physician. 1999;60(6):1699–708.
3. Benson CA. et al. Guidelines for prevention and treatment opportunistic infections in HIV-infected adults and adolescents; recommendations from CDC, the National Institutes of Health, and the HIV Medicine Association/Infectious Diseases Society of America; 2009.
4. Leoung GS. Comprehensive, up-to-date information on HIV/AIDS treatment and prevention from the University of California san Francisco. Pneumocystosis and HIV, University of California San Francisco; 2005. hivinsite.ucsf.edu/InSite?page=kb-05-02-01#S2.2.1X.
5. Silverberg MJ, Lau B, Achenbach CJ, et al. Cumulative incidence of cancer among persons with HIV in North America: a cohort study. Ann Intern Med. 2015;163(7):507–18.
6. Yarchoan R, Uldrick TS. HIV-associated cancers and related diseases. N Engl J Med. 2018;378(11):1029–41.
7. Cohen MS, et al. Acute HIV-1 infection. N Engl J Med. 2011;364(20):1943–54.
8. Wood BR, Spach DH. Acute and recent HIV Infectio. National HIV Curriculum. 2019, www.hiv.uw.edu/go/screening-diagnosis/acute-recent-early-hiv/core-concept/all#citations.
9. Center for Substance Abuse Treatment. Centers for Disease Control and Prevention. FDA-approved HIV screening tests for laboratory use only. http://www.cdc.gov/hiv/pdf/testing/hiv-tests-laboratory-use.pdf. Accessed 28 Aug 2019.
10. Routine Universal Screening for HIV. American Medical Association. https://www.ama-assn.org/delivering-care/ethics/routine-universal-screening-hiv.
11. Marcus JL, et al. Narrowing the gap in life expectancy between HIV-infected and HIV-uninfected individuals with access to care. J Acquir Immune Defic Syndr. 2016;73(1):39.
12. Treatment Improvement Protocol (TIP) Series, No. 37.
13. HIV Criminalization in the United States: A Sourcebook of State and Federal HIV Criminal Law and Practice. https://www.hivlawandpolicy.org/sites/default/files/Arizona%20-%20Excerpt%20from%20CHLP%27s%20Sourcebook%20on%20HIV%20Criminalization%20in%20the%20U.S.pdf. Accessed 29 Aug 2019.

27 Fatigued and Confused

Patrick Sarette

Learning Objectives

1. Describe the normal physiology of the cardiac membrane and how hyperkalemia alters cardiac myocyte function.
2. Review basic renal physiology at the unit of the nephron to explain how common comorbid conditions and medications increased his risk of hyperkalemia.
3. Identify common underlying etiologies that may lead to hyperkalemia (as a framework, consider that elevated serum K+ must either be due to release from the intracellular space, due to impaired excretion (physiologic or medication-mediated), or due to excessive intake).
4. Analyze the progression of ECG findings typically seen in acute hyperkalemia (please provide examples). Correlate changes seen on ECG with cardiac physiology.
5. Describe the medical interventions used in the emergent treatment of hyperkalemia and the rationale behind these interventions.
6. Describe additional pharmacologic interventions that may be used to lower serum potassium in non-emergent treatment.

Setting: Community emergency department.

P. Sarette (✉)
The University of Arizona College of Medicine-Phoenix, Phoenix, AZ, USA
e-mail: pasare@iu.edu

Patient: Mr. James Markovich is a 52-year-old white male presenting to the Emergency Department, accompanied by his wife. They arrive via personal vehicle.

Chief complaint: "I've been really tired and weak lately. Yesterday, I started vomiting, and today, I fell down!"

Stop and Think Based on this chief complaint, generate a broad differential.

Table 27.1 provides a breakdown of various differential diagnoses to consider based on organ system.

Table 27.1 Differential diagnosis by system using VINDICATES

Vascular	Anemia, cardiac dysrhythmia, acute coronary syndrome,
Infectious	Viral syndrome, sepsis
Neoplastic	Cancer
Drug	Sedating medications, alcohol, withdrawal syndromes, organophosphate toxicity
Inflammatory/ idiopathic	Cyclic vomiting syndrome, chronic obstructive pulmonary disease
Congenital	–
Autoimmune	Multiple sclerosis
Trauma	Post-concussive syndrome
Endocrine/ metabolic	Hypothyroidism, hypoglycemia, new-onset diabetic ketoacidosis, electrolyte abnormality, pancreatitis, adrenal insufficiency
PSychiatric	Insomnia

C. A. Standley (ed.), *Biomedical Science and Clinical Foundations*,
https://doi.org/10.1007/978-3-031-98353-5_27

History of Presenting Illness Over the last 2 days, the patient reports progressively worsening fatigue and generalized weakness. Yesterday, he began to experience nausea and non-bloody, non-bilious emesis. Today, he was walking to the kitchen when he began to experience muscle cramping in the bilateral calves and fell. He did not strike his head or lose consciousness. He remembers the entire incident.

ROS

(+) generalized malaise, weakness, nausea, vomiting, muscle cramping, oliguria

(−) fevers, chills, unexplained weight loss, headache, head trauma, chest pain, dyspnea, cough, wheezing, abdominal pain, diarrhea, hematemesis, seizures.

Unless otherwise stated above, other relevant systems are also negative.

Past Medical History: "I have high blood pressure. It's been hard to control, they keep putting me on new medications. I know my doctor is going to get on me about it, so I've started taking a few extra of the pills when my pressure is running high"

Medications: amlodipine 10 mg in the morning, lisinopril 10 mg in the morning, spironolactone 50 mg at night

Allergies: Penicillin (reaction: hives)

Family History: Mr. Markovich was adopted shortly after birth. His family history is unknown.

Social History: Tobacco use: current 1 pack/day for 25 years. Alcohol use: 2 glasses of wine/week. Substance use: marijuana in early 20's, none currently. Medically retired from the military. Sedentary lifestyle at home.

Stop and Think How does the patient history change your differential?

This is a good time to go back to Table 27.1 and revise the proposed differentials based on this new information about the patient. A revised differential list is provided in Table 27.2.

Table 27.2 Revised differential diagnosis by system using VINDICATES

Vascular	~~Anemia~~ (less likely given acute onset and no obvious bleeding), cardiac dysrhythmia, acute coronary syndrome,
Infectious	Viral syndrome, sepsis
Neoplastic	Cancer
Drug	~~Sedating medications~~ (less likely given medication list), ~~alcohol withdrawal syndromes~~ (less likely given occasional alcohol use and no other substance use), ~~organophosphate toxidrome~~ (less likely given no reported exposure, spouse not ill)
Inflammatory/ idiopathic	~~Cyclic vomiting syndrome~~ (acute, first time onset), ~~chronic obstructive pulmonary disease~~ (no prior history, no respiratory symptoms, would be unusual to present with vomiting)
Congenital	–
Autoimmune	~~Multiple sclerosis~~ (would be unusual to have vomiting and oliguria)
Trauma	~~Post-concussive syndrome~~ (no history of head trauma)
Endocrine/ metabolic	Hypothyroidism, hypoglycemia, new-onset diabetic ketoacidosis, electrolyte abnormality, pancreatitis, adrenal insufficiency
PSychiatric	~~Insomnia~~ (would not cause vomiting, oliguria)

Vital Signs

BP: 160/85
HR: 92
RR: 18
Temperature: 37.2 C (98.9 F)
SpO2: 98% on room air
BMI: 27.4 kg/m^2

Physical Exam

General: Well-developed, well-nourished white male, alert and conversant, in no acute distress. Significant other at bedside. Uncomfortable-appearing. Emesis bag with non-bloody, non-bilious emesis.

HEENT: Normocephalic, atraumatic. PERRL—4 mm bilat. Bilateral canals clear without cerumen. Nasal septum midline. Oral mucous membranes dry, uvula midline. Trachea midline. No JVD. Freely ranging neck without meningismus.

Cardiac: Regular rate, regular rhythm.

Respiratory: Lungs clear to auscultation bilaterally. Normal work of breathing without conversational dyspnea.

Abdomen: Soft, non-tender, non-distended. Bowel sounds are present in all four quadrants. Non-peritonitic. Emesis bag with non-bloody, non-bilious emesis.

Musculoskeletal: When attempting to ambulate, patient has an unsteady gait, citing cramping in the bilateral calves and thighs.

Neurologic: GCS 15. CN II–XII bilaterally intact. Sensation intact to light touch in upper extremity and lower extremity dermatomes. 4/5 strength in bilateral deltoids, biceps, triceps, grip, hip and knee flexors/extensors, and foot dorsi/plantar flexion. Bicipital and patellar tendon reflexes 3+ bilaterally. Downgoing toes bilaterally on plantar stimulation.

Integumentary: Warm and dry. No suspicious lesions or rashes.

Psychiatric: Mood and behavior are appropriate to context.

Stop and Think How does the physical exam change your differential? With consideration of your current differential, what labs, imaging, and other objective data would you like to order?

Glucose, EKG (Fig. 27.1), CBC (Table 27.3), CMP (Table 27.4), Lipase (Table 27.5), Thyroid profile (Table 27.6), Chest X Ray.

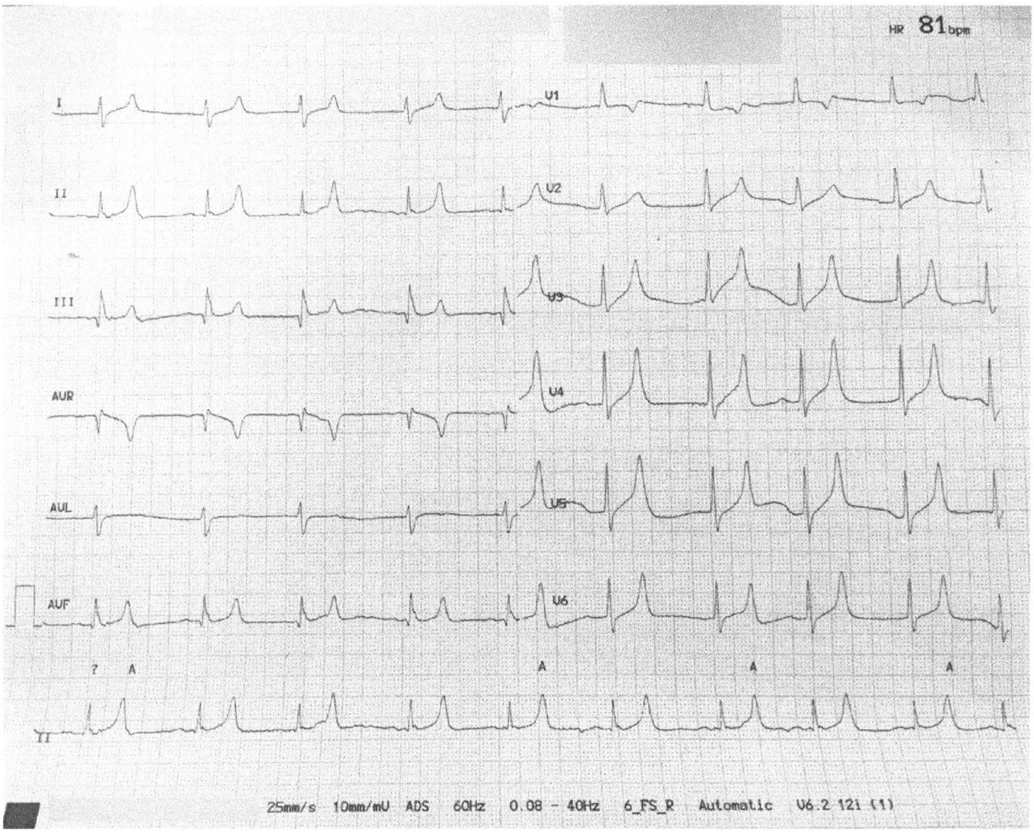

Fig. 27.1 The patient's electrocardiogram. Dr. Michael-Joseph F. Agbayani and Dr. Eddieson Gonzales (Manila, Philippines), CC BY 4.0 https://creativecommons.org/licenses/by/4.0, via Wikimedia Commons. (https://upload.wikimedia.org/wikipedia/commons/6/67/Hyperkalemia_ECG.jpg)

Table 27.3 Complete blood count (CBC)

Component	Patient	Reference
WBC	9.6	3.5–10.5 K/CUMM
RBC	4.8	3.7–5.2 million/CUMM
Hemoglobin	11.2	12.0–15.0 g/dL
Hematocrit	36.2	35.0–49%
Platelets	401	150 K/CUMM
MCV	95	81–99 fL
MCH	31	27.0–34.0 pg
MCHC	34	32.0–36.0 g/dL
RDW	14	11.5–14.5%
MPV	9.1	7.0–12.0 fL

Table 27.4 Complete Metabolic Panel (CMP)

Component	Patient	Reference
Sodium	132	135–145 mmol/L
Potassium	8.9 (no hemolysis noted)	3.5–5.5 mmol/L
Chloride	94	95–105 mmol/L
CO2	29	22–29 mmol/L
BUN	34	7–21 mg/dL
Cr	3.22	0.6–1.2 mg/dL
Glucose	174	70–99 mg/dL (fasting)
Calcium	9.0	8.5–10.5 mg/dL
Protein	7.2	6.2–7.8 g/dL
Albumin	6.2	3.5–5.0 g/dL
Total bilirubin		<1.0 mg/dL
Alkaline phosphatase	113	20–125 U/L
AST	23	13–40 U/L
ALT	21	7–50 U/L

Table 27.5 Lipase

Component	Patient	Reference
Lipase	44	12–50 units/L

Table 27.6 Thyroid profile

Component	Patient	Reference
TSH	3.218	0.27–4.2 uIU/mL
FT4	1.06	0.9–2.3 ng/dL

Point of care glucose (fingerstick): 172 mg/dL.

Electrocardiogram

Chest X-Ray

Impression: "Possible mild pulmonary vascular congestion, otherwise normal chest radiograph."

Critical Actions, Disposition, and Case Resolution

Final diagnosis: hyperkalemia, likely from acute kidney injury and overuse of potassium-sparing diuretics (spironolactone).

Critical illness: Patient is at risk of fatal cardiac dysrhythmias, as evidenced by electrocardiographic changes on ECG.

Medical Optimization: The patient should be placed on cardiac telemetry to monitor for life-threatening dysrhythmias. He will also need calcium to stabilize the cardiac membrane (3 g calcium gluconate or 1 g calcium chloride). Medical temporizing measures, such as insulin (5 U insulin lispro given intravenously with 25 g of D10W solution), as well as 20 mg of nebulized albuterol and 10 g of sodium zirconium cyclosilicate (Lokelma). Repeat ECGs should be obtained at regular intervals to monitor treatment effect.

Consultants: The patient will require a STAT nephrology consult for consideration of emergent hemodialysis to safely and definitively remove extracellular potassium.

Disposition and Case Resolution: The on-call nephrologist agrees to see the patient and initiate emergent hemodialysis. They kindly request that you order 10 mg sodium zirconium cyclosilicate every 8 h and 40 mg intravenous furosemide in the meantime. You call the intensive care unit (ICU) team, and they agree to admit the patient to the ICU for further care, dialysis co-management, and continuous cardiac monitoring.

End of Case

Learning Objective Answers

1. **Describe the normal physiology of the cardiac membrane and how hyperkalemia alters cardiac myocyte function.**

The cardiac myocyte membrane maintains a resting membrane potential of approximately −80 to −90 mV, primarily due to the high permeability of potassium through inward rectifier potassium channels [1, 2]. The Na^+/K^+ ATPase pump actively maintains the electrochemical gradient by extruding 3 Na^+ ions and importing 2 K^+ ions, which helps stabilize the resting potential. During an action potential, the following key phases occur:

1. Phase 0 (Depolarization): Rapid Na^+ influx through voltage-gated sodium channels causes a sharp rise in membrane potential.
2. Phase 1 (Early Repolarization): Transient outward K^+ channels allow brief K^+ efflux.
3. Phase 2 (Plateau Phase): L-type Ca^{2+} channels allow calcium influx, balancing K^+ efflux through delayed rectifier K^+ channels.
4. Phase 3 (Repolarization): Delayed rectifier K^+ channels restore negativity.
5. Phase 4 (Resting Potential): The inward rectifier K^+ current maintains stability until the next stimulus.

Hyperkalemia, defined as an elevated extracellular potassium level (>5.0 mEq/L), disrupts the cardiac electrophysiology of the normal action potential [3]. Firstly, increased extracellular potassium reduces the electrochemical gradient at rest, thus depolarizing the resting membrane potential. This inactivates voltage-gated Na + channels, decreasing the amplitude of depolarization, and slows conduction velocity. Additionally, the high extracellular potassium concentration increases outward potassium conductance, shortening the action potential duration. This can lead to peaked T-waves on ECG due to rapid repolarization [4]. Severe hyperkalemia can cause sinus arrest, AV block, or even ventricular fibrillation due to failure of impulse generation and propagation.

2. **Review basic renal physiology at the unit of the nephron to explain how common comorbid conditions and medications increased his risk of hyperkalemia.**

The nephron is the functional unit of the kidney, responsible for maintaining potassium homeostasis primarily through filtration, reabsorption, and secretion [5]. The nephron begins with the glomerulus, which filters plasma, allowing free movement of potassium into Bowman's space. Approximately 90% of filtered potassium is reabsorbed in the proximal tubule (67%) and loop of Henle (25%). In the distal tubule and collecting ducts, principal cells regulate potassium excretion under the control of aldosterone, which increases Na^+ reabsorption via ENaC (epithelial sodium channels) and enhances K^+ secretion through renal outer medullary K^+ (ROMK) channels. A second cell type, the intercalated cells, can reabsorb K^+ during hypokalemia.

Comorbid conditions, such as chronic kidney disease, associated with reduced nephron mass, can impair potassium secretion, increasing hyperkalemia risk [6]. Additionally, reduced GFR in this condition decreases potassium filtration and thus potassium excretion, leading to hyperkalemia. In heart failure and liver disease, treatment with renin-angiotensin-aldosterone inhibitors reduces aldosterone, impairing potassium excretion. In diabetes, diabetic nephropathy reduces renal function, and insulin deficiency reduces intracellular potassium uptake, increasing serum potassium.

Medications that increase risk of hyperkalemia include:

- ACE inhibitors: decrease aldosterone and reduce potassium excretion
- Aldosterone antagonists: directly block aldosterone and decrease potassium secretion
- NSAIDs: reduce renal perfusion, decrease GFR, and decrease potassium excretion
- Beta blockers: reduce cellular potassium uptake by inhibiting Na+/K+ ATPase
- Potassium-sparing diuretics: Block ENaC, reducing potassium excretion

3. **Identify common underlying etiologies that may lead to hyperkalemia (as a framework, consider that elevated serum K+ must either be due to release from the intracellular space, due to impaired excretion (physiologic or medication-mediated), or due to excessive intake.**

In reality, most critically ill patients presenting with hyperkalemia have a multifaceted underlying etiology. However, causes of hyperkalemia can largely be broken down into three categories:

1. Excess intake of potassium
2. Shift of existing potassium from the intracellular space to the extracellular space
3. Impaired excretion/elimination of potassium

Excess Intake of Potassium

Approximately 90% of oral potassium is absorbed through the GI tract over the time frame of hours [7]. However, due to the relatively low amounts of potassium in food items, combined with the longer absorption time, development of sustained or life-threatening hyperkalemia from dietary intake alone is not common. For example, a banana contains approximately 12 mEq of potassium. With 90% oral availability, this would equate to 10.8 mEq absorbed over the course of several hours. In clinical practice, it is often estimated that every 10 mEq of potassium given will raise serum levels by 0.1 mEq/L. In patients with normal renal function, kaliuresis will compensate for potassium intake to maintain potassium homeostasis. However, other sources of potassium intake, to include intravenous repletion (e.g., potassium chloride) or total parenteral nutrition (TPN), may rapidly raise serum levels if not carefully monitored [8]. For this reason, potassium repletion via the intravenous route often occurs at a rate of 10 mEq/hr or less, and in patients receiving TPN, electrolyte levels are trended and TPN electrolyte content is reviewed daily.

Potassium Shifts Between the Intracellular and Extracellular Spaces

There are certain pathologies and medications which can alter the balance of potassium across the cellular membrane between the intracellular and extracellular compartments. For example, patients who present in diabetic ketoacidosis can have high-normal or even critically elevated serum potassium levels. This is because of the underlying insulin deficiency that is a driving factor in the pathology. Along with modulating cellular uptake of glucose, insulin also shifts potassium into cells by upregulating activity of sodium-potassium ATPase channels. When there is a global deficiency of insulin, there can be less sodium-potassium ATPase-mediated potassium uptake into cells, leading to accumulation in the serum (even though due to other aspects of DKA pathophysiology, there may actually be a total-body potassium deficit).

Another pathology which can lead to large amounts of extracellular potassium is tumor lysis syndrome. This is an oncologic emergency that can occur in patients with a large burden of rapidly dividing tumor cells, such as the case of leukemia or lymphoma. When medical treatment (e.g., radiation, chemotherapy, or immunologic therapy) is initiated, a large number of tumor cells may die at once, lysing open and releasing their contents into the plasma. Electrolyte derangements such as hyperuricemia, hyperphosphatemia, and hyperkalemia may occur. Along similar lines, as myocytes store a large percentage of total-body potassium, rhabdomyolysis due to any cause (e.g., trauma, overexertion, excessive sympathomimetic stimulation) may lead to similar electrolyte derangements, to include hyperkalemia, as seen in tumor lysis syndrome.

Pseudohyperkalemia is a phenomenon that can cause artificially elevated potassium values. It is mechanistically similar to tumor lysis syndrome or rhabdomyolysis in that the derangement is caused by hemolysis and subsequent spilling of intracellular potassium into the serum, but it occurs during or after phlebotomy and specimen collection. Patient fist-clenching, too tight of a phlebotomy tourniquet, mechanical lysis through the blood collecting system, or smaller intravenous catheters can cause the blood collected to become hemolyzed (without reflecting broader systemic hemolysis) and thereby elevate collected serum potassium levels. Often, the laboratory will report the degree of hemolysis, if any, with a collected sample to allow the clinician to better interpret value against the patient's overall clinical condition.

Finally, medications that act on the sodium-potassium ATPase may also alter serum potassium. Digoxin, a cardiac aminoglycoside used in the management of refractory arrhythmias, is a sodium-potassium ATPase poison. As a result, there is decreased pumping of potassium from the extracellular space to the intracellular space. Hyperkalemia is a hallmark electrolyte derangement of digoxin toxicity.

Impaired Potassium Excretion

The kidney is responsible for approximately 90% of potassium excretion, with the remaining 10% being excreted in stool or in sweat. Specifically within the nephron, potassium excretion occurs at the distal collecting tubule. As such, any insult to renal function and specifically the distal collecting system can threaten potassium homeostasis.

Patients with chronic kidney disease, especially those with end-stage renal disease requiring dialysis, are at higher risk of developing hyperkalemia because of decreased baseline renal dysfunction. In patients with end-stage renal disease who have progressed to the point of being anuric, any missed or shortened runs of dialysis should raise concern for hyperkalemia because these patients have no other means of potassium excretion. Acute kidney injury can also predispose patients to hyperkalemia, depending on the underlying impact on renal function. Medications that specifically act at the distal collecting tubule, such as potassium-sparing diuretics, can also raise serum potassium.

4. **Analyze the progression of ECG findings typically seen in acute hyperkalemia (please provide examples). Correlate changes seen on ECG with cardiac physiology**

Cardiac effects of Hyperkalemia

Patients with hyperkalemia are often asymptomatic. They may present with palpitations, nausea, vomiting, muscle cramps, or paralysis. However, the feared effect of hyperkalemia is cardiac dysrhythmia. Increased serum potassium levels will increase the positivity of the extracellular space, thereby raising the resting membrane potential of cardiac myocytes. At first, the increase in the number of myocytes experiencing early depolarization will also lead to a larger amount of simultaneous repolarization. However, as the resting membrane potential becomes higher (less polarized as progressive hyperkalemia continues to contribute to an increase in extracellular positive charge), the number of available voltage-gated sodium channels in Phase 0 decreases, leading to a prolonged depolarization. This in turn leads to a prolonged action potential, further increase in the number of refractory voltage-gated sodium channels, and ultimately, myocyte paralysis.

Electrocardiogram Changes in the Hyperkalemic Patient

The physiologic changes occurring at the myocyte level that are described above created observable electrocardiographic changes in patients [4].

Tall, peaked T-waves. Often the earliest sign of hyperkalemia. Repolarization abnormality. Initially, hyperkalemia will lead to a higher resting potential, predisposing myocytes to earlier depolarization. Peaked T-waves as these many cardiac myocytes simultaneously undergo early repolarization.

P-wave flattening, PR interval prolongation. Progressive atrial paralysis as sodium channels become refractory to depolarization and the atrial myocytes become paralyzed.

Abnormal conduction. Similar to above, eventually conduction between the sinus node and the AV node slows, manifesting as heart block. This can manifest as widening of the QRS complex, new bundle-branch blocks, high-grade heart blocks, and junctional rhythms. Ultimately, the patient can progress to a "sine wave" rhythm, which should be considered a "peri-arrest" rhythm, pulseless electrical activity, asystole, or ventricular fibrillation.

5. **Describe the medical interventions used in the emergent treatment of hyperkalemia and the rationale behind these interventions**

Once the diagnosis of hyperkalemia is made, the clinician must act rapidly to initiate treatment [9]. Treatment can be simplified into three main aims:

1. Stabilize the myocardium
2. Shift the serum potassium intracellularly
3. Eliminate potassium from the body

Stabilization of the Cardiac Myocyte Membrane

Calcium salts, usually calcium gluconate or calcium chloride, are given intravenously to stabilize the cardiac membrane [10, 11]. The onset of action is rapid (on the level of a few minutes), though the duration of action is short (30–60 min), requiring re-dosing as needed. Calcium gluconate is usually given as 30 mL of a 10% calcium gluconate solution (3 g of calcium gluconate) or 10 mL of a 10% calcium chloride solution (1 g of calcium chloride). Calcium chloride should ideally be administered through central access (i.e., central venous catheter, peripherally inserted central catheter), if available, because it can be sclerotic to the vasculature whereas calcium gluconate can be readily administered through peripheral, intravenous line.

As above, hyperkalemia initially results in a higher (more positive) resting membrane potential, increasing the excitability of the cardiac myocyte. Sustained hyperkalemia and a higher resting membrane potential will lead to a decrease in activity of Phase 0 sodium channels required for depolarization, which ultimately decreases cardiac myocyte excitability. Though exact mechanisms are not definitively known, it is hypothesized that calcium acts in these two areas. In vitro research has demonstrated that in calcium solutions, the threshold potential is raised, whereas the resting membrane potential remains unchanged. In short, calcium is thought to reinstate the difference between resting and threshold potential to decrease initial myocyte hyperexcitability. Calcium has also been shown to upregulate the activity of Phase 0 sodium channels and thereby combat the eventually decreased cardiac myocyte activity seen in later phases of hyperkalemia.

Diuresis, in patients who still produce urine, can be an effective way to lower serum potassium. Loop diuretics, such as furosemide, are often first-line agents in attempts to encourage kaliuresis. They may be used in conjunction with thiazide diuretics, such as metolazone, for added diuretic effect. In patients with end-stage renal disease who are known to be anuric, diuretics are a futile effort. However, patients who are still producing urine (even in the setting of acute kidney injury) are usually given diuretics, as effective kaliuresis may negate the need for hemodialysis.

Hemodialysis, or another form of renal replacement therapy, is the most definitive and titratable means of treating hyperkalemia in critically ill patient. A nephrologist can predictably lower the patient's serum potassium over a defined amount of time. However, dialysis is invasive (requiring placement of a temporary hemodialysis catheter), time-consuming, and resource-intensive to initiate. With these limitations in mind, not every patient who presents with hyperkalemia will actually require hemodialysis. The oft-taught "AEIOU" mnemonic for dialysis indications still applies to the hyperkalemic patient; that is, severe **acidosis**, **electrolyte abnormality** (medically refractory hyperkalemia or patient with known end-stage renal disease on dialysis), **intoxication** (if underlying cause of renal failure is a dialyzable toxin), volume **overload** (refractory to diuresis), and life-threatening

uremia. Nevertheless, a nephrologist should be consulted early in the diagnosis of hyperkalemia to guide management (medical or otherwise) and, if necessary, to begin the process of initiating hemodialysis.

6. **Describe additional pharmacologic interventions that may be used to lower serum potassium in non-emergent treatment.**

Shift Serum potassium Intracellularly

Some literature suggests that at physiologic baseline, 98% of total-body potassium is stored intracellularly, with only 2% existing in the extracellular space. In the hyperkalemic patient, there are several temporizing measures that aim to shift extracellular potassium back toward this physiologic norm.

Insulin acts on sodium-proton antiporters that line the cell membrane, increasing the concentration of intracellular sodium. This in turn upregulates sodium/potassium antiporters, which transport sodium ions out of the cell and potassium into the cell. Because of the hypoglycemic effects of insulin, it must be co-administered with dextrose in attempts to maintain euglycemia.

Albuterol, in addition to its beta-2 agonist effects, also upregulates the activity of the sodium-potassium ATPase that has been central to the physiology of hyperkalemia discussed thus far. Time to onset is approximately 30 min, and duration of effect is approximately 2 hours, making albuterol a readily available, relatively quick-acting agent to lower serum potassium. Of note, in the treatment of hyperkalemia, significantly higher doses of albuterol are needed to effectively achieve the desired potassium-lowering effect when compared to doses that are typically used in the treatment of obstructive lung diseases. Whereas 2.5 mg of nebulized albuterol may be given back-to-back for three doses in the initial treatment of asthma, for example, patients with hyperkalemia may require doses up to 20 mg to effectively shift potassium intracellularly.

Sodium bicarbonate, in an isotonic preparation (i.e., 150 mEq of sodium bicarb in 1 L D5W), theoretically acts by three mechanisms to decrease serum potassium, though multiple studies suggest that this is only of benefit in patients with a concomitant metabolic acidosis [12–15]. The first is likely by way of dilution; isotonic bicarbonate is usually administered in the range of 1–2 L. The second is by encouraging uptake of potassium into skeletal muscle. This occurs via H+/K+ exchange (H+ ions exit the myocyte down a pH gradient via a H+/Na + antiporter, leading to increased intracellular Na + that then powers Na+/K+ ATPases) as well as via HCO3-/K+ cotransport (where HCO3- enters the myocyte down a pH gradient via an HCO3-/Na + symporter that then similarly powers an Na+/K+ ATPase). The third mechanism is by optimizing potassium excretion in the distal convoluted tubule, as acidemia downregulates potassium excretion and alkalemia upregulates potassium excretion, though the end goal should be bringing the pH closer toward a physiologic norm (not over-alkalinizing the serum). Isotonic sodium bicarbonate, as opposed to hypertonic preparations, is used to avoid a concept called "solute drag" which may paradoxically worsen hyperkalemia. Taken together, isotonic bicarbonate should be considered in the hyperkalemic patient who is hypovolemic (can tolerate larger resuscitative volumes) who has an underlying metabolic acidosis as a component of the primary pathology (e.g., metabolic acidosis from uremia secondary to renal failure).

Eliminate Potassium from the Body

Sustainable or definitive treatment of hyperkalemia involves removal of the excess extracellular potassium from the body. This can occur via the renal system and urinary excretion, the gastrointestinal tract, or from the serum via renal replacement therapy/hemodialysis.

Potassium-binding agents are cation-exchange resins that work by exchanging sodium ions for potassium ions in intestinal epithelial cells. Examples of these medications include sodium zirconium cyclosilicate or sodium polystyrene sulfonate, which are typically given via oral route [16]. They have a relatively slow onset of action, with time to onset ranging between 2 and 24 h, making them second- or third-line agents in acute hyperkalemia.

In summary, when approaching treatment of the hyperkalemic patient, a calcium salt should be the first agent given with the goal of stabilizing the cardiac membrane against potentially fatal arrhythmogenic effects of hyperkalemia. Then, rapid-acting medications, to include insulin with dextrose and nebulized albuterol, can be tried, with careful attention paid to the expected time of onset and duration of action of the medications given to guide repeat electrocardiographic monitoring for treatment effect. If the patient is acidotic, the clinician can consider the use of isotonic sodium bicarbonate. As hyperkalemia is a medical emergency, discussion should be promptly initiated with a nephrologist to guide further definitive treatment and consideration for hemodialysis.

Exam Questions

1. While rotating on the general medicine wards, you are called down to the ED to evaluate a patient for admission to your service. The patient is a 23-year-old male college student with no known medical history who was competing in his first-ever triathlon event consisting of a 2.4-mile swim, 112-mile bicycle race, and 26.2-mile run for which he had trained for 6 weeks. Halfway through the run, he complained of diffuse muscle aches and nausea. When he went to the restroom, he noticed dark urine. He was brought to your hospital by race staff EMS. He denies fevers, fatigue, weakness, chest pain, abdominal pain, or palpitations. Physical exam is only significant for tenderness to palpation over the shoulders, thighs, and calves. Blood pressure is 125/79. Heart rate is 72. Respiratory rate is 18. Temperature is 37.9 C. SpO2 is 99% on room air. ECG is normal sinus rhythm. Rate of 70, regular. Axis normal. Intervals all within normal limits. No changes in ST-segment or T-wave morphology.

   Urinalysis: tea-colored, 2+ blood on dipstick, RBCs 0/hpf. Select labs shown below:

Value	Patient values	Reference values
Na^+	135	135–145 mEQ/L
K^+	5.5	3.5–5.0 mEQ*L
Cl^-	101	96–106 mmol/L
CO_2	25	23–29 mmol/L
BUN	18	6–20 mg/dL
Cr	1.1	0.6–1.2 mg/dL
Gluc.	95	70–100 mg/dL
Creatine kinase	2500	39–308
Ca^{2+}	8.4	8.5–10 mg/dL
PO_4^{3-}	4.7	2.5–4.5 mg/dL

   The underlying cause of his hyperkalemia is most closely similar to which of the following?

   A. ACE inhibitor-mediated hyperkalemia
   B. Adverse effect of spironolactone
   C. Chronic kidney disease
   D. Primary hypoaldosteronism
   E. Tumor lysis syndrome

Answer: E

Learning Objective: Identify common underlying etiologies that may lead to hyperkalemia (as a framework, consider that elevated serum K+ must either be due to release from the intracellular space, due to impaired excretion (physiologic or medication-mediated), or due to excessive intake).

Explanation: Out of all the answer options, tumor lysis syndrome is the only choice that involves catabolism of cells/spillage of intracellular electrolyte stores. A is incorrect, as ACE inhibitors mediate hyperkalemia by decreasing aldosterone production in the adrenal medulla as well as by reducing the amount of sodium that reaches the distal nephron. B is incorrect, as aldosterone antagonists such as spironolactone function well as potassium-sparing diuretics, reducing the amount of secretion that occurs in the distal nephron. C is incorrect, as CKD may lead to hyperkalemia due to impaired excretion.

While some may argue that rhabdomyolysis can cause an AKI, this patient's BUN and Cr are within normal limits. D is incorrect as primary hypoaldosteronism (Addison's disease) leads to decreased potassium secretion as well as decreased sodium reuptake in the distal nephron.

2. A 63-year-old male patient with a past medical history of chronic kidney disease and hypertension presents to the emergency department complaining of fatigue and generalized weakness. Blood pressure is 129/78, heart rate is 72, respiratory rate is 18, and temperature is 37.1 C. SpO2 is 95% on room air. His ECG shows sinus rhythm with PR prolongation (220 ms) and tall, peaked T-waves. Serum chemistry is as follows:

Sodium: 138 mEq/L
Potassium: 6.5 mEq/L
Chloride: 104 mEq/L
Carbon dioxide: 25 mEq/L
BUN: 40 mg/dL
Creatinine: 2 mg/dL

Vascular access cannot be obtained despite repeated attempts. Which of the following would be the most acceptable next step to treat this patient?

A. Oral administration of a calcium salt
B. Oral administration of an inhibitor that blocks the conversion of angiotensin I to angiotensin II
C. Oral administration of an oral cation-exchange resin
D. Inhaled formulation of a beta-2-adrenergic and an oral cation-exchange resin
E. Oral administration of a medication that binds the chloride binding site of the Na-K-Cl cotransporter in the thick ascending limb of the nephron
F. A cardiac glycoside used as an antiarrhythmic agent acting at the sodium-potassium ATPase pump.

Answer: D

Learning Objective: Describe the medical interventions used in the emergent treatment of hyperkalemia and the rationale behind these interventions (e.g., insulin/glucose, beta blockers).

Explanation: Nebulized albuterol is a good alternative not requiring vascular access that will rapidly shift potassium inside the cell. Sodium polystyrene (Kayexalate) may be given orally or per rectum and can be efficacious as an adjunct to lower serum potassium. A is incorrect, as calcium gluconate given intravenously is indicated for stabilization of the cardiac membrane and does not lower serum potassium levels. B is incorrect, as ACE inhibitors, such as lisinopril, have no role in the management of hyperkalemia and can contribute to elevated serum potassium. C is incorrect, as by itself, sodium polystyrene (Kayexalate) is not indicated in the use of hyperkalemic emergency but may be used as an adjunct. E is incorrect, as loop diuretics, such as furosemide, may be given as IV pushes to aid renal elimination. However, it would not be an appropriate next step in this clinical vignette. F is incorrect, as digoxin is a medication that, in acute toxicity, may precipitate hyperkalemia due to its action of inhibiting normal function of the sodium-potassium ATPase pump.

3. A 42-year-old female patient with a medical history of type 2 diabetes mellitus well-controlled with diet presents to her primary care physician's office for a follow-up visit to discuss a new diagnosis of hypertension. During her recent well-adult visit, she had no new medical problems, a benign physical exam, and lab work (CBC, CMP, lipid panel) that were within normal limits. With shared decision-making, the patient and physician agree to start a first-line antihypertensive agent that would help lower her blood pressure and aid in protecting her kidneys from diabetic nephropathy. Her physician did warn the patient that a common side effect is a dry cough. Which of the following is true with regard to this class of medication?

A. This medication would be contraindicated in a patient with C1-esterase inhibitor deficiency.
B. Over the next few months while taking this medication, the patient's serum renin would be expected to gradually decrease.
C. The location of the kidney most directly affected by this medication is the afferent thick limb of the loop of Henle.
D. Use of this medication is safe during pregnancy.
E. Electrolyte abnormalities are uncommon with the use of this medication.

Answer: A

Learning Objective: Review basic renal physiology in the context of this patient's comorbid conditions and medications and how they increased his risk of hyperkalemia.

Explanation: ACE inhibitors are contraindicated in this case. They (e.g., lisinopril, captopril) prevent the breakdown of bradykinin. In patients with C1-esterase inhibitor deficiency, patients have increased activity of kallikrein, which activates bradykinin, leading to potentially dangerous hereditary angioedema. B is incorrect as by blocking the conversion of angiotensin I to angiotensin II, there would be an expected absence of negative feedback of angiotensin II on renin production, thereby increasing serum renin levels. C is incorrect, as ACE inhibitors primarily exert their effects on the efferent arteriole. They decrease constriction of the efferent arteriole (due to inhibiting the synthesis of angiotensin II, which constricts the efferent arteriole), thereby reducing GFR. D is incorrect, as ACE inhibitors are contraindicated in pregnancy due to concern for deleterious effects on fetal renal development. E is incorrect; as seen in the case, ACE inhibitors increase a patient's risk for hyperkalemia, particularly in the setting of kidney disease.

References

1. Zacchia M, Abategiovanni ML, Stratigis S, et al. Potassium: from physiology to clinical implications. Kidney Dis. 2016;2:72–9.
2. Rosen MR, Janse MJ, Wit AL. Cardiac electrophysiology: a textbook prepared in honor of Brian F. Hoffman; 1990.
3. Weiss JN, Qu Z, Shivkumar K. Electrophysiology of hypo- and hyperkalemia. Circ Arrhythm Electrophysiol. 2017;10(7):e004667.
4. Buttner R, Burns E, Burns RBA. Hyperkalaemia [Internet]. Life in the Fast Lane LITFL. Life in the Fast Lane; 2018 [cited 2024 Jul 20]. Available from: https://litfl.com/hyperkalaemia-ecg-library/,
5. Palmer BF, Clegg DJ. Physiology and pathophysiology of potassium homeostasis. Adv Physiol Educ. 2017;41(4):480–90.
6. Lehnhardt A, Kemper MJ. Pathogenesis, diagnosis and management of hyperkalemia. Pediatr Nephrol. 2011;26:377.
7. Rajendran VM, Sandle GI. Colonic potassium absorption and secretion in health and disease. Compr Physiol. 2018;8:1513.
8. Potassium Supplement (Oral Route, Parenteral Route) [Internet]. 2024 [cited 2024 Jul 20]. Available from: https://www.mayoclinic.org/drugs-supplements/potassium-supplement-oral-route-parenteral-route/description/drg-20070753.
9. Palmer BF, Clegg DJ. Hyperkalemia treatment standard. Nephrol Dial Transplant [Internet] 2024 [cited 2024 Jul 15];39. Available from: https://pubmed.ncbi.nlm.nih.gov/38425037/.
10. Weidmann S. Effects of calcium ions and local anaesthetics on electrical properties of Purkinje fibres. J Physiol. 1955;129:568.
11. Robert T, Joseph A, Mesnard L. Calcium salt during hyperkalemia. Kidney Int [Internet]. 2016 [cited 2024 Jul 15];90. Available from: https://pubmed.ncbi.nlm.nih.gov/27418095/.
12. Blumberg A, Weidmann P, Ferrari P. Effect of prolonged bicarbonate administration on plasma potassium in terminal renal failure. Kidney Int [Internet]. 1992 [cited 2024 Jul 15];41. Available from: https://pubmed.ncbi.nlm.nih.gov/1552710/.
13. Fraley DS, Adler S. Correction of hyperkalemia by bicarbonate despite constant blood pH. Kidney Int [Internet]. 1977 [cited 2024 Jul 15];12. Available from: https://pubmed.ncbi.nlm.nih.gov/24132/.
14. Gutierrez R, Schlessinger F, Oster JR, et al. Effect of hypertonic versus isotonic sodium bicarbonate on plasma potassium concentration in patients with end-stage renal disease. Miner Electrolyte Metab [Internet]. 1991 [cited 2024 Jul 15];17. Available from: https://pubmed.ncbi.nlm.nih.gov/1668124/.
15. Aronson PS, Giebisch G. Effects of pH on potassium: new explanations for old observations. J Am Soc Nephrol [Internet]. 2011 [cited 2024 Jul 15];22. Available from: https://pubmed.ncbi.nlm.nih.gov/21980112/.
16. Rahman S, Marathi R. Sodium polystyrene sulfonate. StatPearls [Internet]. StatPearls Publishing; 2023.

28 Slurred Speech

Abbey Bayless

Learning Objectives

1. Breakdown the pharmacokinetics of methanol and ethylene glycol and how they cause damage to the body.
2. Address what acid-base derangement occurs as a result of this toxicity and how plasma osmolal gap can be used to help interpret lab results.
3. Identify how hepatic oxidation of either methanol or ethylene glycol can be blocked and what substances can do this. Identify what can accelerate elimination of methanol and possibly ethylene glycol.
4. Create a differential for toxic ingestion and how you might initially differentiate the potentials in a clinical setting.
5. Illustrate the major physical exam findings associated with methanol ingestion and how they change over time. Contrast this with ethylene glycol ingestion symptoms.
6. Explain what laboratory testing is available for toxic substances and their limitations (specifically the tests that identify the substance).
7. Summarize risk factors and protective factors for suicide and identify which this patient had.

A. Bayless (✉)
University of Arizona, Anesthesiology Residency, Tucson, AZ, USA
e-mail: abbeycolorafi@arizona.edu

Chief Complaint

I went over to check on my dad earlier today, and he was very tired and acting weird, so I brought him in.

Prompt: What questions do you want to ask the son? What is on your differential?

Important to ask the son:

- Why he went to check on him? Was he just casually going over or was he worried beforehand?
- What is his dad's baseline mental status? How is this different from that?
- What makes this behavior "weird"?
- These questions might help guide our differential.
- When a patient's mental status is altered, having a historian who knows the patient is invaluable and their opinion of the change should be heavily considered in the differential. Listen to whenever a close individual/relative says something is "off" with a patient.

Differential:

- Main complaint is altered mental status. Students should have a broad differential based on this initial CC, especially before knowledge of the patient's medical history (Fig. 28.1). Students should discuss what need to be ruled out ASAP: stroke, brain bleed, MI.

C. A. Standley (ed.), *Biomedical Science and Clinical Foundations*,
https://doi.org/10.1007/978-3-031-98353-5_28

History of Present Illness

- Patient is a 65-year-old male brought to the ED by his son.
- The son provided the chief complaint and most of the history.
- The son had not heard from his dad for a few days and was worried about him. When he got to his dad's house, he found him in the garage.
- "He was very lethargic and just acting weird. His words were slurring, and he was having a hard time answering any of my questions. It seemed like maybe he was drunk, but something seemed off. His clothes were wet, and there was a strange odor coming from them. I immediately drove him to the ER after finding him."

Prompt: What should immediately be done before asking any more questions?

What specific medical history might you want to ask about now?

- His clothes being covered with an unknown substance is very concerning, especially given the altered mental status. His clothes should be removed and he should be given a hospital gown. You are unaware if the substance could be caustic.
- You would want to ask the son further about any known history of alcohol use disorder or any other substances. You should also ask about history of depression, sudden changes in his life, or any prior suicide attempts.

History of Present Illness (Cont.)

- The son shares that his dad has history of alcohol use disorder and has been hospitalized multiple times for it. His dad recently had him "remove all the alcohol bottles from his house because he wanted to get better."
- He denies knowledge of his father's use of any other substances.
- The patient's wife had passed away 1 year ago.
- "I would say he's been depressed this past year but hasn't seen a psychiatrist or anything."

Prompt: How does this change your differential?

This points more towards a possible ingestion/intoxication, especially given history of ETOH use. Recent removal of liquor bottles should sug-

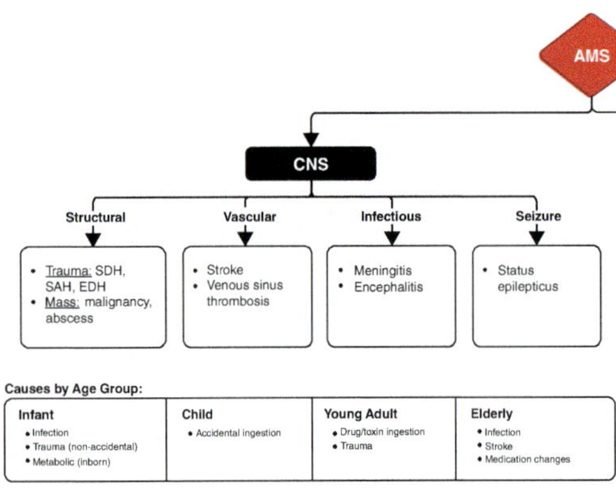

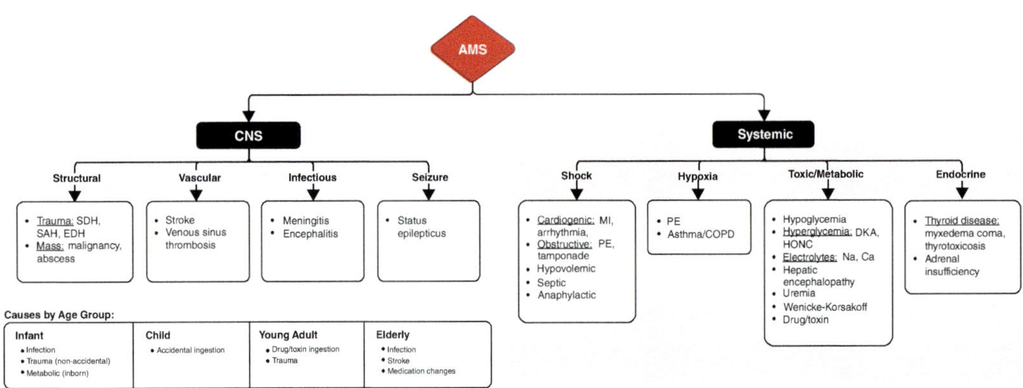

Fig. 28.1 Algorithm for altered mental status [1]

gest this could be a different type of intoxication.

We still don't know about this patient's remaining medical history, so other things still need to be evaluated (i.e. possibility of stroke, MI).

Past Medical History

- Patient has a history of Type 1 DM that is poorly controlled. The son is unsure the last time his father took his insulin.
- Son denies history of myocardial infarction, stroke, TIAs.

Social History

- Mr. Jackson lives alone in a house.
- As mentioned before, his wife passed away 1 year ago from cancer.
- He was a car mechanic for 40 years before retiring.
- He does not smoke. It is unknown how much he usually drinks in a week.
- His son and daughter live nearby and try to check on him often.

Family History

- The patient's father has diabetes.
- The patient's brother has depression.
- His children are all healthy.
- There is no known medical history of stroke or MIs.

Prompt: What would be the sequence of your activities & examination in the ED?

- Mental status exam: what is his level of consciousness?
- Vital signs: is he hypotensive?? Tachycardic? Bradycardic?? Febrile?
- Any sign of trauma?

Testing:
- POC glucose
- CBC & CMP: Electrolyte abnormalities or infection could cause this presentation
- Tox screen
- ETOH levels given history
- ABG
- EKG
- Possible head imaging

Review of Systems (as Reported by Son & Limited Due to Patient's Mental Status)

- General: Admits to poor dietary habits and chronic drinking.
- HEENT: + recent vision changes. No oral lesions.
- Cardio/Pulm: +difficulty breathing.
- GI: + stomach pain.
- GU: No hematuria, dysuria.
- MSK: No recent falls or trauma.
- Psych: + h/o depression. No hallucinations, prior suicide attempts.
- Neuro: + changes in vision, h/a, dizziness, weakness.

Prompt: How has your preliminary diagnosis changed? What are you looking for on physical examination?

- These acute symptoms are pointing towards a toxic ingestion that is now causing physical effects.
- Changes in vision suggest this is something other than ETOH intoxication.
- A stroke would result in a localized weakness, not respiratory/abdominal symptoms.
- Infection could still be part of the picture, but would not expect vision changes due to that.
- With h/o of DM → also worried about DKA → could cause respiratory changes. Vision changes could be due to DM (although less likely).

Physical Exam

- Vital Signs:
- BP: 150/90
- P: 115 beats/min
- RR: 29 breaths/min
- T: 38.5 C
- General: Disheveled. Slurring words and giggling inappropriately when asked questions. Audibly wheezing as he spoke.
- HEENT: Head atraumatic. Optic disk edema present on fundoscopic exam. Pupillary response to light absent bilaterally. No oral ulcers or erythema.
- CV: Tachycardic. Regular rhythm.
- Pulm: Audible wheezing throughout lungs.
- Abdominal: Epigastric pain.
- Genital/Rectal: Negative DRE.
- Extremities: Wide-based gait.

Prompt: How has your preliminary diagnosis changed?

- Very likely some sort of toxic ingestion
- Options to consider:
  - Methanol poisoning
  - Arsenic poisoning
  - Cocaine poisoning
  - Ethylene glycol poisoning
  - CO poisoning
  - Complex partial seizures
- DKA is still possible at this point as well due to abdominal pain, changes in breathing
- Pancreatitis could be occurring as well due to intoxication, presentation of epigastric abdominal pain

Case Update

- Due to apparent respiratory distress and possible toxic ingestion, the medical team decides it is best to intubate.
- This precludes a mental status exam.

Facilitator note from article: Burket et al. [2]

- Management of the airway in the critically ill pharmaceutical-poisoned patient comes with numerous challenges. **The existing literature does not elucidate one specific management strategy for the poisoned patients**. Instead the clinical circumstances should guide the decision to intubate; the specific approach to ETI; the administration of any antidote, paralytic, or sedating medication and decontamination; and the selection of induction or paralytic medications. The specific properties of the pharmaceuticals that were ingested should be taken into consideration when developing an airway management strategy.

LABS

CBC:
- WBC: 9000 cells/mcL (normal 4500–11,000 cells/mcL)
- RBC: 4.0 million cells/mcL (normal 4.5–5.9 million cells/mcL)
- Hb: 11 gm/dL (normal 14–17.5 gm/dL men)
- MCV: 111 fL (normal 80–96 fL)
- PLT: 200,000 (normal 150,000–450,000)

CMP:
- Na: 140 (normal 136–144 mmol/L)
- K: 4 (normal 3.5–5 mEq/L)
- BUN:10 (normal 5–10 20 mg/dL)
- Cr: 4 (normal 0.6–1.5 mg/dL)
- Glucose: 95 (normal 7–110)
- Ca2+: 9.5 (normal 9–10.5 mg/dl)
- Cl: 110 (normal 95–105 mEq/L)
- HCO3: 15 (normal 23–39 mEq/L)
- AST: 120 (normal 0–35 units/L)
- ALT: 60 (normal 4–36 units/L)
- Bilirubin: 0.5 (normal 0.3–1 mg/dL)
- Albumin: 3.0 (normal 3.5–5.0 g/dL)
- Lipase: 50 (normal 0–160 u/L)

Prompt: Interpret the lab findings.

- Macrocytic anemia to be expected with chronic ETOH use and malnutrition.
- Kidney damage evident from lab results.
- Glucose WNL → helps us rule out DKA as cause of acidosis.
- Low HCO3, high CL → thinking **acidosis.**
- AST 2X ALT expected with chronic ETOH use.
- Lipase WNL → **DOES NOT RULE OUT PANCREATITIS** → diagnosis requires 2/3 abd pain in epigastric region, imaging findings, and/or elevated lipase.

ABG:
- pH: 7.20 (normal 7.35–7.45)
- HCO3+: 15 mEq/L (normal 22–26 mEq/L)
- pCO2: 32 (normal 35–45 mmHg)

Prompt: What acid/base derangement is shown here? What is the anion gap?

What can cause this? -metabolic acidosis with anion gap 15.

The acid-base disorder is a metabolic acidosis (Fig. 28.2).

Toxicology Screen
- Acetaminophen: negative
- Salicylate: negative
- Ethylene glycol: negative
- Isopropyl alcohol: negative
- **Serum methanol: elevated**
- Negative for marijuana, methamphetamines, cocaine, benzos, oxycodone, morphine, and PCP.

EKG
The patient's EKG is shown in Fig. 28.3.

Prompt: Interpret the EKG.

Normal sinus rhythm.

Prompt: What is the diagnosis?

Diagnosis: Methanol poisoning with subsequent end organ damage

- Vision loss, Renal damage, Possible GI effects.

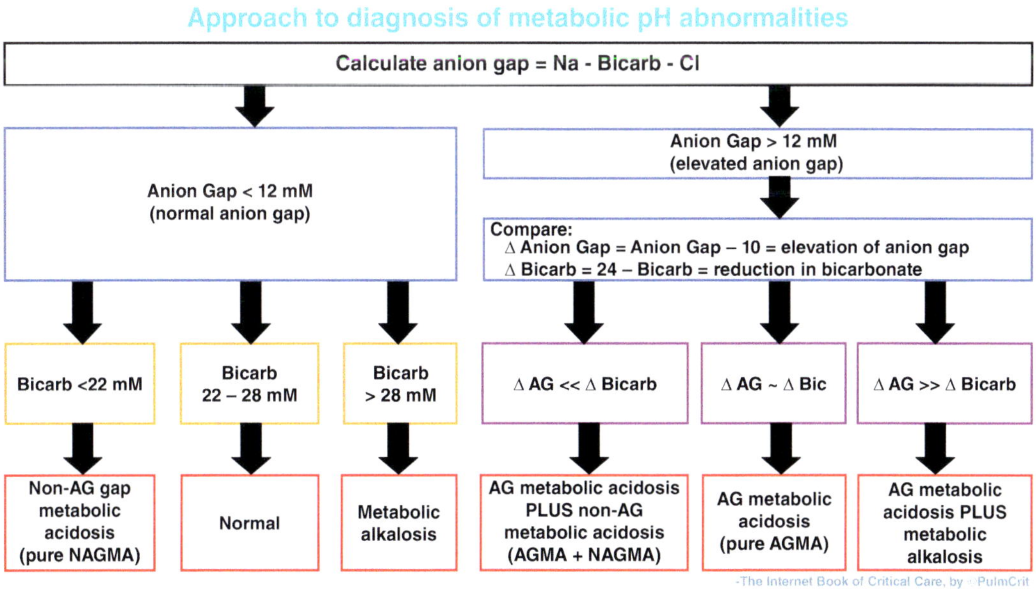

Fig. 28.2 Approach to acid-base disorders [3]

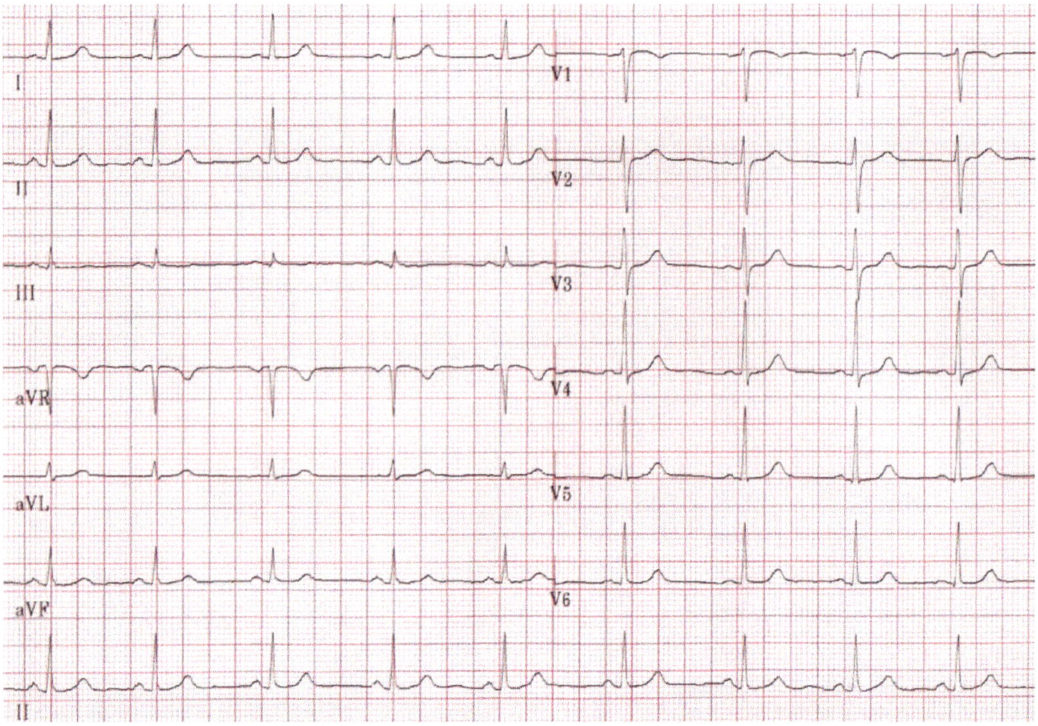

Fig. 28.3 Electrocardiogram. CardioNetworks: Drj, CC BY-SA 3.0 https://creativecommons.org/licenses/by-sa/3.0, via Wikimedia Commons (https://commons.wikimedia.org/wiki/File:Nsr_%28CardioNetworks_ECGpedia%29.jpg) (Source: https://en.ecgpedia.org/wiki/File:Nsr.jpg)

Prompt: What treatment would you give?

Important note: GIVE TREATMENT ASAP If EXPECTED METHANOL TOXICITY and with this storyline (Fig. 28.4). You are not waiting for lab to result.

Initial Treatment

- Always ABCDs first: Secure airway (already done).
- Give fluids, especially if hypotensive.
- Block ETOH dehydrogenase with fomepizole (15 mg/kg IV loading > 10 mg/kg Q 12 H × 4 doses).
- Administer sodium bicarbonate (1–2 mEq/kg bolus followed by infusion).
- For patients with known/suspected methanol poisoning > folic acid 50 mg IV Q6H.
- DIALYSIS!

Prompt: What additional tests might be needed?

- Repeat ABGs scheduled: want to make sure acidosis improves.
- Repeat electrolytes for dialysis: replete as needed.
- MRI, CT abdomen depending on severity of abdominal pain.

MRI Findings from Methanol Poisoning

- Most common MR findings are bilateral putaminal necroses with possible hemorrhage.

Prompt: What test might be done if the patient had ingested ethylene glycol instead?

What would you find?

Treatment
Secure airway as necessary in severely intoxicated patients
Treat hypotension with intravenous crystalloid, followed by standard vasopressors as necessary
Block alchohol dehydrogenase with **fomepizole**, 15 mg/kg IV loading dose, followed by 10 mg/kg q 12 h × 4 doses. If patient requires further treatment after this regimen, increase dose to 15 mg/kg every 12 hours
If fomepizole is unavailable or patient has a known allergy, block alcohol dehydrogenase with ethanol, 10 mL/kg of a 10% ethanol solution, followed by 1 mL/kg of 10% ethanol solution infused per hour. Titrate to serum ethanol concentration of 100 mg/dL.
Administer **sodium bicarbonate,** 1 to 2 meq/kg bolus followed by infusion of 132 meq $NaHCO_3$ in 1 L D5W to run at 200 to 250 mL/hour for patients with pH below 7.3
For patients with know or suspected methanol poisoning, administer **folic acid,** 50 mg IV every six hours
For patients with know or suspected ethylene glycol posioning, administer **thiamine,** 100 mg IV, and administer **pyridoxine,** 50 mg IV
If the diagnosis is uncertain but clinical suspicion is high; the clinician should initiate antidotal treatment wiht alcohol dehydrogenase blockad and consultation for hemodialysis
Hemodialysis is indicated in severe toxicity, which we define as follows:
Metabolic acidosis, regardless of drug level
Elevated serum methanol or ethylene glycol levels (more than 50 mg/dL; or methanol 15.6 mmol/L, ethylene glycol 8.1 mmol/L), unless arterial pH is above 7.3
Evidence of end-organ damage (eg, visual changes, renal failure)

Fig. 28.4 Treatment for methanol poisoning. UpToDate, [4]

Urine Studies

Oxalate Crystals: late and nonspecific finding following ethylene glycol ingestion. Two types possible.

- Needle shaped monohydrate crystals.
- Envelope shaped dihydrate crystals.

Main Take Away

Rapid recognition and early treatment, including alcohol dehydrogenase (ADH) inhibition, are crucial.

End of Case

Learning Objective Answers

LO #1: Break down the pharmacokinetics of methanol and ethylene glycol and how they cause damage to the body.

UpToDate, https://www.uptodate.com/contents/methanol-and-ethylene-glycol-poisoning-pharmacology-clinical-manifestations-and-diagnosis?search=ethylene%20glycol&source=search_result&selectedTitle=1~35&usage_type=default&display_rank=1

Methanol and ethylene glycol, the "parent alcohols," are generally not highly toxic and mainly cause sedation. However, severe toxicity can occur once these alcohols are metabolized. When consumed in large amounts, methanol forms formate, and ethylene glycol produces glycolate, glyoxylate, and oxalate, which accumulate. Once plasma levels exceed approximately 20 mg/dL (6 mmol/L of methanol or 3 mmol/L of ethylene glycol), these metabolites can lead to damage to specific organs:

- Formate can cause retinal damage with optic disc swelling, edema, and possibly permanent blindness. It can also cause ischemic or hemorrhagic injury to the basal ganglia, likely due to mitochondrial dysfunction.
- Ethylene glycol metabolites primarily affect the kidneys, causing reversible acute kidney injury (oliguric or anuric renal failure), which slows down the elimination of ethylene glycol. Kidney damage is mainly from glycolate harming the tubules, though oxalate crystals may also cause blockage. Hypocalcemia,

caused by calcium oxalate formation, is rare in cases of ethylene glycol poisoning.

Like other simple alcohols, both methanol and ethylene glycol are quickly and fully absorbed after oral ingestion, with peak serum concentrations usually reached within an hour (Fig. 28.5). The alcohols are metabolized through a two-step oxidation process involving alcohol dehydrogenase (ADH) and aldehyde dehydrogenase, resulting in toxic metabolites.

LO #2: Address what acid-base derangement occurs as a result of this toxicity and how plasma osmolal gap can be used to help interpret lab results.

Citation for answer:
UpToDate, https://www.uptodate.com/contents/methanol-and-ethylene-glycol-poisoning-pharmacology-clinical-manifestations-and-diagnosis?search=ethylene%20glycol&source=search_result&selectedTitle=1~35&usage_type=default&display_rank=1

When methanol or ethylene glycol is ingested, a significant anion gap metabolic acidosis develops, which worsens central nervous system depression and triggers a cycle of hypoxia and acidosis (Fig. 28.6). A large, unexplained osmolal gap strongly suggests recent exposure to methanol, ethylene glycol, or isopropyl alcohol, provided significant ethanol ingestion is ruled out.

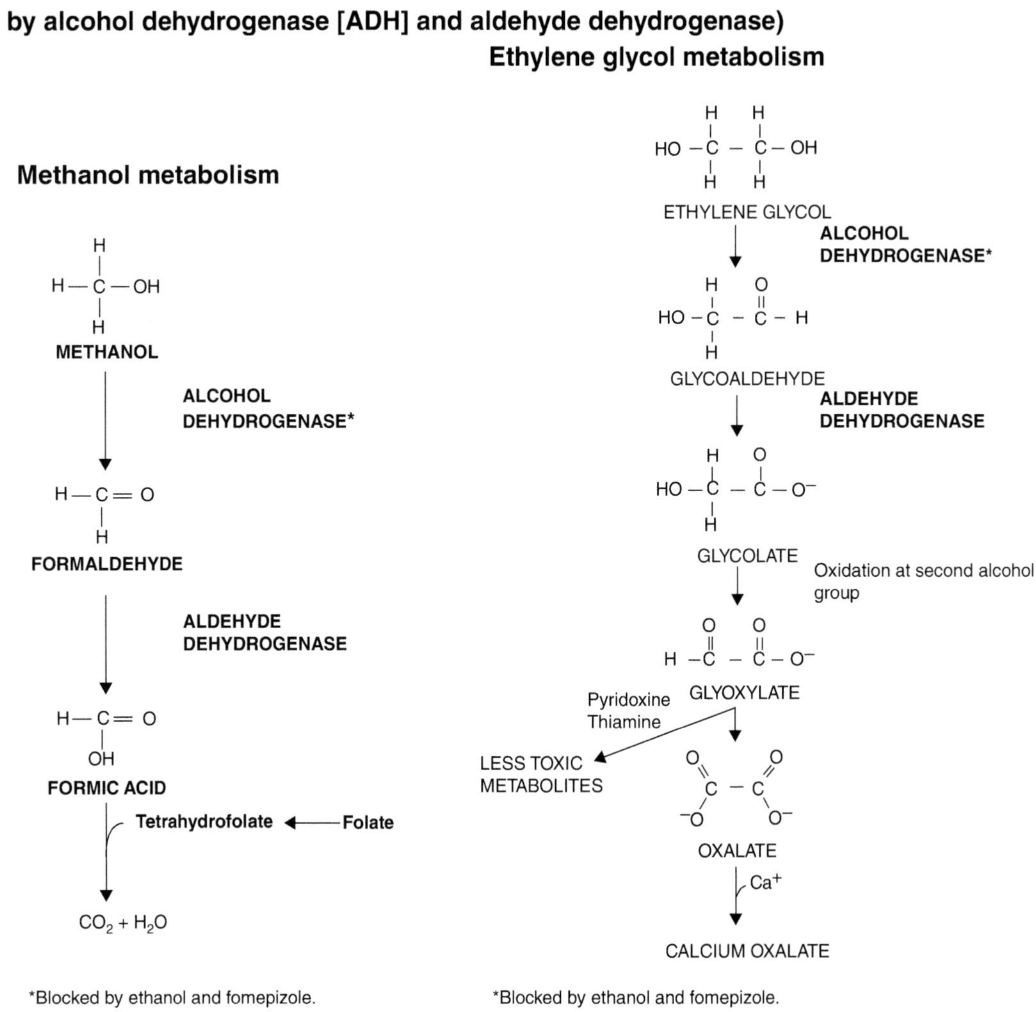

Fig. 28.5 Methanol & ethylene glycol metabolism. UpToDate, [4]

Mechanism of acidosis	Increased AG	Normal AG
Increased acid production	Lactic acidosis	
	Ketoacidosis	
	Diabetes mellitus	
	Starvation	
	Alcohol associated	
	Ingestions	
	Methanol	
	Ethylene glycol	
	Aspirin	
	Toluene (if early or if kidney function is impaired)	Toluene ingestion (if late and if kidney function is preserved; due to excretion of sodium and potassium hippurate in the urine)
	Diethylene glycol	
	Propylene glycol	
	D-lactic acidosis	A component of non-AG metabolic acidosis may coexist due to urinary excretion of D- lactate as Na and K salts (which represents potential HCO_3)
	Pyroglutamic acid (5-oxoproline)	

Fig. 28.6 Acidosis differential UpToDate, [4]

The osmolal gap is the difference between measured osmolality and calculated plasma osmolality. It is calculated as:

Calculated Posm = (2 × plasma [Na]) + [glucose]/18 + [BUN]/2.8 or, using standard units: Calculated Posm = (2 × plasma [Na]) + [glucose] + [urea]

Several points must be considered when interpreting the plasma osmolal gap in suspected toxic alcohol ingestion (Fig. 28.8). It cannot differentiate between ethanol, isopropyl alcohol, methanol, or ethylene glycol, and ethanol treatment can interfere with its value. The gap increases with the parent alcohols but not their metabolites, as these are charged at normal pH. Therefore, the gap becomes less sensitive once the parent alcohol has been metabolized.

The gap may not detect small ingestions, especially soon after consumption. High ethanol levels (over 100 mg/dL) can artificially increase the osmolal gap. In critically ill patients, other factors, such as idiogenic osmoles or conditions like sickle cell crises, may elevate the gap.

A large plasma osmolal gap (over 25) is a strong indicator of recent methanol, ethylene glycol, or isopropyl alcohol exposure. However, dismissing toxic alcohol exposure based on a gap under 10 or assuming a small increase indicates ingestion in a low-probability case is incorrect. Few conditions cause severe high anion gap metabolic acidosis without a high lactate level, though ethylene glycol can elevate lactate levels without fully explaining the acidosis.

A mild form of metabolic acidosis in an alcoholic patient can also be triggered by conditions such as alcoholic ketoacidosis, sepsis, alcohol withdrawal seizures, diabetic ketoacidosis, or salicylate poisoning.

An increased plasma osmolal gap may be observed in individuals with methanol or ethylene glycol poisoning, but it can also occur in cases of alcoholic or diabetic ketoacidosis, isopropyl alcohol ingestion, large amounts of ethanol consumption, and other severe conditions like sepsis, ischemic bowel, or shock (Fig. 28.7).

LO#3: Identify how hepatic oxidation of either methanol or ethylene glycol can be blocked and what substances can do this. Identify what can accelerate elimination of methanol and possibly ethylene glycol.

Source: https://www.uptodate.com/contents/methanol-and-ethylene-glycol-poisoning-pharmacology-clinical-manifestations-and-diagnosis?search=ethylene%20glycol&source=search_result&selectedTitle=1~35&usage_type=default&display_rank=1

The metabolism of ethanol, methanol, and ethylene glycol is shown in Fig. 28.8. Fomepizole is used as an antidote in confirmed or suspected

Fig. 28.7 Differential with elevated plasma/serum osmolal gap UpToDate, [4]

Differential diagnosis of an elevated plasma/serum osmolal gap

With anion gap metabolic acidosis

Major causes of a large osmolal gap

- Ethylene glycol ingestion
- Methanol ingestion
- Propylene glycol infusin

Causes of a smaller osmolal gap

- Severe chronic kidney disease without regular dialysis
- Ketoacidosis (diabetic or alcoholic)
- Lactic acidosis
- Paraldehyde ingestion or injection

Without anion gap metabolic acidosis

- Ethanol
- Isopropanol
- Diethyl ether
- Infusion of mannitol, sorbitol, or glycine
- Pseudohyponatremia (severe hyperlipidemia or hyperproteinemia)

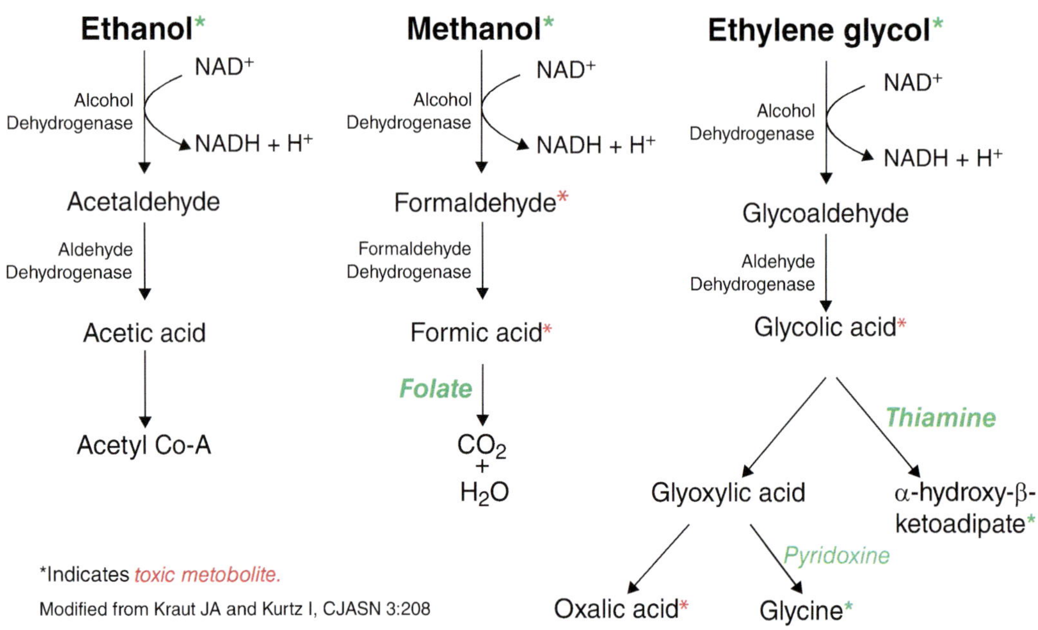

Fig. 28.8 Metabolism of ethanol, methanol & ethylene glycol [6]

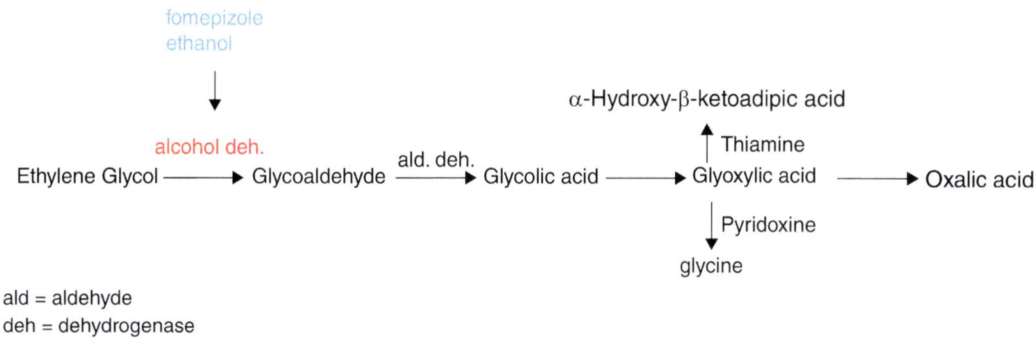

Fig. 28.9 Ethylene glycol metabolism [7]

Fig. 28.10 Treatment of alcohol poisoning [8]

	ETHANOL	FOMEPIZOLE
Advantages	Available in clinical setting Extensive experience in the Netherlands Antidote in different alcohol poisonings Administration orally and intravenously	Minimal adverse effects Registered for ethylene glycol poisoning
Disadvantages	Dose calculations based on blood-alcohol levels Hospitalization in intensive care unit necessary during treatment Not officially registered as antidote	High costs Not available in all clinical settings Limited shelf life Not registered for methanol in the Netherlands Lack of experience in the Netherlands Little experience in other alcohol poisonings

methanol or ethylene glycol poisoning. Fomepizole is a competitive inhibitor of alcohol dehydrogenase, the enzyme that catalyzes the initial steps in the metabolism of ethylene glycol and methanol to their toxic metabolites [5]. If hepatic oxidation is inhibited by an ADH antagonist like ethanol or fomepizole, several changes occur (Fig. 28.9):

- Methanol: Elimination shifts to pulmonary and renal routes, becomes first order, and slows significantly (half-life 48–54 h).
- Ethylene glycol: Elimination becomes almost entirely renal, with a half-life as short as 14 h if kidney function is normal.

Formate, the toxic methanol metabolite, relies partially on tetrahydrofolate for elimination, and its elimination is thought to speed up with folic acid administration.

Pyridoxine and thiamine are involved in minor elimination pathways for glycolate, an ethylene glycol metabolite, but it's unclear how much their supplementation speeds up these pathways.

Advantages and disadvantages of using ethanol and fomepizole in the treatment of methanol poisoning are shown in Fig. 28.10.

LO#4: Create a differential for toxic ingestion and how you might initially differentiate the potentials in a clinical setting.

Stimulated	Depressed	Discordant	Normal
Sympathetics Sympathomimetics	Sympatholytics	Asphyxiants	Nontoxic exposure
Ergot alkaloids	α_1-Adrenergic antagonists	Cytochrome oxidase inhibitors	Psychogenic illness
Methylxanthines	α_2-Adrenergic agonists	Inert gases	Toxic time bombs
Monoamine oxidase inhibitors	ACE Inhibitors	Irritant gases	Slow absorption
Thyroid hormones	Anglotensin receptor blockers	Methermoglobin inducers	Anticholinergics
Anticholinergics	Antipsychotics	Oxidative phosphorylation Inhibitors	Carbamazepine
Antihistamines	β-Adrenergic blockers	AGMA Inducers	Concretion formers
Antiparkinsonian agents	Calcium channel blockers	Alcohol (ketoacidosis)	Extended-release phenytoin sodium capsules (Dilantin Kapseals)
Antipsychotics	Cardiac glycosides	Ethylene glycol	Drug packets
Antispasmodics	Cyclic antidepressants	Iron	Enteric-coated pills
Belladonna alkaloids	Cholinergics	Methanol	Diphenoxylate-atropine (Lomotil)
Cyclic antidepressants	Acetylcholinesterase inhibitors	Salicylate	Opiodis
Muscle relaxants	Muscarinic agonists	Toluene	Salicylates
Mushrooms and plants	Nicotinic agonists	CNS syndromes	Sustained-release pills
Hallucinogens	Opioids	Extrapyramidal reacions	Valproate
Cannabinoids (marijuana)	Analgesics	Hydrocarbon inhalation	Slow distribution
LSD and analogues	GI antispasmodics	Isoniazid	Cardiac glycosides
Mescaline and analogues	Heroin	Lithium	Lithium
Mushrooms	Sedative-hypnotics	Neuroleptic malignant syndrome	Heavy metals
Phencyclidine and analogues	Alcohois	Serotonin syndrome	Salicylate
Withdrawal syndromes	Anticonvulsants	Strychnine	
Barbiturates	Barbiturates		

Fig. 28.11 Various Toxidromes poisoning and drug overdose [9]

Fig. 28.12 Differential with anion gap metabolic acidosis UpToDate, [4]

With anion gap metabolic acidosis
Major causes of a large osmolal gap
▪ Ethylene glycol ingestion ▪ Methanol ingestion ▪ Propylene glycol infusion
Causes of a smaller osmolal gap
▪ Severe chronic kidney disease without regular dialysis ▪ Ketoacidosis (diabetic or alcoholic) ▪ Lactic acidosis ▪ Paraldehyde ingestion or injection
Without anion gap metabolic acidosis
▪ Ethanol ▪ Isopropanol ▪ Diethyl ether ▪ Infusion of mannitol, sorbitol, or glycine ▪ Pseudohyponatremia (severe hyperlipidemia or hyperproteinemia)

- Many different ways to categorize (Fig. 28.11)
  Option 1: Ref: [9]
  Option 2: DDx regarding metabolic acidosis (Fig. 28.12, Table 28.1) (uptodate)
  Option 3: toxic ETOHs (Fig. 28.13, Table 28.1): link 1, link 2, link 3
- LO#5: Illustrate the major physical exam findings associated with methanol ingestion and how they change over time. Contrast this with ethylene glycol ingestion symptoms.
  - Might have some overlap with LO #4

Source

https://www.uptodate.com/contents/methanol-and-ethylene-glycol-poisoning-pharmacology-clinical-manifestations-and-diagnosis?search=ethylene%20glycol&source=search_result&selectedTitle=1~35&usage_type=default&display_rank=1

It is crucial to determine the source and nature of the exposure by interviewing the patient and family and obtaining the original container. Methanol and ethylene glycol are commonly

Table 28.1 Differentiating between different alcohol poisonings

Type of alcohol poisoning	Common sources	Clinical clues	Treatment
Ethanol	Alcoholic beverages, hand sanitizers, mouthwash	CNS depression, ataxia, hypoglycemia (in children), respiratory depression in severe cases	Supportive care (IV fluids, glucose if hypoglycemic, airway protection if needed)
Methanol	Windshield washer fluid, antifreeze, industrial solvents	Anion gap metabolic acidosis, visual disturbances ("snowfield" vision), CNS depression	Fomepizole or ethanol, dialysis in severe cases, bicarbonate for acidosis
Ethylene glycol	Antifreeze, industrial solvents	Anion gap metabolic acidosis, renal failure, CNS depression, hypocalcemia	Fomepizole or ethanol, dialysis in severe cases, calcium supplementation for hypocalcemia
Isopropanol	Rubbing alcohol, disinfectants, hand sanitizers	CNS depression, ketosis without acidosis, fruity breath odor, GI irritation	Supportive care, IV fluids, airway protection if needed

	Containing Fluids	Clinical Findings	Unique Lab Findings
Methanol	Windshield wiper fluid, adulterated ethanol "moonshine"	Blurred ("snowstorm") vision, blindness, basal ganglia hemorrhage leading to Parkinsonism	Lactic acidosis
Ethylene Glycol	Antifreeze	Fluorescent urine, calcium oxalate crystals	Hypocalcemia, wide QRS, prolonged QTc
Propylene Glycol	Diluent in parenteral medications	Hepatic/Renal failure patients at higher risk	Lactic acidosis
Isopropyl Alcohol	Hand sanitizer, rubbing alcohol	May cause acute pancreatitis	Acetonemia (may falsely elevate Cr) [5], does not cause HAGMA

Fig. 28.13 Various Alcohol Toxicities [10]

found in products like automotive coolant/antifreeze, de-icing solutions, windshield wiper fluid, solvents, cleaners, fuels, and other industrial items.

Without proper treatment, an ingestion of about 1 g/kg of methanol or ethylene glycol can be lethal, and serious toxicity can occur from as little as one teaspoon of methanol. However, inhalation or dermal exposure rarely causes toxicity, even after intentional recreational inhalation of substances like carburetor cleaner or lacquer thinner.

It's imperative to determine when the ingestion happened and if ethanol was also consumed. Ethanol inhibits alcohol dehydrogenase (ADH), reducing the formation of toxic metabolites from the parent alcohol. The intent behind the exposure—whether accidental, recreational, suicidal, or homicidal—may become clear only after further investigation, such as interviews with friends or family.

Patients should be questioned about visual symptoms (e.g., blurred vision, scotomata) that suggest methanol poisoning or genitourinary symptoms (e.g., flank pain, hematuria, oliguria) that point to ethylene glycol poisoning.

Physical Examination: A brief initial screening should include vital signs, mental status, and pupil checks to identify immediate needs for stabilization. Patients with large methanol or ethylene glycol ingestions may present with mild CNS effects like inebriation or sedation, similar to ethanol intoxication. If ethanol was co-ingested, these symptoms may worsen. Coma, seizures, deep breathing (Kussmaul-Kien respirations), and hypotension suggest significant metabolism of the parent alcohol into toxic metabolites.

An afferent pupillary defect is a concerning sign of advanced methanol poisoning. Eye exams in methanol poisoning may also show mydriasis, retinal edema, and optic disk hyperemia.

It's important to note that the onset of methanol or ethylene glycol toxicity is delayed when ethanol is co-ingested. Therefore, the possibility of simultaneous ethanol and toxic alcohol consumption should always be considered, especially in alcoholics who may ingest alcohol in various forms.

Ethylene glycol metabolism can result in cranial nerve palsies and tetany, likely due to oxalate-induced hypocalcemia. Oliguria and hematuria may also occur, and cerebral herniation and multi-organ failure are common in severe poisoning cases.

LO #6: Explain what laboratory testing is available for toxic substances and their limitations (specifically the tests that identify the substance).

Source: https://www.uptodate.com/contents/methanol-and-ethylene-glycol-poisoning-pharmacology-clinical-manifestations-and-diagnosis?search=ethylene%20glycol&source=search_result&selectedTitle=1~35&usage_type=default&display_rank=1

Serum concentrations of methanol and ethylene glycol are typically measured using gas chromatography, but this testing is often unavailable and requires sending samples to reference labs. When concentrations are available, clinicians must verify the units used (mmol/L vs. mg/dL) and reference ranges to avoid diagnostic errors.

Enzymatic methods for detecting ethylene glycol can produce false positives, such as in severe acetaminophen toxicity or interference from substances like propylene glycol. These tests should not be relied on in suspected ethylene glycol toxicity cases. While new diagnostic tests are in development, none are widely available yet for rapid confirmation.

Lactate levels may be elevated in ethylene glycol poisoning, either due to actual lactate increases or falsely elevated levels because laboratory instruments can't distinguish between lactate and glycolate, ethylene glycol metabolites. A significant discrepancy in lactate levels between two methods can be a clue to ethylene glycol poisoning. Though high lactate levels often point to other conditions like tissue hypoxia, ethylene glycol should not be excluded based solely on a high lactate reading.

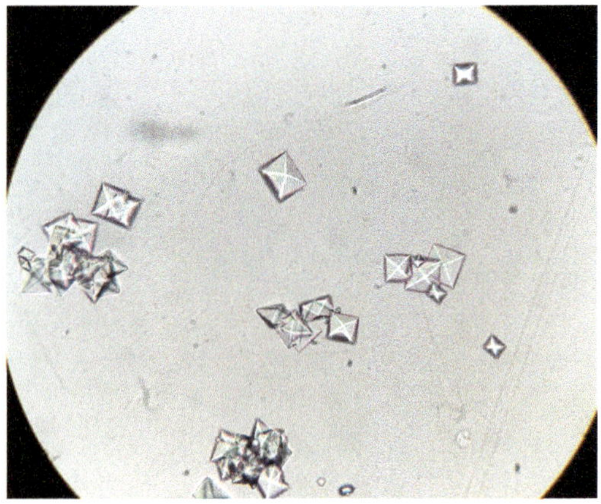

Fig. 28.14 Urinary calcium oxalate dihydrate crystals [11]UpToDate, https://www.uptodate.com/contents/methanol-and-ethylene-glycol-poisoning-pharmacology-clinical-manifestations-and-diagnosis?search=ethylene%20glycol&source=search_result&selectedTitle=1~35&usage_type=default&display_rank=1

Urine testing for oxalate crystals and fluorescence is common but should be interpreted cautiously (Fig. 28.14). Oxalate crystals in the urine are a late and nonspecific sign. Fluorescence, used to detect fluorescein in antifreeze solutions, lacks sensitivity and specificity. Not all ethylene glycol products contain fluorescein, and it only appears briefly in the urine. Furthermore, normal urine and other substances can cause fluorescence.

LO#7: Summarize risk factors and protective factors for suicide and identify which this patient had.

Risk factors and protective factors for suicidality are shown in Figs. 28.15 and 28.16. For this patient, protective factors were the support from kids. Risk factors: h/o depression, recent loss of wife, isolation, chronic condition with DM

Fig. 28.15 Risk and protective factors for suicide [12]

Table 2 – Risk and protective factors for suicide

Risk factors	Protective factors
• Mental illness	• Social support
• Previous suicide attempt	• Connectedness
• Serious physical illness/chronic pain	• Strong therapeutic alliance
• Specific symptoms	• Access to mental health care
• Family history of mental illness and suicide	• Positive attitude to mental health treatment
• History of childhood trauma	• Coping skills
• Shame/despair	• Problem solving skills
• Aggression/impulsivity	• Cultural/religious beliefs
• Triggering event	• Biological/psychological resilience
Access to lethal means	
• Suicide exposure	
• Inflexible thinking	
• Genes: stress and mood	

Fig. 28.16 Risk and protective factors for suicide [13]

Risk factors	Protective factors
INDIVIDUAL-LEVEL	
Prior suicide attempt(s)	Problem-solving skills
Mental disorders (Axis II diagnosis)	Frustraton tolerance
Trauma or abuse history	Self-control
Hopelessness	Reasons for living and optimism
Stressful life events	Perceptions of positive health
Self-harm	Participation in sporing activities
Prior psychiatric hospitalization	–
Family history of suicide	–
Chronic illness and pain	–
Personality traits	–
Biomedical/physical determinants	–
SOCIAL-LEVEL	
Job or financial loss	Family relationships
Socio-economic disadvantage	Partnership
Relationship conflict, discord or loss	Social relationships and social support
Disaster, war and conflict	Religious or spiritual beliefs
Acculturation stress	Employment

(McLean et al., 2008); (Ougrin et al., 2015); (World Health Organization, 2014).

Exam Questions

1. A 70-year-old-male was found in his garage by his son. The patient was described as being "covered in some liquid" and "acting like he was drunk." The patient has a history of depression and alcohol use disorder. Urine studies showed the following (seen in Fig. 28.17). Choose the name of the toxic metabolite causing these symptoms and what inhibitor can be given for immediate treatment purposes.

A. Glycolic acid, naltrexone
B. Glycolic acid, fomepizole
C. Formic acid, naltrexone
D. Formic acid, fomepizole
E. Acetaldehyde, naltrexone
F. Acetaldehyde, fomepizole

Answer: B

Learning Objective #3: Identify how hepatic oxidation of either methanol or ethylene glycol can be blocked and what substances can do this. Identify what can accelerate elimination of methanol and possibly ethylene glycol.

Explanation: Glycolic acid is the toxic metabolite of ethylene glycol (which can cause oxalate crystals seen in image). Fomepizole is an ADH antagonist to block hepatic oxidation of this toxic substance. A is incorrect, as naltrexone is not the immediate treatment for ethylene glycol poisoning. It is used with alcohol use disorder to reduce cravings. C and D are incorrect, as formic acid is the toxic metabolite of methanol, which does not have the urinary findings shown. E and F are incorrect, as acetaldehyde is a byproduct of ethanol, not ethylene glycol, as described by the case.

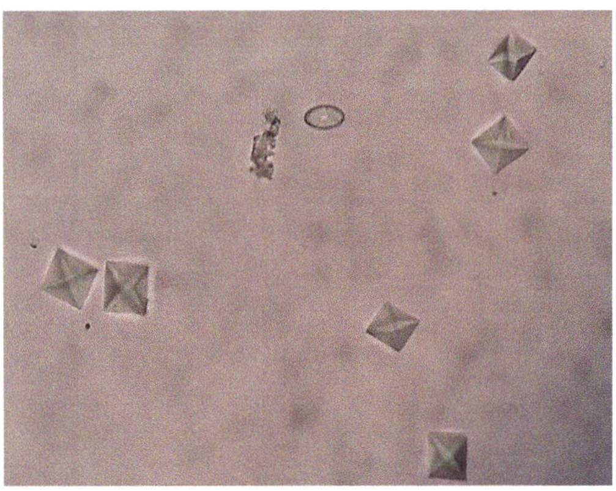

Fig. 28.17 Patient's urine sample under the microscope. Ajay Kumar Chaurasiya, CC BY-SA 4.0 https://creativecommons.org/licenses/by-sa/4.0, via Wikimedia Commons https://commons.wikimedia.org/wiki/File:Calcium_oxalate_crystals_in_Urine_Microscopy.jpg, https://upload.wikimedia.org/wikipedia/commons/4/4f/Calcium_oxalate_crystals_in_Urine_Microscopy.jpg

2. A patient presents to the emergency department after he was found ingesting "a bottle from his cabinet." Contrast the unique organ system that would most likely be affected if it were a methanol versus ethylene glycol ingestion.

Option	Methanol toxicity	Ethanol toxicity
A.	Ototoxicity	Kidney damage
B.	Retinal damage	Retinal damage
C.	Hemorrhage of the basal ganglia	Musculoskeletal damage
D.	Lung damage	Cardiac damage
E.	Retinal damage	Kidney damage
F.	Kidney damage	Musculoskeletal damage

Answer: E

Learning Objective #5: Illustrate the major physical exam findings associated with methanol ingestion and how they change over time. Contrast this with ethylene glycol ingestion symptoms.

Explanation: Methanol is known uniquely for the retinal damage it can cause, while ethylene glycol is known uniquely for the kidney damage it can cause. A is incorrect, as methanol is associated with retinal toxicity, not ototoxicity. B is incorrect, as methanol is only associated uniquely with retinal damage, but ethylene glycol is known uniquely for kidney damage. C is incorrect, as methanol is associated with hemorrhage of the basal ganglia, but ethylene glycol is known uniquely for kidney damage, not MSK damage. D is incorrect, as methanol is uniquely associated with retinal, not lung, damage. Ethylene glycol is associated with kidney damage, not cardiac. F is incorrect, as methanol is known to cause retinal damage, not kidney. Ethylene glycol is associated with kidney damage, not MSK.

3. A patient is brought into the emergency department after ingesting half a bottle of windshield wiper solution. She is expected to have methanol poisoning based on preliminary lab results. Evaluate what acid-base and plasma osmolal gap results you would expect.

Option	pH	HCO3 (mmol/L)	PCO2	NA (mEq/L)	K (mEq/L)	Cl (mEq/L)	Plasma Osmolal Gap (mOsm)
A.	7.30	24	55	140	4	100	35
B.	7.30	24	55	140	4	100	15
C.	7.27	20	32	140	4	110	35
D.	7.50	35	40	140	4	100	10
E.	7.20	15	32	140	4	110	15
F.	7.20	15	32	140	4	110	35

Answer: F

Learning Objective #2: Address what acid-base derangement occurs as a result of this toxicity and how plasma osmolal gap can be used to help interpret lab results.

Explanation: The lab values depicted in option F are consistent with a metabolic acidosis with an anion gap, as expected with methanol poisoning. In addition, the plasma osmolol gap is >25, which is expected. A is incorrect, as this depicts a respiratory acidosis with the PCO2 > 45, which is not expected with methanol poisoning, even though the plasma osmolal gap is greater than 25, which would be expected with methanol poisoning. B is incorrect, as this depicts a respiratory acidosis with the PCO2 > 45, which is not expected with methanol poisoning and the plasma osmolol gap is also <25, which is less likely. C is incorrect as this depicts a metabolic acidosis without an anion gap. Methanol poisoning, is expected to result in metabolic acidosis with an anion gap. The plasma osmolal gap is >25, which is expected. D is incorrect as this depicts a metabolic alkalosis. Methanol poisoning is expected to result in metabolic acidosis with an anion gap. The plasma osmolol gap is also <25, which is less likely. E is incorrect as This depicts a metabolic acidosis with an anion gap, as expected with methanol poisoning. However, the plasma osmolol gap is <25, which is less likely with the large amount of ingestion

References

1. Dr. Tom Fadial: Causes of Altered Mental Status #Diagnosis #EM #IM …, https://www.grepmed.com/images/935/alteredmentalstatus-differential-algorithm-diagnosis-ddxof.
2. Burket GA, Horowitz BZ, Hendrickson RG, Beauchamp GA. Endotracheal intubation in the pharmaceutical-poisoned patient: a narrative review of the literature. J Med Toxicol. 2021;17(1):61–9. https://doi.org/10.1007/s13181-020-00779-3. Epub 2020 May 11. PMID: 32394224; PMCID: PMC7785763.
3. About EMCrit: Diagnosis of metabolic acid-base disorders & Anion-gap metabolic acidosis, https://emcrit.org/ibcc/agma/
4. UpToDate, https://www.uptodate.com/contents/methanol-and-ethylene-glycol-poisoning-pharmacology-clinical-manifestations-and-diagnosis?search=ethylene%20glycol&source=search_result&selectedTitle=1~35&usage_type=default&display_rank=1
5. Brent J. Fomepizole for ethylene glycol and methanol poisoning. New England Journal of Medicine. 2009;360:2216–23. https://doi.org/10.1056/nejmct0806112.
6. About EMCrit: Ethylene glycol & methanol poisoning. https://emcrit.org/ibcc/alcohols/
7. Nov 7, 2005: What is the toxicity and treatment of ethylene glycol? Part II | Tennessee Poison Center | FREE 24/7 Poison Help Hotline 800.222.1222, https://www.vumc.org/poison-control/toxicology-question-week/nov-7-2005-what-toxicity-and-treatment-ethylene-glycol-part-ii
8. Uges D. Treatment of ethylene glycol and methanol poisoning: why ethanol? https://www.semanticscholar.org/paper/Treatment-of-ethylene-

glycol-and-methanol-poisoning-Uges/1211ff3cdaa7b8de5f148002d4c9f89782a25d24
9. Harrison's Manual of Medicine, 18th Ed. Chap 32: Poisoning and Drug Overdose Poisoning and Drug Overdose—Medical Emergencies—Harrisons Manual of Medicine, 18th Ed., https://doctorlib.org/medical/harrisons-manual-medicine/32.html
10. LaFollette R. Taming the SRU. https://www.tamingthesru.com/blog/diagnostics/toxic-alcohols
11. J3D3, CC BY-SA 4.0. https://creativecommons.org/licenses/by-sa/4.0, via Wikimedia Commons. https://upload.wikimedia.org/wikipedia/commons/6/67/Calcium_Oxalate_Detail.png
12. Yu C, Centers D. Suicide prevention: translating evidence into practice. Psychiatric Times. 33; (2016)
13. Méndez-Bustos P, Calati R, Rubio-Ramírez F, Olié E, Courtet P, Lopez-Castroman J. Effectiveness of psychotherapy on suicidal risk: a systematic review of observational studies. Front Psychol. 2019;10 https://doi.org/10.3389/fpsyg.2019.00277.

29 Sudden Disorientation

Andrew Albert

Learning Objectives

1. Describe the anatomy of the portocaval anastomotic network and identify related complications in the setting of portal hypertension.
2. Differentiate clinical signs related to hepatic failure from those related to portal hypertension. List their pathophysiological mechanism.
3. Describe common hematologic abnormalities seen in the setting of liver cirrhosis and elucidate the mechanism by which they occur.
4. Explain the medical and endoscopic treatment approach to patients with bleeding esophageal varices in the setting of cirrhosis.
5. Outline an approach to the resuscitation of an unstable patient with bleeding varices.
6. Discuss prophylactic management measures to decrease the incidence of bleeding in patients with known varices. Include an explanation of prophylaxis employed during a bleeding episode to reduce complications in the acute setting.
7. Describe types of Emergency Medical Services systems. Include an explanation of the various levels of training that EMTs receive and how it impacts the care they are able to provide pre-hospital.

A. Albert (✉)
Department of Emergency Medicine, New York University Langone Health, Brooklyn, NY, USA
e-mail: andrew.albert@nyulangone.org

Chief Complaint

A 45-year-old male presents to the emergency department via Emergency Medical Services (EMS) with altered mental status. The patient is a known alcoholic with a history of Hepatitis C and multiple ED visits for alcohol intoxication.

Additional HPI

He is confused but answers some questions appropriately. He nods his head "yes" when you inquire about recent abdominal pain and he also nods to indicate that he has been vomiting. The patient is unable to provide any further history secondary to altered mental status.

Prompt: What is your differential diagnosis?

Students should anchor their differential on altered mental status and abdominal pain. Patient should be presumed to have chronic liver disease.

Vascular: Hemorrhage secondary to bleeding esophageal varices, acute coronary syndrome
Infectious: Spontaneous bacterial peritonitis (SBP), CNS infections (meningitis, encephalitis, brain abscess)
Neoplastic: Hepatocellular carcinoma, intracranial neoplasm

C. A. Standley (ed.), *Biomedical Science and Clinical Foundations*,
https://doi.org/10.1007/978-3-031-98353-5_29

Drugs: Alcohol intoxication (EtOH and toxic alcohols), alcohol withdrawal syndrome, drug overdose, drug side-effect
Degenerative: Not applicable
Iatrogenic: Not applicable
Inflammatory: Non-infectious encephalitis
Congenital: Not applicable
Autoimmune: Not applicable
Trauma: Intracranial hemorrhage
Endocrine/Metabolic: Hepatic encephalopathy, hypoglycemia, uremia, thyrotoxicosis, myxedema coma, Cushing's syndrome

Another mnemonic to consider specifically for altered mental status is MOVE STUPID:

Metabolic
Oxygen
Vascular
Electrolyte/Endocrine

Seizure
Trauma/Toxin
Uremia
Psychiatric
Infection
Drugs/Withdrawal

Prompt: What other information would you like to obtain from your EMS squad and a review of the medical records?

- Past medical history
  - Important to ask specifically about liver disease status
- Any known ingestions
- By whom and why was EMS called

The Case Continues

The EMS-paramedic squad reports that they have "run" on the patient multiple times recently for alcohol intoxication. They stated that he seemed to be more altered than usual today. His wife called because he had been vomiting, had become progressively more confused, and was no longer easily aroused. EMS found the patient in his home surrounded by a puddle of dark-colored emesis (Fig. 29.1).

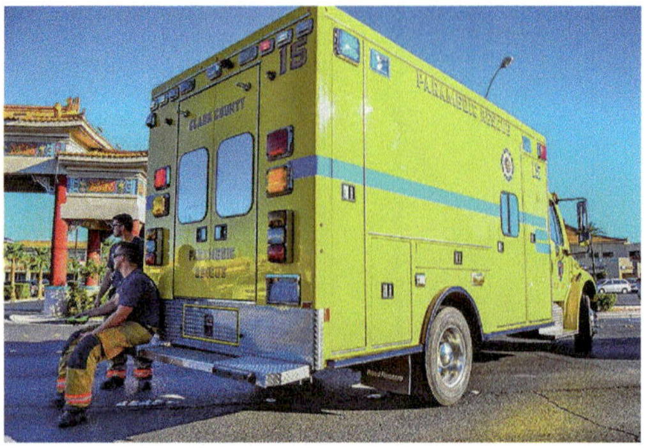

Fig. 29.1 EMS. (From Tomás Del Coro from Las Vegas, Nevada, USA, licensed under CC BY-SA 2.0). (https://creativecommons.org/licenses/by-sa/2.0, via Wikimedia Commons https://commons.wikimedia.org/wiki/File:Clark_County_Paramedic_Rescue_15_%2835247940061%29.jpg)

Past Medical History
- (Obtained from chart review)
- Chronic Hepatitis C
- Alcohol use disorder

Medications
- None currently

Allergies
- NKDA

Social History

Positive for heavy alcohol use and remote history of IV drug use

Review of Systems

Unable to be obtained secondary to altered mental status

Prompt: How does this change your differential diagnosis?

Chronic liver disease and related pathologies should be raised to the top of the differential.

- Consider GI bleed, hepatic encephalopathy, SBP (spontaneous bacterial peritonitis)

Physical Exam

Vitals: T 99.3 °F, P 109, R 18, SpO_2 97% on RA, BP 100/65

General: Somnolent but arouses to painful stimuli, confused, cachectic appearance

HEENT: Conjunctiva pale, mucus membranes are dry, there is dried dark-colored emesis evident on the patient's beard

Neck: No JVD, no thyroidmegaly

Chest: Decreased breath sounds bilateral bases, lungs otherwise clear and symmetric

Cardiac: Tachycardic, regular rate. No murmurs/rubs/gallops

Abdomen: Distended, bowel sounds decreased, no appreciable fluid wave, minimally tender diffusely, no localizing tenderness

Extremities: There is a pink discoloration of the skin of his palms, there are multiple enlarged tortuous appearing superficial veins over the upper chest and extremities (spider angiomas)

Neurologic: Somnolent, arouses to painful stimuli, unable to cooperate with formal neurologic testing

Prompt: What additional physical examination should be performed?

Rectal examination to evaluate for gross blood or melena. Guaiac testing for occult GI bleed should also be considered.

Physical Exam Continued

Digital rectal examination: Performed with RN chaperone present. No gross blood. Dark tarry stools noted consistent with melena. No mass or tenderness.

Prompt: How does the information you obtained from your physical exam change your differential diagnosis?

Students should rank all causes of GI bleeding higher on the differential. Facilitator should encourage discussion of upper vs. lower GI bleed and how physical exam findings suggest one over the other. Briefly, melena is more likely to be a sign of upper GI bleeding as the heme moieties becomes oxidized as it passes through the GI tract changing the color to a dark red/maroon, whereas gross red blood (hematochezia) would be more suggestive of lower GI bleeding.

Prompt: What laboratory tests and additional diagnostics would you like to order based on your differential diagnosis?

Labs: Finger stick blood glucose, CBC, type and cross match, BMP, hepatic panel, PT/INR, ammonia.

This list has been curtailed to focus the students on work up of a GI bleed. A broader workup for the many additional causes of altered mental status may be considered in clinical practice. This might include EKG and troponin to rule out acute coronary syndrome, toxicology labs to rule out ingestions, CT brain to rule out intracranial hemorrhage, blood cultures and urinalysis as well as Chest X-ray to evaluate for any infectious precipitant of altered mentation, etc.

Laboratory Findings

CBC	Result	Reference range (USMLE)
WBC	9500/mm^3	4500–11,000/mm^3
Hemoglobin	7 g/dL	Male: 13.5–17.5 g/dL
Hematocrit	21%	Male: 41%–53%
MCV	82 fL	80–100 fL
Platelet count	94,000/mm^3	150,000–400,000/mm^3
Segmented neutrophil	61%	54–62%
Bands	5%	3–5%
Lymphocytes	30%	25–33%
Monocyte	3%	3–7%
Eosinophil	1%	1–3%
Basophil	0%	0–1%
Blood type	A+	n/a

Prompt: Interpret the complete blood count (CBC) findings.

Depressed hemoglobin, hematocrit, and platelet levels. Patient has a normocytic anemia likely secondary to blood loss. Note that in acute blood loss a normocytic anemia or even normal hemoglobin may be seen as the hemoglobin lab value 'lags' behind the patient's blood loss. Chronic blood loss eventually leads to iron deficiency and a microcytic anemia, which might be seen in chronic blood loss from colorectal cancer, for instance. Additionally, thrombocytopenia is often seen in chronic liver disease. (Learning objective #3)

Additional Laboratory Results

BMP	Result	Reference range (USMLE)
Sodium (Na^+)	136 meq/L	136–145 mEq/L
Potassium (K^+)	3.5 meq/L	3.5–5.0 mEq/L
Chloride (Cl^-)	103 meq/L	95–105 mEq/L
Bicarbonate (HCO_3^-)	23 meq/L	22–28 mEq/L
Blood urea nitrogen (BUN)	39 mg/dL	7–18 mg/dL
Creatinine	1.2 mg/CL	0.6–1.2 mg/dL
Glucose	73 mg/dL	70–110 mg/dL

Prompt: Interpret the basic metabolic panel (BMP) results.

Note elevated BUN:Cr ratio >30, which may be seen in cases of upper GI bleed in patients without pre-existing renal disease.

The physician suspects the patient has signs and symptoms of liver disease and thus, orders a liver panel as well as coagulation studies.

Hepatic function panel	Result	Reference range (USMLE)
Albumin	3.0 g/dL	3.5–5.5 g/dL
Alkaline phosphatase	25 U/L	20–70 U/L
Alanine aminotransferase (ALT)	16 U/L	8–20 U/L
Aspartate aminotransferase (AST)	10 U/L	8–20 U/L
Bilirubin: total	1.2 mg/dL	0.1–1.0 mg/dL
Bilirubin: direct	0.2 mg/dL	0.0–0.3 mg/dL
Protein	5.6 g/dL	6.0–7.8 g/dL
Ammonia	25 μmol/L	20-65 μmol/L
Additional hematologic		

Hepatic function panel	Result	Reference range (USMLE)
Partial thromboplastin time, activated (PTT)	45 s	25–40 s
Prothrombin time (PT)	20 s	11–15 s
INR	2.0 s	0.9–1.1 s

Prompt: Interpret the hepatic function panel and the coagulation study results.

Findings are overall consistent with cirrhosis. For instance, low aminotransferase values suggests that there are few surviving functional hepatocytes in the cirrhotic liver (note, that while still in the normal range, the value is low for what you would expect a patient with chronic liver disease to have). Decreased hepatic synthetic function is evidenced by low albumin (and total protein) as well as coagulopathy with elevated INR. Ammonia within reference range makes hepatic encephalopathy less likely, although this diagnosis is primarily made on clinical grounds and ammonia within reference range does not definitively exclude this diagnosis.

Prompt: What is your provisional diagnosis for this patient?

GI Bleed, likely upper. Liver cirrhosis.

Prompt: What is the most likely cause of this patient's GI bleeding?

This should stimulate discussion of GI bleed in chronic liver disease. This patient likely has an upper GI bleed based on the history reported by EMS and findings on physical exam. In the setting of cirrhosis, the upper GI bleed is most likely secondary to bleeding esophageal varices, consistent with advanced cirrhosis. Other common causes of upper GI bleeding include Mallory-Weiss tear, gastritis, peptic ulcer disease, Dieulafoy lesion, ateriovenous malformation (AVM), etc.

Prompt: The patient remains minimally responsive. His blood pressure is 90/50 and pulse is 110.

Is this patient in shock?

Yes. This patient is in hemorrhagic shock. Students should be able to identify that the abnormal vital signs in combination with evidence of

Class of haemorrhagic shock				
	I	II	III	IV
Blood loss (mL)	Up to 750	750 – 1500	1500 – 2000	> 2000
Blood loss (% blood volume)	Up to 15	15–30	30–40	> 40
Pulse rate (per minute)	< 100	100–120	120–140	> 140
Blood pressure	Normal	Normal	Decreased	Decreased
Pluse pressure (mm Hg)	Normal or increased	Decreased	Decreased	Decreased
Respiratory rate (per minute)	14–20	20–30	30–40	>35
Urine output (mL/hour)	>30	20–30	5–15	Negligible
Central nervous system/ mental status	Slightly anxious	Mildly anxious	Anxious, confused	Confused, lethargic

Fig. 29.2 Classification of hemorrhagic shock. (https://lifeinthefastlane.com/wp-content/uploads/2011/06/Class-of-haemorrhagic-shock-JPEG2.jpg)

end-organ damage (altered mental status) suggest that this patient is in shock. According to the classical stages of hemorrhagic shock taught in advanced trauma life support (ATLS) (Fig. 29.2), this patient would be classified as being in stage two or three of hemorrhagic shock.

Prompt: What initial treatment directed at stabilizing this patient would you like to initiate?

Students may discuss initial volume resuscitation with IV fluids or blood products. Either would be a reasonable immediate approach, although this patient will likely ultimately need a blood transfusion.

The Case Continues

The patient receives 30 cc/kg of IV Lactated Ringers solution and BP improves minimally to 100/60. You call the blood bank at your hospital to request preparations to be made for a blood transfusion.

Prompt: What kind of blood can this patient receive while you are waiting for type-matched blood to arrive?

Type-matched blood refers to blood that has been matched to the patient's blood type based on laboratory testing methods. The traditional universal donor that this patient may receive prior to type-matched blood becoming available is blood type O, Rh negative (note that blood type O, Rh positive blood may be used for emergency transfusions in adult male patients whereas female patients of childbearing age must receive blood type O, Rh negative products).

Prompt: In addition to blood transfusion, what additional medications should be given to this patient with presumed bleeding esophageal varices and liver cirrhosis?

Patients with acute variceal bleeds should receive IV octreotide (somatostatin analogue whose mechanism of action is to reduce splanchnic blood flow thereby potentially reducing rate of hemorrhage). In the setting of cirrhosis, patients with upper GI bleeding should also receive antibiotics (typically ceftriaxone) to prophylaxis against spontaneous bacterial peritonitis and gut translocation of bacteria into the bloodstream. Available evidence supports that antibiotic administration in variceal GI bleeding is the most effective treatment to reduce mortality in this patient population outside of resuscitation and hemorrhage control.

Prompt: What are the definitive management options for this patient's condition?

Endoscopic interventions such as banding, ligation, and sclerotherapy are invasive options to identify and treat any actively bleeding lesions.

Prompt: What emergency measures can be taken to temporarily achieve hemorrhage control while awaiting definition management?

A Sengstaken-Blakemore tube or Minnesota tube may be placed in an attempt to temporarily tamponade upper GI bleeding. Note that the patient usually requires a definitive airway to be established (placement of endotracheal tube) prior to placement of either of these devices.

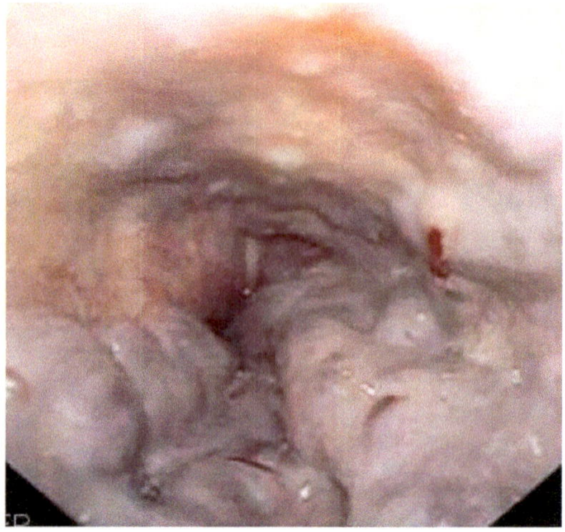

Fig. 29.3 Endoscopic view of esophageal varices. (https://commons.wikimedia.org/wiki/File:Esophageal_varices_-_wale.jpg)

Next Steps

The patient's vitals are P 95 and BP 110/65 after you administer 2 L of IV fluids and two units of packed RBCs. He also receives IV octreotide and ceftriaxone while in the emergency department. The gastroenterology service is consulted for the next steps in management. The patient is ultimately transferred to the endoscopy suite where GI performs emergent endoscopic ligation of two actively bleeding esophageal varices in the distal esophagus (Fig. 29.3).

End of Case

Learning Objective Answers

Learning Objective #1: Describe the anatomy of the portocaval anastomotic network and identify related complications in the setting of portal hypertension.

The portocaval anastomotic network is a series of connections between the venous blood supply of the liver (portal venous blood vessels) and that of the systemic circulation (caval venous network) (Fig. 29.4). The portal venous system is the destination for the majority of the intestinal venous drainage. In brief, the union of the superior mesenteric vein with the splenic vein forms the portal vein. The inferior mesenteric vein joins the splenic vein prior to its confluence with the superior mesenteric vein. Portal hypertension is defined as a hepatic-portal venous pressure gradient greater than 6 mmHg [1]. Cirrhosis is the most common cause of portal hypertension in the United States. Alternative causes of portal hypertension include right-sided heart failure, hepatic or portal venous thromboembolism, and Budd-Chiari syndrome to name a few.

Portal hypertension results in the reversal of the normal blood flow through the portal system, which results in a reversal of flow and congestion in the vessels that feed the portal vein. In the setting of portal hypertension, some of the intestinal blood flow is selectively shunted away from the normal route of the portal vein and instead returns to the systemic system via a series of portocaval anastomoses (Fig. 29.5). This anastomotic network includes the esophageal, rectal, periumbilical, retroperitoneal, and intrahepatic vessels. Reversal of blood flow through this anastomotic network may lead to a variety of complications such as esophageal varices, internal hemorrhoids, and a caput medusae (visible engorgement of superficial epigastric veins on the anterior abdominal wall). As evidenced by this case, esophageal varices can rupture and lead to life-threatening hemorrhage.

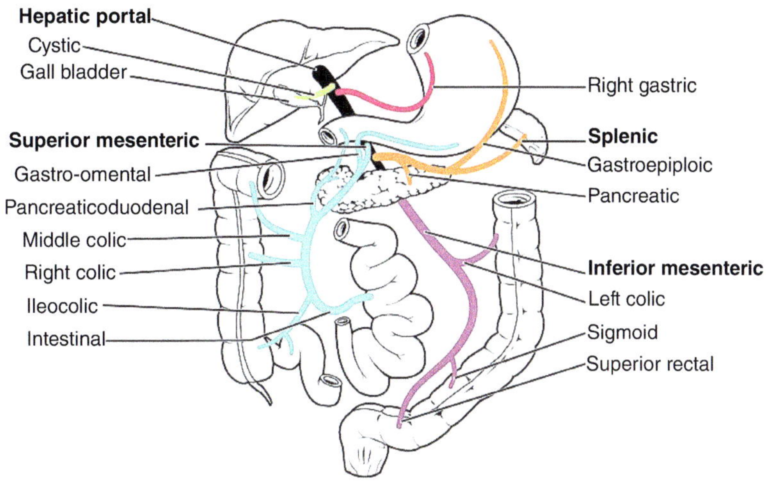

Fig. 29.4 Portal venous system and splanchnic venous system. (https://commons.wikimedia.org/wiki/File:2138_Hepatic_Portal_Vein_System.jpg)

Learning Objective #2: Differentiate clinical signs related to hepatic failure from those related to portal hypertension. List their pathophysiological mechanism.

There are a variety of clinical signs that can be seen in chronic liver disease. Generally, signs are related either to liver failure itself or to portal hypertension. (italic show what this patient has)

Findings related to hepatic failure	
Sign	Pathophysiology
Palmar erythema (red-pink discoloration of palms)	Elevated circulating levels of estrogen
Jaundice	Decreased excretion of bilirubin
Encephalopathy	Decreased hepatic excretion of ammonia
Pitting edema/anasarca	Decreased synthesis of albumin leads to decreased capillary oncotic pressure
Gynecomastia	Decreased degradation of estrogen
Spider angiomas	Decreased degradation of estrogen
Asterixis	Mechanism unclear
Coagulopathy	Decreased synthesis of coagulation factors

Findings related to portal hypertension	
Sign	Pathophysiology
Splenomegaly	Increased splenic blood flow
Caput medusae	Increased flow through superficial epigastric veins
Esophageal varices	Increased flow through esophageal vessels
Hemorrhoids	Increased flow through rectal venous plexus
Ascites	Due to hypoalbuminemia in addition to being a direct result of portal hypertension

Learning Objective #3: Describe common hematologic abnormalities seen in the setting of liver cirrhosis and elucidate the mechanism by which they occur.

Cirrhosis leads to a “rebalancing” of the normal hemostatic mechanisms. Patients with cirrhosis may have abnormalities in all of the major stages of hemostasis including primary hemostasis (platelet activation and adhesion), secondary hemostasis (generation of a stable cross-linked fibrin clot), and fibrinolysis (degradation of cross-linked fibrin clots). In addition to deficiencies in thrombogenesis, patients with cirrhosis may also have prothrombotic defects. Standard coagulation tests do not reliably assess the myriads of hemostatic abnormalities seen in cirrhosis.

Coagulation factor defects: The liver is the site of production for the majority of the numbered coagulation factors (e.g., factors I, II, V, VII, IX, X, and XII) (Fig. 29.6). Notable exceptions include factor VIII, which is produced by blood vessel endothelial cells, and a portion of factor XIII produced by the bone marrow.

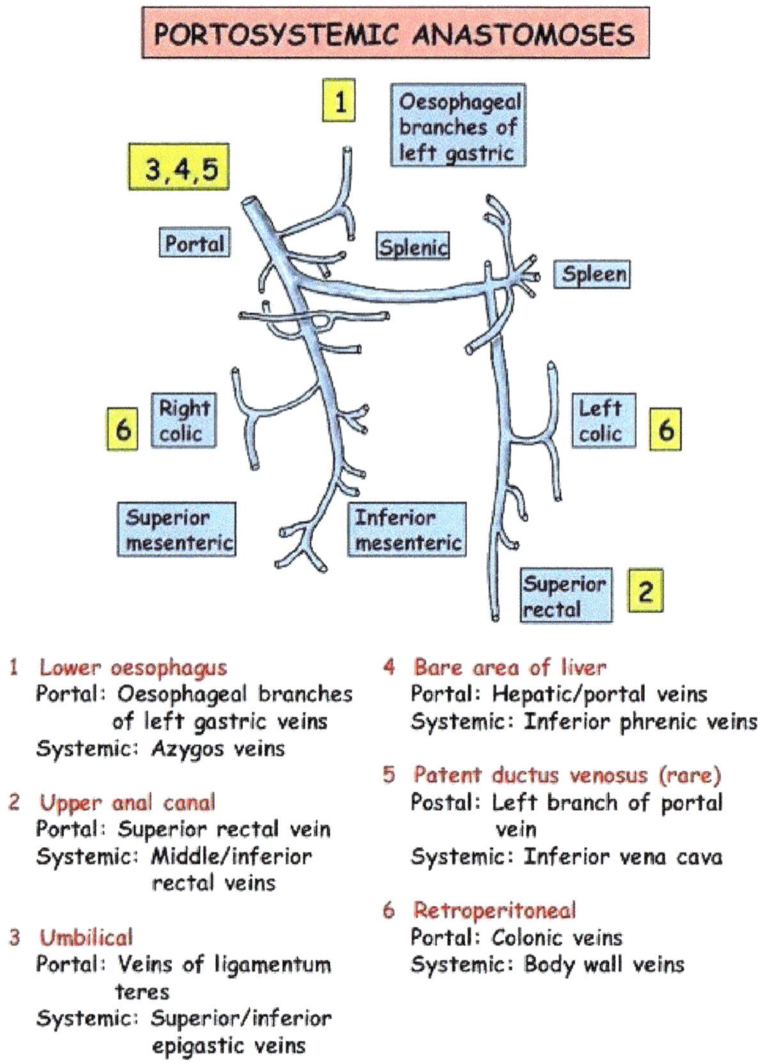

Fig. 29.5 Schematic of portosystemic anastomotic network. (https://i.pinimg.com/736x/40/cc/36/40cc36e6635b2f51403ef8f7947907e2.jpg)

Additionally, the liver is responsible for the post-translational modification of these proteins that renders them hemostatically active. Students should recall the Vitamin K-dependent coagulation factors that undergo gamma carboxylation in the liver including factors II, VII, IX, and X.

Thrombocytopenia: Patients with liver disease often exhibit varying degrees of thrombocytopenia. Proposed mechanisms include impaired production of platelets and decreased hepatic synthesis of thrombopoietin. Additionally, causes of chronic liver disease including Hepatitis C Virus and chronic alcohol abuse may independently suppress the bone marrow leading to thrombocytopenia. Patients with portal hypertension significant enough to result in splenomegaly may also have an element of splenic sequestration of platelets contributing to their thrombocytopenia.

Platelet dysfunction: In addition to quantitative platelet disorders, the platelets that are produced in patients with advanced liver disease often also have qualitative abnormalities. Impaired platelet function is due to coexisting uremia, prevalent endothelial abnormalities,

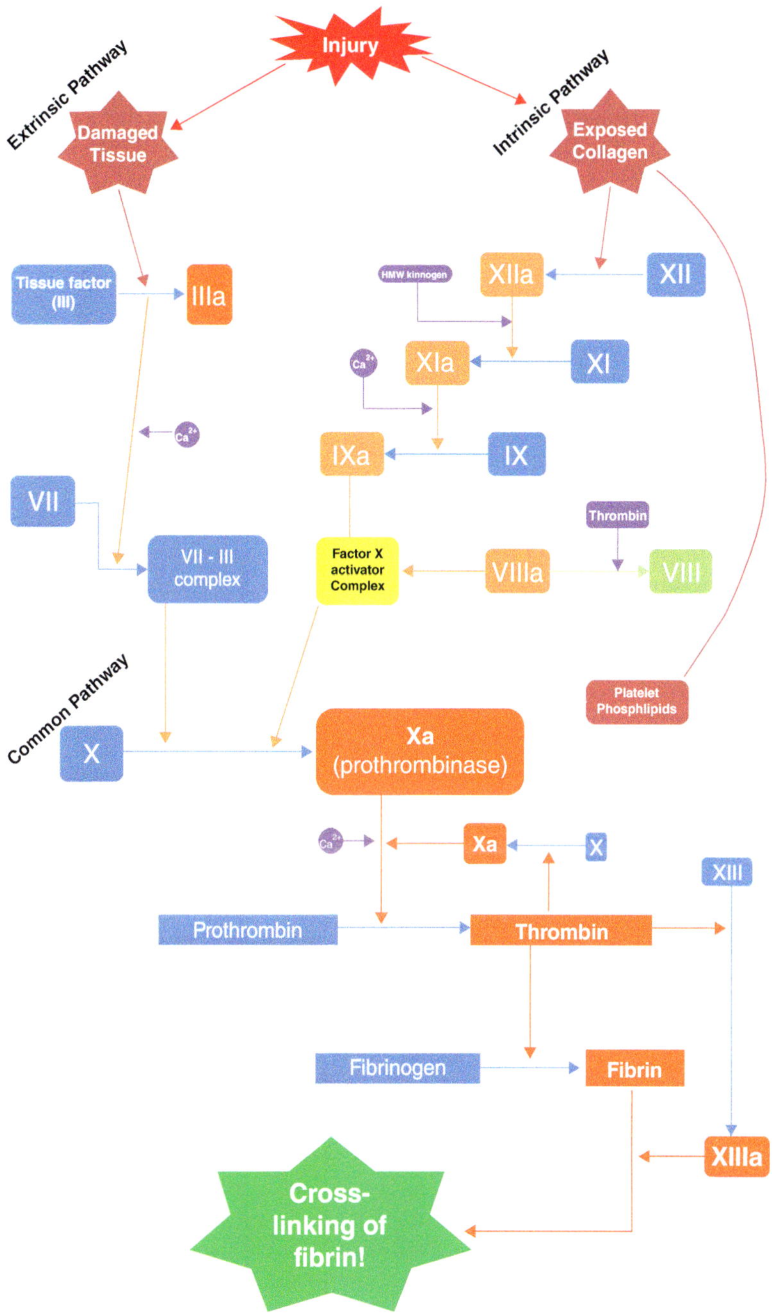

Fig. 29.6 Coagulation cascade. (https://almostadoctor.co.uk/encyclopedia/clotting-cascade; https://almostadoctor.co.uk/encyclopedia/clotting-cascade)

nitric oxide metabolism defects, and infections. Infectious causes range the spectrum from covert low-grade endotoxemia, which is estimated to have a prevalence as high as 30%, to overt sepsis.

Increased fibrinolysis: Hyperfibrinolysis seen in advanced liver disease promotes premature dissolution of mature clots and also impairs their formation in the first place due to the rapid turnover of clots. Possible mechanisms of hyperfibrinolysis in cirrhosis include increased levels of tissue plasminogen activator (tPA), decreased levels of alpha 2 antiplasmin, coagulation factor XIII, and elevated levels of fibrin breakdown products (e.g., D-dimer), which also interfere with coagulation.

Prothrombotic abnormalities: The liver, in addition to being the site of clotting factor production, also is responsible for producing inhibitors of coagulation such as protein C, protein S, and antithrombin. Advanced liver disease leads to a prothrombotic state through quantitative defects in coagulation inhibitors. Although patients with advanced liver disease will often have abnormalities in clotting laboratory studies such as increased aPTT and PT/INR, these results are often not reflective of the abnormal balance between procoagulants and anticoagulants in this patient population.

Learning Objective #4: Explain the medical and interventional treatment approach to patients with bleeding esophageal varices in the setting of cirrhosis.

Bleeding esophageal varices are a significant cause of mortality in patients with cirrhosis. It is estimated that variceal hemorrhage is responsible for approximately 1/3 of cirrhosis-related deaths. Furthermore, compared to other causes of upper GI bleeding, variceal hemorrhage is much more likely to require intervention to control hemorrhage as only 50% resolve without intervention. Treatment of acute variceal hemorrhage follows a three-pronged approach consisting of resuscitation, medical management, and definitive endoscopic therapies. The most immediate demand on the treating clinician is the need to perform rapid hemodynamic resuscitation of the actively bleeding patient (this should be covered in more detail in Learning Objective #5).

Medical management of acute variceal hemorrhage is primarily directed at reducing portal blood flow and thereby ameliorating the rate of hemorrhage. The vasoactive medications indicated for acute variceal hemorrhage include vasopressin, terlipressin, and somatostatin analogues such as octreotide. Although terlipressin (not available in the United States) is the only medication that has been shown to reduce mortality, the group of vasoactive medications as a whole has been shown to decrease morbidity and improve hemostasis. A recent meta-analysis demonstrated a decrease in seven-day mortality, transfusion requirement, and hospital length of stay with the use of vasoactive medications compared to placebo [2].

The mechanism through which vasopressin acts is via constricting of mesenteric arterioles thereby decreasing portal venous inflow. Vasopressin alone can achieve hemostasis initially in 60–80% of patients. However, there is a significant concern for complications associated with extrasplanchnic vasoconstriction with vasopressin use (e.g., myocardial, cerebral, and bowel ischemia), which limits its effective use in the United States. Terlipressin is a sustained-release synthetic analogue of vasopressin that carries less risk of extrasplanchnic vasoconstriction and similar hemostatic benefits as vasopressin; however, it is not available in the United States.

Octreotide is a somatostatin analogue that indirectly leads to splanchnic vasoconstriction and decreased portal flow by inhibiting the release of vasodilatory hormones such as glucagon. Octreotide is initially given as a 50 mcg bolus followed by a continuous infusion at 50 mcg/hr. The infusion is continued for 3–5 days to reduce the risk of immediate rebleeding. Its effects include rapid but short-lived decreases in portal flow, portal pressure, azygos flow, and intravariceal pressures. Initial hemostasis rate of treatment with octreotide is 63% when used alone and 100% in combination with endoscopic therapy. Although octreotide improves hemostatic measures, a mortality benefit has never been demonstrated with its use.

Interventional approaches to acute variceal hemorrhage management include balloon tamponade and endoscopic therapies (Fig. 29.7). The most commonly used balloons are the Sengstaken-Blakemore tube and the Minnesota tube. These measures are temporary; however, successful tamponade of bleeding lesions has been observed in 30–90% of cases in which they were utilized. Endoscopic treatments are the definitive treatment of choice for this condition. The goal time frame for endoscopy is within 12 h of the initial presentation. The initial endoscopic therapy of choice is

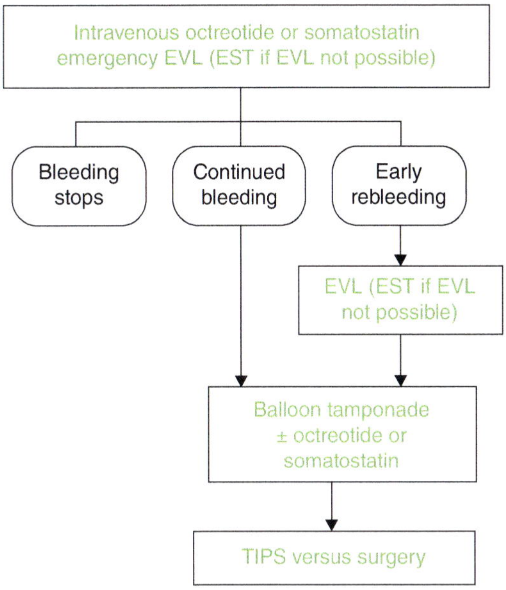

Fig. 29.7 Depiction of stepwise general treatment strategy for variceal bleeding. (https://www.uptodate.com/contents/image?imageKey=GAST%2F59327&topicKey=GAST%2F1260&source=outline_link)

endoscopic variceal ligation (EVL) in which small elastic bands are placed around the varix [3]. If EVL fails, endoscopists can utilize endoscopic sclerotherapy by injecting a sclerosant material directly into the lesion. Most studies report success rates of approximately 90% [4].

Learning Objective #5: Outline an approach to the resuscitation of an unstable patient with bleeding varices.

Recognition of patients in need of resuscitation is the first step in successfully caring for critically ill patients. In this case, the patient's hemodynamic compromise was suggested by his initial vital signs as well as the trajectory of his clinical course throughout the case. Shock, regardless of its form, can be simply defined as inadequate tissue perfusion to meet the demands of vital organs. Altered mental status in this case was a sign of end-organ damage from the patient's hemodynamic instability. We can therefore classify this patient as being in hemorrhagic shock based on his hemodynamic instability and signs of end-organ damage.

Initial resuscitation should focus on the A-B-C's (i.e., securing the airway, breathing, and circulation). It would be reasonable to perform endotracheal intubation in cases of massive hematemesis in an attempt to protect the airway; however, its utility in ameliorating aspiration risk is not entirely proven. Restoration of intravascular volume is critically important in patients with acute variceal bleeding. Intravenous access with two large bore peripheral IVs or intraosseous access would be most useful. If there is diagnostic uncertainty, it would be reasonable to initiate resuscitation with IV isotonic crystalloid solutions (i.e., normal saline or Lactated Ringers); however, these patients are hypovolemic from blood loss, and thus many authors would suggest that immediate replacement of blood products would be prudent. Blood loss should be replaced with packed red blood cells and clotting factors as needed with fresh frozen plasma (containing all coagulation factors). If coagulopathy cannot be corrected with the use of FFP alone, recent data have suggested a potential role for recombinant human factor VIIa [5]; however, the data regarding its potential benefits are mixed. Monitoring of platelet values is also important as some patients will have thrombocytopenia at presentation due to their liver disease and platelet counts are additionally anticipated to drop within 48 h of bleeding. Most sources suggest a platelet transfusion if values fall below 50,000/mm^3.

Monitoring resuscitative efforts is critical. This would generally involve placing the patient on cardiac monitoring with continuous pulse rate readings and frequent blood pressure checks. Resolution of tachycardia and improvement of blood pressure are encouraging signs of a successful resuscitation. Clinical signs that might suggest a successful resuscitation include improvement in mental status and evidence of improvement in peripheral perfusion.

Learning Objective #6: Discuss prophylactic measures to decrease the incidence of bleeding in patients with known varices. Include an explanation of prophylaxis employed during a bleeding episode to reduce complications in the acute setting.

The prevention of variceal hemorrhage can be achieved through a couple of mechanisms. Primary prophylaxis in this instance refers to the prevention of a first variceal bleed in patients with known varices. Available prophylactic measures include pharmacologic and endoscopic therapies. Nonselective beta-blockers are the mainstay of pharmacologic primary prophylaxis in patients with medium to large varices or advanced cirrhosis. Propranolol and nadolol are commonly utilized agents [6]. Nonselective beta blockers work to decrease portal blood flow by blocking the beta receptor-mediated adrenergic dilatory tone in mesenteric vessels. The resultant unopposed alpha-adrenergic activity leads to vasoconstriction and decreased flow through mesenteric vessels. A meta-analysis demonstrated that patients treated with beta-blockers had low rates of bleeding (12 vs. 23%) and fewer bleeding-related deaths (5 vs. 10%) compared to controls.

Endoscopic variceal ligation is an alternative to pharmacologic prophylaxis. Typical use of EVL is for patients who are intolerant or have contraindications to beta blockers. The data suggests that EVL is similarly effective in reducing the rate of first variceal hemorrhage to beta blockers; however, the invasiveness of the procedure and possible complications has generally rendered EVL a second-line therapy.

Prophylaxis during an acute variceal bleeding episode generally refers to the antibiotic use. Bacterial infections existing at the time of admission are evident in up to 20% of patients hospitalized with cirrhosis and an acute variceal bleeding episode. Furthermore, 50% will additionally develop an infection during the course of hospitalization. Common sites include the urinary tract, respiratory infections, bacteremia, and spontaneous bacterial peritonitis. Spontaneous bacterial peritonitis is defined as a bacterial infection of the ascitic fluid without an apparent source. Diagnosis is made by laboratory examination of aspirated ascitic fluid.

The prevalence of infections in this patient population and the increased mortality associated with them suggests a potential role for antibiotic prophylaxis [7]. A number of trials examining this question have indeed found an overall reduction in infectious complications and decreased mortality with antibiotic prophylaxis. There is data to suggest that the risk of recurrent bleeding may also be reduced by antibiotic use. The optimal choice of antibiotic agent and duration of therapy is unclear. The majority of studies utilized either a quinolone-class antibiotic (e.g., ciprofloxacin, ofloxacin, etc.) or cephalosporins (most commonly ceftriaxone in the United States). Ceftriaxone, with its broad spectrum of coverage, was shown to be superior to norfloxacin in a single randomized controlled trial. Most sources suggest 7 days of prophylactic coverage unless a focus of infection has been identified in which case treatment should be tailored to the identified infection. The American Association for the Study of Liver Diseases recommends short-term (<7d) antibiotic prophylaxis in patients with cirrhosis and GI hemorrhage with ciprofloxacin or ceftriaxone in patients with advanced cirrhosis or in areas with high rates of quinolone-resistant organisms.

Learning Objective #7: Describe types of Emergency Medical Services systems. Include an explanation of the various levels of training that EMTs receive and how it impacts the care they are able to provide pre-hospital.

The three most common forms of EMS are city or county, private, and volunteer [8]. The regional government usually operates City/County EMS systems. Advantages include integration into the fire department and the potential for an integrated dispatch system. Budget concerns are frequently cited as disadvantages of such a system. Private EMS companies, where they exist, generally provide some 911 coverage and are available for interfacility transport. However, they often do not operate 911 coverage if an EMS system run by the regional government is already in place. Job turnover tends to be higher in private EMS systems than government-run programs. Volunteer EMS is most often seen in rural communities. The scope of practice of volunteer EMS practitioners tends to be broader than in the aforementioned systems as distances between hospitals and transfer times are often greater in the rural setting.

The scope of practice for EMS providers spans first responders, Emergency Medical Technician-Basic (EMT-B), EMT-Intermediate (EMT-I), and EMT-P (EMT-Paramedic). Providers at each level of training have varying scopes of practice as detailed below (Table 29.1):

Exam Questions

1. A 45-year-old white male with a history of chronic alcohol use presents with hematemesis. On exam, vital signs are stable. The patient has hepatosplenomegaly but an otherwise nontender abdomen. The patient undergoes endoscopy and is diagnosed with bleeding esophageal varices. Endoscopic ligation of the vessel is unsuccessful. Creating an

Table 29.1 Scope of practice delineation for pre-hospital medical providers. https://www.uptodate.com/contents/image?imageKey=PEDS%2F78718&topicKey=EM%2F5796&rank=1~112&source=see_link&search=emergency%20medical%20services; https://www.uptodate.com/contents/image?imageKey=EM%2F83593&topicKey=EM%2F5796&rank=1~112&source=see_link&search=emergency%20medical%20services

Provider (current designation)	Provider (future designation)	Scope of practice
First responder	Emergency medical responder (EMR)	Ensure environment is safe to enter and provide care Gather initial history Appropriate physical examination Basic cardiopulmonary resuscitation Operate an automated external defibrillator Oxygen administration Provide bag-mask ventilation Administer unit dose auto-injectors (e.g. epinephrine) Provide manual C-spine and fracture stabilization Assist uncomplicated delivery of newborn
Emergency medical technician-basic (EMT-B)	Emergency medical technician (EMT)	As for first responder and: Access and extricate trapped victims Apply traction splint Perform spine immobilization (C-spine and backboard) Apply tourniquet Apply pneumatic antishock garment if indicated Irrigate eyes Provide basic burn management Administer limited types of oral medications (e.g. aspirin, glucose paste)
Emergency medical technician-intermediate (EMT-I)	Advanced emergency medical technician (AEMT)	As for first responder, EMT-B and: Insert esophageal-tracheal or multi-lumen airway Obtain peripheral IV and IO access Administer limited medications (e.g., nitroglycerine SL, IM or SC epinephrine, IV dextrose, IM or IV naloxone, IV fluids) Administer inhaled beta agonists
Emergency medical technician-paramedic (EMT-P)	Emergency medical technician-Paramedic (EMT-P)	As for first responder, EMT-B, EMT-I and: Orotracheal/nasotracheal intubation Surgical airway IV and IO access Chest decompression Advanced rhythm interpretation and manual defibrillation Synchronized cardioversion and transcutaneous pacing Comprehensive pharmacologic intervention Advanced newborn resuscitation

anastamosis between which of the following vessels would result in improvement in the patient's condition?

A. Splenic vein – Superior mesenteric vein
B. L testicular vein – L renal vein
C. Splenic vein – L renal vein
D. Portal vein – superior mesenteric vein
E. Azygos vein – R renal vein

Answer: C

Learning Objective: Describe the anatomy of the porto-caval anastamotic network and identify related complications in the setting of portal hypertension.

Explanation: Option C is a porto-caval anastamosis, which would allow decompression of the hepatoportal pressure gradient and cause resultant improvement in portal hypertension. A is incorrect, as this would be a portal-portal anastamosis. B is incorrect as this would be a caval-caval anastomosis. D is incorrect as this would be a portal-portal anastomosis. E is incorrect as this would be a caval-caval anastomosis.

2. A 50-year-old female with a history of IV drug use presents with hematemesis. She also has a long-standing history of Hepatitis C. On initial presentation vital signs are P 105 and BP 90/60. The patient receives two units of packed RBCs. The patient receives Octreotide in an attempt to control the hemorrhage. What is the mechanism by which this medication reduces portal hypertension?

   A. Inhibiting vasodilatory hormones thereby decreasing portal blood flow.
   B. Dilating mesenteric arterioles thereby decreasing portal venous inflow.
   C. Dilating lead renal vein thereby promoting increased flow in the splenic vein.
   D. Creation of a shunt between the hepatic and portal veins thereby decompressing portal venous pressure

Answer: A

Learning Objective: Explain the medical and endoscopic treatment approach to patients with bleeding esophageal varices in the setting of cirrhosis.

Explanation: Octreotide binds to somatostatin receptors and inhibits hormone secretion particularly vasodilatory hormones like glucagon while directly constricting the smooth muscle of the mesenteric blood vessels to reduce portal blood flow. B is incorrect as while vasopressin could be used to control hemorrhage, its mechanism of action is to constrict mesenteric arterioles to decrease portal venous inflow. C is incorrect as this describes the transjugular inhepatic portal shunt procedure (TIPS) and isn't how octreotide works. D is incorrect as dilation of the renal vein would not change splenic vein flow as the two vessels are not connected.

3. A 60-year-old male with a history of cirrhosis presents with hematochezia. He has no complaints of vomiting or hematemesis. He additionally has a history of diverticulitis. On exam his vital signs are stable and his abdomen is flat and nontender. In addition to standard resuscitative measures, the patient should additionally receive which of the following antibiotics as a prophylactic measure?

   A. Ceftriaxone
   B. Amoxicillin
   C. Nitrofurantoin
   D. Acyclovir

Answer: A

Learning Objective: Discuss prophylactic management measures to decrease incidence of bleeding in patients with known varices. Include an explanation of prophylaxis employed during an acute bleeding episode to reduce complications in the acute setting.

Explanation: The American Association for the Study of Liver Disease recommends a cephalosporin or ciprofloxacin for prophylaxis in cirrhotic patients with GI bleed. B and C are incorrect as these antibiotics would not provide an adequately broad spectrum of coverage in this case. D is incorrect as acyclovir is an antiviral medication, which would not prophylaxis against bacterial infections.

References

1. Sanyal AJ, Shiffman ML. The pharmacologic treatment of portal hypertension. Annu Rev Gastrointest Pharmacol. 1996;242
2. Wells M, Chande N, Adams P, et al. Meta-analysis: vasoactive medications for the management of acute variceal bleeds. Aliment Pharmacol Ther. 2012;35:1267.
3. Li L, Yu C, Li Y. Endoscopic band ligation versus pharmacological therapy for variceal bleeding in cirrhosis: a meta-analysis. Can J Gastroenterol. 2011;25:147.
4. Laine L, Cook D. Endoscopic ligation compared with sclerotherapy for treatment of esophageal variceal bleeding. A meta-analysis. Ann Intern Med. 1995;123:280.
5. Bendtsen F, D'Amico G, Rusch E, et al. Effect of recombinant Factor VIIa on outcome of acute variceal bleeding: an individual patient based meta-analysis of two controlled trials. J Hepatol. 2014;61:252.
6. Hayes PC, Davis JM, Lewis JA, Bouchier IA. Meta-analysis of value of propranolol in prevention of variceal haemorrhage. Lancet. 1990;336:153.
7. Chavez-Tapia NC, Barrientos-Gutierrez T, Tellez-Avila F, et al. Meta-analysis: antibiotic prophylaxis for cirrhotic patients with upper gastrointestinal bleeding – an updated Cochrane review. Aliment Pharmacol Ther. 2011;34:509.
8. http://www.ems.gov/education/EMSCoreContent.pdf (Accessed on September 19, 2017).

Additional Reading

9. https://www.uptodate.com/contents/general-principles-of-the-management-of-variceal-hemorrhage?source=history_widget#H10
10. https://www.uptodate.com/contents/methods-to-achieve-hemostasis-in-patients-with-acute-variceal-hemorrhage?source=history_widget#H62477588
11. https://www.uptodate.com/contents/primary-and-pre-primary-prophylaxis-against-variceal-hemorrhage-in-patients-with-cirrhosis?source=search_result&search=esophageal%20varices&selectedTitle=1~116#H4

Part XII

Anaphylaxis

30 Painful Sting

Cynthia A. Standley

Learning Objectives

1. Define anaphylaxis, its common triggers (e.g., food, medications, insect stings), and how it is different from other allergic reactions.
2. Recognize the signs and symptoms of anaphylaxis, including respiratory, cardiovascular, and skin manifestations.
3. Describe the fluid shifts that occurred in this patient because of her allergic reaction, and explain these in terms of oliguria, edema, dyspnea, and cyanosis.
4. Explain the determinants of vascular smooth muscle tone and the mechanism of action and side effects of the vasoactive substances used in this case.
5. Discuss the reflex mechanisms that maintain arterial blood pressure. Describe why pressure falls in this patient and what mechanisms are activated to return pressure to normal.
6. Describe the pathophysiology of the depressed myocardial function and ischemia in this patient and how an intra-aortic balloon pump helped remedy this situation.
7. Explain the importance of patient education regarding anaphylaxis triggers and emergency action plans. Advise patients on the proper use of epinephrine auto-injectors.

C. A. Standley (✉)
Department of Bioethics and Medical Humanism, University of Arizona College of Medicine-Phoenix, Phoenix, AZ, USA
e-mail: cstand@arizona.edu

Chief Complaint

I'm having trouble breathing after being stung by a bee.

Prompt: *What are you most concerned about?*

When someone is having trouble breathing after a bee sting, the most immediate concern is a life-threatening allergic reaction called anaphylaxis. This is a severe, potentially fatal allergic reaction that can cause difficulty breathing, swelling of the throat and tongue, hives, and a sudden drop in blood pressure. Time is critical with anaphylaxis, so fast action can save a life.

History of Present Illness

A 45-year-old female presents to the emergency room with a diffuse skin rash, dyspnea, cyanosis, and an audible wheeze. The patient had made an emergency visit to her physician's office after being stung by a bee. At the physician's office, the patient's pulse became imperceptible, and blood pressure declined to a point where it could not be recorded. EMS was called, and she received intramuscular and IV epinephrine, as well as hydrocortisone, during transport. She arrives at the ED with persistent dyspnea, cyanosis, wheezing, and a diffuse skin rash.

C. A. Standley (ed.), *Biomedical Science and Clinical Foundations*,
https://doi.org/10.1007/978-3-031-98353-5_30

Prompt: *Why were these drugs immediately administered?*

This patient is most likely experiencing an anaphylactic attack. Functionally, the patient is hypovolemic because a pulse is not detected. First line treatment for anaphylaxis is immediate intramuscular epinephrine [1] to stimulate cardiac beta-1 receptors and increase contractility of the heart, stimulate beta-2 receptors to cause bronchodilation, and stimulate alpha-2 receptors to cause vasoconstriction in periphery. Hydrocortisone is a glucocorticoid that is used to reestablish the integrity of capillary endothelium to prevent leakage of fluid. It is also inflammatory as it antagonizes histamine.

Past Medical History

History of prior bee sting sensitivity (previously sensitized)
No history of heart disease
No known chronic illnesses

Past Surgical History

No prior surgeries reported

Medications

None reported prior to this event
Received IV epinephrine, intramuscular epinephrine, and hydrocortisone en route to ED.

Allergies

Bee stings
No known drug allergies reported.

Family History

No known history of cardiovascular disease or anaphylaxis in family

Social History

Occupation: Botanist (high likelihood of recurrent bee exposure)
Non-smoker
No history of alcohol or drug use reported

Review of Systems

General: Acute distress, cyanosis present

Skin: Diffuse erythematous rash, possible urticaria

ENT: Possible oropharyngeal swelling; voice changes not reported

Neurological: No loss of consciousness reported, but may have experienced presyncope or altered mental status due to hypotension

Respiratory: Dyspnea, wheezing, stridor, increased respiratory effort

Cardiovascular: Hypotension, history of imperceptible pulse prior to EMS intervention

Gastrointestinal: No nausea, vomiting, or abdominal pain reported

Prompt: *What can you interpret from the review of systems and how does that help prioritize your differentials?*

The review of systems provides critical information that helps guide clinical prioritization and differential diagnoses. The primary diagnosis to consider here is anaphylaxis leading to anaphylactic shock. This is supported by history (bee sting), respiratory distress, hypotension, rash, and rapid onset. Other possible considerations (less likely but critical to rule out):

- Severe Asthma Attack**:** If the patient had a history of asthma, bronchospasm could have worsened post-sting. However, the acute hypotension is not typical of asthma alone.

- Acute Angioedema (hereditary or ACE-Inhibitor Related): Could mimic anaphylaxis but usually lacks urticaria and has a different triggering mechanism.
- Pulmonary Embolism: Hypotension + dyspnea is concerning, but no deep venous thrombosis (DVT) risk factors or sudden pleuritic chest pain.
- Toxic Shock Syndrome: Rapid cardiovascular collapse but no infectious source or prolonged exposure risk.

Physical Examination

General Appearance: Anxious, in severe respiratory distress; cyanotic, diaphoretic, and gasping for air; sitting upright, using accessory muscles to breathe

Vital Signs: Temp 98.6 °F (37 °C), HR 130 bpm, BP 80/59 mmHg, Resp rate 26 breaths/min, O_2 Sat 89%

HEENT: Swollen face and lips; possible conjunctival injection; edema of the tongue, soft palate, and possibly larynx; no obvious airway obstruction, no visible foreign body; no jugular venous distention

Skin: Diffuse urticaria across the trunk and extremities; cool, clammy skin

Cardiovascular: Normal S1, S2, presence of S3; no murmurs or pericardial rubs noted; pulses weak or thready; Capillary refill is prolonged, indicating poor perfusion.

Pulmonary: Decreased chest expansion; severe bronchospasm with wheezing bilaterally, hemoptysis, bilateral pulmonary rales; diminished breath sounds in lower field; no signs of pneumothorax

Abdomen: No distention; normal bowel sounds; soft, non-tender; no hepatosplenomegaly

Neurologic

- **Mental status:** Alert but anxious
- **Cranial nerves:** Normal
- **Motor & sensory:** No focal deficits
- **Reflexes:** Normal

Prompt: *Summarize the key exam findings and their importance.*

The heart rate is tachycardic, likely due to compensatory response to hypotension or epinephrine administration. Blood pressure is hypotensive due to anaphylactic shock. Respiratory rate is tachypneic with signs of respiratory distress. Hemoptysis (bloody sputum) is likely related to increased pulmonary capillary pressure, as these vessels (near the esophagus) may burst due to enhanced transmural pressure. Low oxygen saturation and cyanosis suggest hypoxia. Swollen face and lips indicate angioedema, extravasation of fluid from vessels into interstitial fluid (ISF). Cool, clammy skin suggests shock. Third heart sound (S3) suggests cardiac dysfunction or early pulmonary edema. Weak or thready pulses consistent with shock state. Capillary refill prolonged indicating poor perfusion. Bilateral pulmonary rales (crackles) suggest fluid leakage into alveoli (possible non-cardiogenic pulmonary edema). No signs of acute GI pathology.

This examination strongly supports anaphylaxis with airway compromise, shock, and possible pulmonary complications, demanding aggressive intervention.

Prompt: *Explain the significance of the third heart sound.*

The third heart sound (S3) occurs when blood enters the ventricle during the rapid filling phase due to decreased end systolic volume. [2] S3 occurs early in diastole, following opening of the AV valves. This sound is normal in children due to sound of chordae tendinea tightening and reflecting expansion of the chamber. However, in adults, this sound implies LV contractile dysfunction and indicates volume overload due to congestive heart failure.

Treatment

The patient was given promethazine intramuscularly. The patient was normotensive at the time of arrival, but she rapidly became hypotensive and oliguric. Aggressive treatment was initiated at this point.

Prompt: *What is promethazine?*

Antihistamine, anti H1 receptor, will eliminate hives and edema

EKG

Electrocardiogram showed widespread T wave inversion in Leads I, II, III, aVL, aVF, V5, and V6 and non-specific ST changes.

Prompt: *Interpret the EKG findings.*

T wave inversion in Leads II, III, and aVF indicates that the inferior aspect of the heart is affected, while T wave inversion in Leads I, aVL, V5 and V6 indicates that the lateral aspect of the heart is affected. [3] Thus, this patient is experiencing inferiorlateral myocardial ischemia. The T wave inversion is due to myocardial ischemia. Poor coronary artery perfusion and increased myocardial demand contribute to an ischemic heart condition. If the blood supply to the heart becomes insufficient, causing inadequate oxygen supply, an energy deficiency occurs. Unlike depolarization of the cardiac myocardium, which is largely passive, repolarization requires the expenditure of a great deal of cellular energy. Whether the T wave is upright or inverted depends on where the ischemia is. In normal hearts, repolarization begins in the epicardium and progresses toward the endocardium, producing a positive T wave. In subepicardial ischemia, there is a delay in the repolarization of the subendocardial cardiac cells. Because of this, repolarization begins at the endocardium and progresses in the reverse direction, from endocardium to epicardium, slowing when it reaches the ischemic area. This produces a prolonged QT interval and a symmetrically negative deep T wave. Inverted T waves produced by myocardial ischemia are classically narrow and symmetric.

Non-specific ST changes are very common. They tend to be elevated in the leads facing the zone of injury and depressed in opposite leads. Because this patient has two zones of injury, the ST changes are non-specific in determining the anatomic distribution of the injury.

Table 30.1 Course of Treatment in the Patient from Time of Admission

	Time from Admission (hours)						
	0	10	12^B	24	36	72^{B*}	Reference Value
Inotropic Agent	E	E + DB	E + DB	DB	DB	NE + DA	
MAP (mmHg)	75	78	80	80	80	60	90–100
Mean PAP (mmHg)	27	30	26	24	22	21	10–22
PCWP (mmHg)	14	24	18	16	16	18	6–15
CVP (mmHg)	8	15	12	12	10	11	6–8
CO (L/min)	4.5	3.0	3.0	4.7	4.65	5.0	4–6
HR (bpm)	150	140	125	115	115	90	60–100
SV (ml)	30	21.4	24.0	40.9	40.4	55.6	75–80
SVR (mmHg/L/min)	14.9	21.0	22.7	14.5	15.1	9.8	17
PVR (mmHg/L/min)	2.9	2.0	2.7	1.7	1.3	0.6	1–2
LVEF		0.15			0.29		55–75
pH	7.29	7.31		7.39			7.4
PO_2 (mmHg)	44	118		109			80–100
PCO_2 (mmHg)	25	32		39			33–44
HCO_3^- (mEq/L)	12	15		23			22–24
Hemoglobin (g/dL)	14			12		12	14–19

E epinephrine, *DB* dobutamine, *NE* norepinephrine, *DA* dopamine, *MAP* mean arterial pressure, *PAP* pulmonary artery pressure, *PCWP* pulmonary capillary wedge pressure, *CVP* central venous pressure, *CO* cardiac output, *HR* heart rate, *SV* stroke volume, *SVR* systemic vascular resistance, *PVR* pulmonary vascular resistance, *LVEF* left ventricular ejection fraction. ^{B}after insertion of the balloon, ^{B*}after removal of the balloon

Course of Treatment and Diagnostic Evaluation

Table 30.1 follows the hemodynamic and hematologic variables of this patient during the course of treatment.

The Case Continues

When the hypotension developed, the patient was administered crystalloid solutions and epinephrine infusions. The patient was intubated and ventilated with positive end-expiratory pressure. A pulmonary artery catheter was inserted, and a high-dose epinephrine infusion was continued to maintain blood pressure. Within 10 h after admission, respiratory function stabilized, but cardiovascular function continued to deteriorate. Two-dimensional echocardiography and radionuclide ventriculography confirmed profound myocardial dysfunction. Dobutamine was added with no improvement.

Prompt: *What is a cystalloid solution? How does this help the patient?*

Hypotension in anaphylaxis is due to a shift in intravascular volume, so aggressive fluid resuscitation is important. Crystalloid solutions (like saline or lactated Ringer's) are the preferred choice for this, as they are readily available and effective in restoring blood volume. Albumin or hypertonic solutions are not indicated [4].

The Case Continues

Just after 10 h postadmission, the patient was experiencing cardiovascular collapse. An intraaortic balloon pump was inserted to provide temporary circulatory support. Urine began to flow immediately at a rate in excess of 1 ml/kg/h. Twelve hours after balloon insertion, epinephrine treatment was discontinued, and the acidosis was resolved. The patient was extubated at 30 h, and the balloon was removed after 72 h. The patient was closely monitored for any complications and allowed to go home the following day.

End of Case

Learning Objective Answers

1. **Define anaphylaxis, its common triggers (e.g., food, medications, insect stings), and how it is different from other allergic reactions. Describe how being previously sensitized to an allergen can lead to anaphylaxis upon re-exposure.**

Anaphylaxis is a severe, potentially life-threatening allergic reaction that can occur rapidly, involving multiple body systems, and requires immediate medical attention. The immune system overreacts to a substance (allergen) it perceives as harmful, leading to the release of chemicals that cause a cascade of reactions.

Common triggers include foods. Peanuts, tree nuts, shellfish, milk, eggs, soy, wheat, and sesame seeds are common culprits. Certain medications, including antibiotics (like penicillin) and nonsteroidal anti-inflammatory drugs (NSAIDs), can trigger anaphylaxis in susceptible individuals. Insect venom from stings or bites from bees, wasps, hornets, and other stinging insects can cause anaphylaxis. Another common culprit is latex, found in gloves, balloons, and other products.

Anaphylaxis differs from other allergic reactions in that it is life-threatening. Other allergic reactions are typically milder and more localized. [1, 4, 5] Anaphylaxis develops rapidly, within minutes of exposure, affecting multiple body systems, while other allergic reactions may develop more slowly and are confined to a specific area such as the skin or airways. Mild allergic reactions might present with localized symptoms such as a runny nose or skin rash, whereas anaphylaxis can involve severe respiratory distress, cardiovascular collapse, and gastrointestinal symptoms. Allergic reactions can be treated over the counter with antihistamines and other medications, while anaphylaxis requires immediate medical attention. Recognizing these differences is crucial, as anaphylaxis requires immediate medical intervention to prevent fatal outcomes.

The patient in this case had a severe anaphylactic reaction to the venom in a bee sting after having previously been sensitized. This occurred via a two-step immunological process: sensitization followed by re-exposure to the allergen. [6, 7] Upon previously having been stung by a bee, components from the venom, such as phospholipase A_2, hyaluronidase, and melittin, enter the bloodstream. These proteins are recognized as foreign by the immune system, leading to the production of specific immunoglobulin E (IgE) antibodies. These IgE antibodies bind to high-affinity receptors (FcεRI) on the surface of mast cells and basophils, effectively "sensitizing" the individual to bee venom.

Upon the next bee sting, the previously formed venom-specific IgE antibodies on mast cells and basophils recognized and bound to the venom allergens. This cross-linking of IgE receptors triggered degranulation of these cells, releasing mediators such as histamine, leukotrienes, and prostaglandins. These substances caused vasodilation, increased vascular permeability, bronchoconstriction, and other systemic effects characteristic of anaphylaxis.

2. **Recognize the signs and symptoms of anaphylaxis, including respiratory, cardiovascular, and skin manifestations.**

Recognizing the signs and symptoms of a life-threatening anaphylaxis episode across various systems is crucial for prompt intervention. [4] Most immediate is the recognition of bronchoconstriction, which causes shortness of breath, wheezing, and tightness in the chest. Swelling of the throat (angioedema) and tongue can lead to hoarseness, stridor (a high-pitched, wheezing sound), and difficulty swallowing, potentially progressing to complete airway obstruction. Cardiovascular manifestations include the heart beating faster in response to low blood pressure. This is recognized by a rapid pulse. The significant drop in blood pressure is due to widespread vasodilation and can lead to the signs of dizziness, light-headedness, or loss of consciousness. Raised, itchy welts on the skin are common in an anaphylactic reaction. Recognizing these symptoms is vital for the timely administration of treatments, such as epinephrine, to prevent progression and potentially fatal outcomes.

3. **Describe the fluid shifts that occurred in this patient as a result of her allergic reaction, and explain these in terms of oliguria, edema, dyspnea, and cyanosis.**

Fluid extravasation can be significant in the patient with anaphylaxis. [7] The initial perturbation of fluid balance in this patient was the histamine-induced loss of capillary integrity and histamine-bradykinin-induced vasodilation. The pores between the capillary endothelial cells become enlarged, allowing large proteins (most notably albumin) to leak from the vascular space into the interstitial fluid (ISF). Water follows in the same direction. This causes two things:

- ISF hydrostatic pressure increases as a result of the fluid leak and vasodilation.
- ISF oncotic pressure increases as a result of the protein leak.

As the ISF oncotic pressure increases, more fluid leaks, and the cycle repeats. Therefore, the major fluid shift is from the plasma to the ISF.

Additionally, as plasma oncotic pressure decreases (i.e., proteins are escaping to the ISF), water will start to shift from erythrocytes (presumably still trapped within the compromised capillary) into the plasma space in order to reestablish isosmotic compartments. This is a minor compensatory mechanism.

As far as the clinical signs and symptoms are concerned, oliguria means decreased urine output. This occurs as vascular volume becomes so depressed that arterial blood pressure falls tremendously. Such low perfusion pressure signals renal perfusion to slow (eventually it will cease). Autoregulation fails, and the kidneys stop producing urine.

Edema is due to the increase in ISF volume. This occurs for reasons described above. In addition, lymphatic recycling cannot keep pace with fluid leakage into the ISF for two reasons:

- ISF volume increases to a point where lymphatic pumping is less than needed even if the lymphatic vessels are patent, and
- The lymphatic vessels are squeezed shut (i.e., lymphatic vessel transmural pressure approaches 0 mmHg) because of the tremendous ISF pressure.

Dyspnea, the subjective difficulty of breathing, occurs in this patient because of the following:

- Cardiac output from the right heart is compromised due to depressed functional plasma volume. In the face of low pulmonary perfusion, there is less oxygenation of blood.
- Systemic and exogenous vasoconstrictors are attempting to vasoconstrict pulmonary arterioles (her PAP is increased, Table 30.1).
- Pulmonary alveolar hypoxia will further vasoconstrict pulmonary arterioles.
- Pulmonary edema decreases pulmonary capillary/arterial transmural pressure, forcing them closed.
- Bronchoconstriction is present.

Cyanosis occurs because of deficient oxygenation of blood due to depressed pulmonary perfusion.

4. **Explain the determinants of vascular smooth muscle tone and the mechanism of action of endogenous vasoactive substances such as catecholamines and histamine.**

Vascular smooth muscle tone determines the degree of constriction or dilation of blood vessels. It is regulated by various factors, including intracellular calcium levels, membrane potential, and the influence of endogenous vasoactive substances such as catecholamines and histamine. [8] The contraction of vascular smooth muscle cells (VSMCs) is primarily driven by the concentration of intracellular calcium ions (Ca^{2+}). An increase in intracellular Ca^{2+} binds to calmodulin, activating myosin light chain kinase (MLCK), which phosphorylates myosin light chains, leading to muscle contraction. Conversely, a decrease in intracellular Ca^{2+} results in muscle relaxation.

The membrane potential of VSMCs influences the opening and closing of voltage-dependent calcium channels (VDCCs). Depolarization of the membrane opens VDCCs, allowing Ca^{2+} influx and promoting contraction.

Hyperpolarization closes these channels, reducing Ca^{2+} entry and causing relaxation. Various ion channels, including potassium channels, play a crucial role in setting and regulating membrane potential, thereby affecting vascular tone.

Catecholamines (epinephrine, norepinephrine) bind to adrenergic receptors on VSMCs, leading to different responses. Activation of alpha-1 adrenergic receptors causes vasoconstriction by increasing intracellular Ca^{2+} through the phospholipase C pathway. Activation of beta-2 adrenergic receptors leads to vasodilation by increasing cyclic AMP (cAMP), which inhibits MLCK, resulting in muscle relaxation. The overall effect of catecholamines on vascular tone depends on the distribution and density of these receptor subtypes in different vascular beds.

Histamine's effects contribute to the regulation of vascular tone during inflammatory responses and allergic reactions. Histamine binds to histamine receptors on VSMCs and endothelial cells. Activation of histamine H1 receptors on endothelial cells leads to the release of nitric oxide (NO), causing vasodilation. Activation of histamine H2 receptors on VSMCs increases cAMP, leading to relaxation.

The regulation of vascular smooth muscle tone by these endogenous substances directly impacts fluid balance. Vasoconstriction increases vascular resistance and blood pressure, while vasodilation decreases resistance and blood pressure. During anaphylactic reactions, massive histamine release leads to widespread vasodilation and increased vascular permeability, resulting in fluid shifting from the intravascular to the interstitial space, causing hypotension and edema. Thus, understanding the mechanisms controlling vascular tone is essential for comprehending the fluid dynamics observed in this pathological condition.

5. **Discuss the reflex mechanisms that maintain arterial blood pressure. Discuss why pressure falls in this patient and what mechanisms are activated to return pressure to normal**.

Arterial blood pressure is meticulously regulated by a combination of neural and hormonal mechanisms to ensure adequate tissue perfusion. The primary reflex mechanism maintaining arterial blood pressure is the baroreceptor reflex, a rapid negative feedback loop involving stretch-sensitive mechanoreceptors in the carotid sinus and aortic arch that adjust heart rate and blood vessel tone to maintain stable blood pressure. [9] An increase in blood pressure stretches these receptors, increasing their firing rate, which signals the brainstem's cardiovascular control center to reduce sympathetic outflow and enhance parasympathetic activity, leading to vasodilation and a decrease in heart rate and contractility and ultimately a reduction in blood pressure to restore it back to normal. The reverse of this process happens when blood pressure drops. The baroreceptor reflex is a rapid mechanism that provides short-term adjustments to blood pressure in response to sudden changes, such as standing up or exercising.

While the baroreceptor reflex is the primary short-term mechanism, other reflexes, such as the chemoreceptor reflex (sensitive to changes in blood oxygen and carbon dioxide levels) and the Bainbridge reflex (responds to changes in atrial stretch), also contribute to blood pressure regulation. Peripheral chemoreceptors in the carotid and aortic bodies respond to hypoxia, hypercapnia, and acidosis by stimulating respiratory centers and sympathetic pathways, leading to increased ventilation and vasoconstriction to maintain oxygen delivery and blood pressure.

Long-term blood pressure regulation is influenced by factors like blood volume, kidney function, and hormonal systems, such as the renin-angiotensin-aldosterone system (RAAS). The RAAS responds to decreased renal perfusion by releasing renin, which catalyzes the formation of angiotensin II, a potent vasoconstrictor. Angiotensin II elevates blood pressure by increasing systemic vascular resistance and stimulating aldosterone secretion, promoting sodium and water retention to augment blood volume and thus blood pressure.

In anaphylaxis, these regulatory systems are challenged [9, 10]. Anaphylaxis triggers a rapid release of mediators from mast cells and basophils, leading to vasodilation and increased vascular permeability, reducing systemic vascular resistance and arterial blood pressure. In response to hypotension during anaphylaxis, the body initiates compensatory mechanisms. Decreased arterial pressure reduces baroreceptor firing, enhancing sympathetic outflow, which increases heart rate and peripheral vasoconstriction. The adrenal medulla secretes epinephrine and norepinephrine to support vasoconstriction. Reduced renal perfusion stimulates renin release, leading to angiotensin II production and aldosterone secretion, promoting vasoconstriction and sodium and water retention to restore blood volume. In summary, while the body employs several reflex mechanisms to maintain arterial blood pressure, the overwhelming mediator release during anaphylaxis can surpass these compensatory responses, leading to significant hypotension that often requires prompt medical treatment.

6. **Describe the pathophysiology of the depressed myocardial function and ischemia in this patient and how an intra-aortic balloon pump helped remedy this situation.**

Bee sting venom allergies are primarily considered a Type I hypersensitivity reaction, mediated by venom allergen-specific IgE antibodies. [11] The allergen induced massive vasodilation, which decreased vascular functional volume and thus cardiac output, inducing a relative hypovolemia. [7] The decreased vascular functional volume also decreased peripheral vascular resistance, which then decreased arterial blood pressure. This decreased perfusion pressure to the coronary arteries, causing myocardial ischemia and contractile dysfunction.

The drop in blood pressure was dramatic. As a result, perfusion of the coronary arteries was compromised, resulting in a depression in the overall contractile state of the heart. This is evidenced by the observed decreases in cardiac output, stroke volume, and ejection fraction (Table 30.1). The poor perfusion pressure also resulted in ischemia, as evidenced by the EKG abnormalities noted. Leukotrienes and platelet-activating factor from the immune response may have also contributed to the cardiac depression.

When the vasoconstrictors and inotropic agents were not exerting beneficial effects on the heart or the vasculature, the patient was inserted with an intra-aortic balloon pump. The intended use of this balloon is to salvage the failing myocardium by reducing the load on the heart. [12] A plastic balloon connected to a catheter is inserted in the thoracic aorta via the femoral artery and alternately inflated in diastole immediately following aortic valve closure and deflated during systole (generally synchronized with the EKG). The augmentation of diastolic pressure, to a level higher than systolic pressure, increases coronary perfusion as well as that of other tissues. The balloon deflates at the end of diastole, immediately before LV contraction, abruptly decreasing the afterload and improving LV ejection and the work of the LV.

The intra-aortic balloon is a particularly attractive therapeutic option because it decreases myocardial oxygen demand while simultaneously increasing oxygen supply and maintaining aortic pressure. This is the only method that will augment diastolic aortic pressure without increasing oxygen demand, as is the case with catecholamine-mediated vasoconstriction.

Weaning from the intra-aortic balloon should begin in 24–48 h of reperfusion or medical stabilization. This is accomplished by gradually reducing the proportion of cardiac cycles during which the balloon inflates. When the patient's own circulation can be maintained at a pumping frequency of every fourth or greater cardiac cycle, the balloon can usually be removed successfully. It should not be completely stopped *in situ* because of the danger of thrombus formation.

7. **Explain the importance of patient education regarding anaphylaxis triggers and emergency action plans. Advise patients on the proper use of epinephrine auto-injectors.**

Patient education on anaphylaxis triggers, emergency action plans, and epinephrine auto-injector use is crucial for preventing and managing severe allergic reactions. Educating patients about their specific triggers (e.g., food, medications, insect stings) allows them to take proactive steps to avoid exposure and reduce the risk of anaphylaxis.

Recognizing their symptoms quickly allows them to take steps in the case of an anaphylactic reaction, such as using an epinephrine auto-injector or seeking immediate medical attention.

An epinephrine auto-injector (e.g., EpiPen) is a pre-filled, disposable auto-injector device containing epinephrine, used to treat potentially life-threatening allergic reactions by rapidly reversing symptoms like difficulty breathing and swelling. [13] Patients must be trained on how to use an EpiPen correctly, including proper injection technique, dosage, and when to seek medical attention after injection. The device is designed to be easy to use, even for someone with little or no medical experience. EpiPens are injected into the outer thigh muscle, after which it is crucial to seek medical attention. Even if symptoms improve after epinephrine administration, patients should still call 911 or go to the emergency room due to the risk of biphasic anaphylaxis (a second reaction occurring hours later). Patients should always have access to their auto-injector and should carry two doses in case symptoms persist or worsen. Additionally, patients should check expiration dates regularly and store their EpiPen at room temperature, avoiding extreme heat or cold.

Exam Questions

1. A 45-year-old woman is brought to the emergency department with sudden onset of dyspnea, generalized urticaria, and swelling of her lips and tongue after being stung by a bee. On examination, she is cyanotic with an audible wheeze, hypotensive (BP: 78/50 mmHg), and tachycardic (HR: 120/min). Which of the following is the most appropriate immediate treatment?
   A. Epinephrine intramuscularly
   B. Diphenhydramine intravenously
   C. Albuterol nebulizer
   D. Intravenous corticosteroids
   E. Intravenous fluids alone

Answer: A

Learning Objective: #7 Explain the importance of patient education regarding anaphylaxis triggers and emergency action plans. Advise patients on the proper use of epinephrine auto-injectors.

Explanation: The patient is experiencing anaphylaxis. Epinephrine is the first-line treatment and should be administered intramuscularly (IM) as soon as possible. B is incorrect, as while H1 antihistamines like diphenhydramine help alleviate cutaneous symptoms (e.g., urticaria, pruritus), they do not address the life-threatening airway compromise or hypotension. They are adjunctive but not first-line treatments. C is incorrect, as while albuterol is useful for bronchospasm, it does not treat the underlying vasodilation and shock seen in anaphylaxis. It may be used as an adjunct but not as a first-line treatment. D is incorrect, as corticosteroids are used to prevent late-phase anaphylactic reactions. E is incorrect, as while IV fluids help with hypotension, they do not address the underlying pathophysiology of anaphylaxis.

2. A 62-year-old man with a history of peanut allergies is admitted to the intensive care unit with anaphylactic shock following accidental ingestion of a peanut-containing dessert. He is found to have severe left ventricular dysfunction with an ejection fraction of 25% on echocardiography. Despite inotropic support, his blood pressure remains low, and signs of end-organ hypoperfusion persist. An intra-aortic balloon pump (IABP) is placed to stabilize the patient. Which of the following best describes a beneficial effect of intra-aortic balloon counterpulsation in this patient?
   A. Decreases diastolic pressure in order to decrease afterload on the LV
   B. Increases systolic pressure to aid movement of fluid from the extravascular space into the vascular space
   C. Increases diastolic pressure in order to more efficiently perfuse the coronary circulation
   D. Serves to increase pulse pressure

Answer: C

Learning Objective: #6 Describe the pathophysiology of the depressed myocardial function and ischemia in this patient and how an IABP helped remedy this situation.

Explanation: During diastole, balloon inflation increases diastolic pressure, which enhances coronary perfusion by improving blood flow to the coronary arteries. This is particularly important in patients with left ventricular dysfunction and ischemia, where maintaining adequate coronary perfusion is critical. A is incorrect because IABP increases diastolic pressure (not decreases it) to enhance coronary perfusion. B is incorrect because the balloon does not directly increase systolic pressure. Instead, it reduces systolic afterload to assist cardiac output. D is incorrect, as while the balloon increases diastolic pressure, it does not significantly raise systolic pressure, meaning pulse pressure may stay the same or even slightly decrease rather than increase.

3. A 58-year-old woman experienced an anaphylactic reaction after receiving an intravenous contrast agent for a CT scan. She was promptly treated with epinephrine, IV fluids, and antihistamines, and her symptoms resolved. Her renal function remains within normal limits, and she maintains a stable sodium intake. Over the long term, what is the most likely outcome for her blood pressure?
   A. Exactly return to normal
   B. Return to about 75% of normal
   C. Become hypertensive
   D. Will remain 50% below normal
   E. We don't know what will happen to her blood pressure

Answer: A

Learning Objective: #5 Discuss the reflex mechanisms that maintain arterial blood pressure. Describe why pressure falls in this patient and what mechanisms are activated to return pressure to normal.

Explanation: This patient had an anaphylactic reaction, which likely led to transient vasodilation and hypotension, followed by successful treatment and recovery. Since no permanent physiological changes have occurred in the systems that regulate BP, it is expected that her BP will return to baseline after her recovery. B is incorrect—this option suggests persistent hypotension, which would occur if there were ongoing issues like adrenal insufficiency, autonomic dysfunction, or chronic heart failure. However, none of these conditions are present in this patient, so her BP should normalize. C is incorrect, as since her kidneys are intact, her sodium intake is stable, and no chronic pathologic changes have been mentioned, there is no reason to expect sustained hypertension. D is incorrect, as a chronic 50% drop in BP would indicate severe autonomic dysfunction, adrenal insufficiency, or cardiogenic shock, none of which apply to this patient. E is incorrect, as while some degree of uncertainty always exists in medicine, the patient's normal renal function, sodium intake, and absence of chronic cardiovascular pathology strongly predict a return to baseline BP.

References

1. Pflipsen MC, Vega Colon KM. Anaphylaxis: recognition and management. Am Fam Physician. 2020;102(6):355–62.
2. Silverman ME. The third heart sound. In: Walker HK, Hall WD, Hurst JW, editors. Clinical methods: the history, physical, and laboratory examinations. 3rd ed. Boston: Butterworths; 1990. Chapter 24.
3. Belic N, Gardin JM. ECG manifestations of myocardial ischemia. Arch Intern Med. 1980;140(9):1162–5.
4. McLendon K, Sternard BT. Anaphylaxis. [Updated 2023 Jan 26]. In: StatPearls [Internet]. Treasure Island (FL): StatPearls Publishing; 2025 Jan-. Available from: https://www.ncbi.nlm.nih.gov/books/NBK482124/
5. Dribin TE, Motosue MS, Campbell RL. Overview of allergy and anaphylaxis. Emerg Med Clin North Am. 2022;40(1):1–17.
6. Burzyńska M, Piasecka-Kwiatkowska D. A review of honeybee venom allergens and allergenicity. Int J Mol Sci. 2021;22(16):8371.
7. Nuñez-Borque E, Fernandez-Bravo S, Yuste-Montalvo A, Esteban V. Pathophysiological, cellular, and molecular events of the vascular system in anaphylaxis. Front Immunol. 2022;13:836222.
8. Tykocki NR, Boerman EM, Jackson WF. Smooth muscle ion channels and regulation of vascular tone in resistance arteries and arterioles. Compr Physiol. 2017;7(2):485–581.

9. Shahoud JS, Sanvictores T, Aeddula NR. Physiology, arterial pressure regulation. [Updated 2023 Aug 28]. In: StatPearls [Internet]. Treasure Island (FL): StatPearls Publishing; 2025 Jan-. Available from: https://www.ncbi.nlm.nih.gov/books/NBK538509/
10. Peavy RD, Metcalfe DD. Understanding the mechanisms of anaphylaxis. Curr Opin Allergy Clin Immunol. 2008;8(4):310–5.
11. Abbas M, Moussa M, Akel H. Type I hypersensitivity reaction. [Updated 2023 Jul 17]. In: StatPearls [Internet]. Treasure Island (FL): StatPearls Publishing; 2025 Jan-. Available from: https://www.ncbi.nlm.nih.gov/books/NBK560561/
12. Khan TM, Siddiqui AH. Intra-aortic balloon pump. [Updated 2023 Apr 24]. In: StatPearls [Internet]. Treasure Island (FL): StatPearls Publishing; 2025 Jan-. Available from: https://www.ncbi.nlm.nih.gov/books/NBK542233/
13. Sicherer SH, Kelso JM, Feldwig AM Patient education: Using an Epinephrine autoinjector (Beyon the Basics). UpToDate 2025. Accessed at https://www.uptodate.com/contents/using-an-epinephrine-autoinjector-beyond-the-basics

Part XIII

Pediatrics

31 Persistent Cough

Paul R. Standley

Learning Objectives

1. Describe motifs and domains found in the CFTR protein and the six classes of mutations responsible for cystic fibrosis.
2. Describe the normal function and regulation of the CFTR protein in ion transport.
3. Describe the composition and production of mucus and demonstrate how defects in the CFTR protein (particularly the ΔF_{508} mutation) upset chloride transport, leading to thickened mucus and increased sweat NaCl.
4. Describe newborn screening tests for CF, how the sweat chloride test is performed, interpret a positive test, and relate this to CFTR function.
5. Describe the clinical manifestations of cystic fibrosis in the respiratory, gastrointestinal, reproductive, and endocrine organ systems as they present in infants, children, and adults.
6. Discuss the role of CFTR modulators and symptom-related therapies in the treatment of CF patients.
7. Describe the incidence and prevalence of CF in the United States and how it varies by race/ethnicity.

P. R. Standley (✉)
Department of Basic Medical Sciences, University of Arizona College of Medicine-Phoenix, Phoenix, AZ, USA
e-mail: standley@arizona.edu

Chief Complaint

Mr. and Mrs. Bobelu state "Our 13-month-old boy, Scott, has had a really bad cough for the past three weeks."

Prompt: *Given these data, list possibilities for this presentation.*

Using the vindicators mnemonic, diagnostic possibilities are provided in parentheses.

V –vascular *(e.g., heart failure)*
I – infectious/idiopathic *(see below*)*/immune *(e.g., immunodeficiency, post-viral syndrome)*
N – neoplastic *(e.g., tumor pressing on tracheal carina, other respiratory tumor)*
D – drug reaction
I – *iatrogenic/intoxication*
C – congenital/ cardiac *(chest deformity, CF)*
A – autoimmune/allergic *(e.g., allergic/asthmatic cough)*
T – traumatic *(foreign body)*
E – endocrine/metabolic *(e.g., gastrointestinal reflux, malnutrition)*
R – *Renal/Respiratory*
S – *pSychiatric,(psychogenic cough or tic)*

**1. Viral (coronavirus, parainfluenza virus, respiratory syncytial virus, etc.)*
2. Bacterial (strep pneumo, h.flu, pertussis, moraxella catarrhalis, etc)

C. A. Standley (ed.), *Biomedical Science and Clinical Foundations*,
https://doi.org/10.1007/978-3-031-98353-5_31

3. *Fungal (coccidiomycosis, candida albicans, etc.)*
4. *Other (n/a for this case)*

History of Present Illness

Scott is a 13-month-old boy of Native American origin, who has been coughing as long as the family can recall, perhaps more than 6 months. The cough has worsened in the past three weeks. During this time, Scott began waking in the middle of the night with coughing that lasted for nearly an hour before falling back to sleep. The coughing seemed to be worse upon waking in the morning and again upon waking from his daily afternoon nap. Lately, Scott seems to be coughing hard enough to bring up thick phlegm.

Mrs. Bobelu is concerned that Scott does not appear to be growing as fast as the other children they interact with at the park near their home.

Mr. Bobelu states that the smell of Scott's diaper at changing time is very foul and is getting worse, but both parents assumed this was normal. Also, he has had diarrhea, which has not resolved for several months.

Prompt: *How have these data modified your differential?*

Students should realize that this is a chronic (>4 wk duration) cough that is acute-on-chronic worsened. Students should be able to narrow differential diagnosis based upon the list above; should include consideration of systemic illness (acute/chronic infectious vs. metabolic/endocrine vs. genetic, for example)

Past Medical History

- Term infant was delivered at home without complications.

Family History

- Mother has asthma.
- Father has mild HTN (hypertension) and mild diabetes.
- Maternal grandmother (deceased) had diabetes.
- Paternal grandfather was treated for tuberculosis when he was young, but died from an unknown cause. He used to make furniture and coughed a lot as he got older, although he did not smoke.

Social History: Lives with parents, no siblings; father smokes outside of the house; one pet at home (dog). Both parents grew up on the Zuni Pueblo south of Gallup, New Mexico, and moved to Phoenix for work after graduating from college four years ago. On one of their regular visits to Zuni, Scott was taken to a Traditional Practitioner for Blessing and Naming ceremonies.

Medications: none

Allergies: No known drug allergies

Review of Systems

The child has no history of fever, vomiting, or difficulty breathing, but he has a persistent, productive cough. He has a good appetite with poor weight gain. There is no history of rashes. Developmentally, he is meeting motor milestones, although he appears small for his age.

Prompt: *Why was this condition not detected at birth?*

Delivery at home may explain why Scott's condition wasn't detected via mandatory newborn screening.

Physical Examination

Vital Signs

T 37.0 °C (98.6 °F)	(reference 36.6–37.9)
R 36 breaths/min	(reference 20–30)
P 128 bpm	(reference 70–110)
BP 92/60 mmHg	(reference 90–105/55–70)

General: Interactive child, coughing during examination with a slight increase in breathing effort.

HEENT: Conjunctiva clear and sclera anicteric, oropharynx is clear, significant and purulent nasal secretions

Chest: No deformities. Symmetrical excursion. Upon auscultation, bilateral rhonchi with wheezing

Cardiovascular: Regular rate and rhythm, tachycardic, S1 and S2, no murmur

Abdominal: Abdomen is soft, but distended without tenderness to palpation, no masses or organomegaly, bowel sounds present

Musculoskeletal: Appropriate muscle tone and movement for stated age.

Skin: No cyanosis of lips or nail beds. Warm and dry without rashes or lesions. Hair has normal texture.

Developmental Milestones: Appropriate for stated age

Length: 27 inches

Weight: 17 lb

Prompt: *Is Scott's size within the expected range?*

No, reference normal growth chart [1]. Our patient is in the less-than-2 percentile for both height and weight.

Prompt: *What is meant by developmental milestones?*

Developmental milestones help determine if a child is undergoing typical development versus if a child has delayed in a given area or over multiple areas in the process of aging development. Milestones are social/emotional, gross and fine motor, language, and cognitive.

Prompt: *Has your differential changed based on the physical exam?*

Wheezing is generally associated with reactive airway disease such as COPD or asthma. It can also be heard in acute bronchitis, foreign body aspiration, or CHF. Rhonchi are generally coarse sounds heard in specific lobes that tend to correspond to underlying infection [2].

Laboratory

- *Blood Tests:*

The following tests were ordered: a complete blood count (Table 31.1), complete metabolic profile (Table 31.2), and sputum bacteriological analysis, including culture and antibiotic susceptibility testing (Table 31.3).

*BACTERIOLOGY FINAL REPORT
Collection sample: SPUTUM
Comment on specimen: GOOD SPECIMEN SUBMITTED

3+ (MODERATE) GRAM-POSITIVE COCCI
CULTURE RESULTS: >10,000 CFU/ml STAPHYLOCOCCUS AUREUS

Grading system: 1+= rare, <1/field, 2+ = few, 1-10/field, 3+= moderate, 11-25/field, 4+= many, >25/field. Based on an average of ten fields. Moderate levels of Staph must be interpreted in the clinical context.

Prompt: *Is the patient experiencing an active infection?*

Table 31.1 Complete blood count (CBC)

CBC profile	Patient	Reference Ranges
WBC	8.7 K/ul	6.0–14.0
RBC	4.4 M/ul	3.7–4.9
HGB	13.3 g/dl	10.5–14
HCT	35.7%	32–42
MCV	79.4 fl	72–88
MCH	28.1 pg	24–30
MCHC	34.3 g/dl	32–36
RDW	13.4%	11–16
PLT	239 K/ul	150–440
GRAN %	58.7%	54–62
LYMPH %	29.6%	25–33
MONO %	5.2%	3–7
EOS %	2.1%	1–3
BAS %	0.2%	0–0.75

Table 31.2 Complete metabolic panel

Blood chemistry	Patient	Reference Ranges
GLUCOSE	80 mg/dL	60–100
CREATINE	.25 mg/dL	.03–.50
BUN	11 mg/dl	5–18
NA	138 mmol/L	134–143
K	3.9 mmol/L	3.3–4.6
CL	102 mmol/L	98–106
CO_2	27 mmol/L	23–33
CA	9.9 mg/dL	8.8–10.8
MAG	2.2 mg/dL	1.6–2.6
PROTEIN	7.3 g/dL	6.1–7.9
ALBUMIN	3.8 gm/dl	3.4–4.2
ALKPHOS	240 U/L	145–420
AST	42 U/L	20–60
ALT	31 U/L	5–45
T BILI	0.6 mg/dL	.2–1

Table 31.3 Antibiotic susceptibility test results

SUSC	
CLINDAMYCIN S	Cost per day PO $2.60 IV $3.48
ERYTHROMYCIN S	Cost per day PO $0.44 IV $3.40
OXACILLIN S	
PENICILLIN S	Cost per day PO $0.11 IV $2.76
RIFAMPIN S	Cost per day $0.88
TETRACYCLINE S	Cost per day $0.10
TRIM/SULF S	Cost per day PO $0.11 IV $8.25
VANCOMYCIN S	Cost per day PO $10.62 IV $7.41
GENTAMICIN S	Cost per day $0.62
LEVOFLOXACIN S	

Patient doesn't exhibit elevated neutrophils or show signs of fever, so may be colonized rather than experiencing active infection. Lab results are not consistent with an active infection.

You ask Mr. and Mrs. Bobelu if they noticed any changes in the smell or taste of Scott's skin. They replied that they thought Scott's skin tasted salty, as if he had been sweating a lot.

Prompt: Are there other tests you are considering at this point?

Sweat chloride test based upon salty taste of skin.

Genetic screen for congenital disorders such as cystic fibrosis.

Sweat Chloride Test #1	75 mEq/L	(normal: <39)
Sweat Chloride Test #2	71 mEq/L	(normal: <39)

Prompt: *What is the significance of a high sweat chloride level?*

This is part of a learning objective, but the positive sweat chloride test is the gold standard for diagnosing cystic fibrosis.

Prompt: What type of follow-up might be in order?

There are numerous issues to follow up on, and they form the core of multiple learning issues below. Examples include:

- Is this disease treatable; yes partially with medications, physical therapy, diet supplements, etc.
- Is this disease curable; no, it is not but morbidity and mortality has been greatly reduced over the past 50 years due to new and emerging treatments.
- Is it the lack of prenatal care that caused this disease; no although it may have been screened for earlier had such care been available.

Genotyping of CFTR mutations by mass spectroscopy:	
Reason for Test: Identification of mutations associated with cystic fibrosis (CF) and related conditions	
Pattern of inheritance: Autosomal Recessive	
Result/ Interpretation	c.1521-1523delCTT (p.Phe508del) [Legacy: delta F508]: Disease-causing CFTR mutation.
	This mutation is present in apparent homozygosity (2 copies) (see caveats below in Additional Test Information). No further diagnostic testing will be performed. Genetic counseling is recommended.
	These molecular results should be evaluated in conjunction with the test sensitivity and the patient's clinical presentation.
Clinical Sensitivity:	This analysis will detect approximately 95% of CFTR mutations and will identify both causative mutations in approximately 90% of clinically diagnosed patients. This analysis will not detect complex gene rearrangements, large gene deletions, or deep intronic mutations that may affect splicing (other than those specifically listed). Polymorphisms that may be detected will not be reported. This test is only validated for inherited gene alterations associated with the phenotypes(s) specified above.
Analytic Sensitivity:	At least 99% accuracy for nucleotides evaluated; our analysis parameters are not designed to detect mosaicism.

Prompt*:* Interpret the genotype results and identify next steps.

Based on the genotype results, the diagnosis is delta 508 mutation in the CFTR causing cystic fibrosis. Next steps include counseling parents, providing resources, ruling out other known cystic-fibrosis co-morbidities, prescribing appropriate medications and other treatments such as physical therapy (if needed), nutritional supplementation, etc. as described in the learning objectives below.

Imaging

- *Chest x-ray impression:*

Scott's film shows hyperinflation and bronchiectasis (bronchial cuffing and ring shadows) with multiple nodular densities seen with mucous impaction present bilaterally.

Mrs. Bobelu is distraught. She had not mentioned it before, but her cousin had "fibrosis" and died from a severe pneumonia when they were teenagers. She loves Scott dearly and does not want this to happen to him. She has many questions and wants to know what she and her husband can do to save their child's life.

Prompt: How will you talk with them about Scott's diagnosis?

- Consider any cultural context
- Use principles of clear communication as appropriate: decrease medical jargon, have the patient repeat back what you have told them
- Validate concerns and feelings
- Use NEURSing approach: Name it, Express/ Emotion, Understand, Respect, Support

This can be used as a prompt to get the students questioning the consequences of this mutation over the course of the patient's life.

Prompt: What organ systems are involved beyond pulmonary and GI?

This is covered in a learning objective, but in addition to the lungs and GI track, the pancreas is involved also and underlies the need for diet supplementation as described below

Prompt: What is the prognosis?

This is covered in a learning objective, but depends in large part upon the CFTR mutation present. Some mutations are mostly benign while others are incompatible with life. Overall, for the most common variants: three decades ago, the average person with cystic fibrosis would live only to the age of 30, but now 50 years is typical, and some patients with CF live into their 80s

Prompt: What treatments are available?

This is covered in a learning objective, but mainly fall into these categories:

- Drugs that target gene changes and improve how the CFTR protein works.
- Antibiotics to treat and prevent lung infections.
- Anti-inflammatory drugs to lessen swelling in the airways in the lungs.
- Mucus-thinning drugs, such as hypertonic saline, to help cough up mucus.
- Bronchodilators to keep airways open by relaxing the muscles around the bronchial tubes.
- Pancreatic enzyme capsules taken by mouth to help the digestive tract absorb nutrients.
- Stool softeners to prevent constipation or bowel obstruction.
- Acid-reducing medicines to help pancreatic enzymes work better.

Mrs. Bobelu also wonders if there are any tests that could have been done during her pregnancy to determine if Scott had this mutation.

Prompt: How would you respond to this?

Potential benefits of knowing include having parents who are informed of the risk for CF in the newborn. They can watch for potential signs or symptoms of the disease and/or can have the newborn tested after delivery.

Potential harms of knowing include causing added stress or tension for a couple testing positive for the carrier status.

Couples who test positive for carrier status could decide to not have children, due to the risk of having a child with the disease. Depending on what state they live in, they could have early prenatal genetic testing when they do get pregnant, and terminate the pregnancy when CF is suspected. They could undergo in vitro fertilization and perform genetic testing prior to embryo implantation.

Identification of one mutation (or none) does not necessarily mean that they do not have CF; they could have a mutation that has not been identified yet. Two positive sweat chloride tests is still the gold standard for diagnosis.

Prompt: What mechanisms are in place to detect common disease conditions in infants?

National Health Resources and Administration Recommended Uniform Screening Panel [3].

The goal here is to make the students aware that screening test are done routinely and that they are quite extensive. Scott's CF wasn't detected earlier, likely due to his being born at home rather than in a hospital setting. The above link takes you to the NHRA site which includes the currently recommended screening tests for newborns. Arizona Department of Health currently tests for 31 of these disorders, including CF.

Prompt: What social determinants of health could potentially play a role in this case?

The patient is Native American and we hear some of the social background involved. Could discuss some of the potential and real barriers to care that affect many Native Americans such as limited access to care while living on reservations as well as the poverty level in some of these communities. The insurance status is not discussed but that could also be an issue in terms of coverage whether they are able to pay for the care involved with a new diagnosis of a chronic condition. They have in the social history described cultural practices such as blessing ceremonies; how does that play in and shape health literacy or even comfort with conventional medicine as part of this patient's care? Below is a list of some of the key questions that can be discussed depending on your personal comfort level and knowledge as SDOH considerations for any case.

- What would be additional considerations if this patient is underinsured or without health insurance coverage? How might this impact patient care and future health outcomes for them?
- Consider the education level and health literacy of the patient.
- Transportation: does the patient have the ability to come to follow-up visits? What would change if there are transportation issues?
- How might access and barriers to care affect this patient if they belonged to a vulnerable

and stigmatized population, e.g. undocumented, LGBTQ+, sexual assault survivor, formerly incarcerated?
- How can you assess a patient's access to and ability to purchase healthy foods?
- How might this patient handle the diagnosis and subsequent interventions with a limited support system?
- How might a patient's income and/or employment affect access to care and follow-up?
- How would you assess this person's living situation and whether it presented any barriers to care or risks to the patient?
- How would you assess the safety of the patient's relationships and rule out any abuse or harmful relationships that could affect this person's ability to stay healthy and safe?
- How would you discuss any cultural beliefs or perspectives that may affect this patient's care and how could you communicate effectively with this patient in a culturally humble and respectful manner?

End of Case

Learning Objective Answers

A comprehensive review of cystic fibrosis, which includes discussion of many of the pertinent learning objectives, has been published by Grasemann et al. [4].

1. **Describe motifs and domains found in the CFTR protein and the six classes of mutations responsible for cystic fibrosis.**

Key Points
1. CFTR is a member of the ATP binding cassette (ABC) superfamily and is present in the plasma membrane of epithelial cells
2. CFTR consists of three major types of domains: The first type consists of membrane-spanning domains 1 and 2 (MSD1 and MSD2), each with six membrane-spanning regions. The second type consists of the two nucleotide-binding domains (NBD1 and NBD2) that bind ATP to control gating. The third is the regulatory domain, R, which is phosphorylated by protein kinase A (PKA) and modulates CFTR function.
3. Gating of the CFTR is controlled by hydrolysis of ATP bound to NBD1 and NBD2, which is regulated by the phosphorylation state of the R domain.
4. Six classes of mutation are associated with CF—see list and figure below.

The cystic fibrosis transmembrane conductance regulator (CFTR) is a 1480 amino-acid-membrane-bound glycoprotein with a molecular mass of 170,000. It functions both as a cyclic AMP-regulated chloride channel and, as its name implies, a regulator of other ion channels. The fully processed form of CFTR is found in the plasma membrane in normal epithelia. It is a member of the ATP-binding cassette (ABC) superfamily of proteins. The protein is comprised of two six-span membrane-bound regions (MSD1 and MSD2), each connected to a nucleotide-binding domain (NBD1 and NBD2), respectively, which bind ATP (Fig. 31.1). The two NBDs form an intramolecular dimer with two ATP molecules at the interface. Gating (opening and closing) of the CFTR channel is thought to be mediated by the hydrolysis of one of the ATP molecules. Notably, ATP hydrolysis is not required for the

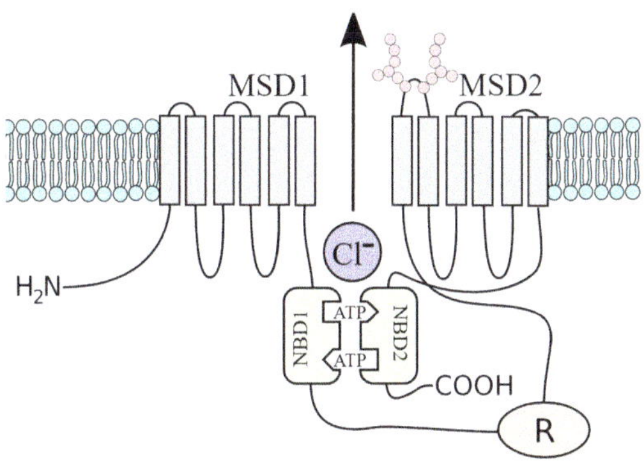

Fig. 31.1 The domains and motifs of the CFTR. (Adapted from Rogan et al. [5]. Kuebi = Armin Kübelbeck, CC BY-SA 3.0 <https://creativecommons.org/licenses/by-sa/3.0>, via Wikimedia Commons. https://upload.wikimedia.org/wikipedia/commons/8/83/CFTR_protein_structure_scheme_02.svg)

movement of Cl^- ions through the channel: ion transport is a passive process that occurs once the channel is open.

Between these two units is a regulatory (R)-domain, a unique feature of CFTR within the ABC superfamily, which is comprised of many charged amino acids and is the target of cellular kinases (PKA) and phosphatases.

The location of the CFTR gene is at cytogenetic location 7q31.2, meaning on the long (q) arm of chromosome seven at position 31.2. This corresponds to base pairs 116,907,252 to 117,095,950. This means that the gene spans nearly 200,000 base pairs, providing a relatively large target for mutations that can disrupt expression, splicing, or coding of the protein. The most common cause of cystic fibrosis is the phenylalanine 508 mutation (ΔF_{508}), which is responsible for 70% of cases of cystic fibrosis. This is a *deletion* mutation in which three nucleotides (TTT), coding for phenylalanine (F), at position 508 of the protein, are deleted. However, different CFTR mutations lead to varied molecular consequences (see below). Currently, more than 1900 different mutations in the CFTR gene have been identified.

Classes of Mutations Responsible for CF

Class I: Mostly nonsense, a few frameshift mutations—no functional CFTR made.

Class II: Amino acid deletion, some missense—defective folding/transport to the cell surface. The ΔF508 mutation falls into this category.

Class III: Missense mutation, affecting gating of CFTR at the cell surface, resulting in reduced time in the "open" state.

Class IV: Missense mutation, affecting conductance of the CFTR channel, even when open, does not transport Cl^- efficiently.

Class V: Altered splicing, reduced levels of CFTR.

Class VI: Missense mutation—the rarest type of mutation, CFTR gets to the plasma membrane but is turned over more rapidly

2. **Describe the normal function and regulation of the CFTR protein in ion transport.**

Key Points

1. CFTR allows Cl^- ion transfer. The gate is controlled by the R domain, which regulates hydrolysis of ATP bound to the nucleotide-binding domains. ATP hydrolysis controls the opening and closing of the gate. The movement of Cl^- ions does not require input energy.
2. CFTR activity is controlled by posttranslational modification of the R Domain. Specifically, protein kinase A (PKA), which is activated by cyclic AMP, phosphorylates the regulatory domain of CFTR, which triggers ATP hydrolysis by the NBDs and allows the transport of chloride through the channel.

Proper function of the CFTR chloride channel requires the activity of three domains. The first two domains are the nucleotide-binding domains (NBD), which bind ATP and regulate the opening and closing of the channel. Channel opening requires that ATP bound at one of the NBDs is hydrolyzed. Importantly, the flow of chloride through the open channel does not require input of metabolic energy (ATP) because the net movement of chloride is down its electrochemical gradient. The 2nd domain is the regulatory (R) domain that is phosphorylated by protein kinase A (PKA). PKA is activated by cyclic AMP (cAMP), which is created upon activation of certain G protein-coupled receptors. If the R domain is not phosphorylated or ATP is not available, the gateway for chloride's passage into the cell is blocked.

The following link is to a movie that provides an overview of the CFTR protein, the mutations that can impair its activity, and some potential therapeutic strategies that may be able to restore CFTR function in patients: http://www.youtube.com/watch?v=_j99-xgOIaw [6]

3. **Describe the composition and production of mucus and demonstrate how defects in the CFTR protein (particularly the ΔF_{508} mutation) upset chloride transport, leading to thickened mucus and increased sweat NaCl.**

Key Points

1. Mucus is 95% water, composed of glycosylated proteins (glycoproteins) called mucins and inorganic salts.
2. It is secreted by goblet cells present on the mucus membranes in the body.
3. In the respiratory epithelium, the ΔF508 mutation prevents chloride transport and increases the electrochemical gradient for Na^+, which moves into cells along with water. Resultant extracellular dehydration thickens the mucus, which blocks airways and other ducts in the body lined by mucus membranes
4. In sweat ducts, lack of Cl^- transport into cells leads to chloride accumulation outside the skin surface along with Na^+, thus increasing the "saltiness" of the skin.

Mucus is a slippery secretion of the lining of various mucus membranes in the body. Mucus is produced by goblet cells in the mucous membranes that cover their surfaces. It is 95% water and mucins, which are highly glycosylated proteins (glycoproteins) that polymerize to form a gel-like consistency. In addition, mucus contains inorganic salts, antimicrobial compounds, and enzymes. Phlegm is a type of mucus that is restricted to the respiratory tract, while the term mucus refers to secretions of the nasal passages as well.

There are a number of defects in the CFTR that are possible, ranging from those that mildly inhibit chloride transport to those that completely block it. The ΔF_{508} mutation that Scott possesses results in the inability of the translated CFTR to be processed properly in the ER (and thus is a Class II mutation), and, therefore, functional transporters are not inserted into the membrane. The lack of chloride transport out of airway epithelial cells results in an increased membrane potential (negative within the cell due to increased negatively charged chloride within the cells). This, in turn, increases the electrochemical gradient for Na (positively charged and in higher concentration in the ECF vs. ICF) to move into the cells. Since the cytoplasm becomes hyperosmotic with this Na influx, water moves (via aquaporins) from the airway into the cell to regain osmotic homeostasis. This extracellular (airway) dehydration results in a dehydrated, thick mucus. Mucus with this property results in blunted ciliary movement, stagnation, and optimal growth surfaces for a variety of harmful microorganisms, most notably *H. influenza*. There are mucus-thinning drugs (mucolytics) that are used to hydrolyze mucins, thereby making them flow more freely and thereby ameliorating the dehydrated mucus problems.

The students should be able to describe the reasons why CF patients have increased Cl^- levels on their skin (and a positive sweat chloride test). Essentially the same as above, but in this case, Cl- is trapped outside the cell, so Na+ follows it.

[Note: lack of postural movements during sleep further slows ciliary action and posture-induced mucus mobilization, thereby exacerbating systems during sleep].

4. **Describe newborn screening tests for CF, how the sweat chloride test is performed, interpret a positive test, and relate this to CFTR function.**

Key Points:

1. Screening: Newborns are screened for elevated levels of immunoreactive trypsinogen (IRT) in blood. This leaks out from damaged pancreatic cells. All 50 states include this in their newborn screening guidelines.
2. Sweat chloride test: Application of electric current allows penetration of pilocarpine. This stimulates the production of sweat. The collected sweat is tested for the amount of chloride. If the amount seems to be elevated, the test is repeated at a subsequent visit to the doctor. Two tests indicating elevated NaCl in the sweat confirm a diagnosis of CF.

The following is adapted from Kaye [7].

Screening *Methodology*

Determination of immunoreactive trypsinogen (IRT) concentrations from dried blood spots serves as the basis for the first tier in all newborn screening programs for CF. IRT concentration is high in the blood of infants with CF, presumably from leakage of the protein into the circulation after exocrine pancreatic injury. Two approaches can be taken if the IRT concentration is high. The more common approach is to perform mutation analysis from the dried blood spot for a set of CF mutations. Another approach is based on persistent elevation of IRT concentration, which requires a second dried blood spot taken 2–3 weeks after birth. The value at which the initial IRT concentration is considered abnormal varies from program to program. If mutation analysis is performed from the first dried blood spot, a second specimen is not required. Thus, the IRT cutoff can be set to include a substantial fraction of the newborn population. In some programs, the top 5% of all IRT concentrations are considered abnormal, and mutation analysis is performed. In other programs, the cutoff is set at the top 1%. Programs that are based on persistent elevation of IRT set the cutoff value for IRT at a higher concentration (0.5% of newborn infants) than programs that perform mutation analysis. Diagnosis through persistent elevation of IRT concentration can identify infants with CF who do not carry mutations included in most mutation analysis panels.

Timing

Because IRT concentration is frequently high immediately after birth, specificity is improved if the test is performed after the first day of life.

Sensitivity and Specificity

The sensitivity of most CF screening programs, whether based on genotyping or persistent elevation of IRT concentration, is approximately 95%. The specificity of programs that rely on persistent elevation of IRT concentration without genotyping is approximately 99.5% after the first measurement of IRT concentration. The specificity of programs that perform genotyping after the initial elevation of IRT may be as high as 99.9%.

The Sweat Chloride Test

The sweat chloride test is a common and simple test used to evaluate a patient who is suspected of having CF. The goal of this test is to painlessly stimulate the patient's skin to produce a large enough amount of sweat, which may then be absorbed by a special filter paper and analyzed for the content of chloride. To produce the necessary volume of sweat, a technique called iontophoresis is employed. The technique requires the application of a minute (painless) electrical current that allows the penetration of a medication (typically pilocarpinium ions) that maximizes sweat stimulation. The patient's forearm is commonly used. However, in small infants, the back may also serve as an appropriate area to perform this procedure. The entire test lasts approximately 30-60 min. The sweat is collected on a specialized filter paper and placed under negative pressure to efficiently extract skin surface sweat. After determining that enough sweat has been collected to ensure test reliability (as noted by a colored solvent front moving from the skin surface into the filter paper), the amount of chloride in the sweat is measured. The normal sweat chloride values are 10–35 mE/L. Patients with CF usually have a sweat chloride value greater than 60 mEq/L. To ensure accuracy, the test is repeated once more and, if elevated, is considered a true indication of elevated Cl^- on the skin and a diagnosis of CF can be made. Intermediate values between 35 and 60 mEq/L may be seen in some CF patients (and in some normal children) and also necessitate repeat testing. In a severely malnourished patient with CF, the sweat chloride level may be normal. However, once the malnutrition is corrected, the test becomes positive. There are a few rare conditions that produce a false positive sweat chloride test. Such situations include diseases of the adrenal, thyroid, or pituitary glands, rare lipid storage diseases, and infection of the pancreas. Generally, however, these children are easily differentiated from patients with CF by their clinical condition, and molecular tests for CF can be done to clarify the diagnosis.

To understand what the sweat test results mean, a chloride level of:

- Less than or equal to 29 mEq/L => CF is unlikely regardless of age
- Between 30 and 59 mEq/L => CF is possible and additional testing is needed

- Greater than or equal to 60 mEq/L => CF is likely to be diagnosed

When sweat chloride test results fall between the range of 30–59 mEq/L, the sweat test is usually repeated.

Because of the large number of CF mutations, DNA analysis is not used for primary diagnosis. Because of widespread newborn screening in all 50 states, most cases are identified soon after birth. The final diagnosis of CF rests on a combination of clinical criteria, including analyses of sweat Cl^- values and genetic testing.

See learning objective 3 for an explanation of why sweat chloride is elevated in CF patients.

For newborns and infants younger than six months of age:

- ≤29 mEq/L : Normal (CF very unlikely)
- 30–59 mEq/L: Intermediate (Possible CF)
- ≥60 mEq/L: Abnormal (Diagnosis of CF)

For infants ≥6 months, children, and adults:

- ≤39 mEq/L : Normal (CF very unlikely)
- 40–59 mEq/L: Intermediate (Possible CF)
- ≥60 mEq/L: Abnormal (Diagnosis of CF)

Rationale for and Benefits of Newborn Screening

The principal benefit of newborn screening and early diagnosis is improved height and weight at least through adolescence, demonstrated in a well-controlled clinical trial. Improvement in height and weight likely occurs from early institution of pancreatic enzyme, fat-soluble vitamin, and salt supplementation, as well as the general nutritional follow-up that is part of care at a CF center. In addition, it is likely that early diagnosis and attention to nutrition can help patients avoid severe nutritional complications. Severe nutritional complications of CF in infancy include anemia from vitamin E deficiency, zinc deficiency, linoleic acid deficiency, hypoelectrolytemia, and protein-calorie malnutrition. In addition, vitamin E deficiency as symptomatic diagnosis of CF is associated with cognitive deficits. Another benefit of screening is that parents of children identified through screening have been shown to have greater trust in the medical establishment than parents whose children are identified only after symptoms appear.

5. **Describe the clinical manifestations of cystic fibrosis in the respiratory, gastrointestinal, reproductive, and endocrine organ systems as they present in infants, children, and adults.**

Key Points

Infancy:

Respiratory tract:
1. Frequent pneumonia infections

Gastrointestinal tract:
1. Meconium ileus, a bowel obstruction in the newborn due to inspissated/hard stool that cannot pass
2. Failure to thrive due to malabsorption from pancreatic insufficiency

Reproductive:
1. Absence of the vas deferens in the embryologic development of males

Childhood:

Respiratory tract:
1. Frequent pneumonias, cough, and shortness of breath
2. Asthma
3. Bronchiectasis (destruction of the lungs due to frequent infections)
4. Chronic sinusitis with need for surgical intervention

Gastrointestinal tract:
1. Distal intestinal obstruction syndrome (DIOS) from impacted stool
2. Pancreatic insufficiency with malabsorption of nutrients and calories
3. Liver injury due to inspissated bile and resulting liver failure/cirrhosis
4. Gall stones

Endocrine system:
1. Diabetes due to pancreatic insufficiency

Adults

Same as children with the following additions:

Respiratory:

Recurrent sinus infections requiring sinus surgeries for debridement

Coughing up blood (hemoptysis) due to lung destruction from chronic infections

Reproductive tract:

Infertility of males (97% of males are infertile due to vas deferens absence.)

Having ongoing medical care by a team of doctors, nurses, and respiratory therapists who specialize in CF is important. These specialists often are located at major medical centers or CF Care Centers.

It is standard to have CF checkups every 3 months. Patients should get an annual flu shot and stay up to date on other vaccinations. Encourage patients to take all medicines as prescribed. In between checkups, patients should contact the doctor if any of the following occur:

- Blood in mucus, increased amounts of mucus, or a change in the color or consistency of mucus
- Decreased energy or appetite
- Severe constipation or diarrhea, severe abdominal pain, or vomit that is dark green
- Fever

Transition of Care

Better treatments for CF allow people who have the disease to live longer now than in the past. Thus, the move from pediatric care to adult care is an important step in treatment.

Encourage patient education for both the child and the parents about the disease. Encourage the child to take an active role in treatment. This will help prepare the child for the transition to adult care.

CF Care Centers can help provide age-appropriate treatment throughout the transition period and into adulthood. They also will support the transition to adult care by balancing medical needs with other developmental factors, such as increased independence, relationships, and employment.

Lifestyle Changes

In between medical checkups, encourage patients to practice good self-care and follow a healthy lifestyle.

Patients should adopt a healthy diet that includes a variety of fruits, vegetables, and whole grains.

Other lifestyle changes include:

- Not smoking and avoiding tobacco smoke
- Washing hands often to lower risk of infection
- Exercising regularly and staying hydrated
- Doing chest physical therapy

Other Concerns

Although CF requires daily care, most people who have the disease are able to attend school and work.

Adults who have CF can expect to have normal reproductive lives. Most men who have the disease are infertile (unable to have children). However, modern fertility treatments may help them.

Women who have CF may find it hard to get pregnant, but they usually can have children.

- Although CF can cause fertility problems, men and women who have the disease should still have protected sex to avoid sexually transmitted infections.

Emotional Issues

Living with CF may cause fear, anxiety, depression, and stress. Provide patients with resources for counseling and support groups in the area.

Support from family and friends also can help relieve stress and anxiety.

6. **Discuss the role of CFTR modulators and symptom-related therapies in the treatment of CF patients.**

Key Points

1. CFTR modulators:
   (a) Potentiator drugs improve gating of CFTR present in the plasma membrane, allowing for more efficient transport of chloride, e.g., ivacaftor. Useful for about

5% of CF but not effective *alone* for ΔF508, so used in combination therapy.
   (b) Corrector drugs: improve folding of CFTR and delivery to the plasma membrane and thus improve chloride transport, e.g., lumacaftor, elexacaftor, and tezacaftor.
   (c) Combination therapy: A potentiator and a corrector—approved for use with ΔF508. Approved for a growing number of genotypes, but some are still not eligible.
2. Symptomatic treatment
   (a) Inhalers and nebulizers to deliver medicine to the airways—combinations of hypertonic saline, DNAse, beta-agonists, and antibiotics.
   (b) Postural drainage and chest percussion—to move secretions out from the small airways.
   (c) Antibiotics—to treat frequent lung and other infections.
   (d) GI disease: high-caloric diet, exogenous pancreatic enzymes, and vitamin supplements.
   (e) Lung transplantation—when forced expiratory volume in one second (FEV1) is 30% of expected or with hypercarbia.

CFTR Modulators

Potentiators—Improve gating of the CFTR, increasing the length of time that CFTR is in the "open" configuration and thus enhancing chloride transport. Effective on many class III and some class IV mutations. Ivacaftor (Kalydeco) was the first FDA-approved CFTR modulator in the US. It is approved for patients with missense (class III) mutations, such as G551D, G178R, S549N, S549R, G551S, G1244E, S1251N, S1255P, and G1349D, and the class IV mutation R117H. Ivacaftor has been approved for 97 different mutations, but this represents less than 5% of CF cases. In 2017, it was approved for the treatment of CF caused by 23 different mutations.

Correctors: Improve folding/transport of CFTR so that it can reach the plasma membrane. Correctors are usually administered in combination with a potentiator. Orkambi was the first of these combination drugs and consists of the corrector lumacaftor in conjunction with ivacaftor. Orkambi was approved by the FDA on July 2, 2015 for use in CF patients >=12 years of age with the ΔF508 mutation and has now been approved for use in patients two years and older. Orkambi is made by Vertex, is expensive, and may or may not be covered by various insurance companies. The next generation correctors include elexacaftor and tezacaftor. Combination therapy, with tezacaftor and ivacaftor (Symdeko), was approved in 2018 and is now favored over Orkambi for patients >12 with two copies of ΔF50. In 2019, the FDA approved a triple combination (Trikafta) that includes elexacaftor, tezacaftor, and ivacaftor for individuals above 12 with at least one copy of ΔF508.

Symptom-Related Treatments:

The major objectives of symptom-related therapy for CF are to promote clearance of secretions and control infection in the lung, provide adequate nutrition, prevent intestinal obstruction, and educate the patient and family about the disease.

Lung Disease: Because a major goal of treatment is to preserve lung function, it is important to get an accurate baseline assessment after diagnosis as soon as possible. Furthermore, patients are typically seen every 2–3 months to monitor lung function and assess for bacterial infections. Patients should be immunized against common respiratory pathogens: influenza, rubeola, and pertussis.

Inhalation Therapy: To deliver medication and hydrate the lower respiratory tract (LRT), inhalers and nebulizers are used. Inhalers/nebulizers are used to deliver normal saline. In addition, beta-agonists can be added if the patient's airway is constricted. Antibiotics can also be administered via inhalers (tobramycin, azithromycin, and Cayston). Recombinant human DNase (pulmozyme) is also delivered in this fashion in a single daily dose and improves pulmonary function and decreases exacerbations by digesting DNA present in the mucus. Hypertonic saline has been reported to have benefits and is approved for use.

Airway Clearance Therapy: Usually involving chest percussion combined with placing the patient in positions favorable for drainage of mucus (postural drainage and percussion). Also called CPT for chest physical therapy, this is designed to help move secretions out of the small airways that are most severely affected by CF. Frequency depends on the severity of symptoms but can be as much as four times/day, with each session 20–40 min. Forced expirations, coughing, or ""huffing," following treatment, help to move secretions. CPT can be done manually or with the use of mechanical percussion vests.

Antibiotic Therapy: More than 95% of patients with CF die of complications resulting from bacterial lung infection. For this reason, antibiotics are the principal agents available for treating lung infection, and their use should be guided by sputum culture results. Treatment varies from intermittent short courses with a single antibiotic to essentially continuous treatment with multiple antibiotics. Dosages are typically higher than for non-CF patients due to the higher clearance rate and lean body mass of CF patients. Antibiotics can be given orally, by aerosol, or by IV. Antibiotic choice should be guided by in vitro susceptibility testing. Azithromycin, aztreonam, inhaled tobramycin, and levofloxacin have all received FDA approval.

Lung Transplantation. If the above therapies are unsuccessful, lung function will decline. In this case, the only option is a double lung transplant. Referral usually occurs when a patient's FEV1 is 30% of expected or when they develop hypercarbia (elevated CO_2 in blood).

Gastrointestinal Disease: Maintenance of adequate nutrition is critical for the health of the patient with CF. Treatment involves dietary adjustment, supplementary vitamins (AquaADEKs®), and replacement of pancreatic enzymes (numerous manufacturers). Many, if not most, CF patients require a higher-than-normal caloric intake. Most (90%) of patients with CF benefit from pancreatic enzyme replacement. Capsules generally contain between 4000 and 29,000 units of lipase. The dose of enzymes (typically no more than 2500 units/kg/meal) should be adjusted on the basis of weight gain, abdominal symptomatology, and character of stools. Replacement of fat-soluble vitamins, particularly vitamins A, D, E, and K, is usually required. Hyperglycemia most often becomes manifest in adults and typically requires insulin treatment. In contrast to most patients with diabetes, CF patients with diabetes are encouraged to remain on a high-caloric diet due to their difficulties in getting adequate nutrition

7. **Describe the incidence and prevalence of CF in the United States and how it varies by race/ethnicity.**

Key Points:

1. Commonest in individuals of European ancestry, 1 in 3300 births, and least common in Asian Americans
2. Ethnicity: Twice as common in Zuni Native Americans as in populations of European descent.
3. Of the 1900 mutations, ΔF508 is the most common.
   - CF is most common in individuals of European descent, with an incidence of 1 in 3300 births.
   - It is least common in Asian Americans, with an incidence of 1 in 32,100.

Many people, including trained physicians, mistakenly believe that only individuals of European descent are at risk for CF; however, CF affects people of all ethnicities. Of special note, the incidence in the Pueblo Native Americans is similar to that of individuals of European descent but in Zuni Native Americans, it is approximately twice as high as in the general population of European ancestry. Notably, the ΔF508 is a rare mutation in this population. A study by Kessler [8] examined six Zunis and found all had the R1162X mutation. In addition, analysis of 585 Zunis found 39 to carry one allele of the R1162X mutation, which indicates a carrier frequency of 6.7%. This is important to know in Arizona as members of both these tribes live in the southwestern United States (although more in New Mexico than Arizona).

There are over 1900 identified mutations of the CFTR gene, which result in phenotypic CF.

- ΔF508 is the single most common mutation in all ethnicities.
  - It is seen in 70% of people of European descent with CF.
  - It is present in almost half of Hispanic and African American patients with CF.
- Up to 15% of cases can be traced to another 20 common mutations.
- The remainder of the cases are rare, more "unique" mutations.

- The standard screen tests for ΔF508 and ~160 other common mutations, with sensitivities outlined above. The sensitivity is the highest (above 90%) in Ashkenazi Jews; Pueblo and Zuni Indians; Celtic Bretons; and French Canadians from Quebec. This ethnic variation in sensitivity underscores the importance of discussing the limitations of the test patients; a group with poor screening sensitivity may be falsely reassured by a negative screen.

Exam Questions

1. A 12-year-old female with cystic fibrosis presents with a cough associated with thick phlegm. Which of the following best describes the mechanism responsible for thick phlegm production?
   A. Airway mucus dehydration
   B. Loss of airway ciliary action
   C. Nonproductive cough
   D. Overproduction of mucus

   Answer: A

   Learning Objective: Describe the composition and production of mucus and demonstrate how defects in the CFTR protein upset chloride transport, which leads to thickening of mucus and increased NaCl in sweat.

   Explanation: "Airway mucus dehydration" is correct and occurs due to Na and water movement from the airway lumen into the airway epithelial cells. B is incorrect since ciliary action (which is depressed in CF) does not affect the viscosity of phlegm. C is incorrect as nonproductive cough is not associated with mucus production. D is incorrect since it is dehydration of mucus and not its clearing from the airway that leads to its increased viscosity.

2. Your patient is a five-month-old who is not growing appropriately for her age and is suspected of having cystic fibrosis. Which of the following is the best test to diagnose cystic fibrosis?
   A. CFTR gene mutation test
   B. Chest X-ray
   C. Pancreatic enzymes
   D. Sputum culture
   E. Sweat chloride test

   Answer: E

   Learning Objective: Describe how the sweat chloride test is performed, interpretation of a positive test, and relate this to CFTR function.

   Explanation: The sweat test can be done in one day and is inexpensive and has a sensitivity of 83% and specificity of 98% in diagnosing CF.

   A is incorrect as although genetic testing is required to determine which of hundreds of mutations the patient expresses, it is expensive and requires several days to weeks to complete. B is incorrect as it is nonspecific for CF. C is incorrect as deficiencies in pancreatic enzymes are not specific for CF. D is incorrect as a sputum culture fails to measure Cl transport dysfunction.

3. A 12-month-old female patient with cystic fibrosis has a sweat chloride level of 80 mEq/L (normal <39 mEq/L). Which of the following best describes the ionic mechanism resulting in this chloride level?
   A. Reduced Cl^- efflux from sweat duct epithelial cells.
   B. Reduced Cl^- influx into sweat duct epithelial cells.

C. Excessive Na^+ efflux from sweat duct epithelial cells.
D. Excessive Na^+ influx into sweat duct epithelial cells.

Answer: B

Learning Objective: Describe the normal function and regulation of the CFTR protein in ion transport.

Explanation: In sweat gland epithelial cells, the CFTR principally directs Cl flux from the duct into the duct epithelial cells (opposite to the scenario in airway epithelial cells). The problem in CF is that Cl^- cannot be reabsorbed into the sweat duct epithelial cells due to a defective CFTR. Thus, "reduced Cl- influx" accurately describes the mechanism. A is incorrect, as in CF, the issue is not about Cl- leaving the cell (efflux), but rather that it cannot enter the cell from the lumen. C and D are incorrect since the CFTR does not conduct Na (only Cl).

References

1. https://www.cdc.gov/growthcharts/who-growth-charts.htm
2. https://www.physio-pedia.com/Auscultation
3. https://www.hrsa.gov/advisory-committees/heritable-disorders/rusp
4. Grasemann H, Ratjen F. Cystic Fibrosis. New Engl J Med. 2023;389:1693–707.
5. Rogan MP, Stoltz DA, Hornick DB. Cystic fibrosis transmembrane conductance regulator intracellular processing, trafficking, and opportunities for mutation-specific treatment. Chest. 2011:1480–90. https://upload.wikimedia.org/wikipedia/commons/archive/8/83/20150324213200%21CFTR_protein_structure_scheme_02.svg; https://commons.wikimedia.org/wiki/File:CFTR_protein_structure_scheme_02.svg.
6. Ferreira M. https://www.youtube.com/watch?v=_j99-xgOIaw
7. Kaye CI. Introduction to the newborn screening fact-sheets. Pediatrics. 2006;118:1304–12.
8. Kessler D, Moehlenkamp C, Kaplan G. Determination of cystic fibrosis carrier frequency for Zuni native Americans of New Mexico. Clin Genet. 1996;49:95–7.

Part XIV

Simulations

32 Sterral Pain

Jacob K. Lythgoe

Overview

The nurse/facilitator will introduce the case by giving the patient's name, age, and a one-sentence history before allowing the student doctors into the room. The student doctors will obtain the remainder of the history from the simulation operator or live patient model as they ask questions and progress through the case. Physical exam findings can be given to the student doctors during their examination if not simulated. Simulated vital signs can be displayed on the in-room monitor and adjusted as the case progresses and interventions are attempted. The chest radiograph and EKG can be displayed on the monitor once they have been ordered. Additional tests, such as bloodwork, can be added to the simulation if desired, or the nurse/facilitator can state the results will not be available before the end of the simulation. Following the simulation, a debrief meeting with the team is recommended to allow them to self-reflect, discuss what went well and could be improved, and review the learning objectives.

Learning Objectives

By the end of the simulation, students will be able to:

Factual Knowledge

(a) Define obstructive shock and cardiac tamponade. Explain the compensatory mechanisms that attempt to increase myocardial oxygen when cardiac perfusion is limited.

Conceptual Knowledge

(a) Compare and contrast the four major types of shock.
(b) Create a differential diagnosis for obstructive shock.
(c) Describe initial management strategies for patients in shock.

Procedural Knowledge

(a) Explain when a Focused Assessment with Sonography in Trauma (FAST exam) would be performed and demonstrate its use in a simulated clinical scenario.
(b) Explain when ultrasound-guided pericardiocentesis would be performed and demonstrate its use in a simulated clinical scenario.

J. K. Lythgoe (✉)
Department of Radiology, University of Vermont Medical Center, Burlington, VT, USA

C. A. Standley (ed.), *Biomedical Science and Clinical Foundations*,
https://doi.org/10.1007/978-3-031-98353-5_32

Metacognitive Knowledge

(a) Self-reflect on how the simulation went, how effectively the team worked together, and what gaps in learning remain.

Theme Objective

(a) Discuss factors that affect a patient's access to care (such as availability, affordability, or accommodation) and how they interact with patient characteristics (such as beliefs, culture, language, or literacy) to form potential healthcare barriers.

Scenario Setup

- 1 simulation operator
- 1 nurse/facilitator
- 1 live patient model for ultrasound scanning practice
- 4–6 student doctors
- Estimated 30 min for the case
- Previous exposure to ultrasound/FAST exam is recommended

Materials Required

- Simulation mannequin or live patient model
- Computer and monitor for displaying simulated vital signs and images
- Ultrasound machine
- Pericardiocentesis training mannequin
- Pericardiocentesis kit

Case Walkthrough

1. Doctors will be called in to evaluate the patient.
2. Facilitator briefly introduces the case: "The patient arrived in the emergency department via ambulance following a motor vehicle accident that occurred approximately 15 minutes ago. EMTs reported that the patient was awake and alert at the scene of the accident."

Chief complaint: Chest pain			
Patient Name	Charlie Thompson	**DOB/ Age**	35
Height/ Weight	6'/180 lbs	**Sex**	Male

3. Doctors may ask for the initial vital signs to be displayed on the monitor (See "Primary Vitals").

Primary Vitals:			
Heart rate	Blood pressure	Respiratory rate (RR)	Pulse oximetry (SpO_2)
120 bpm	100/75 mmHg	28	89% on RA 91% on supplemental O_2 (if given)

4. Doctors will obtain a directed history and perform a physical exam. The facilitator can confirm positive physical exam findings if asked, or after the physical exam:

History of Present Illness (HPI):
Charlie Thompson is a 35-year-old male that presents to the Emergency Department via ambulance with chest pain following a motor vehicle accident 15 min ago. He is also complaining of difficulty breathing. He states that his chest hit the steering wheel. The pain is localized to his sternum, is dull and achy, and is 4–5/10. The pain does not radiate, but it hurts more when pressure is applied to the sternum.

Medical and surgical history:	
Past Medical History (PMH)	Hypertension Asthma Gluten Intolerance
Past Surgical History (PSH)	Tonsillectomy, age 6 Appendectomy, age 22
Family History (FH)	Mother: HTN. Died from a heart attack at 54 Father: Recently diagnosed with ALS Brother: Healthy No children
Social History (SH)	Marital Status: Single Education: College graduate Occupation: Information Technology- sedentary Tobacco Use: None Alcohol Use: 1–2 beers nightly Drug use: None
Allergies	Seasonal
Medications	Claritin as needed Lisinopril 5 mg daily Albuterol inhaler, PRN. Uses it 1–2 times per week

Review of Systems (ROS):	
Pertinent positives:	Chest pain, difficulty breathing, lightheadedness.
Pertinent negatives:	Fever, chills, headache, abdominal pain, broken bones, back pain, loss of bowel/bladder control, numbness, tingling, burning, or shooting pains.

Physical exam:		
Constitutional/General	**Respiratory**	**Integumentary/Skin**
Sternal pain with pressed Awake and Alert	tachypneic Diminished lung sounds	Clammy skin Diaphoretic
Head/Eyes/Ears/Nose/Throat	**Cardiovascular**	**Neurological**
normal	tachycardic Muffled heart sounds 1+ weak, thready pulses	normal
Neck	**Abdomen**	**Psychiatric/Endocrine**
JVD	normal	normal
Musculoskeletal	**Genitourinary**	
normal	normal	

5. Doctors may order the following tests during the simulation. Test results can be made available for review on the in-room monitor after a short delay:
   (a) EKG:
      (i) EKG demonstrates electrical alternans (Fig. 32.1a) and low-voltage QRS complexes (Fig. 32.1b).
   (b) Chest Radiographs:
      (i) A prior normal chest radiograph can be available for comparison (Fig. 32.2a).
      (ii) The chest radiograph taken in the Emergency Department demonstrates new cardiomegaly and is otherwise normal (Fig. 32.2b).
   (c) Ultrasound FAST exam:
      (i) Facilitator may PROMPT the doctors if ultrasound is not proposed: “Is there a non-invasive test we can do at the bedside to get more immediate information?”
      (ii) Simulation should be paused when facilitator is ready for the FAST exam.
      (iii) Live model and ultrasound machine enter the room for the exam when indicated by the facilitator to practice scanning a normal FAST exam.
      (iv) Abnormal ultrasound findings appear on the monitor for review: still ultrasound images demonstrate an abnormal pericardial effusion (Fig. 32.3a and 32.3b) and right ventricular diastolic collapse (Fig. 32.4a and 32.4b).
   (d) Any additional tests will not come back before the end of the simulation.
6. Doctors may or may not put the patient on supplemental oxygen due to tachypnea and hypoxia.
   (a) If so, SpO_2 increases, but the patient continues to feel short of breath.
7. If doctors administer IV fluids for hypotension, the patient’s condition will worsen (change to “Secondary Vitals,” see below).
   (a) Patient develops lightheadedness and generalized weakness.

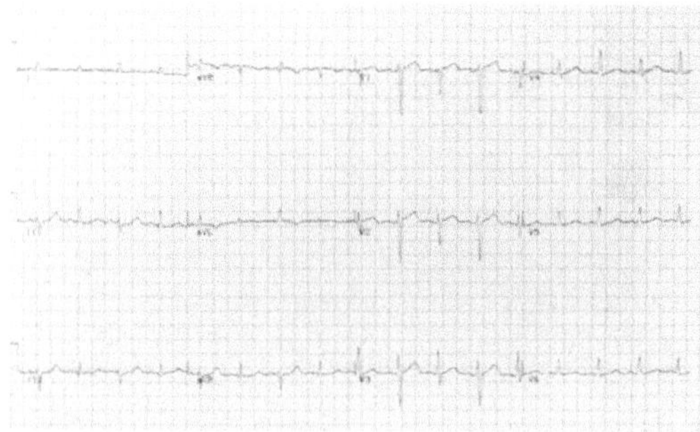

Fig. 32.1a EKG demonstrates alternating amplitudes of the QRS complexes in at least one lead. This is known as electrical alternans, a sign of massive pericardial effusion. (With permissions from the University of Vermont Medical Center (UVMMC) Department of Cardiology)

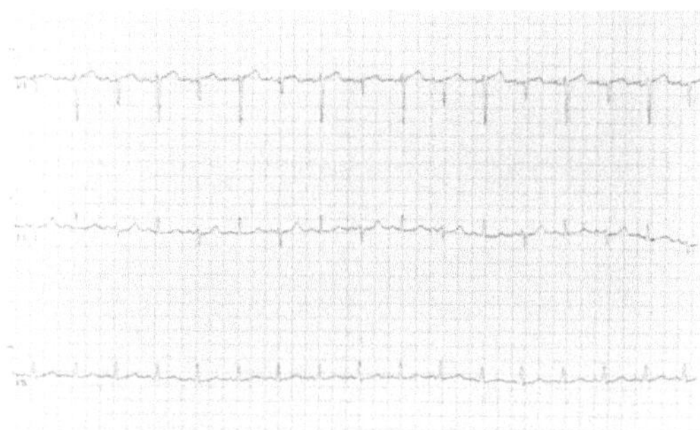

Fig. 32.1b EKG demonstrates low voltage QRS complexes, a non-specific finding which can be seen with pericardial effusion or cardiac tamponade. (With permissions from the UVMMC Department of Cardiology)

   (b) Facilitator can prompt the team, “The fluids seem to have made him worse! What do you think could be going on?”
8. Diagnosis: Cardiac Tamponade
   (a) After FAST exam is performed and abnormal findings have been presented, a diagnosis of pericardial effusion and cardiac tamponade should be made.
   (b) The patient decompensates regardless of whether treatment with IV fluids was ordered (see “Secondary Vitals”).
   (c) Patient develops lightheadedness and generalized weakness.

Secondary vitals (decompensated, pre-treatment):

Heart rate	Blood pressure	Respiratory rate (RR)	Pulse oximetry (SpO_2)
180	75/60	33	80% on room air 80% if on supplemental O_2

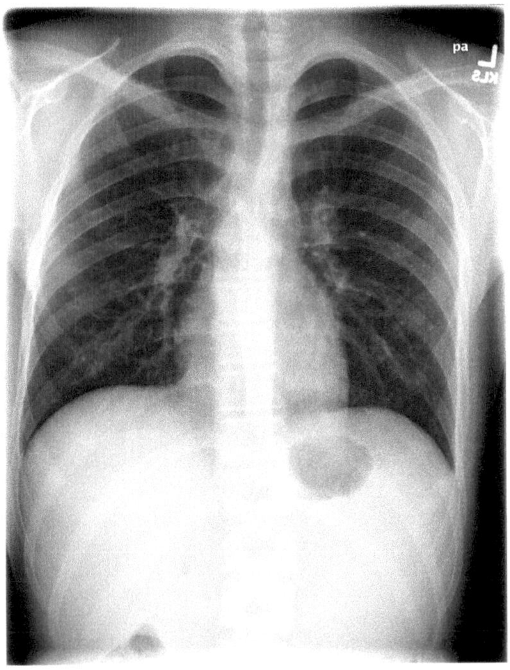

Fig. 32.2a Normal chest radiograph of the patient taken 1 month prior to the accident. (With permissions from the UVMMC Department of Radiology)

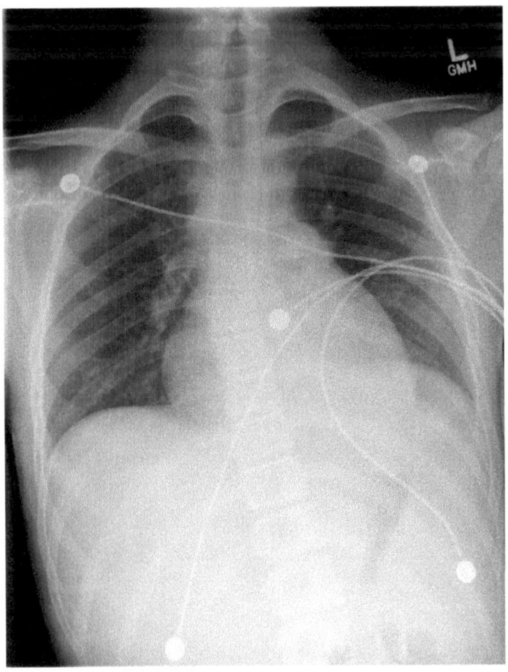

Fig. 32.2b Abnormal chest radiograph of the same patient taken in the ED on the day of the accident demonstrates new enlargement of the cardiac silhouette. (With permissions from the UVMMC Department of Radiology)

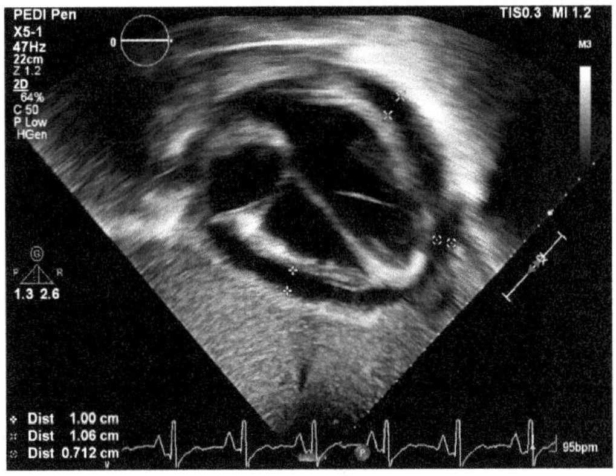

Fig. 32.3a Non-annotated ultrasound image of the cardiac atria and ventricles demonstrates abnormal pericardial fluid surrounding the heart. (With permissions from the UVMMC Department of Radiology)

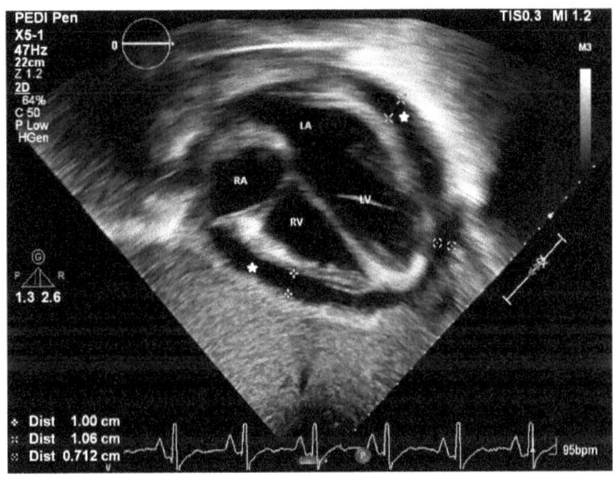

Fig. 32.3b Annotated ultrasound image of the cardiac atria and ventricles demonstrates abnormal pericardial fluid (stars) surrounding the heart. (With permissions from the UVMMC Department of Radiology)

9. Doctors should evaluate for causes of shock and identify obstructive shock.
   (a) If appropriate, the facilitator may pause simulation for discussion on types of shock.
10. Treatment: Ultrasound-guided pericardiocentesis
   (a) Simulation will be paused for the doctors to perform pericardiocentesis on the simulation trainers.

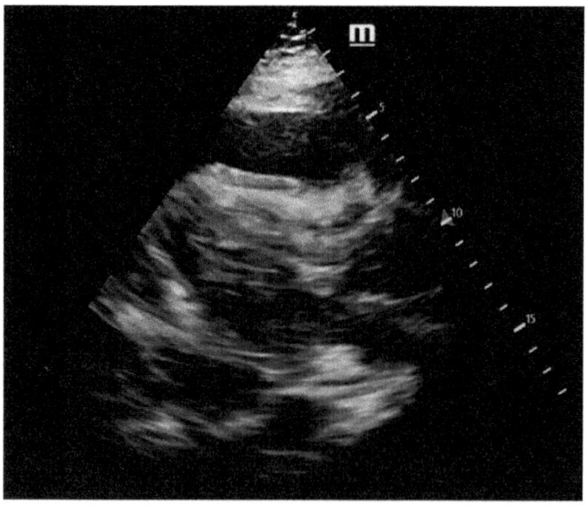

Fig. 32.4a Non-annotated ultrasound image obtained during diastole demonstrates abnormal pericardial fluid and collapse of the right ventricle. (With permissions from the UVMMC Department of Radiology)

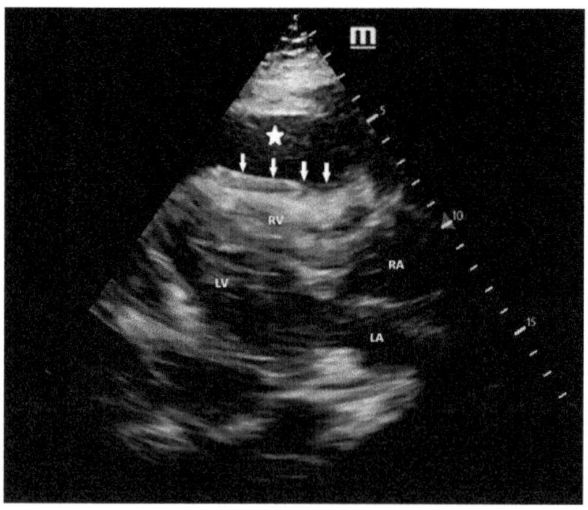

Fig. 32.4b Annotated ultrasound image obtained during diastole demonstrates abnormal pericardial fluid (star) and collapse of the right ventricle (arrows). (With permissions from the UVMMC Department of Radiology)

11. After pericardiocentesis, the patient will stabilize and rapidly feel better.
    (a) Proceed to tertiary vital signs.

Tertiary vitals (post-treatment, in recovery):			
Heart rate	Blood pressure	Respiratory rate (RR)	Pulse oximetry (SpO_2)
90 bpm	100/60 mmHg	20	94% on supplemental oxygen

12. Doctors will call the cardiothoracic surgery team, ending the scenario.
13. If time permits and if the scenario is appropriate to the level of training, the doctors may simulate the call and provide an oral summary to the surgical team for handoff.

Learning Objective Answers

Factual Knowledge

(a) Define obstructive shock and cardiac tamponade. Explain the compensatory mechanisms that attempt to increase myocardial oxygen when cardiac perfusion is limited.
   (i) Obstructive shock is a category of shock that occurs due to extracardiac causes leading to decreased left ventricular cardiac output. Etiologies can be vascular (pulmonary embolism and severe pulmonary hypertension) or mechanical (cardiac tamponade, tension pneumothorax, or constrictive pericarditis). This decrease in cardiac output results in decreased blood pressure and decreased oxygen delivery to end organs. The carotid sinus detects the decrease in blood pressure and tries to compensate by releasing epinephrine, constricting peripheral blood vessels, and increasing heart rate to maintain end-organ perfusion.

Conceptual Knowledge

(a) Compare and contrast the four major types of shock.
   (i) See Fig. 32.5. Categories of Shock.
(b) Create a differential diagnosis for obstructive shock.
   (i) Obstructive shock is due to extracardiac causes of decreased left ventricular cardiac output. Causes can be pulmonary

Shock	Inadequate organ perfusion and delivery of nutrients necessary for normal tissue and cellular function. Initially may be reversible but life threatening if not treated promptly.					
	CAUSED BY	SKIN	PCWP (PRELOAD)	CO	SVR (AFTERLOAD)	TREATMENT
Hypovolemic	Hemorrhage, dehydration, burns	Cold, clammy	↓↓	↓	↑	IV fluids
Cardiogenic	Acute MI, HF, valvular dysfunction, arrhythmia	Cold, clammy	↑or↓	↓↓	↑	Inotropes, diuresis
Obstructive	Cardiac tamponade, pulmonary cmbolism, tension pneumothorax	Cold, clammy	↑or↓	↓↓	↑	Relieve obstruction
Distributive	Sepsis, anaphylaxis	Warm	↓	↑	↓↓	IV fluids, pressors
	CNS injury	Dry	↓	↑	↓↓	

Fig. 32.5 Categories of Shock. (With permissions from Le et al. [1], no changes were made)

vascular or mechanical in nature. Examples include:

1. Pulmonary vascular:
   (a) Pulmonary embolism
   (b) Severe pulmonary hypertension
2. Mechanical compression
   (a) Cardiac tamponade
   (b) Tension pneumothorax
   (c) Restrictive cardiomyopathy
   (d) Constrictive pericarditis
   (e) Dynamic hyperinflation (severe asthma or COPD)

(c) Describe initial management strategies for patients in shock.

(i) Shock that is not quickly diagnosed and treated can rapidly become life-threatening to your patient. The first step in treating shock is securing the airway and ensuring adequate oxygenation, followed by obtaining peripheral, intraosseous, or central venous access. The patient should be very closely monitored and evaluated to establish a specific diagnosis. Further treatment should be targeted to the underlying cause of the shock. In patients with distributive or hypovolemic shock, immediate fluid resuscitation is important for maintaining blood pressure and organ perfusion. If tension pneumothorax is suspected, a chest X-ray will confirm the diagnosis, and immediate needle decompression will relieve the obstruction. For obstructive shock due to suspected cardiac tamponade, a diagnosis can quickly be confirmed by cardiac ultrasound during the FAST exam. Pericardiocentesis should be urgently performed to relieve the obstruction.

Procedural Knowledge

(a) Explain when a FAST exam would be performed and demonstrate its use in a simulated clinical scenario.

(i) The FAST exam is a bedside ultrasound examination used to quickly identify intraperitoneal and intrapericardial fluid. It is a rapid and inexpensive exam that is highly specific. The FAST exam is indicated in cases of undifferentiated shock, hypotension, and blunt and/or penetrating abdominal and/or thoracic trauma. It can be used in the emergency room to rapidly identify internal bleeding in patients that are hemodynamically unstable, cannot be transported, or cannot otherwise undergo a CT scan. The FAST exam is performed in 5 anatomic locations: right upper quadrant, left upper quadrant, suprapubic, anterior thoracic, and subxiphoid.

(b) Explain when ultrasound-guided pericardiocentesis would be performed and demonstrate its use in a simulated clinical scenario.

(i) Pericardiocentesis is a procedure performed in the setting of obstructive shock secondary to cardiac tamponade. A needle is inserted into the pericardial space using a subxiphoid approach to remove accumu-

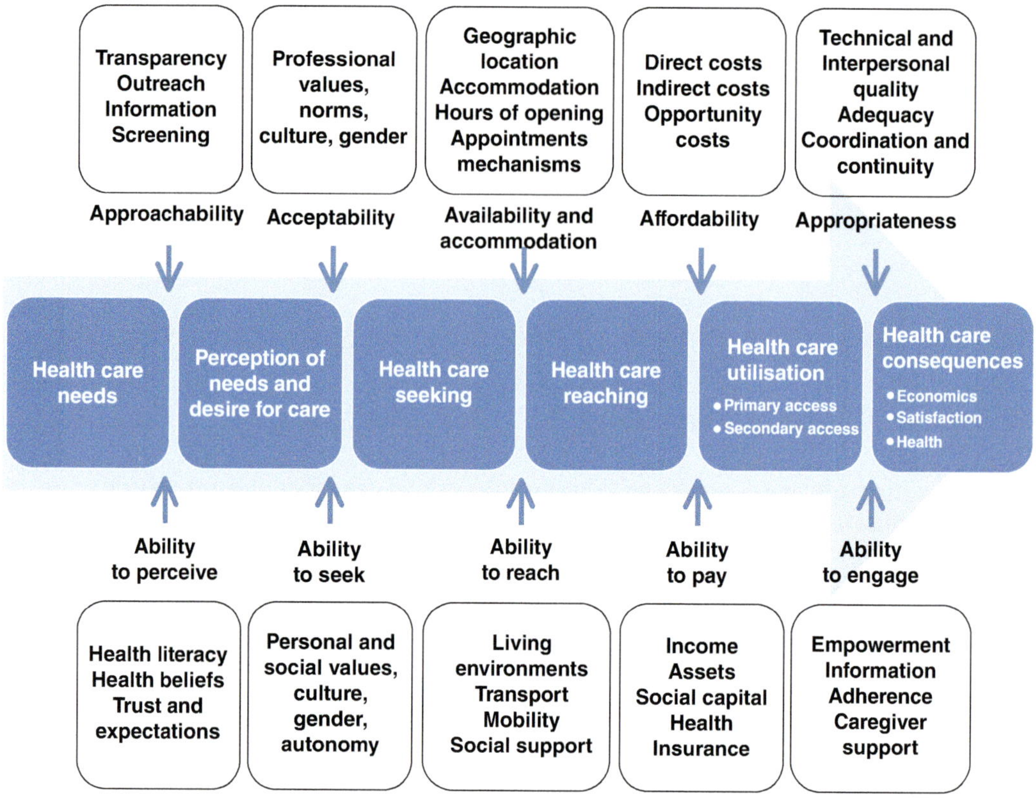

Fig. 32.6 Examples of factors affecting patient care that could form potential barriers to healthcare. (With permissions from Levesque et al. [2], no changes were made)

lated pericardial fluid and relieve pressure compressing the heart. It can be done blindly, if necessary, but is typically done under ultrasound or fluoroscopic visualization. Ultrasound is inexpensive and readily available, and direct visualization may reduce the risk of complications. Pericardiocentesis is a temporary measure meant to stabilize the patient until the patient can be evaluated by the cardiothoracic surgery team for potential surgical creation of a pericardial window.

Metacognitive Knowledge

(a) Self-reflect on how the simulation went, how effectively the team worked together, and what gaps in learning remain.

Theme Objective

(a) Discuss factors that affect a patient's access to care (such as availability, affordability, or accommodation) and how they interact with patient characteristics (such as beliefs, culture, language, or literacy) to form potential healthcare barriers.
   (i) See Fig. 32.6 for examples.

Exam Questions

1. A 22-year-old male is brought to the ED after he was hit by a car while walking. He is pale, hypotensive, and tachycardic on physical exam and loses consciousness shortly after arrival. Which of the following imaging

modalities is the most appropriate at this time for this patient?

A. Ultrasonography
B. CT scan
C. X-ray
D. MRI

Answer: A

Learning Objective: Explain when a FAST exam would be performed and demonstrate its use in a simulated clinical scenario.

Explanation: Bedside ultrasonography can be used to perform a FAST exam, which is used to identify the presence of free fluid in the peritoneum or the pericardium. It can be performed at the bedside and can be used on hemodynamically unstable patients without moving the patient, including during a code. It is also fast and cost-effective. B is incorrect, as CT is not an option for hemodynamically unstable patients that cannot be moved, such as this patient. It can be very useful for detecting free air and delineating the extent of solid organ injuries but should wait to be performed until after the patient has been stabilized. C is incorrect, as while portable X-ray is fast and useful for ruling out pneumothorax or hemothorax, it would not reveal the presence or absence of internal bleeding. Moreover, it is not appropriate for this hemodynamically unstable patient who just lost consciousness. D is incorrect, as MRI is not appropriate for patients who cannot spend extended periods of time inside the scanner. This hemodynamically unstable patient needs immediate treatment and would not be able to undergo the scan.

2. A 62-year-old male presents with 3 days of progressive dyspnea. He is a lifetime smoker with a 4-month history of lung adenocarcinoma. On exam, he is found to be tachypneic, hypotensive, and tachycardic with electrical alternans on EKG. Which of the following additional findings would most likely be found in this patient?
   A. Bilateral rhonchi
   B. Pulmonary arteriolar hyperplasia
   C. Peripheral edema
   D. Pulsus paradoxus

Answer: D

Learning Objective: Create a differential diagnosis for obstructive shock.

Explanation: This patient has cardiac tamponade secondary to adenocarcinoma invading the pericardium. Cardiac tamponade commonly presents with the classic findings of Beck's triad: hypotension, muffled heart sounds, and JVD. Tachycardia and tachypnea can also be seen. EKG findings include low-voltage QRS complexes and electrical alternans. Pulsus paradoxus is defined as a decrease in systolic blood pressure of greater than 10 mmHg with inspiration and is highly indicative of cardiac tamponade. A is incorrect: Chronic obstructive pulmonary disease is common in older adults with a long history of smoking and follows a chronic course. Exacerbations present with dyspnea, hypoxemia, bilateral rhonchi, and sputum production. Electrical alternans is not seen in COPD. B is incorrect: Pulmonary fibrosis is a slowly progressive, chronic condition caused by pulmonary arteriolar hyperplasia. While dyspnea and hypoxemia are common findings, electrical alternans and hypotension are not expected in pulmonary fibrosis. C is incorrect: Heart failure exacerbations present with dyspnea, hypoxemia, jugular venous distension, and lower extremity edema. EKG findings are typically normal or indicative of ischemia, and electrical alternans would not be seen.

3. A 43-year-old male presents to the emergency department complaining of 3 days of chest pain that is worse when lying on his back. On physical exam, he is found to be hypotensive and tachycardic with an elevated jugular venous pressure. Which of the following is the most likely cause of this patient's hypotension?
   A. Tearing of the aortic tunica intima
   B. Systemic peripheral vasodilation
   C. Fluid collection in the pericardial space
   D. Increased intracranial pressure
   E. Disruption of sympathetic pathways

Answer: C

Learning Objective: Compare and contrast the four major types of shock.

Explanation: This patient has acute pericarditis complicated by cardiac tamponade and obstructive shock. Obstructive shock due to cardiac tamponade occurs when increased intrapericardial pressure compresses the heart during diastole and prevents ventricular filling. Other findings include distant heart sounds, tachycardia, and jugular venous distension. A is incorrect: Aortic dissection commonly presents as tearing chest pain radiating to the back, typically in hypertensive or normotensive patients. Hypotension is a complication that can occur in aortic dissection if the tear ruptures or extends proximally into the pericardium. B is incorrect: Hypotension due to peripheral vasodilation occurs in anaphylactic shock. Hypotension is accompanied by difficulty breathing, angioedema, and urticaria and is due to a severe allergic reaction. D is incorrect: The Cushing reflex is a response to increased intracranial pressure that causes systemic hypertension, not hypotension, to maintain brain perfusion. In addition to hypertension, bradycardia and irregular breathing are other common features. E is incorrect: Neurogenic shock presents as sudden hypotension, bradycardia, and flushing of the skin, typically following trauma to the central nervous system.

References

1. Le T, Bhushan V, et al. First Aid for the USMLE Step 1, a Student-to-Student Guide. 2017; p 299.
2. Levesque JF, Harris M, Russell G. Patient-centred access to health care: conceptualising access at the interface of health systems and populations. Int J Equity Health. 2013;12:18. https://doi.org/10.1186/1475-9276-12-18.

33 Intractable Vomiting

Jennifer Kirkpatrick

Learning Objectives:
Participants should be able to:

- Recognize the emergent nature of the patient presenting in diabetic ketoacidosis (DKA).
- Communicate effectively with the team to obtain necessary diagnostic tests and execute necessary treatments.
- Communicate effectively with the patient and family member to keep them informed of the patient's condition and the risks and benefits of diagnostic and therapeutic interventions.
- Order the necessary diagnostic workup and initiate appropriate therapy for the patient presenting with DKA.

Case Scenario: Intractable Vomiting (DKA)

Patient Name: Megan Brooks

CC:
"My daughter has been throwing up and isn't acting right."

HPI:
The patient is a 14-year-old female brought into the pediatric ED after her mother noticed that she was unusually lethargic after returning home from work. She had been having some nausea and vomiting for the past two days, and was complaining of abdominal pain. She did not have any known fevers. The patient's mother assumed she picked up a stomach bug from one of her friends. She was noted feeling thirsty, so the mother has been giving her sports drinks at home. She did seem very tired over the past few days and reported feeling weak this morning, so she was allowed to stay home from school. Her mother relays that due to work and Megan spending more time with her friends, she is unsure if there have been any additional symptoms, though it does seem that her clothes appear to be fitting more loosely recently, but she assumed her daughter was trying to lose weight due to peer pressure. She has otherwise been well.

ROS:
Positive for nausea, vomiting (about 8 episodes since yesterday), abdominal pain, fatigue, lethargy, and weight loss.

PMH:
None. The patient is previously healthy. Immunizations up-to-date (UTD). She was born full-term via an uncomplicated normal spontaneous vaginal delivery (NSVD).

Medications:
None

J. Kirkpatrick (✉)
Department of Emergency Medicine, The Permanente Medical Group, Sacramento, CA, USA
e-mail: Jennifer.t.kirkpatrick@kp.org

C. A. Standley (ed.), *Biomedical Science and Clinical Foundations*,
https://doi.org/10.1007/978-3-031-98353-5_33

Allergies:
None

Family History:
Mother has a history of high blood pressure. Father is not involved in patient's life and has an unknown family history.

Social History:
Attends the local high school. No known history of drug or alcohol use.

Physical Examination:

Vital Signs:

HR	BP	RR	O_2 Sat	Temp	Weight	Notes
120 bpm	100/66 mmHg	26/min	99% RA	37 °C	48 Kg	Initial
128 bpm	96/60 mmHg	26/min	97% RA			Second labs
98 bpm	105/68	18/min	98% RA			After initiation of therapy

General: Ill-appearing, adolescent female, lying in bed, somnolent. Knows her name, but not oriented to person or time.

HEENT: Normocephalic/atraumatic Extraocular muscles intact normocephalic/atraumatic extraocular muscles intact (NC/AT), EOMI. PERRLA. Trachea midline. No jugular venous distention (JVD). No cervical lymphadenopathy (cervical LAD). No pharyngeal edema or erythema. Mucous membranes are dry. Fruity breath odor present.

Neck: Supple, no tenderness. No rigidity.

Resp: Tachypneic, labored, deep breathing. Lungs clear to auscultation bilaterally clear to auscultation bilaterally (CTAB).

CV: Tachycardic, regular. No murmurs, gallops, or rubs.

Abd: Soft, nondistended. Moderately diffusely tender to palpation + normal bowel sounds.

Back: No midline or Costovertebral angle (CVA) ttp.

Skin: No rashes or lesions. Capillary refill >3 s. Poor skin turgor.

Extremities: Cool to touch. Pedal pulses are thready.

Neuro: Somnolent. Oriented to name, but not to time or place. Uncooperative for the neuro examination. 2+ reflexes. No focal deficits noted.

Scenario Development

1. The participant will enter the room to see the patient.
2. The participant will get the history from the patient's mother.
3. The participant should ask for the patient to be placed on the cardiac monitor.
4. The participant should order a peripheral IV line and ask for blood to be drawn.
5. The participant should perform a physical examination, which should include:
   - Head, eyes, ears, nose, thorat (HEENT) exam
   - Skin exam
   - Heart and lung exam
   - Abdominal exam
   - Neurologic exam
   - Assessment of pulses
6. The participant should order the following tests:
   - Fingerstick glucose
   - Urine or serum hCG
   - CBC
   - BMP
   - Urine dip/UA
   - ABG or VBG
   - CT head
7. The participant should begin treatment
   - 0.9% NaCl bolus at 10 cc/kg after hypovolemia is noted on examination.
   - Reassessment should be made for improvement in perfusion.

After the return of laboratory studies, the participant should order

- IV insulin at 0.05–0.1 units/kg/hr
- KCl 40 mEq/L in IV fluids

8. The participant should ask the vital signs to be checked every 5 min.
9. The participant should call the pediatric intensive care unit (PICU) to admit the patient.
10. The case will end once the PICU physician comes down to admit the patient.

Scenario Props

- Female manikin
- Cardiac monitor
- Oxygen saturation monitor
- Blood pressure cuff
- Peripheral IV
- Nasal cannula
- Oxygen source (wall or tank)
- Nonrebreather
- Bag-valve mask
- IV fluids
- Endotracheal tube with stylet and syringe
- Mac or Miller blade size of 3 or 4
- Labs showing elevated glucose, decreased Na+, increased BUN/Cr, decreased HCO_3^- and Cl^-, urine ketones, and glucose. ABG should also show a metabolic acidosis with respiratory compensation
- Medications: Insulin, IV fluids, KCl-containing IV fluids, IV mannitol, IV lorazepam
- Phone to call consults

Personnel Props

- Female patient
- Mother
- ED Nurse
- PICU physician

Participant's Name(s) ______________________
____

Medical Student Simulation-Based Training

Case: DKA

1 = Observed/Performed correctly
0 = Omitted/Failed to perform correctly
X = No opportunity to perform/Not required

Hits = obtains without prompting (full points)
IG = Instructor-/Confederate-Guided (subtract 1 point)
Wgt = How much the critical action is weighted (3 = always done, 2 = sometimes done, 1 = optional)

Event	Critical response	Hits	IG	Wgt
14-year-old female brought in by mother for nausea, vomiting, abdominal pain, and lethargy.	The participant obtains a complete history and performs a comprehensive physical examination.			**3**
	The participant asks for an IV, vital signs, and cardiorespiratory monitoring.			**3**

Event	Critical Response	Hits	IG	Wgt
The patient is examined and noted to be tachypneic, somnolent, and with signs of poor perfusion	The participant places the following orders:			
	Fingerstick glucose			**3**
	CBC			**3**
	BMP			**3**
	ABG or VBG			**3**
	Urinalysis			**3**
	Serum or urine hCG			**2**
	IV fluid bolus			**3**

Event	Critical response	Hits	IG	Wgt
The participant receives results showing evidence of diabetic ketoacidosis	The participant administers IV insulin ***after*** return of K+			**3**
	The participant orders fluids with IV KCl			**3**
	The participant communicates results and plan with the patient's mother			**3**

Event	Critical response	Hits	IG	Wgt
The nurse says, "What is the plan for her?"	The participant calls the PICU team for admission.			**3**

Event	Critical response	Hits	IG	Wgt
The patient becomes unresponsive and then has a seizure	The participant administers an IV benzodiazepine such as lorazepam			**3**
	The participant intubates the patient			**3**
	The participant administers IV mannitol			**3**

Total # of (Weighted) Hits: ______________

____

Number of Instructor-Guided Hits: ________

____

General Comments and Suggestions ________

____

____

____

____

____

____

____

____

____

____

____

Labs

Point-of-Care Testing:

Urine pregnancy test: Negative

Fingerstick glucose: Too high to read

Urine dip: Glucose +++, ketones +++

CBC			
WBC	7.0	K/ul	4.0–10.5
Hb	14.2	g/dl	12.5–17.0
Hct	42.5	%	36.0–50.0
PLT	190	K/ul	150–450

BMP			
Na+	134	meQ/L	135–145
K+	4.6	meQ /L	3.5–5.1
Cl-	97	meQ /L	98–110
CO_2	11	meQ/L	20–32
Glu	592	mg/dL	65–99
BUN	40	mg/dL	6–24
Creat	1.4	mg/dL	0.76–1.24

ABG		
pH:	7.05	7.35–7.45
PCO_2:	28 mm/Hg	35–45 mm Hg
PO_2:	98 mm/Hg	80–100 mm/Hg
HCO_3^-:	12 mEq	22–26 mEq/L
O_2 sat:	98%	95–100%
B.E.	-17	–2 to +2 mEq/L

Radiology

Chest X-ray

Normal, if ordered for cough

Debriefing Notes

- Recognize DKA as an endocrine emergency, especially in a previously healthy pediatric patient coming in with weight loss, nausea, vomiting, abdominal pain, and lethargy.
- Realize that up to 40% of patients with T1DM present in DKA at the time of diagnosis.
- General treatment guidelines for DKA include: IV fluids (bolus and maintenance) to correct for hypovolemia, insulin, potassium supplementation, and assessing for the presence of/treating intercurrent infection or illness.
- Continue insulin until metabolic acidosis/elevated anion gap resolves. Once glucose levels

fall (to a level of 300 mg/dL in children), add dextrose to IV fluids to minimize the risk for hypoglycemia.

- When evaluating for electrolyte abnormalities, potassium levels may be normal or high, but recognize that there is typically a total body potassium deficit as cells pump out K^+ ions in exchange for H+ ions going in to compensate for the acidosis. In pediatric DKA, K^+-containing fluids are administered once the serum K^+ is <5 mEq/L. If hypokalemia is present on labs, K^+ should be repeated before insulin is started, as it will further shift K^+ intracellularly.
- Recognize that cerebral edema is a feared complication of DKA and keep a high index of suspicion if your patient suffers a sudden change in mental status or exhibits focal neurologic signs after initially improving.
  - If cerebral edema develops, address ABCs and give IV mannitol at 0.5–1 g/kg, given over 10–15 min.

Exam Questions

See Exam Questions in Chap. 13

34 Lightheaded and Fatigued

Soham Gupta

Learning Objectives:

- The participants should take the following concrete actions to successfully manage the simulated patient:
  - Review EMS transport run sheet for information.
  - Obtain a SAMPLE history and focused physical examination.
  - Recognize unstable vital signs and determine the severity of patient illness.
  - Obtain and interpret EKG.
  - Generate an appropriate differential diagnosis.
  - Order appropriate laboratory workup.
  - Perform bedside transthoracic echocardiogram (TTE) and correctly interpret the mechanical cause of cardiogenic shock.
  - Administer inotrope (dobutamine) for hypotension.
  - Add loop diuretics and BiPAP for pulmonary edema.
  - Admit the patient to the Cardiac Intensive Care Unit and provide a case presentation to the cardiologist.
- Knowledge, Skills, and Attitudes:
  - Recognize the patient is in a critical condition with unstable vital signs.
  - Provide hemodynamic support.
  - Make the correct diagnosis of decompensated heart failure and later cardiogenic shock.
  - Order the correct laboratory analysis and imaging for the patient.
  - Acknowledge the patient's concerns and address them in a thoughtful and comprehensive manner.
  - Advocate for the patient and expedite his care.

S. Gupta (✉)
Oregon Health and Science University, Resident Physician, Multnomah Pavilion, Portland, OR, USA

Scenario Timeline

- 5 min: Introduction and role assignment
- 25 min: Simulation session
- 25 min: Debrief and didactics

Case Scenario: Decompensated heart failure progressing to cardiogenic shock

Patient Name: Mark Johnson

Chief Complaint: Lightheadedness and fatigue

History of Present Illness: A 66-year-old male patient comes into the emergency department with progressively worsening shortness of breath and cough that has become more productive in the last week. He is unable to speak for long periods of time and frequently catches his breath. Shortness of breath is worse when supine. Past

C. A. Standley (ed.), *Biomedical Science and Clinical Foundations*,
https://doi.org/10.1007/978-3-031-98353-5_34

medical history is significant for a "murmur," but the patient does not know what type because he does not see a cardiologist and rarely sees his primary care provider. The patient states he has had trouble going on his morning walks for 2 months and has had significant lightheadedness in the past week.

Initial Vitals: Blood pressure of 145/95 mmHg, a pulse of 110/min, and respirations of 26/min, SpO_2: 88%

Past Medical History: Hypertension

Review of Systems

Positive: Racing heart, fatigue, syncope, headache, shortness of breath, lower extremity swelling, waking up at night

Negative: Denies all other symptoms, including chest pain

Past Surgical History: Appendectomy at age 35

Medications: Lisinopril for hypertension, 10 mg oral daily

Allergies: PCN (penicillin) (rash)

Vaccines: Up to date

Family History: Father and brother with prostate cancer; Mother with Alzheimer's disease; son is healthy.

Social History

Tobacco 1 ppd × 20 years

No alcohol or drug use

Married. 1 son. Lives in Arizona, has no recent travel, worked in mining near Tucson for 35 years, and is now retired. No pets.

Physical Exam

General: Well-developed obese patient, sitting propped up on multiple pillows. Appears uncomfortable due to shortness of breath but is awake and oriented ×4.

HEENT: NC/AT, PERRLA, TMs clear bilaterally, moist mucous membranes. Neck supple.

Trachea midline. +JVD.

Resp: Tachypneic. Crackles at bilateral lung bases.+ mild wheezing. No stridor.

CV: Tachycardic rate, regular rhythm, soft, high-pitched, early diastolic decrescendo murmur heard best at the 3rd intercostal space on the left sternal border. 2+ bilateral LE edema to the mid-shin.

Abd: Soft, non-tender to palpation, no guarding or rebound.

Ext: Symmetric pulses at 1+. Capillary refill 2–3 s. 2+ bilateral LE edema to the mid-shin. No cyanosis.

Skin: Warm, diaphoretic. No rashes. No petechiae. No purpura.

Neuro: CN 2–12 intact. No focal deficits noted. A&O × 4.

Psych: Normal affect. No suicidal ideation (SI) or homicidal ideation (HI). Good insight.

Scenario Development

1. On the day of the simulation event, faculty should arrive at their assigned simulation room 30 min before the start of the case. There will be a simulation staff member assigned as the simulation operator/controller and a simulation nurse assigned to each room.
2. Faculty should meet with the simulation operator and simulation nurse to review the case, the mannequin, and the equipment available in the resuscitation room.
3. All of the students will meet in a conference room 15 min prior to the simulation scenario start time. They will receive a brief orienta-

tion from the Simulation Center staff, and they will be divided up into their resuscitation teams for the scenario.

4. In each team, students will be assigned the following roles and will wear name tags with their assigned roles:
   - Team Leader
   - History and Physical Exam
   - Medications and Procedures
   - Results and Data Analysis

If there are multiple simulation sessions back-to-back, students will be instructed to switch roles between sessions.

5. During the case, the simulation controller (sim ops) will be the voice of the patient and will be controlling the patient/mannequin's vital signs from behind the one-way mirror.
6. After the orientation, the students will be escorted into the hallway outside of their assigned simulation bay. They will be asked to wait there until the simulation nurse or faculty facilitator calls them into the room to help the patient.
7. The participants will be asked to discuss what their game plan will be for the case while they wait for the case to begin.
8. The RN should be standing by the patient's bed awaiting instructions from the participants.
9. The faculty facilitator will be sitting in the control room wearing a two-way microphone so that he/she can communicate with the RN who is in the control room. The faculty facilitator can give the RN questions to ask the participants throughout the case.
10. When the RN and facilitator are ready, the RN will walk outside of the room and say to the participants, "We need you to come in and see your patient. He isn't looking so good..."
11. The participants will be provided with the patient's chief complaint and the patient's vital signs en route and informed that they are the first to evaluate the patient.
12. The participant should immediately order:
    - The patient is to be placed on continuous vital monitoring.
    - Oxygen is to be administered given the patient's obvious shortness of breath and halting speech.
    - In general, a nonrebreather face mask with high-flow 100% O_2 is used because the concentration of delivered oxygen is greater than with nasal cannula; however, since this patient is in potential respiratory failure (accessory muscle use and tachypnea), they should be given noninvasive positive-pressure ventilation with BiPAP as soon as possible.
    - IV access given hemodynamic instability (a single normal IV is okay at this time as the patient is not hypotensive; if they want to place 2 large-bore PIVs, ask students what they want to give through that level of access).
    - EKG (given his tachycardia).
    - Chest X-ray given difficulty breathing.
    - CBC/CMP with troponins, BNP.
    - The participants should perform a focused history including all SAMPLE criteria and physical exam with a particular focus on respiratory and cardiovascular auscultation and examination of the peripheries; jugular venous distension should also be evaluated to the extent possible on the mannequin.
    - The patient should be asked if they have any chest pain as part of history taking or the review of systems (they do not have any chest pain).
13. The participant will recognize that the patient has signs of significant aortic regurgitation on the exam. Can be prompted by the RN to identify the murmur if they do not identify it independently.
14. EKG returns quickly (Fig. 34.1):
15. Students should now be prompted to identify what they think the diagnosis is, a full differential diagnosis, and what they want to rule out with future testing

Educator Note—From UpToDate

Acute decompensated heart failure is a heterogeneous condition, and successful management often relies on identifying the cause of decompensation [2]. The search for specific causes is an essential first step in the evaluation of these

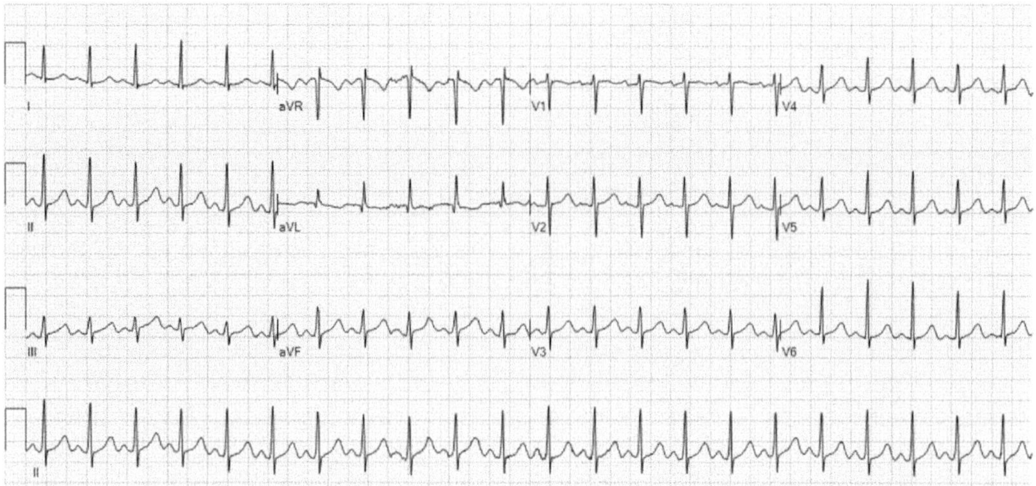

Fig. 34.1 Patient's EKG—Sinus Tachycardia
Caption: Students should identify this as sinus tachycardia [1]

Source: Ewingdo. "ECG Sinus Tachycardia 132 BPM." *Wikimedia Commons*, commons.wikimedia.org/wiki/File:ECG_Sinus_Tachycardia_132_bpm.jpg

patients. These include acute coronary syndrome (ACS), hypertensive emergency, rapid arrhythmias or severe bradycardia/conduction disturbance, acute mechanical causes such as acute valve regurgitation or acute pulmonary embolism, infection, including myocarditis, and tamponade. The acronym CHAMPIT (ACS, hypertension, arrhythmia, mechanical causes, pulmonary embolus, infection, and tamponade) was suggested as a useful reminder of the etiologic considerations by the European Society of Cardiology.

16. Ask what further laboratory and diagnostic testing is requested at this time to narrow the differential:
    - Can get CBC, CMP, BMP, troponins, urinalysis, and CXR at this point if not already ordered.
    - Should also get a transthoracic echocardiogram at this time to identify ejection fraction and characterize the severity of the likely aortic regurgitation at this time.
    - Students should be asked if they want to initiate any symptomatic treatment at this time while we wait for results (Fig. 34.2).
    - They should identify a diuretic to administer immediately as well as balanced vasodilator like nitroprusside to administer if transferred to the ICU
    - Diuretic (one of the following):
      - Furosemide
      - Bumetanide—1 mg intravenously
      - Torsemide—10–20 mg intravenously

If there is little or no response to the initial dose, the dose should be doubled at two-hour intervals as needed up to the maximum recommended doses.

Nitroprusside:

Because of its very potent hemodynamic effects and the potential to excessively lower blood pressure, the use of nitroprusside requires close hemodynamic monitoring, typically with an intra-arterial catheter. The initial dose of 5–10 mcg/min is titrated up every five minutes as tolerated to a dose range of 5–400 mcg/min.

*** Facilitator's notes on diuretic use***

Limited clinical trial data have shown a mortality benefit from diuretic therapy in patients with chronic HF. Although the safety and efficacy of diuretics to treat ADHF have not been

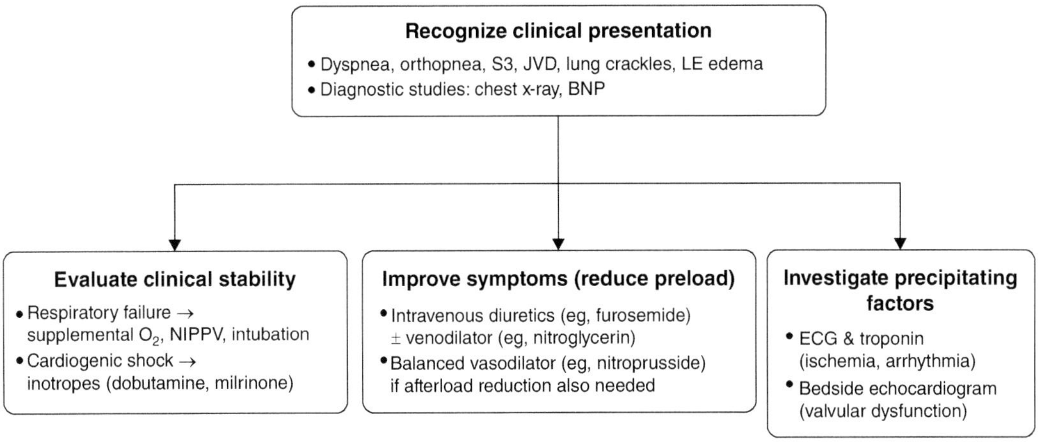

Fig. 34.2 The Initial Management of Acute Decompensated Heart Failure (ADHF) [2]
Caption: Students should evaluate initial clinical stability, give appropriate pharmacological treatment, and identify causes of heart failure
Source: Meyer, Theo. "Approach to Diagnosis and Evaluation of Acute Decompensated Heart Failure in Adults." *UpToDate*, www.uptodate.com/contents/approach-to-diagnosis-and-evaluation-of-acute-decompensated-heart-failure-in-adults

established in randomized trials, extensive observational experience has demonstrated that they effectively relieve congestive symptoms and are essential for the successful treatment of most patients with ADHF and volume overload.

Patients with ADHF and evidence of volume overload, regardless of etiology, should be

promptly treated with intravenous diuretics as part of their initial therapy. As noted in the 2022 American College of Cardiology Foundation/American Heart Association (ACC/AHA) HF guidelines, patients admitted with significant fluid overload should receive diuretic therapy without delay in the emergency department or outpatient clinic, as early intervention may produce better outcomes.

*** Facilitator's notes on nitroprusside use***

In contrast to nitroglycerin, nitroprusside causes balanced arterial and venous dilation. Thus, while it can be used to decrease LV filling pressures, it will cause a concomitant decrease in systemic vascular resistance. In patients in whom systemic resistance is elevated, the resulting decrease in afterload can increase stroke volume without lowering blood pressure; whereas if systemic vascular resistance is not elevated, nitroprusside may cause hypotension. Likewise, arterial dilation and afterload reduction can be of value in patients with depressed stroke volume due to elevated LV afterload, such as acute aortic regurgitation [3], acute mitral regurgitation, acute ventricular septal rupture, or hypertensive emergency.

17. CXR (Fig. 34.3) and TTE (Fig. 34.4) come back in that order.

Echocardiogram Measure of Left Ejection Fraction: 34%
Shows significant regurgitation at the aortic valve.

Other laboratory tests are listed at the end of this case; of relevance are the troponins and BNP. Stress the increased BNP and normal troponins and ask students what an elevated BNP can mean.

18. Change patient vitals to the following: BP: 82/46, P: 140, R: 36, T: 97 degrees F, SpO2: 79%

While students are identifying the TTE, they will be provided with a verbal prompt that the patient is feeling lightheaded (the patient's words should become progressively more incoherent to any follow-up questions.)

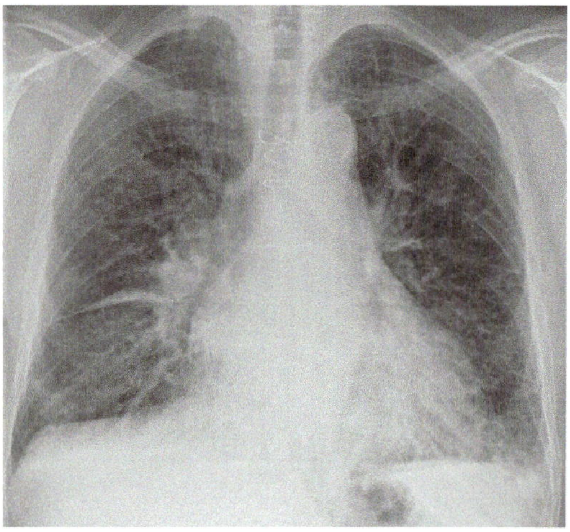

Fig. 34.3 Chest X-Ray showing Chronic Congestive Heart Failure
Caption: Students should be able to identify congestive heart, with an enlarged cardiac silhouette, especially of the left ventricle, as well as perihilar pulmonary congestion
Source: By Mikael Häggström—Own work, CC0, https://commons.wikimedia.org/w/index.php?curid=61595287; https://upload.wikimedia.org/wikipedia/commons/c/ca/Chest_radiograph_of_a_lung_with_Kerley_B_lines.jpg

Students should have the following response:

- Increase oxygenation flow/evaluate airway and work of breathing
- Find breathing to be very shallow and make the decision to intubate
- Should be examining treatment for cardiogenic shock from mechanical factors on their devices
- Should reexamine the patient and find that there is worse crackling in the lungs, prompt students to ensure the patient is properly intubated with correct tube placement if they do not re-auscultate the patient independently
- Now that the patient is hypotensive, they need to administer an inotropic agent (can use dopamine, dobutamine, or milrinone—dosing and specifics in facilitators notes) [4].

Note to facilitators

Temporary intravenous inotropic support was recommended for patients with cardiogenic shock to maintain systemic perfusion and pre-

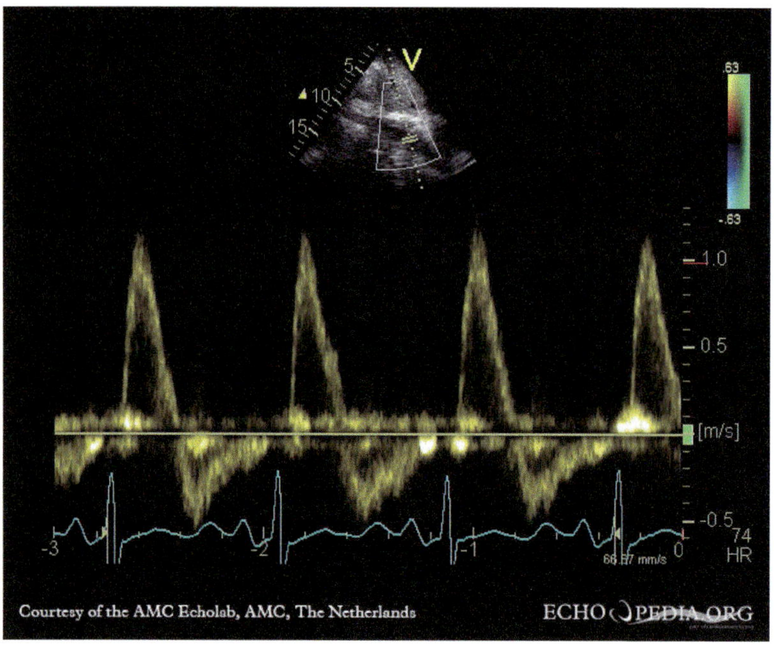

Fig. 34.4 Transthoracic Echocardiogram with Aortic Regurgitation
Caption: Echocardiogram showing aortic regurgitation
Source: CardioNetworks: Secretariat, CC BY-SA 3.0 <https://creativecommons.org/licenses/by-sa/3.0>, via Wikimedia Commons; https://upload.wikimedia.org/wikipedia/commons/2/22/Severe_aortic_regurgitation_E00186_%28CardioNetworks_ECHOpedia%29.jpg

serve end-organ performance until definitive therapy (e.g., coronary revascularization, mechanical circulatory support, or heart transplantation) is instituted or resolution of the acute precipitating problem has occurred (Table 34.1).

Note: Inotropes are not indicated for the treatment of ADHF in the setting of preserved systolic function!

19. Given the patient's increasing hemodynamic instability, the RN should prompt where we should send the patient, with the correct answer being the cardiac ICU.
20. The students will call the cardiac intensivist for emergent evaluation.
21. The preceptor will enter and ask who is in charge of the clinical scenario.
22. The team leader should summarize the case and recommend that the patient be taken to the cardiac ICU immediately.
23. The participants will go back into a debriefing room for a formal debrief.

Table 34.1 Use of Inotropic Agents in Heart Failure with Reduced Ejection Fraction

Agent	Tradename	Dose	Range	Uses
Dopamine	Inotropin	2–5 μg/kg/min	2–20 μg/kg/min	An alternative to norepinephrine in septic shock in highly selected patients (i.e., those with absolute or relative bradycardia and a low risk of tachyarrhythmias). More adverse effects (i.e., tachycardia, arrhythmias particularly at doses > 20 μg/kg/min) and less effective than norepinephrine for reversing hypotension in septic shock. Lower doses (i.e., 1–3 μg/kg/min) should not be used for renal protective effect and can cause hypotension during weaning. Must be diluted so use of a pre-diluted solution is preferred.
Dobutamine	Dobutrex	2–5 μg/kg/min	2–10 μg/kg/min	Initial agent of choice in cardiogenic shock with low cardiac output and maintained blood pressure. Add-on to norepinephrine for cardiac output augmentation in septic shock with myocardial dysfunction or ongoing hypoperfusion despite adequate intravascular volume and vasopressor agents. Increases cardiac contractility and rate; may cause hypotension and tachyarrhythmias. Must be diluted so use of a pre-diluted solution is preferred.
Milrinone	Primacor	0.125–0.25 μg/kg/min	0.125–0.75 μg/kg/min	Alternative for short-term cardiac output augmentation to maintain organ perfusion in cardiogenic shock refractory to other agents. Increases cardiac contractility and modestly increases heart rate at high doses; may cause peripheral vasodilation, hypotension, and/or ventricular arrhythmia. . Renally cleared; dose adjustment in renal impairment needed Must be diluted so use of a pre-diluted solution is preferred.

Source: Colucci, Wilson. "Inotropic Agents in Heart Failure with Reduced Ejection Fraction." *UpToDate*, www.uptodate.com/contents/inotropic-agents-in-heart-failure-with-reduced-ejection-fraction?search=Fab%2Bfragment&topicRef=3472

Scenario Props

- High Fidelity Patient Simulator (Male) with lung crackles, aortic regurgitation murmur, LE edema and JVD
- Capnography equipment
- Blood pressure cuff
- Peripheral IVs × 2
- Oxygen Source (wall or tank)
- BiPAP
- IV fluids (NS or LR)
- CXR pulmonary edema
- EKG sinus tachycardia
- TTE showing aortic regurgitation and Heart Failure with Reduced Ejection Fraction (HFrEF)
- Labs showing: elevated BNP, normal troponins
- Medications: inotropes, balanced vasodilator (nitroprusside), diuretics (ex. furosemide)
- Transthoracic echocardiogram machine
- Phone to call consults

Personnel

- Patient (male)
- Nurse
- Cardiac ICU attending

Laboratory Values
Complete Blood Count (CBC)
WBC 9.5 Latest Range: 4.0–10.0 × 103/μL
RBC 4.9 Latest Range: 4.30–5.90 × 106/μL
HEMOGLOBIN 15.0 Latest Range: 13.0–17.0 gm/dL
HCT 44.0 Latest Range: 39.0–51.0%
MCV 92.7 Latest Range: 81.0–99.0
MCH 31.0 Latest Range: 27.0–33.0
MCHC 33.5 Latest Range: 32.5–36.5%
RDW 12.0 Latest Range: 11.6–14.8%
PLATELET COUNT 380 Latest Range: 150–400 × 103/μL

Differential
NEUT% 60 Latest Range: 40.0–74.0%
LYMPH% 36 Latest Range: 12.0–40.0%
MONO% 4.0 Latest Range: 4.0–12.0%
EOSIN% 0.0 Latest Range: 0.0–8.0%
BASO% 0.3 Latest Range: 0.0–2.0%

Comprehensive Metabolic Panel (CMP)
GLUCOSE 90 Latest Range: 60–99 mg/dL
SODIUM 142 Latest Range: 133–145 meq/L
POTASSIUM 4.0 Latest Range: 3.5–5.3 meq/L
CHLORIDE 110 Latest Range: 98–108 meq/L
CO2 36 Latest Range: 23–32 meq/L
BUN 10 Latest Range: 7–23 mg/dL
CREATININE 1.0 Latest Range: 0.6–1.3 mg/dL
CALCIUM 9.3 Latest Range: 8.5–10.3 mg/dL
TOTAL PROTEIN 7.3 Latest Range: 6.1–7.9 g/dL
ALBUMIN 4.0 Latest Range: 3.5–5.5 g/dL
BILIRUBIN TOTAL 0.8 Latest Range: 0.1–1.4 mg/dL
BILIRUBIN DIRECT 0.2 Latest Range: 0.0–0.4 mg/dL
PHOSPHORUS 2.7 Latest Range: 2.4–4.7 mg/dL
ALK PHOSPHATASE 78 Latest Range: 0–135 IU/L
SGOT 28 Latest Range: 0–41 IU/L
SGPT 42 Latest Range: 0–63 IU/L
BNP: 1200 Latest Range: 0–100 (pg/mL)
TROPONINS: 0.01 Latest range: 0–0.04 ng/mL

MAGNESIUM 2.0 Latest Range: 1.7–2.8 mg/dL

LACTATE 1.0 Latest Range: 0.5–1.0 mmol/L

Urine Drug Screen
MARIJUANA SCREEN NEGATIVE No range found
COCAINE MET SCREEN NEGATIVE No range found
AMPHETAMINE SCREEN NEGATIVE No range found
METHAMPHETAMINE SCRN, UR NEGATIVE No range found
BARBITURATE SCREEN NEGATIVE No range found
OPIATES SCREEN NEGATIVE No range found
PHENCYCLIDINE SCREEN NEGATIVE No range found
METHADONE SCREEN NEGATIVE No range found
BENZODIAZEP SCRN NEGATIVE No range found

TRICYCL ANTIDEPRESS SCRN, UR NEGATIVE No range found

Urinalysis
Color Clear
Spec Grav 1.010
Glucose Neg
Ketones Neg
Blood Neg
Nitrites Neg
Leuk Esterase Neg
pH 7.0
Protein 40
Urobilinogen Neg
RBC Neg
WBC Neg

Coagulation Panel
PTT 30 Latest Range: 30–45 s
PT 12 Latest Range: 12–15 s
INR 1.0 Latest Range: 0.8–1.2
Blood Type
A negative

Debriefing Notes:

- If a patient appears critically ill, think and act simultaneously.
- Remember that you should always take a complete history and perform a full physical exam.
- Always address abnormal vital signs.
- Don't wait for laboratory studies to call a consultant if you need them. Use your physical exam and bedside tools.
- Consider high-risk diagnosis for heart failure; ACS must still be ruled out despite more chronic symptoms.

Notes and Reference Material for Evaluators
Adapted from UpToDate Article "Approach to diagnosis and evaluation of acute decompensated heart failure in adults [2]"

Since ADHF frequently presents with the sudden onset of respiratory distress that may or may not be associated with chest discomfort or a previous history of heart disease, other medical conditions must be excluded:

- Pulmonary embolism—The sudden onset of dyspnea, pleuritic chest pain, and cough may be caused by a pulmonary embolism. Establishing the diagnosis may depend upon the characteristics of the ECG and the differences in the appearance of typical chest radiograph findings in the two conditions.
  In addition to being part of the differential diagnosis, venous thromboembolism is more common in patients with HF and, in patients with ADHF, is associated with a worse prognosis.
- Pneumonia—Pneumonia can present with acute shortness of breath, hypoxemia, and an inconclusive pulmonary examination. Chest radiograph findings may differ, but some cases of bibasilar pneumonia may be similar to HF, although evidence of upper zone redistribution is not present with pneumonia. Fever and leukocytosis may suggest an infectious process.
- Asthma—Reactive airways disease can cause acute shortness of breath, cough, and fatigue. In addition, patients with ADHF may present with wheezing that can simulate asthma. The chest radiograph can be helpful in differentiating these conditions.
- Noncardiogenic pulmonary edema (NCPE)—NCPE is invariably associated with an underlying disease, which may or may not be readily apparent. The diagnosis of NCPE often depends on pretest probabilities: acute respiratory distress in a patient with documented sepsis (ie., peritonitis) or pancreatitis should raise the strong possibility that the respiratory failure is due to NCPE. The approach to the management of long-term HF therapy in patients with ADHF includes the following:
- Determine if the patient is stable—In patients with ADHF, the patient's stability determines whether long-term therapy can be continued or initiated. While the degree of stability required for long-term HF therapy is ultimately based on a clinical judgment influenced by many factors, stable patients who can tolerate continuation of their chronic HF therapy in the hospital typically have the following features:

- Heart rate less than 100 bpm
- Absence of cardiogenic shock
- No requirement for intravenous (IV) diuretics or intravenous vasodilators in the preceding six hours
- No requirement for IV inotropes in the preceding 24 h
- Normal or improving kidney function
- Long-term therapy in stable patients—Patients with ADHF who are stable may continue or initiate long-term therapy for HF:
  - Continuation of therapy—In patients with ADHF who exhibit signs of clinical stability at presentation, long-term therapy can be continued during the inpatient admission if it is unlikely to cause harm. However, patients who continue their long-term HF medications should be frequently evaluated for signs of instability to determine whether any component of such therapy should be discontinued or have its dose reduced.

The rationale for starting long-term HF treatment prior to discharge is primarily based on the known benefits of long-term therapy (e.g., reduction of readmission risk) and the observation that adherence to therapy is increased among patients who are prescribed therapy at the time of discharge.

Exam Questions

1. A 65-year-old female undergoes a right lung biopsy for prospective lung cancer and develops shortness of breath and chest pain an hour after the procedure. The patient has a past medical history of hypertension, diabetes mellitus type 2, a recent infection treated with ceftriaxone, and a 20-pack-year smoking history. Vitals are blood pressure of 78/40 mm Hg, pulse of 122, and respiratory rate of 28. On physical exam, the patient is diaphoretic, and skin is cool. Pulmonary catheterization shows a decreased cardiac index and an elevated pulmonary capillary wedge pressure. What type of shock is this patient experiencing?
   A. Hypovolemic shock
   B. Cardiogenic shock
   C. Obstructive shock
   D. Distributive shock

   Answer: B
   Explanation: This patient likely had an acute myocardial infarction following the procedure, leading to cardiogenic shock. The differentiating factor is a decreased cardiac output, which makes septic shock less likely, and increased pulmonary capillary wedge pressure, which is suggestive of increased left atrial pressure due to lack of forward blood flow from a compromised left ventricle.

2. A male patient with end-stage renal disease comes to the hospital for the placement of an arteriovenous fistula for ongoing hemodialysis. The patient feels well without fever or signs of infection at the fistula site. How will afterload, preload, and cardiac output change in this patient following the placement of this fistula?
   A. Afterload: Decreased, Preload: Decreased, Cardiac Output: Decreased
   B. Afterload: Decreased, Preload: Decreased, Cardiac Output: Increased
   C. Afterload: Decreased, Preload: Increased, Cardiac Output: Increased
   D. Afterload: Increased, Preload: Increased, Cardiac Output: Increased

   Answer: C
   Explanation: The creation of an arteriovenous fistula allows blood to bypass systemic capillaries with the highest resistance in the peripheral vasculature. This results in decreased systemic vascular resistance and thus afterload and corresponding increased cardiac output. The increased venous return results in increased preload. This can progress to high-output heart failure if the fistula is too large.

3. A 72-year-old male patient comes into the emergency department with progressively worsening shortness of breath and cough that has become more productive in the last week. He is unable to

speak for long periods of time and frequently catches his breath. Shortness of breath is worse when supine. The patient does not see a doctor regularly and cannot relate past medical history. On physical exam, the patient has lung crackles, jugular venous distension, accessory muscle use for respiration, and bilateral lower extremity edema. Heart sounds are normal. Patient vitals are blood pressure: 160/100 mmHg, pulse of 120/min, and respirations of 32/min. What is the next best step in treatment?

A. Dobutamine
B. Pericardiocentesis
C. Oral anticoagulation
D. Normal saline
E. Noninvasive positive-pressure ventilation

Answer: E

Explanation: This patient's dyspnea, orthopnea, jugular venous distension, lung crackles, and lower extremity edema are suggestive of acute decompensation of heart failure. The patient should be placed on noninvasive positive-pressure ventilation as soon as possible to decrease work of breathing. In patients who are not in cardiogenic shock, like this patient with elevated blood pressure, inotropes like dobutamine are not given. Saline would worsen the patient's symptoms, and diuretics are preferred instead. Oral anticoagulation is not needed urgently, as pulmonary embolism is less likely given the progressive course of this patient's symptoms. Pericardiocentesis is not needed, as cardiac tamponade is less likely given the patient's hypertension.

References

1. Ewingdo. "ECG Sinus Tachycardia 132 Bpm." *Wikimedia Commons*, commons.wikimedia.org/wiki/File:ECG_Sinus_Tachycardia_132_bpm.jpg.
2. Meyer T. "Approach to diagnosis and evaluation of acute decompensated heart failure in adults." *UpToDate*, www.uptodate.com/contents/approach-to-diagnosis-and-evaluation-of-acute-decompensated-heart-failure-in-adults.
3. Zoghbi W. *Clinical Manifestations and Diagnosis of Chronic Aortic Regurgitation in Adults*, www-uptodate-com/contents/clinical-manifestations-and-diagnosis-of-chronic-aortic-regurgitation-in-adults?search=clinical+manifestations+and+diagnosis+of+chronic+aortic+regurgitation+in+adults&source=search_result&selectedTitle=1~150&usage_type=default&display_rank=1. Accessed 24 Jan 2025.
4. Colucci W. "Inotropic agents in heart failure with reduced ejection fraction." *UpToDate*, www.uptodate.com/contents/inotropic-agents-in-heart-failure-with-reduced-ejection-fraction?search=Fab%2Bfragment&topicRef=3472.

Facilitator Note: *Abnormal values are in bold below.*

Scenario Development

1. The group will be waiting in the hall and be called in by a nurse urgently asking for help with a patient who is actively seizing.
2. The nurse will introduce the patient with "This is Mr. Williams, he was in the waiting room of the ED when all of a sudden he started shaking – I think he's having a seizure!"
3. The group should recognize that Mr. Williams is having a seizure and immediately begin workup and management, including [1]:
   (a) ABCs
   (b) Place the patient on a monitor
   (c) Obtain IV access—two large bore IVs
   (d) Place patient on oxygen
   (e) Fingerstick blood glucose! (**NOTE:** the patient will NOT stop seizing despite medications until a fingerstick is done and the patient is given an amp of D50)
   (f) Begin ordering medications
4. The nurse will obtain IV access successfully and report that vitals are:
   (a) **BP 140/95 mmHg**
   (b) **Pulse 122 bpm**
   (c) **RR 23 breaths/min**
   (d) **O_2 saturation 88% on RA**
   (e) Temperature 99.4 F

Facilitator Note: *Ask the participants about these abnormal values – does the patient need supplemental oxygen? Invasive (intubation) or non-invasive (nasal cannula or face mask)? Start with non-invasive.*

5. The participants can order and administer various anti-epileptic drugs to the patient. (They do not need to know exact dosages.) However, the patient **WILL NOT** stop seizing until the participants obtain a glucose level, recognize low sugar, and administer an amp of D50.

Facilitator Note: *If participants are having trouble – stop and ask them, what are possible reasons this patient might be seizing? If they haven't yet, suggest they ask the nurse for any history she has from triage or the computer.*

6. Once the participants get (1) finger stick glucose, (2) recognize low sugar, and (3) give an amp of D50, the patient will stop seizing. New vital signs will be generated:
   (a) BP 125/85 mmHg
   (b) Pulse 90 bpm
   (c) RR 17 breaths/min
   (d) O_2 saturation 99% on face mask or nasal cannula
      (i) *Participants should recognize his initial low O_2 saturation and put on oxygen if not already done so during seizure (NC or NRB mask will improve O_2 sats to high 90 s)*
   (e) Temp 99 F
7. Participants should perform a full history and physical once the seizure has stopped; may also start to order labs (Tables 35.1, 35.2, 35.3, 35.4, and 35.5)
   (a) History—see above
   (b) Physical
      (i) General: slightly confused initially, postictal, progressively more alert, and oriented as time passes
      (ii) HEENT: small laceration on forehead from hitting head on a chair while seizing in the waiting room, PERRLA, trachea midline, no JVD
      (iii) Resp: CTAB, no wheezing, normal work of breathing
      (iv) CV: tachycardic, no murmurs, rubs, or gallops
      (v) Abd: appropriately healing inguinal hernia repair scar, +BS, soft, nondistended
      (vi) GU: normal external genitalia, no rashes
      (vii) Ext: DP, PT pulses symmetric, capillary refill 2 s

Table 35.1 Complete blood count (CBC)

Component	Patient results	Reference range
WBC	**11.9**	4.0–10.0 × 10^3/mL
RBC	5.3	4.3–5.9 × 10^6/mL
Hemoglobin	15.0	13–17 gm/dL
HCT	46.1	39–51%
Platelets	342	150–400 × 10^3/mL
MCV	89.4	81–99
MCH	31.2	27–33
MCHC	33.7	32.5–36.5%
RDW	12.5	11.6–14.8%
Neut%	62	40–74%
Lymph%	27	12–40%
Mono%	7	4–12%
Eosin%	3	0–8%
Baso%	1	0–2%

Only abnormality is slightly elevated WBC from physiologic stress

Table 35.2 Complete metabolic profile (CMP)

Component	Patient results	Reference range
Sodium	135	133–145 mEq/L
Potassium	5.2	3.5–5.3 mEq/L
Chloride	106	98–108 mEq/L
CO_2	24	23–32 mEq/L
BUN	17	7–23 mg/dL
Creatinine	1.0	0.6–1.3 mg/dL
Glucose	**40**	60–99 mg/dL
Calcium	8.7	8.5–10.3 mg/dL
Total protein	7.2	6.1–7.9 g/dL
Albumin	4.9	3.5–5.5 g/dL
Bilirubin	1.1	0.1–1.4 mg/dL
Alkaline phosphatase	56	0–135 IU/L
AST	32	0–41 IU/L
ALT	35	0–56 IU/L

Note low glucose

Table 35.3 Urinalysis (UA)

Component	Patient results	Reference range
Color	Yellow	Colorless, light yellow, yellow
Clarity	Clear	Clear
Specific gravity	1.022	1.005–1.035
Glucose	Negative	Negative
Ketones	**1+**	Negative
Blood	Negative	Negative
Nitrite	Negative	Negative
Leukocyte esterase	Negative	Negative
pH	6.6	5–7
Protein	Negative	Negative
Urobilinogen	0.4	0.2–1 mg/dL
RBC	0	0–2/HPF
WBC	0	0–2/HPF
Squamous epithelial	1	0–1/HPF

Patient has small ketones in urine from being diabetic and having decreased PO intake over the last few days

Table 35.4 Creatine kinase (CK)

Component	Patient results	Reference range
CK	**5023**	30–135 U/L
CK-MB	**50**	0–7.5 ng/mL

Table 35.5 Coagulation panel

Component	Patient results	Reference range
PT	**17 s**	12–15 s
INR	**1.6**	0.8–1.2
aPTT	39	30–40

(viii) Skin: moist, diaphoretic, no rashes or ecchymosis
(ix) Neuro: slightly confused initially, mentation improves with time
(x) Psych: nervous, confused

(c) Labs available:
(i) CBC (Table 35.1), CMP (Table 35.2), fingerstick glucose, UA (Table 35.3), UDS, CK (Table 35.4), coagulation panel (Table 35.5)

Facilitator: *After participants have done a full history and physical, lab results will be provided. Review them with the participants and have them explain abnormal values. After reviewing labs, the patient will complain of weakness.*

8. As the patient becomes clearer/returns to baseline while participants review lab results, he complains of left-sided weakness. Participants should ask for/perform a neurological exam.
   (a) Nurse or facilitator tells students that the patient's strength is 4/5 in the left upper and lower extremities. Reflexes normal throughout. This weakness is new according to the patient. Speech is normal. Remainder of exam normal.

9. Participants should be concerned about stroke symptoms and begin a workup. Should be concerned about hemorrhagic stroke given evidence of head laceration and patient's medication history (Xarelto)
10. The following data may be provided to the participants (if previously requested)
    (a) EKG—sinus tachycardia
    (b) CXR—no acute cardiopulmonary abnormalities
    (c) Head CT shows no evidence of ischemia or acute bleed
    (d) If they request KUB or abdominal CT, neither show any acute process, CT may show evidence of recent surgery (hx of inguinal hernia repair)

Facilitator Note: *Ask participants, did Mr. Williams have a stroke? Or what is going on?*

11. Participants may choose to treat as ischemic stroke with tPA or other thrombolytics—if so let participants treat the patient and admit to ICU
    (a) **NOTE:** if patients chose this route, allow them to push medications and call for admission and give report—then have patient complain of abdominal pain and bleeding at surgical scar site
    (b) Participants should recognize the patient is bleeding and stop all anticoagulation and thrombolytic infusion
    (c) Once participants recognize bleeding and stop medications, allow the case to close for debrief—will discuss contraindications to tPA use, including this patient being on Xarelto
12. If participants recognize Todd's paralysis and recognize that thrombolytics are contraindicated in this patient, allow participants to call for admission and summarize patient, the case will close.

Facilitator Note:
END OF CASE: in order for the case to close, participants must recognize the seizure was due to hypoglycemia and push at least 1 amp of D50. They must also recognize and verbalize the patient has Todd's paralysis, which only requires supportive care. Alternatively, if they push acute stroke medications (tPA, etc.), allow complications to arise (nurse reports patient is bleeding from surgical site). Case will close once participants recognize bleeding and choose to stop administering medications.

Scenario Props

- Patient simulator (male)
  - Patient should have a small 2-inch laceration on R forehead
  - Patient should have a healing scar from his right open inguinal hernia repair
  - Patient should be wearing a type 1 diabetes medical alert necklace under the gown
- Cardiac monitor
- Oxygen saturation monitor
- Blood pressure cuff
- Peripheral IVs (2)
- Oxygen source (wall)
- O_2—nasal cannula and nonrebreather mask
- IV fluids
- CXR normal
- EKG—sinus tachycardia
- Head CT normal
- Medications: IVFs, benzodiazepines (lorazepam, diazepam, midazolam), phenytoin, valproic acid, barbiturates (phenobarbital, pentobarbital), propofol, D50, heparin, tPA

Personnel

- Simulated patient (male)
- Nurse
- Facilitator
- SIM operator

Labs

UDS—Negative

Facilitator Note: *Ask participants about why these lab values are abnormal. CK levels tend to be elevated after seizures, but can also be high for other reasons, such as intense exercise.*

Facilitator Note: *Ask participants about these lab values. Why are they elevated?*

These lab results are outside of the normal range but appropriate for the patient given that he is on an anticoagulant—Xarelto

Fingerstick glucose—33 mg/dL

EKG: Sinus tachycardia

CXR: Normal

Head CT: Normal

Debriefing Notes

- As always when first approaching patients, ABCs!
- First priority is to STOP the seizure! The longer the patient remains seizing the harder it may be to stop and the worse neurological outcomes for the patient
- Always get a fingerstick glucose in a seizing patient ASAP
- Consider "reversible" causes of seizures—drugs, infection, alcohol withdrawal
- Recognize that Mr. Williams has felt "off" and nauseous—if he continued to take his insulin despite decreased PO intake, this could cause hypoglycemia
- When taking history be sure to ask about alcohol consumption—alcohol withdrawal can be extremely dangerous
- Initial antiepileptic is typically a benzodiazepine, such as lorazepam
- Don't forget to stick to an organized and systematic approach—even when a patient situation may be chaotic
- Recognize signs and symptoms of stroke—"FAST"
  - F—face drooping
  - A—arm weakness
  - S—slurred speech
  - T—TIME—call 911 (time is brain)
- Common stroke mimics:
  - Todd's paralysis
    - Brief period of temporary paralysis following a seizure, usually occurs on one side of the body
    - May affect speech and vision
    - Treatment is supportive—usually resolves in 24–48 h
  - Bell's palsy
    - Facial nerve palsy
    - Can differentiate from stroke with forehead movement—stroke patients should be able to raise eyebrows because of innervation from the opposite hemisphere. Stroke is associated with a supranuclear lesion.
    - See Fig. 35.1
- Contraindications to tPA:
  - Intracranial hemorrhage on CT
  - Presentation suggests subarachnoid hemorrhage
  - Neurosurgery, head trauma, stroke in past 3 months
  - Uncontrolled HTN—SBP > 185 or DBP > 110

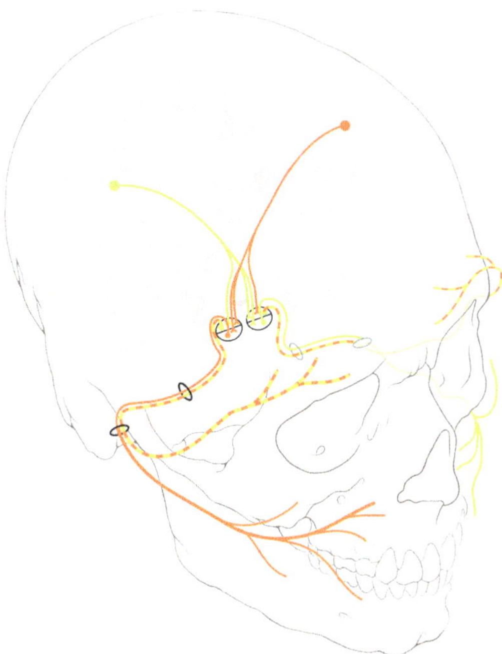

Fig. 35.1 Pathway of cranial nerve VII. (Patrick J. Lynch, medical illustrator, CC BY 2.5 <https://creativecommons.org/licenses/by/2.5>, via Wikimedia Commons (https://upload.wikimedia.org/wikipedia/commons/2/25/Cranial_nerve_VII_bells_palsy.svg))

- Active internal bleeding
- Abnormal glucose (<50 or >400)
- Endocarditis
- Surgery in the last 14 days
- GI or urinary bleeding within the last 21 days
- Bleeding issues: platelet less than 100,000; has received heparin within 48 h; current use of anticoagulants and INR >1.7; use of direct thrombin inhibitor or **Xa inhibitors (our patient was on Xarelto)**

Learning Objectives Answers:

1. **List the possible causes and differentials for seizures.**

Epilepsy

- Seizure may be the first presentation of a patient with epilepsy
- Patient with a history of epilepsy noncompliant with medications, or medication levels are at incorrect dosage

Other conditions that can cause/precipitate seizures [2, 3]:

- Electrolyte disturbances
  - Hyponatremia (in cases such as SIADH or psychogenic polydipsia)
  - Hypercalcemia (in cases such as hyperparathyroidism)
- Hypoglycemia
- Drug withdrawal: alcohol, benzodiazepines, barbiturates
- Drug overdoses: isoniazid, antidepressants, sympathomimetics, antihistamines, anticonvulsants
- Trauma
- Intracranial neoplasms or masses
- Intracranial bleeding
- CNS infections
- Eclamptic seizures in pregnant patients

Conditions that can mimic seizures

- Pseudoseizures
- Syncope (important: NO post-ictal state in patients with syncope)
- Dystonic reactions
- Rigors

2. **Describe the initial workup and management of seizures.**
   - As always: ABCs first!
     - Administer oxygen via face mask
     - For patients who are cyanotic or require intubation use rapid sequence intubations but use short-acting paralytics so that ongoing seizure activity is not masked and missed
   - Obtain IV access ASAP
   - First line treatment is benzodiazepines: usually IV lorazepam (if IV access cannot be obtained both lorazepam and midazolam can be given IM)
     - Lorazepam 0.1 mg/kg IV, usually given as 2 mg IV dose initially
     - Large doses or repeat doses may be required
   - Secondary medications include levetiracetam (Keppra), phenytoin, fosphenytoin, valproic acid
   - Check for reversible causes! Glucose, electrolyte levels, etc.
   - If the patient continues to seize despite drug therapy, the patient may require continuous infusion of antiepileptic medications
     - Drugs for continuous therapy include pentobarbital, midazolam, propofol
     - The patient will need to be intubated as treatment will cause respiratory depression
3. **Identify the various antiepileptic drugs that can be given in an acute seizure and explain their mechanisms of action.**
   - Benzodiazepines: increases the frequency of GABA Cl-channel opening
   - Barbiturates: increased duration of GABA Cl-channel opening
   - Phenytoin: increases Na^+ channel inactivation
   - Valproic acid: increases Na^+ channel inactivation, increased GABA concentration by inhibiting GABA transaminase
   - Propofol: potentiates $GABA_A$ receptors
4. **Describe the initial workup and management of stroke-like symptoms and discuss other disease states that mimic stroke and explain how to differentiate them from stroke.**

H+P and other workup [4]:

- Time of onset of symptoms
- Last seen normal time (did patient wake up with symptoms, i.e., "wake up stroke")
- Activity at onset
- Relevant PMH
- Current medications
- Contraindications to tPA (review above—students should know the contraindications)
- Vitals: BP, HR, temperature
- Glucose and EKG
- Labs: check PT/INR and platelets
- Administer NIH Stroke Scale questionnaire

Disease states that mimic stroke:

- Todd's paralysis after seizure! Differentiate with history and physical. This can sometimes be tricky though because patients may seize due to a stroke. Differentiating requires a thorough history, physical, and clinical judgment.
- Bell's Palsy: the difference between Bell's Palsy and a stroke is the patient's ability to move their forehead [5].
- In Bell's Palsy, the entire half of the face is paralyzed (including the forehead) because of a peripheral facial nerve lesion (Figs. 35.1 and 35.2). In stroke, the pathology occurs centrally, so innervation from the contralateral (healthy) side of the brain is still intact and can move the forehead facial muscles.

5. **Describe the management of Todd's paralysis.**
   - Management is supportive care, addressing the underlying cause, and ensuring patient safety.
   - Symptoms typically resolve in 24–48 h.
   - Since Todd's paralysis follows a seizure, optimizing antiepileptic drug (AED) therapy is essential to reduce seizure frequency and prevent recurrent episodes.
   - Educating the patient and caregivers about the transient nature of the condition and the importance of medication adherence is essential.

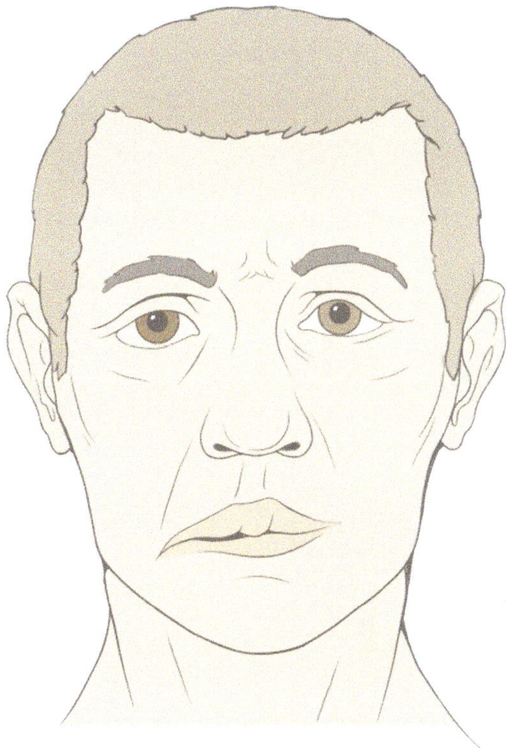

Fig. 35.2 Bell's Palsy leads to facial paralysis on one side of the face. (Patrick J. Lynch, medical illustrator, CC BY 2.5 <https://creativecommons.org/licenses/by/2.5>, via Wikimedia Commons (https://upload.wikimedia.org/wikipedia/commons/3/33/Bells_palsy_diagram.svg))

6. **Recognize and explain the psychosocial impact seizures have on patients—include physician responsibility in reporting seizure episodes.**
   - Patient with epilepsy often suffers from personal injury after seizures such as falls, car accidents, and fractures.
   - Employment status is often impacted by epilepsy.
   - Newly diagnosed patients with epilepsy can suffer a loss of independence, especially if their ability to drive is taken away [6].
   - Patients with epilepsy have a higher chance of poor health behaviors, like increased alcohol consumption, smoking, and less exercise.
   - The US has the Epilepsy Foundation, which maintains a searchable database of driver's license eligibility by state—each

state has different rules, including various requirements for physician reporting [7, 8].

Exam Questions

1. A 37-year-old woman presents to the emergency department with a 3-month history of fatigue, polyuria, nausea, abdominal pain, and increased feelings of depression. Last month she was diagnosed with a kidney stone for the first time. While interviewing her she begins to seize. Which electrolyte/metabolic abnormality is most likely responsible for her seizure?
   A. Hyponatremia
   B. Hypoglycemia
   C. Hypernatremia
   D. Hypercalcemia
   E. Hypokalemia

Answer: D

Learning Objective: #1. List the possible causes and differential for seizures.

Explanation: This patient's history of a kidney stone, along with her symptoms of fatigue, polyuria (from nephrogenic diabetes insipidus due to calcium-induced renal tubular dysfunction), nausea, and depression, strongly suggests hypercalcemia. The patient likely has hyperparathyroidism and elevated calcium levels, resulting in a seizure. A is incorrect as while hyponatremia can cause seizures, it typically presents with neurological symptoms such as confusion, headache, nausea, and altered mental status rather than kidney stones or polyuria. B is incorrect as while hypoglycemia can cause seizures, this patient's chronic history of symptoms (fatigue, polyuria, kidney stone) is not characteristic of hypoglycemia, which typically presents as sudden-onset symptoms such as sweating, tremors, palpitations, and confusion. C is incorrect as while hypernatremia can cause seizures, it typically presents with significant thirst, dehydration, and altered mental status rather than nephrolithiasis. E is incorrect as hypokalemia is associated with muscle weakness, arrhythmias, and cramps, not seizures.

2. A 21-year-old with a history of epilepsy reports 3 days of flu-like symptoms. For the past 2 days he hasn't been able to eat or drink without experiencing postprandial emesis, including not being able to keep down his anticonvulsants. EMS is called to his apartment after a friend witnessed him seizing. En route to the hospital, they administer two doses of lorazepam. Lorazepam stopped his seizures via which of the following mechanisms of action?
   A. Na^+ channel inactivation
   B. Increased duration of GABA Cl- channel opening
   C. Increased frequency of GABA Cl- channel opening
   D. Potentiation of $GABA_A$ receptors

Answer: C

Learning Objective: #3: Identify the various anti-epileptic drugs that can be given in an acute seizure and explain their mechanism of action

Explanation: Lorazepam is a benzodiazepine, which acts by increasing the frequency of chloride (Cl^-) channel opening at GABA A receptors. This enhances the inhibitory effects of GABA, leading to neuronal hyperpolarization and decreased excitability, thereby stopping seizures. A is incorrect as while sodium channel blockers are used for seizure prevention, they are not the primary mechanism by which lorazepam works. B is incorrect—this is the mechanism of action of barbiturates; lorazepam increases the frequency of channel opening, not the duration. D is incorrect as while many drugs potentiate GABA A receptors, including both benzodiazepines and barbiturates, the specific mechanism by which benzodiazepines stop seizures is by increasing the frequency of chloride channel opening.

3. Of the following patients, which one is most likely having a stroke?
   A. A 73-year-old woman with a history of HTN and DM wakes up with difficulty speaking.
   B. A 37-year-old man who presents with complete left sided facial paralysis.
   C. A 60-year-old woman who seizes in her nursing home and develops left sided weakness.
   D. A 58-year-old man who experiences double vision and difficulty speaking for 25 min.

Answer: A

Learning Objective: #4: Describe the initial steps in workup and management of stroke-like symptoms and discuss other disease states that mimic stroke and explain how to differentiate them from stroke.

Explanation: This scenario is highly suggestive of an ischemic stroke, particularly a wake-up stroke (when symptoms are first noticed upon awakening). The sudden onset of difficulty speaking (likely aphasia or dysarthria) strongly suggests an acute cerebrovascular event. B is most likely Bell's Palsy, a peripheral facial nerve (CN VII) palsy, not a stroke. C is likely Todd's Paralysis, a postictal focal neurological deficit that can mimic stroke but resolves within 24 h. D is likely a TIA, a short duration ischemic attack, not an actual stroke.

References

1. Zonnoor B. "Seizure Assessment in the Emergency Department." Accessed via: http://emedicine.medscape.com/article/1609294-overview?pa=LSvYfTgfymktKRUTBNKyF4PEGhotpWBAdUpMGs7sdRo5Vh9sQIoGNXPye%2FcV4DlPFGHIYZD5hjoQjaAWrmGYmychrzF%2F7vlnSF6AEX%2F09M8%3D#a11
2. Nickson C. "Seizure DDx". Life in the Fast Lane (LITFL). Accessed via: https://lifeinthefastlane.com/resources/seizure-ddx/
3. Donaldson R, Ostermayer D, Swartz J, et al. "Seizure". WikiEM. https://wikem.org/wiki/Seizure
4. Barrow Neurological Institute Stroke Education Manual. https://www.barrowneuro.org/resource/stroke-education-manual/
5. Figure: "Stroke vs Bell's Palsy". Evidence Based Medicine Consult.
6. "Overview of the management of epilepsy in adults". UptoDate. Accessed via: https://www.uptodate.com/contents/overview-of-the-management-of-epilepsy-in-adults
7. "Driving restrictions for patients with seizures and epilepsy". UptoDate. Accessed via: https://www.uptodate.com/contents/driving-restrictions-for-patients-with-seizures-and-epilepsy?source=sec_link#H8
8. Epilepsy Foundation. Access via: http://www.epilepsy.com/

Index

C. A. Standley (ed.), *Biomedical Science and Clinical Foundations*,
https://doi.org/10.1007/978-3-031-98353-5